CRITICAL CARE NURSING
OF THE ONCOLOGY PATIENT

Edited by
Meghan Routt, MSN, ANP/GNP-BC, AOCNP®
Lisa Parks, MS, ANP-BC

Oncology Nursing Society
Pittsburgh, Pennsylvania

ONS Publications Department
Publisher and Director of Publications: William A. Tony, BA, CQIA
Senior Editorial Manager: Lisa M. George, BA
Assistant Editorial Manager: Amy Nicoletti, BA, JD
Acquisitions Editor: John Zaphyr, BA, MEd
Associate Staff Editors: Casey S. Kennedy, BA, Andrew Petyak, BA
Design and Production Administrator: Dany Sjoen
Editorial Assistant: Judy Holmes

Library of Congress Cataloging-in-Publication Data
Names: Routt, Meghan, editor. | Parks, Lisa, 1958- editor. | Oncology Nursing
    Society, issuing body.
Title: Critical care nursing of the oncology patient / edited by Meghan
    Routt, MSN, ANP/GNP-BC, AOCNP and Lisa Parks, MS, ANP-BC.
Description: Pittsburgh, Pennsylvania : Oncology Nursing Society, [2018] |
    Includes bibliographical references and index.
Identifiers: LCCN 2017048449 (print) | LCCN 2017047705 (ebook) | ISBN
    9781635930146 (pbk.) | ISBN 9781635930153 ()
Subjects: | MESH: Critical Care Nursing--methods | Neoplasms--nursing |
    Nursing Care--methods
Classification: LCC RC266 (ebook) | LCC RC266 (print) | NLM WY 154 | DDC
    616.99/40231--dc23
LC record available at https://lccn.loc.gov/2017048449

Publisher's Note

This book is published by the Oncology Nursing Society (ONS). ONS neither represents nor guarantees that the practices described herein will, if followed, ensure safe and effective patient care. The recommendations contained in this book reflect ONS's judgment regarding the state of general knowledge and practice in the field as of the date of publication. The recommendations may not be appropriate for use in all circumstances. Those who use this book should make their own determinations regarding specific safe and appropriate patient care practices, taking into account the personnel, equipment, and practices available at the hospital or other facility at which they are located. The editors and publisher cannot be held responsible for any liability incurred as a consequence from the use or application of any of the contents of this book. Figures and tables are used as examples only. They are not meant to be all-inclusive, nor do they represent endorsement of any particular institution by ONS. Mention of specific products and opinions related to those products do not indicate or imply endorsement by ONS. Websites mentioned are provided for information only; the hosts are responsible for their own content and availability. Unless otherwise indicated, dollar amounts reflect U.S. dollars.

ONS publications are originally published in English. Publishers wishing to translate ONS publications must contact ONS about licensing arrangements. ONS publications cannot be translated without obtaining written permission from ONS. (Individual tables and figures that are reprinted or adapted require additional permission from the original source.) Because translations from English may not always be accurate or precise, ONS disclaims any responsibility for inaccuracies in words or meaning that may occur as a result of the translation. Readers relying on precise information should check the original English version.

Printed in the United States of America

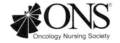

Innovation • Excellence • Advocacy

Contributors

Editors

Meghan Routt, MSN, ANP/GNP-BC, AOCNP®
Nurse Practitioner
Methodist ElderCare Physician Services
Columbus, Ohio
Chapter 21. The Older Adult With Cancer in the Intensive Care Unit

Lisa Parks, MS, ANP-BC
Hepatobiliary Nurse Practitioner
Division of Surgical Oncology
The James Cancer Hospital
The Ohio State University Wexner Medical Center
Columbus, Ohio
Chapter 4. Hepatic, Pancreatic, and Biliary Cancers; Chapter 6. Gastrointestinal Cancers; Chapter 10. Oncologic Emergencies

Authors

Kathleen Blazoff, RN, ANP-BC, ACHPN
Nurse Practitioner, Palliative Care
St. John Providence Hospital and Medical Center
Southfield, Michigan
Chapter 20. Palliative Care in the Intensive Care Unit

Leanne M. Boehm, PhD, RN, ACNS-BC
Postdoctoral Fellow
Vanderbilt University School of Nursing
Nashville, Tennessee
Chapter 13. Delirium

Katherine A. Brown-Saltzman, MA, RN
Co-Director
UCLA Health Ethics Center
Assistant Clinical Professor
University of California, Los Angeles School of Nursing
Los Angeles, California
Chapter 22. Ethics Concepts, Complexities, and Controversies

Cindy Byrd, DNP, RN, ACNP-BC
Advanced Practice Manager, Critical Care/Surgical Intensive Care Unit
The James Cancer Hospital
The Ohio State University Wexner Medical Center
Columbus, Ohio
Chapter 2. Lung Cancer; Chapter 11. Respiratory Failure

Cynthia Chernecky, PhD, RN, AOCN®, FAAN
Professor
Augusta University
Augusta, Georgia
Chapter 18. Vascular Access

Yelena Drexler, MD
Assistant Professor of Medicine
Montefiore Medical Center/Albert Einstein
  College of Medicine
Bronx, New York
*Chapter 8. Renal Failure and Obstructive
Uropathy*

Brenda Freymiller, BSN, MBA, RN, CWON, CWS
Wound and Skin Director
Intermountain Healthcare
Salt Lake City, Utah
Chapter 16. Wounds and Critical Care

Anthony T. Gerlach, PharmD, BCPS, FCCP, FCCM
Specialty Practice Pharmacist, Surgical
  Critical Care
Department of Pharmacy
The Ohio State University Wexner Medical
  Center
Clinical Associate Professor
The Ohio State University College of
  Pharmacy
Columbus, Ohio
Chapter 17. Pharmacology

Ladan Golestaneh, MD, MS
Associate Professor of Medicine
Montefiore Medical Center/Albert Einstein
  College of Medicine
Bronx, New York
*Chapter 8. Renal Failure and Obstructive
Uropathy*

Aimee S. Hoskins, BSN, RN
Research Nurse Specialist III, Delirium and
  Cognitive Impairment Study Group
Vanderbilt University Medical Center
Nashville, Tennessee
Chapter 13. Delirium

Christine Hull, RN, MSN, OCN®
Registered Nurse
Inova Loudoun Hospital
Leesburg, Virginia
Chapter 19. Transitions in Care

Catherine Hydzik, MS, CNS, AOCN®
Clinical Nurse Specialist
Memorial Sloan Kettering Cancer Center
New York, New York
Chapter 5. Gynecologic Cancers

Patricia Jakel, RN, MN, AOCN®
Advanced Practice Nurse—Solid Tumor
University of Los Angeles Health
Santa Monica Medical Center
Santa Monica, California
*Chapter 22. Ethics Concepts, Complexities,
and Controversies*

Donald D. Kautz, RN, PhD, CRRN, ACNS-BC
Associate Professor Emeritus
University of North Carolina Greensboro
  School of Nursing
Greensboro, North Carolina
*Chapter 15. Early Mobility in the Intensive
Care Unit*

Lisa Koser, DNP, RN, ACNP-BC, CPNP-AC
Acute Care Nurse Practitioner, Trauma,
  Critical Care and Burn
The James Cancer Hospital
The Ohio State University Wexner Medical
  Center
Columbus, Ohio
Chapter 11. Respiratory Failure

Neelja Kumar, MD
Assistant Professor of Medicine
Montefiore Medical Center/Albert Einstein
  College of Medicine
Bronx, New York
*Chapter 8. Renal Failure and Obstructive
Uropathy*

Denise Macklin, BSN, RN, VA-BC
Consultant
Satellite Beach, Florida
Chapter 18. Vascular Access

Ainsley Malone, MS, RD, LD, CNSC, FAND, FASPEN
Nutrition Support Dietitian
Mt. Carmel West Hospital
Columbus, Ohio
Chapter 14. Nutritional Support

DaiWai M. Olson, PhD, RN, CCRN, FNCS
Associate Professor
Neurology and Neurotherapeutics, Neuro-
logical Surgery
University of Texas Southwestern Medical
Center
Dallas, Texas
*Chapter 1. Brain Cancer and Neurocritical
Care*

Carol Pavlish, PhD, RN, FAAN
Associate Professor
University of California, Los Angeles School
of Nursing
Los Angeles, California
Professor Emerita, St. Catherine University
St. Paul, Minnesota
*Chapter 22. Ethics Concepts, Complexities,
and Controversies*

Karen M. Perialis, MSN, RN, ANP-BC, OCN®
Adult Nurse Practitioner
Memorial Sloan Kettering Cancer Center
New York, New York
Chapter 5. Gynecologic Cancers

Alex A. Rollo, BS
Medical Student
University of Texas Southwestern Medical
Center
Dallas, Texas
*Chapter 1. Brain Cancer and Neurocritical
Care*

Catherine Sargent, MS, RN, BC, AOCNS®
Infusion Unit Supervisor
Mercy Fitzgerald Hospital
Darby, Pennsylvania
Chapter 9. Cardiovascular Complications

**Brenda K. Shelton, DNP, APRN-CNS, RN,
CCRN, AOCN®**
Clinical Nurse Specialist
Sidney Kimmel Comprehensive Cancer
Center at Johns Hopkins Hospital
Affiliate Faculty, Johns Hopkins University
School of Nursing
Baltimore, Maryland
*Chapter 3. Hematologic Malignancies;
Chapter 9. Cardiovascular Complications*

Laetitia Simeral, RN, MSN, CRNP
Nurse Practitioner
Abramson Cancer Center at Pennsylvania
Hospital
Philadelphia, Pennsylvania
Chapter 7. Bone and Soft Tissue Sarcomas

**William H. Tettelbach, MD, FACP, FIDSA,
FUHM, CWS**
Medical Director
Intermountain Healthcare
Salt Lake City, Utah
Program Director, Hyperbaric Medicine
Fellowship
Adjunct Assistant Professor, Duke University
School of Medicine
Durham, North Carolina
Chapter 16. Wounds and Critical Care

**Yolanda Michelle VanRiel, PhD, RN-BC,
OCN®, CNE, ANEF**
Associate Professor of Nursing
MSN Nursing Education Concentration
Program Coordinator
University of North Carolina Greensboro
School of Nursing
Greensboro, North Carolina
*Chapter 15. Early Mobility in the Intensive
Care Unit*

**Anna Vioral, PhD, MEd, RN, OCN®,
BMTCN®**
Director, Oncology Education and Research
Allegheny Health Network
Pittsburgh, Pennsylvania
Chapter 12. Sepsis

Disclosure

Editors and authors of books and guidelines provided by the Oncology Nursing Society are expected to disclose to the readers any significant financial interest or other relationships with the manufacturer(s) of any commercial products.

A vested interest may be considered to exist if a contributor is affiliated with or has a financial interest in commercial organizations that may have a direct or indirect interest in the subject matter. A "financial interest" may include, but is not limited to, being a shareholder in the organization; being an employee of the commercial organization; serving on an organization's speakers bureau; or receiving research funding from the organization. An "affiliation" may be holding a position on an advisory board or some other role of benefit to the commercial organization. Vested interest statements appear in the front matter for each publication.

Contributors are expected to disclose any unlabeled or investigational use of products discussed in their content. This information is acknowledged solely for the information of the readers.

The contributors provided the following disclosure and vested interest information:

Leanne M. Boehm, PhD, RN, ACNS-BC: American Association of Critical-Care Nurses, research funding; Sigma Theta Tau International Iota Chapter, employment or leadership position

Anthony T. Gerlach, PharmD, BCPS, FCCP, FCCM: Merck Research Laboratories, research funding; Society of Critical Care Medicine Council, employment or leadership position

Ladan Golestaneh, MD, MS: AbbVie Inc., research funding; Relypsa, Inc., consultant or advisory role

Patricia Jakel, RN, MN, AOCN®: Genentech, Inc., consultant or advisory role

Ainsley Malone, MS, RD, LD, CNSC, FAND, FASPEN: Academy of Nutrition and Dietetics Positions Committee, American Society for Parenteral and Enteral Nutrition, employment or leadership position

DaiWai M. Olson, PhD, RN, CCRN, FNCS: *Journal of Neuroscience Nursing*, Neuroscience Nursing Research Center, employment or leadership position; NeurOptics, Inc., research funding

Carol Pavlish, PhD, RN, FAAN: American Association of Critical-Care Nurses, research funding

Karen M. Perialis, MSN, RN, ANP-BC, OCN®: Memorial Sloan Kettering Cancer Center, research funding

William H. Tettelbach, MD, FACP, FIDSA, FUHM, CWS: MiMedx Group, research funding

Anna Vioral, PhD, MEd, RN, OCN®, BMTCN®: American Society of Clinical Oncology, employment or leadership position, consultant or advisory role; Celgene Corporation, honoraria

Contents

Preface xiii

Chapter 1. Brain Cancer and Neurocritical Care 1
  Introduction 1
  Symptom Monitoring 1
  Primary Brain Tumors 4
  Metastatic Brain Tumors 8
  The Blood–Brain Barrier 9
  Monitoring the Brain 10
  Diagnosing Neurologic Disease 11
  Multimodal Brain Monitoring 14
  Therapy and Treatment 19
  Summary 20
  References 20

Chapter 2. Lung Cancer 23
  Introduction 23
  Types of Lung Cancer 23
  Diagnosis and Treatment 24
  Postoperative Care 28
  Postoperative Respiratory Failure 31
  Summary 34
  References 34

Chapter 3. Hematologic Malignancies 37
  Introduction 37
  Diagnostic Tests 37
  Hematologic/Immunologic Therapeutics 38
  Hematologic/Immunologic System Cancers 57
  Nonmalignant Hematologic/Immunologic Disorders 57
  Respiratory Complications 77
  Hematologic/Immunologic Disorders Related to Cancer Treatment 90
  Selected Hematologic/Immunologic Disorders 94
  Summary 97
  References 97

Chapter 4. Hepatic, Pancreatic, and Biliary Cancers 105
  Introduction 105
  Hepatocellular Carcinoma 105

Cholangiocarcinoma 109
Cholangitis 109
Pancreatic Cancer 111
Summary 113
References 113

Chapter 5. Gynecologic Cancers 117
Introduction 117
Overview of Gynecologic Cancers 117
Treatment Modalities 126
Common Complications in Gynecologic Cancers 132
Suggested Reading 148
Summary 148
References 149

Chapter 6. Gastrointestinal Cancers 153
Introduction 153
Common Complications in Gastrointestinal Cancers 154
Complications After Complete Cytoreduction With Heated Intraperitoneal Chemotherapy 156
Summary 161
References 161

Chapter 7. Bone and Soft Tissue Sarcomas 163
Introduction 163
Pathophysiology 163
Treatment 164
Chemotherapy Side Effects 165
Radiation Side Effects 167
Nursing Implications 168
Summary 168
References 168

Chapter 8. Renal Failure and Obstructive Uropathy 171
Introduction 171
Types of Renal Disease 172
Common Electrolyte Derangements 182
Renal Replacement Therapy 187
Summary 188
References 189

Chapter 9. Cardiovascular Complications 195
Introduction 195
Cardiac Injury Related to Cancer 197
Selected Cardiovascular Disorders 216
Summary 240
References 240

Chapter 10. Oncologic Emergencies 245
Introduction 245
Metabolic Emergencies 245
Infectious Emergencies 258
Cardiovascular Emergencies 260
Neurologic Emergencies 262
Hematologic Emergency: Hyperviscosity Syndrome 264

Summary 265
References 265

Chapter 11. Respiratory Failure 269
Introduction... 269
Causes of Respiratory Failure 269
Noninvasive Ventilation in Acute Respiratory Failure... 273
Mechanical Ventilation... 278
Summary 281
References 281

Chapter 12. Sepsis.. 283
Introduction... 283
Definitions.. 284
Epidemiology... 285
Etiology and Risk Factors 286
Pathophysiology.. 288
Neutropenic Sepsis 291
Hematopoiesis... 291
Assessment Criteria 295
Diagnostic Evaluation 296
Treatment Management Strategies.. 297
Nursing Implications 302
Summary 304
References 304

Chapter 13. Delirium 309
Introduction... 309
Etiology, Prevalence, and Subtypes 309
Outcomes Associated With Intensive Care Unit Delirium................................... 311
Monitoring for Intensive Care Unit Delirium 311
Management Recommendations 312
Script for Interprofessional Communication: The Brain Roadmap 314
Interprofessional Care Approach: The ABCDEF Bundle...................................... 316
Summary 319
References 319

Chapter 14. Nutritional Support 323
Introduction... 323
Metabolic Response to Stress 323
Nutrition Status and Assessment 324
Nutrition Care Pathway 324
Malnutrition Diagnosis.. 325
Nutritional Support Interventions.. 326
Timing and Route of Feeding... 326
Enteral Formulas 327
Complications of Enteral Nutrition.. 328
Parenteral Nutrition 330
Complications of Parenteral Nutrition 331
Summary 332
References 333

Chapter 15. Early Mobility in the Intensive Care Unit 337
Introduction... 337

Complications of Immobility 338
Progressive Mobility 338
Barriers and Solutions to Progressive Mobility..................................... 339
Mobility Teams... 339
Summary 340
References 341

Chapter 16. Wounds and Critical Care... 343
Introduction.. 343
Wounds and Critical Care.. 343
Wound Assessment 344
The Healing Process 346
Pressure Injuries 347
Other Types of Pressure Injuries... 351
Pressure Injury Prevention.. 353
Preventive Skin Care 354
Preventive Therapies and Devices... 356
Moisture-Associated Skin Damage 357
Skin Tears 360
Wound Cleansing and Dressing Selection... 363
Summary 367
References 367

Chapter 17. Pharmacology 373
Introduction.. 373
Pharmacokinetics and Pharmacodynamics 373
Fluid Resuscitation 377
Vasopressors... 377
Inotropes... 379
Analgesics and Sedatives... 380
Neuromuscular Blocking Agents 383
Anticoagulants.. 384
Histamine-2 Antagonists and Proton Pump Inhibitors 385
Summary 385
References 385

Chapter 18. Vascular Access... 389
Introduction.. 389
Central Venous Catheter Characteristics... 390
Principles of Flow 390
Catheter Types.. 391
Central Venous Catheter Care and Maintenance 393
Extraluminal Catheter Tract... 393
Skin Integrity.. 394
Dressings... 394
Intraluminal Fluid Pathway.. 395
Summary 398
References 403

Chapter 19. Transitions in Care... 407
Introduction.. 407
The Meaning of Transition... 408
The Time Has Come.. 408

Ethical Responsibilities 409
Admitting Diagnoses and Complications.. 410
Noninvasive and Mechanical Ventilation 411
Potential Pitfalls During Transition 411
Summary 412
References 413

Chapter 20. Palliative Care in the Intensive Care Unit 415
Introduction... 415
Identifying Palliative Care Needs.. 416
Symptom Management... 417
The Family Meeting 422
Spirituality 423
End-of-Life Care 423
Case Study 425
Summary 427
References 428

Chapter 21. The Older Adult With Cancer in the Intensive Care Unit................... 433
Introduction 433
Physiology 433
Polypharmacy 438
Frailty 439
Older Adult Failure to Thrive 440
Summary 440
References 441

Chapter 22. Ethics Concepts, Complexities, and Controversies........................... 443
Introduction: Case Study—Part 1 443
Ethics Concepts in Clinical Practice 445
The American Nurses Association Code of Ethics and Ethical Principles 447
A Closer Look at Autonomy 448
Ethical Complexities 451
Ethical Controversies in Clinical Practice 453
Addressing Treatment Decisions and Nonbeneficial Treatment/Futility 456
The Importance of Resilience in High-Intensity Environments 458
Summary 460
References 461

Index... 467

Preface

The care of patients with cancer has evolved over the past 10 years. Patients who are in intensive care units today would not have been alive a decade ago; patients on medical-surgical floors in the present would have been in intensive care units in the past; and patients discharged home today would still be in the hospital in yesteryears. In this ever-changing environment, it is important that nurses understand the entire continuum of cancer care. The idea that a cancer diagnosis is incompatible with aggressive treatment is outdated; therefore, many more patients with cancer are requiring care in a an intensive care unit after treatment.

Traditionally, oncology nurses and critical care nurses have viewed patients through their own respective lenses, which are not always compatible and certainly require different competencies in providing patient care. The most optimal strategy in caring for critically ill patients with cancer is leveraging the strengths of both specialties as well as working collaboratively throughout the transition from the medical-surgical floor to the intensive care unit and back to the medical-surgical floor. Many cancer centers are developing oncology-specific intensive care units. Nurses staffing these new units may be oncology nurses with little critical care training or critical care nurses with little oncology training. It is our hope that this book will serve as a reference for nurses working in these settings and empower them to consider themselves as both oncology nurses and critical care nurses. As more complex cases of patients with cancer transition from the intensive care setting to the progressive care unit or medical-surgical floor, this text will become a valuable reference for nurses who care for these patients. Understanding previous nursing treatments and the complications of the critically ill will enable nurses to better create a nursing care plan. As editors, we hope that our readers will find this text helpful.

Meghan M. Routt
Lisa S. Parks

CHAPTER 1

Brain Cancer and Neurocritical Care

Alex A. Rollo, BS, and DaiWai M. Olson, PhD, RN, CCRN, FNCS

Introduction

Neurocritical care monitoring has applications for all individuals involved in the care of patients with cancer. Independent of specializations in the oncology spectrum, monitoring brain function becomes a primary focus when patients are admitted to intensive care units with altered mental status. Monitoring information has special value for nurses who are responsible for ongoing monitoring of neurologic function and identifying any subtle neurologic changes. This chapter will provide an overview of neurocritical care in the oncology setting. To adequately understand the interplay between the critical care of the brain and the broader treatments of brain tumors, this chapter will also review the major categories of brain tumors. Location predominantly determines brain cancer treatment and monitoring, specifically the primary location (if the cancer has metastasized) and the anatomic location of the tumor in the brain. In the case of metastases, each primary organ is characterized by tumor aggressiveness, localization in the brain, and ideal treatment tactics based on molecular signatures of the original cell population.

Symptom Monitoring

Advanced neurologic monitoring, or *multimodal neurologic monitoring*, is a broad term used to describe the critical care of patients with a known or suspected brain injury, including various forms of seizures, speech deficits, confusion, delirium, peripheral loss of mechanical/motor function, or even subtle changes (e.g., slight eyelid droop). These signs and symptoms can be early indicators of brain complications. Identification of any sign of brain dysfunction triggers the need for diagnostic testing, which can result in early detection of brain metastasis or the worsening of treatment side effects. Prompt treatment based on test results can prevent the occurrence of irrevocable secondary brain damage (Bader, Littlejohns, & Olson, 2016).

Tumor localization within the brain dictates the likely symptoms and monitoring. For example, a tumor located in or near the ventricles might occlude the flow of cerebrospinal fluid (CSF), requiring methods of measuring intracranial pressure (ICP) or possibly the insertion of an external ventricular drain (EVD) to alleviate the increased pressure (see Figure 1-1) (Olson et al., 2015). It is important to distinguish between primary neoplasms of the central nervous system (CNS) and brain metastases encountered in late-stage cancer of other organs. The type of lesion will affect treatment options. The differentiation of brain tumor etiology and treatment plans involves several different diagnostic methodologies.

Diagnosis

The diagnostic process typically begins with the patient's primary complaint, which may be the patient's description of symptoms or a description of the patient's presenting condition (neurologic examination) by a family member or another practitioner (e.g., nurse, referring physician). Initial symptoms may be noticed at home, during an office visit, or in the emergency department. If the patient's chief complaint and presenting symptoms are consistent with neurologic dysfunction, diagnostic imaging is typically ordered. The choice procedure for neurologic assessment is magnetic resonance imaging (MRI) because of its high anatomic definition of normal neurologic structures and absence of any radiation. Computed tomography (CT) scans are often ordered to rule out acute hemorrhage (see Figure 1-2).

The presence of abnormalities can be accurately detected and localized when using diagnostic imaging. The pathologic significance of these findings (malignant vs. benign) can be characterized using the various imaging techniques available with an MRI. When a more definitive diagnosis is required (tissue diagnosis for tumor type), a biopsy of the lesion may be performed using a CT scan or MRI to guide the biopsy needle directly into the lesion. Imaging and biopsy results are used to determine the most appropriate treatment, such as surgery, chemotherapy, radiation, or a combination. Depending on the level and extent of injury, the focus of nursing care is toward monitoring for secondary brain injury.

Treatment

The goals of monitoring are to provide early detection at each stage of treatment and to act as a marker of success or failure following each intervention. Because of the variety of treatment options available, it is imperative to understand which monitoring method will provide the most meaningful information to guide the most appropriate treatment. Because of the complexity and inter-

Figure 1-1. External Ventricular Drain Set to Drain Cerebrospinal Fluid and Monitor Intracranial Pressure

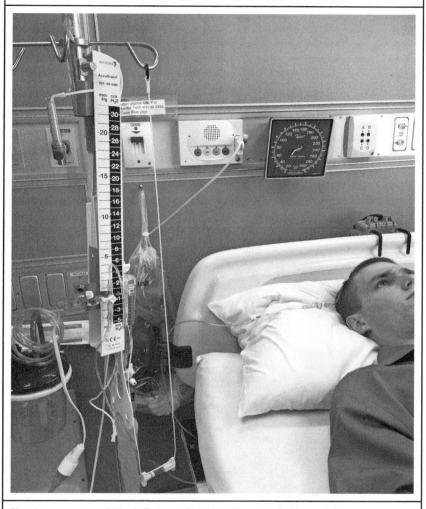

Note. Image courtesy of Alex A. Rollo and DaiWai M. Olson. Used with permission.

connectedness of the human brain, it is especially important to remember that even minimal cerebral edema or changes in tumor size can result in catastrophic changes to a patient's prognosis.

It is important to reaffirm that any cancer treatment, even beyond the scope of primary or metastatic brain tumors, can have complications or side effects that may require the services of a neurocritical care unit (NCCU). For example, long-

Figure 1-2. Computed Tomography Scan Showing Intracerebral Hemorrhage

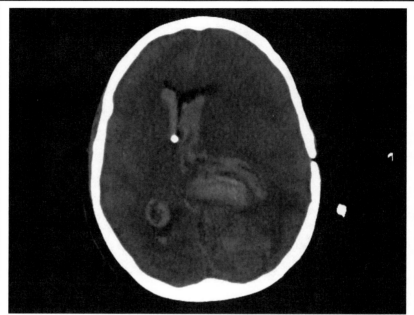

Note that the bone appears bright white. Blood (hemorrhage) appears white and non-uniform. The small white circle (dot) marks the location of the external ventricular drain.

Note. Image courtesy of Alex A. Rollo and DaiWai M. Olson. Used with permission.

term use or large doses of chemotherapy agents treating late-stage lung cancer can adversely affect the ability of oxygen to reach the brain. Reduced cerebral oxygenation may lead to cerebral ischemia and result in permanent brain damage or death. Awareness of neurocritical care is essential not only for nurses caring for patients being treated for brain cancer, but also for nurses involved in the general treatment of all cancer types.

Primary Brain Tumors

Primary CNS tumors begin in the CNS tissues (i.e., brain, meninges, and spinal cord). Primary brain tumors, including neoplasms of the meninges, neural sheaths, and glial cells, occur at a rate of 21.42 per 100,000 age-adjusted persons in the United States (Ostrom, Gittleman, et al., 2014). These tumors can be benign (nonmalignant) or malignant based on their rate of growth, tendency to spread, and histologic appearance. The cells that characterize the tumor will define its treatment. Some of the most common benign primary brain tumors originate from astrocytes (support cells), oligodendrocytes (myelin sheaths for neurons), ependymal cells (lining the ventricles), cells of the meninges (cushion the brain), and the pituitary (secretes hormones) (Ostrom, Gittleman, et al., 2014).

Although laypeople may use the term *benign* to describe something non-threatening, a benign brain tumor does not always mean a favorable prognosis. A tumor's location within the brain and rate of growth affect prognosis. For example, a rapidly growing benign tumor in the pons can easily compromise critical brain stem vasculature. Similarly, a benign intraventricular tumor can cause an obstruction of ventricular CSF flow and result in obstructive hydrocephalus.

Nonmalignant Tumors

Pituitary Adenomas

Pathophysiology: Pituitary adenomas account for 22.7% of nonmalignant tumors (Ostrom, Gittleman, et al., 2014). Despite being benign, pituitary adenomas can have far-reaching effects through their influence on the secretion of adrenal hormones, such as adrenocorticotropic hormone (ACTH), growth hormone (growth factor), prolactin (PRL; milk production/secretion), thyroid-stimulating hormone, and sex hormones (luteinizing hormone and follicle-stimulating hormone). The specific effects of pituitary adenomas can vary depending on the cell within the pituitary that begins the monoclonal expansion, because each hormone is synthesized by a specific cell type (Arafah & Nasrallah, 2001).

Symptoms: Symptoms can result from an excess of one of the hormones listed in Table 1-1 (e.g., unexpected milk secretion in prolactinomas). Although the overproduction of these hormones may wreak havoc on the body and pituitary tumors may impinge on surrounding brain structures, they seldom advance to malignant cancers or spread to other areas of the CNS. A possible explanation for this is that the trophic effects of these hormones intrinsically restrain cells from indefinitely proliferating (Melmed, 2011).

Diagnosis and treatment: Prolactinomas are pituitary tumors most easily diagnosed and monitored with a combination of an MRI and assays for hormones. PRL is the most common hormone oversecreted by pituitary tumors, and prolactinomas are indicated when a patient presents with PRL that is greater than 250 ng/ml (Glezer & Bronstein, 2015). Elevated PRL also can be seen in pregnancy, primary hypothyroidism, and renal failure. An MRI is often used to confirm the presence of a mass in the anatomic location of the pituitary gland. Prolactinomas are usually treated with dopamine agonists, which often will cause shrinkage and a drop in PRL levels (Freda & Wardlaw, 1999).

Somatotroph adenomas are growth hormone–secreting tumors that comprise up to 20% of pituitary tumors. They often result in acromegaly and are

Table 1-1. Common Pituitary Tumors

Tumor	Primary Hormone	Prevalence	Symptoms
Prolactinoma	Prolactin	40%–45%	Galactorrhea, amenorrhea, hypogonadism, infertility, erectile dysfunction
Somatotroph adenoma	Growth hormone	15%–20%	Acromegaly: Enlargement of hands, feet, forehead, jaw, and nose; joint paint, deepening voice
Corticotroph adenoma	Adrenocorticotropic hormone	10%–12%	Weight gain, high blood pressure, rounded face, fatigue, short-term memory and concentration issues, hirsutism, and irregular menstruation
Gonadotroph adenoma	Follicle-stimulating hormone and luteinizing hormone	15%	Mass effects more common: Vision loss, hypopituitarism, headaches

Note. Based on information from Arafah & Nasrallah, 2001.

treated with a combination of dopamine agonists and somatostatin analogs (Arafah & Nasrallah, 2001). Transsphenoidal surgery, a minimally invasive method of accessing the pituitary area through the nose and sphenoid bone, is the gold standard treatment for this tumor type (Glezer & Bronstein, 2015).

Corticotroph adenomas are nearly as common as growth hormone–secreting tumors. Cushing syndrome, caused by ACTH-secreting tumors, presents with an overproduction of glucocorticoids. Symptoms include central obesity, osteoporosis, easy bruising, hypertension, muscle wasting, and psychiatric symptoms. Cushing syndrome is diagnosed when ACTH levels are in the high-normal range and plasma cortisol levels are at a level lower than expected. ACTH-secreting tumors often are too small to be seen on an MRI and are usually found and excised during transsphenoidal surgery (Freda & Wardlaw, 1999).

Meningiomas

Pathophysiology: Meningiomas are tumors originating from the arachnoid cells lining and cushioning the brain. More than 97% of meningiomas are benign, and they are the most common type of primary brain tumor (36.1%) (Ostrom, Gittleman, et al., 2014).

Diagnosis: Although an MRI is preferable for the diagnosis of meningiomas, a CT scan is more widely available and, incidentally, is often how meningiomas and other tumors are first discovered. For example, a patient who has a brain CT scan after a car crash might be found to have an asymptomatic meningioma.

Treatment: Although symptomatic meningiomas are often treated with radiosurgery or surgery, an MRI also can be used in conjunction with an endovascular meningioma embolization, a procedure that occludes the vessel supplying the tumor by placing 350–500 mcm diameter plastic particles with a catheter (Saloner, Uzelac, Hetts, Martin, & Dillon, 2010).

Malignant Tumors: Gliomas

Pathophysiology

Gliomas are tumors that originate from astrocytes, oligodendrocytes, microglia, or ependymal cells. They are the most common primary malignancy of the brain and have an incidence of 4.67 to 5.73 per 100,000 age-adjusted persons (Ostrom, Gittleman, et al., 2014). The World Health Organization distinguishes gliomas based on the cell of origin and grades them from I (low-grade pilocytic astrocytoma) to IV (high-grade glioblastoma) (Ostrom, Bauchet, et al., 2014). Grade I pilocytic astrocytoma, the most common tumor in children, and grade II diffuse gliomas are most accurately diagnosed using a conventional MRI.

Diagnosis

When required, biopsies are obtained using an MRI. Treatment monitoring also uses a conventional MRI. When characterization of a high-grade glioma (III or IV) is required, metabolic imaging with positron-emission tomography (PET) and 2-[^{18}F]fluoro-2-deoxy-D-glucose (FDG) is used (Pedersen & Romner, 2013).

Treatment

The treatment for low-grade gliomas (grade II) is typically a combination of surgery and adjuvant radiation. Recently, temozolomide (TMZ) chemotherapy has been used for salvage therapy; however, interest has grown in larger cohort studies of low-grade gliomas treated with a combination of procarbazine, lomustine, and vincristine (Pedersen & Romner, 2013).

Grade II gliomas almost invariably transform to more malignant tumors, such as anaplastic gliomas (grade III) or glioblastoma multiforme (GBM; grade IV) (Stupp, Brada, van den Bent, Tonn, & Pentheroudakis, 2014). Although GBM accounts for more than 45% of malignant primary brain tumors, it is responsible for only 15.4% of all primary brain tumors (Ostrom, Gittleman, et al., 2014). Patients with GBM present nearly 50% of the time with a primary complaint of a headache, usually with unilateral localization and progressive severity, and 20%–40% present with a seizure, often with a focal onset (Omuro & DeAngelis, 2013). Obtaining a brain MRI is essential to help with staging because GBM metastases outside the CNS are rare. First-line treatment is almost always surgical resection, and biopsies may be tested with a methylation-specific polymerase chain reaction, as an epigenetically silenced methyl-guanine methyl transferase (*MGMT*) gene is associated with a decreased ability to recover from DNA damage. Methylated MGMT increases the tumor's sensitivity to alkylating agent chemotherapy, nearly doubling median survival from 13 to 23 months with postsurgical TMZ treatment (Stupp et al., 2014).

Nursing Implications

Because of the fast rate of growth in GBM as well as the increased risk of thromboembolic events, patients should be assessed regularly for performance status and neurologic function. An increased risk of stroke and deep vein thrombosis is attributed to a tumor-induced hypercoagulable state, neurologic deficits, immobilization, and steroid use. ICP monitoring should be considered with a change in neurologic status. Cerebral and tumor-associated edema may be alleviated with steroids such as dexamethasone. Steroid treatment is usually followed with rapid tapering and discontinuation after surgical resection to avoid toxicity. Radiation often follows surgery, and 4–12 weeks after completion of radiation treatment, an MRI is used to evaluate the tumor's initial response (Stupp et al., 2014). A pseudoprogression may be observed in 60% of patients, as radiation therapy may result in increased contrast enhancement (Stupp et al., 2014).

Metastatic Brain Tumors

Most brain tumors originate in other tissues and metastasize to the brain (secondary or metastatic brain tumor), making early recognition of the primary tumor that much more vital. Metastatic brain tumors are estimated to occur at a rate of 7–14 per 100,000 age-adjusted persons (Fox, Cheung, Patel, Suki, & Rao, 2011); however, true incidence is difficult to measure because many brain metastases are identified during autopsy (Fox et al., 2011). Up to 40% of all systemic cancers originating outside of the brain eventually will metastasize to it, and the incidence of metastatic brain cancer is as high as 10 times that of primary brain cancer (Patchell, 2003).

Lung cancer (primarily small cell and adenocarcinoma) is the most common source of brain metastases. Brain metastasis secondary to lung cancer is thought to be related to the advanced progression of the disease before presentation of symptoms. In fact, a diagnosis of lung cancer often follows with the presentation of neurologic symptoms of brain metastases. Equally important, 91% of patients with lung cancer with a working diagnosis of localized disease have been found to have brain metastases within one year of their initial diagnosis for lung cancer (Schouten, Rutten, Huveneers, & Twijnstra, 2002).

Nurses caring for patients with cancer should note that other primary cancers have significantly high rates of metastasis to the brain. Breast cancer is the second most common cause of secondary brain tumors, followed by skin cancer (melanoma), and then cancer of the gastrointestinal tract (colorectal) (Langley & Fidler, 2013). Many attribute the rising incidence of secondary brain tumors to the improved efficacy of cancer treatment options, which has resulted in increased survival time of patients with cancer but also has allowed more time for cancer cells to enter the bloodstream and metastasize to the brain.

The process of metastasizing to the brain requires cancer cells to overcome several barriers, beginning with normal cells being converted to cancer cells in the host organ. After the cancer cells attach to the extracellular matrix, the malignant cells rapidly degrade the matrix by producing proteolytic enzymes and pro-inflammatory cytokines. The degradation process allows the cancer cells to enter the bloodstream (Ridley et al., 2003). The entry can occur either by penetrating the thin-walled endothelium of small vessels or by circulating in the lymphatic system until entry to the blood vessels is achieved.

After entering the bloodstream, the cancer cells must overcome the predisposition of cells toward apoptosis (normal cell death) and avoid host immunity (death from natural killer cells). Cancer cells also can seed the venous capillary bed of the lungs before reaching the arterial circulation through the left heart. This process is the basis for the strong correlation between lung cancer and brain metastasis, as the lung capillary bed is the last site for metastatic localization before the metastatic cells enter the left heart and are then transported via the arterial system to the brain (Gavrilovic & Posner, 2005).

The Blood–Brain Barrier

The blood–brain barrier (BBB) is an important concept for neurologic nursing, as it plays a role in every aspect of brain function, from nutrition and metabolism to proper medication dosing and duration. The BBB is the final barrier against cancer cells gaining access to the brain and is formed by junctions between endothelial cells, the basement membrane, and the end-feet processes of astrocytes. These structures combine to limit the access of water-soluble, charged, and large objects to CNS tissues.

Metastatic cancer cells use a class of proteins called selectins to attach to the endothelial wall of vessels and upregulate other proteins, known as integrins, to aid in extravasation into the extracellular matrix of the brain (Preusser et al., 2012). Once tumor cells have breached the BBB and have entered the CNS, the cells still must adapt to the unique environment of the brain. In fact, some cancers, such as melanoma and certain breast cancers, do not immediately adapt to the environment, but they enter a dormant phase that can last years past eradication of the primary tumor before maturing into an active secondary brain tumor (Preusser et al., 2012).

Although the BBB provides protection from a plethora of potential pathogens, it is also agnostic to preventing entry to the CNS. Most chemotherapy agents are water soluble. This makes it difficult for the chemotherapy agent to pass through the tight junctions of the BBB, therefore providing a sanctuary for tumorigenesis and growth. Most current treatments will not be able to reach the tumor until it has developed its own leaky vasculature (i.e., a breakdown in the BBB). This breakdown is typically through the process of angiogenesis, or the natural formation of new blood vessels.

One experimental technique to provide reversible BBB disruption is the addition of concentrated solutions into the carotid artery. This method works by osmotically drawing water out of the endothelial cells of brain vessels, resulting in cell shrinkage and cracks in the tight junctions, allowing chemotherapy agents to leak into the CNS. The vessels eventually resume their normal BBB function after the hypertonic bolus enters venous drainage (Kroll & Neuwelt, 1998).

Monitoring the Brain

A thorough nursing history is crucial in almost every aspect of nursing care. This is especially true with neurologic disease (Olson, Meek, & Lynch, 2004). Because many brain tumor symptoms are episodic in nature and the likelihood of interviewing the patient during the episode is low, a detailed history is paramount for early diagnosis (Gates, 2010). Symptoms that should alert a caregiver to the possibility of a brain tumor include headache, cognitive difficulties, personality changes, gait disorder, hemiparesis (single-sided weakness), aphasia (difficulty understanding speech or speaking), or a visual field defect.

Mild neurologic deficits (by history or examination) that progressively and steadily worsen are a hallmark of brain tumors. The classic headache associated with a brain tumor is most evident in the morning but improves during the day. Although headaches occur in 50% of patients with brain tumors, the pattern of a steadily worsening headache is seen in a minority of cases (Hauser & Josephson, 2010). Seizure is the second most common symptom leading to a diagnosis of an underlying brain tumor and is seen in more than 70% of low-grade gliomas, 38% of all primary CNS tumors, and 18%–20% of metastatic brain tumors (Hauser & Josephson, 2010; Lynam et al., 2007). In a cohort of 200 pediatric patients with brain tumors, 41% experienced a headache as their first symptom, followed by vomiting (12%), unsteadiness (11%), and visual difficulties (10%). The 42 patients in the study that were aged 3 years or younger were more likely to present with behavioral problems (48%) over headache (12%) or seizure (7%) (Wilne, Ferris, Nathwani, & Kennedy, 2006).

When taking a history, one should question patients about the symptoms immediately before, during, and after the episode that brought them to the hospital. Important qualifying information can be gathered concerning abnormal body movement (e.g., head, limbs), duration of any episodes (including loss of consciousness), and in the case of pain, whether it is dull or sharp, radiates, or if any action relieves it. A thorough personal and family history should also be gathered to better understand the potential etiology of the symptoms; however, these findings can only suggest the cause and should never rule out other pathologic processes (Gates, 2010).

A neurologic examination should fully investigate the primary complaint and explore the patient's mental status, cranial nerves, sensory and motor systems, reflexes, cerebellum, meninges, and system survey (Bader et al., 2016). Any irregular findings on neurologic examination can point to a brain tumor or at least neural involvement. An observant caregiver checking the cognitive status or reflexes of a patient with cancer could identify and aid in the early treatment of brain metastasis.

Diagnosing Neurologic Disease

Computed Tomography Scan

A CT scan creates a series of cross-sectional images of a patient from the rotation of an x-ray beam and an associated detector. The resulting tomographic images (slices) are a map of the comparative attenuation of the x-ray signal by the patient's body tissue, which has various densities (e.g., fat, muscle, bone, tumor). A CT scan lacks the sensitivity and high resolution of an MRI and delivers significant, undesirable radiation to the brain; however, CT devices cost less, have fewer restrictions, and are more readily available than MRIs. A CT scan is indicated over an MRI in any patient with metal cardiac or cochlear implants or implanted electronic devices (e.g., a pacemaker) that could interfere with the magnetic resonance signal or create a safety hazard for the patient. A CT scan is often used as the first imaging choice in the initial evaluation of altered mental status, suspected acute stroke, hemorrhage, or trauma (Hauser & Josephson, 2010).

Magnetic Resonance Imaging

When a brain tumor is suspected, an MRI is the preferred method of diagnosis because of its high resolution and absence of ionizing radiation, which is inherent to a CT scan. MRI images are created by passing a strong, alternating magnetic field over the brain, causing hydrogen atoms (protons) to momentarily transition from a low- to a high-energy state. When the hydrogen protons return to their resting state (relax), an energy wave is emitted. The magnitude of the energy emitted is unique to the object being imaged. Its characteristics are used to differentiate the various structures of the brain. In conventional applications, two relaxation rates are measured, with T1 being the time in milliseconds for 63% of the protons to return to their resting state and T2 being the time for 63% to dephase because of the interaction of other protons (Hauser & Josephson, 2010). See Table 1-2 for definitions of the common terms used in brain MRI scanning.

Table 1-2. Common Magnetic Resonance Imaging Terms	
Term	**Working Definition**
Blood-oxygen-level dependent (BOLD)	BOLD is a functional magnetic resonance imaging (MRI) scanning technique used to differentiate active brain.
Diffusion-weighted imaging (DWI)	DWI is an MRI technique used to weight the signal by the amount of diffusion of water molecules in selected voxels.
Fluid-attenuated inversion recovery (FLAIR)	FLAIR is an MRI technique that nulls the effect of fluid on the image.
Functional MRI (fMRI)	fMRI observations are made to assess how different parts of the brain respond to stimuli.
Magnetic resonance angiogram (MRA)	MRA is a technique used to show the blood vessels.
Magnetic resonance spectroscopy (MRS)	MRS is a technique used to study the magnetic resonance spectrum of a tissue (e.g., glioma).
Pixel	A pixel is the smallest part of a digital image. Its name derives from picture (pix) and element (el).
T1	T1 is the time in milliseconds for 63% of the protons to return to their resting state.
T1-weighted	T1-weighted are images where much of the contrast is due to differences in T1 tissue.
T2	T2 is the time for 63% of the protons to dephase due to the interaction of other protons.
T2-weighted	T2-weighted are images where much of the contrast is due to differences in T2 tissue.
Voxel	A voxel is a three-dimensional volume element corresponding to a pixel.

Common MRI sequences used to diagnose brain tumors include T1-weighted, T1-weighted with gadolinium contrast enhancement, T2-weighted, and T2-weighted with fluid-attenuated inversion recovery (FLAIR). T1-weighted is used for baseline structural analysis, while T1-weighted with gadolinium contrast enhancement highlights tumor borders caused by the leakiness of the BBB in the region. T2-weighted brightens the edema region surrounding the tumor, and FLAIR enhances this by separating the edema from the CSF (Bauer, Wiest, Nolte, & Reyes, 2013).

Newer magnetic resonance techniques have gained popularity in noninvasive exploration of the morphologic, functional, and metabolic properties

of brain tumors, such as diffusion-weighted imaging (DWI), magnetic resonance spectroscopy (MRS), and perfusion-weighted imaging (PWI) (Bauer et
al., 2013). DWI is useful in grading gliomas, measuring brain injury following tumor resection, mapping white matter tracts, and differentiating cacogenic
(leaky vessels) from cytotoxic edema. MRS is a powerful technique that provides a signature spectrum (fingerprint) that noninvasively characterizes tissue
type (biopsy signature for benign vs. malignant) and can also provide metabolic
information, such as lactate levels or information to help monitor oxygen levels. PWI offers a measure of tumor angiogenesis as well as the permeability of
capillaries, both of which are important markers of malignancy and prognosis
(Cha, 2006).

Positron-Emission Tomography

PET detects photons when a positron is emitted from a radioactive agent
interacting with an electron. The most commonly used positron-emitting iso-
tope is fluorine-18, and the most commonly used imaging agent is FDG, a glucose analog that mimics glucose uptake in metabolically active tissue. It can
reveal regional differences between the metabolic activity in normal tissue and
fast-growing tumors (Hauser & Josephson, 2010). PET imaging has the advantage of pinpointing small, metabolically active tumors that an MRI might over-
look; however, its usage is limited by the already high metabolism of glucose
in healthy brain tissue. Although PET may not be used in the initial diagnosis
of most brain tumors, it can aid in differentiating recurrent tumor from radiation necrosis. High uptake in a previously low-grade tumor that had low uptake
establishes the diagnosis of anaplastic transformation. Currently, high interest exists in the future of novel PET tracers, such as [18F]fluoro-methionine and
[18F]fluorodopa to target tumors that FDG may miss, 3'-deoxy-3'-[18F]fluorothy-
midine to evaluate tumor cell proliferation, and [18F]fluoromisonidazole for the
imaging of tumor hypoxia (Chen, 2007).

Combined PET/MRI machines are being developed to perform integrated
metabolic/anatomic imaging with a single machine; however, MRI alone is the
superior option for almost any brain tumor indication when available. Although
PET/MRI is a hopeful possibility in development, its availability has been largely
limited by cost (Buchbender et al., 2012).

Electroencephalogram

The presence of seizure can be accurately ruled out by electroencephalography
(EEG). Patients with both primary and secondary brain tumors may have seizure
as their presentation. Seizure is considered a medical emergency and should be
treated immediately. Status epilepticus is defined as a seizure that lasts longer than
five minutes (Brophy et al., 2012). On stabilization, patients who present with seizures and are found to have brain tumors via MRI analysis may undergo a video

encephalography prior to surgical resection. The purpose of a long presurgical EEG evaluation is to ensure that the chosen surgically removed section of brain will result in a seizure-free outcome, as concern exists that the source of epilepsy may be outside of the tumor. However, mounting evidence suggests that certain cancers, such as low-grade gliomas and glioneuronal tumors, have a high enough correlation with seizure symptoms that EEG may not be necessary prior to surgery (Kennedy & Schuele, 2013).

Multimodal Brain Monitoring

The concept of multimodal brain monitoring has become widespread. Robust agreement exists that the brain has electrical, chemical, and biologic functions. As such, the tools required to monitor the brain must include electrical, chemical, and biologic monitors. In concert, tasks traditionally relegated to subjective human observation have been replaced by technological advancement. The practice of evaluating for the presence of stroke simply by examination has been augmented by radiologic imaging. The subjective pupillary examination has been replaced by automated pupillometry (Olson et al., 2016). Assessing for central cyanosis as a surrogate for the adequacy of cerebral perfusion has been replaced by sensors capturing infrared light. Seizure is now captured on video and linked to cerebral electrical signals. Monitoring the brain has become simultaneously easier and more complex.

Cerebral Cellular Metabolism

A fundamental understanding of cerebral cellular metabolism is helpful to appreciate the purpose and methodology of continuously monitoring the brain. A primary function of metabolism (cellular respiration) is to produce energy in the form of adenosine triphosphate (ATP), a high-energy molecule used by much of the cellular machinery throughout the human body. ATP production requires glucose and greatly benefits from oxygen. When oxygen is available, ATP is produced primarily by the citric acid cycle (aerobic), which creates far more ATP than glycolysis (anaerobic). If no oxygen is present, cells are forced to depend on anaerobic metabolism for ATP production. The by-products of anaerobic metabolism are lactate and pyruvate.

In stark terms, the brain is an oxygen and glucose hog. The brain is one of the most metabolically active organs in the human body and requires a large supply of ATP. The sodium-potassium (Na^+/K^+) pump maintains the osmotic and electrochemical gradient of cells and is entirely dependent on a constant supply of ATP. Without a steady supply of aerobic ATP production, the Na^+/K^+ pump slows down, and sodium begins to leak into the cells of the brain. As sodium goes into the cell, it draws in water and the cell swells (cerebral edema). Unless reversed, the process of swelling will eventually lead to cell death. This is a primary example of cytotoxic cerebral edema.

The brain stores neither oxygen nor glucose, making it entirely dependent on the oxygen and glucose concentrations in the blood reaching the brain and the extent of delivery throughout the vasculature of the brain. Brain tumors can obstruct this delivery. Both cancer and cancer therapy can drastically affect oxygen being carried in the blood (oxygen bound to hemoglobin) and, ultimately, the blood supply to the brain (cerebral perfusion); continuous monitoring of these and other factors is vital to the well-being of patients with cancer.

To this end, critically ill and hospitalized patients with cancer should always have some form of continuous measure of blood oxygen content. Systemic oxygen is best measured by oxygen saturation (SaO_2), an expression of the percentage of all hemoglobin binding sites in the blood bound to oxygen. Normal SaO_2 is greater than 90%.

Pulse Oximetry

Pulse oximetry is a highly reliable and the least invasive method of estimating SaO_2. The abbreviation SpO_2 may be used to denote the source of measurement (e.g., pulsatile flow in the finger) of SaO_2. Pulse oximetry is a direct measure of SaO_2 and works by passing light at different wavelengths (usually red and infrared) through an ear or finger and measuring the difference in absorption sensed on the other side, which corresponds to the concentration of saturated to unsaturated hemoglobin (Aoyagi, 2003).

Arterial Blood Gas

Alternatively, SaO_2 can be calculated from an arterial blood gas (ABG) sample. In the critically ill patient, this is most commonly accomplished by inserting a catheter into an artery (arterial line). An arterial line allows for direct measurement of blood pressure, serves as a conduit for obtaining blood samples (lab samples), and measures ABGs (acid–base concentration, partial pressure of oxygen, partial pressure of CO_2 [$PaCO_2$], bicarbonate, and the base excess/deficit in the blood). When available, this method of monitoring for systemic hypoxemia and hypercapnia is by far the most reliable (Le Roux et al., 2014).

End-Tidal Carbon Dioxide

End-tidal carbon dioxide ($ETCO_2$) is broadly used in caring for the critically ill patient with known or suspected brain injury. $ETCO_2$ can be measured noninvasively by a capnometer and expressed as a percentage or in mm Hg. $ETCO_2$ reflects circulation, metabolism, and ventilation. In the absence of illness or injury, $ETCO_2$ will approximate $PaCO_2$ within 2–5 mm Hg, with normal values in the range of 35–40 mm Hg. In impaired pulmonary function, such as in lung cancer or chemotherapy-related pulmonary fibrosis, the gradient between these two values may fluctuate over time (Oddo & Bösel, 2014). Higher $ETCO_2$ values generally correlate with hypoventilation or respiratory acidosis, whereas lower values correlate with hyperventilation or respiratory alkalosis. Although originally developed for mechanically ventilated patients, $ETCO_2$ is now available for patients with mask and/or nasal oxygen delivery systems. $ETCO_2$ is increasingly being used as an adjunct monitor for oversedation in patients with narcotic infusion (e.g., patients with cancer using patient-controlled analgesia pumps).

Partial Pressure of Brain Tissue Oxygen

Although SaO_2 and $ETCO_2$ monitoring may provide the nurse with indirect but key aspects of cerebral perfusion, it may become beneficial to directly measure the brain oxygen level. Regional brain tissue oxygen tension is measured as the partial pressure of brain tissue oxygen ($PbtO_2$), which is measured by directly inserting a catheter into the subcortical white matter and often monitored alongside ICP (Oddo & Bösel, 2014). The normal range of $PbtO_2$ is 25–35 mm Hg, with values lower than 20 considered abnormal and at risk of ischemia; however, $PbtO_2$ is not only a marker of ischemia or cerebral blood flow, and values vary with probe location (Le Roux et al., 2014).

Venous Oxygen Saturation

An alternative to $PbtO_2$ monitoring is the insertion of a central venous catheter into the jugular bulb. The catheter can be used to sample the by-products of intracranial circulation by measuring the venous oxygen saturation, or $SjvO_2$ (Oddo & Bösel, 2014). $SjvO_2$ values can detect both ischemia and hyperemia, but position, clot formation, and human error can make this method less reliable than $PbtO_2$ monitoring (Le Roux et al., 2014).

Near-Infrared Spectroscopy

Near-infrared spectroscopy (NIRS) is an enticing alternative to the invasive methods of measuring brain tissue oxygen level. NIRS is noninvasive and works similarly to the rather reliable pulse oximeter. By using the near-infrared spectrum (700–1100 nm), photons from multiple sources can travel several centimeters or more into the brain tissue. These photons can penetrate the skull and refract or scatter to surface signal sensors (Scheeren, Schober, & Schwarte, 2012). Like SaO_2, hemoglobin molecules saturated with oxygen will absorb specific portions of the spectrum. Algorithms have been developed to produce a digital display that reflects the oxygen content available in the region of the brain corresponding to the NIRS sensor. Four commercially available models exist, including FORE-SIGHT® by CAS Medical Systems, Inc., EQUANOX™ by Nonin Medical, Inc., INVOS™ by Medtronic, and NIRO® by Hamamatsu Photonics K.K. (Oddo &

Bösel, 2014). Although great potential exists for future improvements on this and similar noninvasive measurements, medical consensus is that NIRS has limitations in adult use and minimal clinical use (Le Roux et al., 2014).

Intracranial Pressure Monitoring

ICP is a well-established cornerstone in multimodal neurocritical care monitoring. For the neurologically injured patient, ICP provides another vital measurement, particularly in the setting of advanced or fast-growing brain tumors. ICP is most often measured invasively via an EVD connected to a strain-gauge transducer or via a fiber-optic pressure monitor placed into the intraparenchymal tissue. ICP monitoring via EVD is accomplished by inserting a catheter through a coronal burr hole into either of the lateral ventricles. The EVD catheter is advantageous in that it allows the nurse to drain CSF out of the ventricles. Draining CSF may aid in reducing ICP in the setting of obstructive hydrocephalus (Reddy et al., 2011). Additionally, an EVD provides an entry point for intrathecal (into CSF) administration of therapeutic agents (Raboel, Bartek, Andresen, Bellander, & Romner, 2012). ICP monitoring and CSF drainage have been associated with a known risk of complications, including infection (Olson, Zomorodi, James, et al., 2013).

Alternatively, ICP micro transducers can be used when EVD is not desired. This group comprises fiber-optic, strain-gauge, and pneumatic devices most commonly placed into the parenchyma. The prototypical fiber-optic micro transducer is the Camino® Intracranial Pressure Monitor, which uses a fiber-optic cable and a mirror that is moved depending on ICP. Piezoelectric strain gauges, such as the MicroSensor™ ICP Transducer by Codman and Shurtleff, Inc., Neurovent-P® by Raumedic, Inc., and the Pressio® sensor by Sophysa, Ltd., measure the resistance changes in a sensor that bends under pressure. Pneumatic sensors, such as the pressure sensors by Spiegelberg GmbH & Co. KG, measure ICP using a small balloon. Although research is limited, lower risk of infection exists with intraparenchymal ICP monitoring compared to EVD monitoring. Fiber-optic ICP monitoring has been associated with infection in two studies, while the Spiegelberg sensor has caused few errors with no infection. The MicroSensor ICP Transducer and Neurovent-P showed no infection or technical errors in efficacy studies (Raboel et al., 2012).

Cerebral Perfusion Pressure

As ICP rises or blood pressure drops, cerebral perfusion pressure (CPP) drops. A rapid or excessive decrease in CPP may lead to cerebral ischemia. CPP is defined as the mean arterial pressure (MAP) minus the ICP (CPP = MAP − ICP) and is used as a surrogate marker of the adequacy of tissue blood perfusion. When brain vasculature is healthy, it regulates blood flow by controlling the size of arterioles, or cerebral autoregulation. This can only occur when MAP is within

50–150 mm Hg, cerebrovascular feedback mechanisms are intact, and ICP is approximately normal (Raboel et al., 2012).

Treating Elevated Intracranial Pressure

The treatment for elevated ICP is typically dichotomized based on mechanism of injury (traumatic vs. nontraumatic brain injury). The guidelines for monitoring and treating elevated ICP in nontraumatic injury (e.g., neoplasm) advocate for a stepwise approach; however, approaches vary from institution to institution (Helbok, Olson, Le Roux, & Vespa, 2014). Although no definitive evidence exists to support a best practice for ICP management, most strategies employ CSF drainage, osmotic diuretic (mannitol), hypertonic saline, temperature management (hypothermia), and in cases of refractory intracranial hypertension, surgical resection or hemicraniectomy (Bader et al., 2016). Fluid volume replacement and vasopressive medications to enhance CPP have also been advocated (Helbok et al., 2014).

Cerebral Blood Flow

The measurement of cerebral blood flow is another neurocritical parameter to keep in mind. Although continual measurement in a single location can be made with thermal diffusion flowmetry or laser Doppler flowmetry probes, their use is limited by invasiveness, small field of view, and placement uncertainty (Le Roux et al., 2014). Noninvasive transcranial Doppler and transcranial color-coded duplex sonography are far preferred for monitoring larger regions of the brain. Although primarily used to predict vasospasm in the aftermath of subarachnoid hemorrhage in the NCCU, measurement of the rate of blood flow into regions where a tumor may be compressing can be of great use in treating a critically ill patient with a brain tumor (Miller & Armonda, 2014).

Continuous Electroencephalography

The wide availability of EEG monitoring has extended the use of EEG beyond a single-time, limited observation. Continuous EEG monitoring is increasingly being used in the NCCU for several days at a time to evaluate for seizure and determine the success or failure of treatment regimens. High-speed computing and microprocessors have helped further the field of electrical signal monitoring. Consciousness, neurofunction, and hypnosis monitoring have been developed to acquire and transform raw EEG signals. The bispectral index and SedLine® monitoring systems both rely on computerized algorithms (fast Fourier transform) to analyze components of the EEG signal and produce a highly reliable numeric interpretation of an individual's level of consciousness, ranging from 0 (no brain activity) to 100 (maximal activity). This technology has been validated intraoperatively and in critical care as an adjunct to subjective sedation assessment (Olson, Zomorodi, Britz, et al., 2013).

Therapy and Treatment

Nursing Care

The type and intensity of therapy provided for patients with cancer and brain injury vary widely. The role of the nurse as clinician, educator, and patient advocate cannot be overstated. An accurate and comprehensive neurologic examination is fundamental in providing the medical team, patients, and families with information to determine prognosis and treatment options. Because nurses often have unique relationships with patients and their families, the contributions of nursing toward education and patient advocacy are essential elements of care.

Surgery

Surgery can be curative or palliative and is indicated for removal of mass (e.g., hematoma, neoplasm), repair (e.g., aneurysm clipping), or alleviation of pressure (e.g., decompressive hemicraniectomy). The most common postsurgical complications are cerebral edema and hemorrhage. After undergoing surgical resection of a brain tumor, patients should be observed closely for 12–24 hours in an intensive care unit to detect and rapidly treat postoperative complications (Ziai, Veralas, Zeger, Mirski, & Ulatowski, 2003). Beyond cerebral edema, other common postoperative complications include pulmonary issues, dysphagia/vocal cord paresis, seizures, cerebral edema, and cardiac arrhythmias (Ziai et al., 2003).

Radiation

Although acute brain injury days to weeks after irradiation is rare in modern radiation therapy, early delayed brain injury occurs one to six months after treatment and involves transient demyelination and somnolence (Greene-Schloesser et al., 2012). These can result in serious complications but are usually self-limiting and reversible.

Late delayed brain injury occurs after six months and is described by irreversible and progressive vascular abnormalities, demyelination, and white matter necrosis, which can lead to dementia and death (Greene-Schloesser et al., 2012). Two schools of thought delineate on how this occurs. One proposes that radiation damages the vasculature of the brain, leading to ischemic damage to the white matter, while the other attributes the death of oligodendrocytes (myelin loss) and astrocytes (physical support) to the collapse of brain infrastructure and vasculature.

Regardless, radiation-induced cognitive impairment, including dementia, occurs in 50%–90% of patients with brain tumors who survive more than six months after irradiation (Greene-Schloesser et al., 2012). Symptoms include loss of verbal and spatial memory, attention, and problem-solving ability. Occasionally, patients who receive more than 3 Gy progress to dementia with progressive memory loss, ataxia, and urinary incontinence (Greene-Schloesser et al., 2012).

Chemotherapy

Neurotoxic side effects are very common and are often dose limiting in the treatment of cancer. Vinca alkaloids, cisplatin, and taxanes are most commonly peripherally neurotoxic, while methotrexate, cytarabine, and ifosfamide are known for central neurotoxicity (Verstappen, Heimans, Hoekman, & Postma, 2003). Cognitive or neurologic deficits after chemotherapy, such as "chemobrain," have been identified as a real phenomenon (Frank, Vance, Triebel, & Meneses, 2015). The exact pathophysiology, identification, and treatment of chemobrain have yet to be identified (Wang et al., 2015).

Summary

Nursing care of patients with cancer is multidimensional. Spanning the continuum from cure to care to palliation, nurses must carefully consider the tools best suited for each individual patient. The NCCU environment is rapidly evolving. New treatment modalities and methods of assessment are being developed every year. Nurses providing care to patients with cancer and acute neurologic injury benefit from understanding these evolving options.

References

Aoyagi, T. (2003). Pulse oximetry: Its invention, theory, and future. *Journal of Anesthesia, 17,* 259–266. doi:10.1007/s00540-003-0192-6

Arafah, B.M., & Nasrallah, M.P. (2001). Pituitary tumors: Pathophysiology, clinical manifestations and management. *Endocrine-Related Cancer, 8,* 287–305. doi:10.1677/erc.0.0080287

Bader, M.K., Littlejohns, L.R., & Olson, D.M. (Eds.). (2016). *AANN core curriculum for neuroscience nursing* (6th ed.). Glenview, IL: American Association of Neuroscience Nurses.

Bauer, S., Wiest, R., Nolte, L.-P., & Reyes, M. (2013). A survey of MRI-based medical image analysis for brain tumor studies. *Physics in Medicine and Biology, 58,* R97. doi:10.1088/0031-9155/58/13/R97

Brophy, G.M., Bell, R., Claassen, J., Alldredge, B., Bleck, T.P., Glauser, T., ... Vespa, P.M. (2012). Guidelines for the evaluation and management of status epilepticus. *Neurocritical Care, 17,* 3–23. doi:10.1007/s12028-012-9695-z

Buchbender, C., Heusner, T.A., Lauenstein, T.C., Bockisch, A., & Antoch, G. (2012). Oncologic PET/MRI, part 1: Tumors of the brain, head and neck, chest, abdomen, and pelvis. *Journal of Nuclear Medicine, 53,* 928–938. doi:10.2967/jnumed.112.105338

Cha, S. (2006). Update on brain tumor imaging: From anatomy to physiology. *American Journal of Neuroradiology, 27,* 475–487.

Chen, W. (2007). Clinical applications of PET in brain tumors. *Journal of Nuclear Medicine, 48,* 1468–1481. doi:10.2967/jnumed.106.037689

Fox, B.D., Cheung, V.J., Patel, A.J., Suki, D., & Rao, G. (2011). Epidemiology of metastatic brain tumors. *Neurosurgery Clinics of North America, 22,* 1–6. doi:10.1016/j.nec.2010.08.007

Frank, J.S., Vance, D.E., Triebel, K.L., & Meneses, K.M. (2015). Cognitive deficits in breast cancer survivors after chemotherapy and hormonal therapy. *Journal of Neuroscience Nursing, 47,* 302–312. doi:10.1097/JNN.0000000000000171

Freda, P.U., & Wardlaw, S.L. (1999). Diagnosis and treatment of pituitary tumors. *Journal of Clinical Endocrinology and Metabolism, 84,* 3859–3866. doi:10.1210/jcem.84.11.6202

Gates, P. (2010). *Clinical neurology: A primer.* Sydney, Australia: Elsevier Australia.

Gavrilovic, I.T., & Posner, J.B. (2005). Brain metastases: Epidemiology and pathophysiology. *Journal of Neuro-Oncology, 75,* 5–14. doi:10.1007/s11060-004-8093-6

Glezer, A., & Bronstein, M.D. (2015). Prolactinomas. *Endocrinology and Metabolism Clinics of North America, 44,* 71–78. doi:10.1016/j.ecl.2014.11.003

Greene-Schloesser, D., Robbins, M.E., Peiffer, A.M., Shaw, E.G., Wheeler, K.T., & Chan, M.D. (2012). Radiation-induced brain injury: A review. *Frontiers in Oncology, 2,* 73. doi:10.3389/fonc.2012.00073

Hauser, S., & Josephson, S. (Eds.). (2010). *Harrison's neurology in clinical medicine* (3rd ed.). Columbus, OH: McGraw-Hill Education.

Helbok, R., Olson, D.M., Le Roux, P.D., & Vespa, P. (2014). Intracranial pressure and cerebral perfusion pressure monitoring in non-TBI patients: Special considerations. *Neurocritical Care, 21*(Suppl. 2), s85–s94. doi:10.1007/s12028-014-0040-6

Kennedy, J., & Schuele, S.U. (2013). Long-term monitoring of brain tumors: When is it necessary? *Epilepsia, 54,* 50–55. doi:10.1111/epi.12444

Kroll, R.A., & Neuwelt, E.A. (1998). Outwitting the blood-brain barrier for therapeutic purposes: Osmotic opening and other means. *Neurosurgery, 42,* 1083–1099. doi:10.1097/00006123-199805000-00082

Langley, R.R., & Fidler, I.J. (2013). The biology of brain metastasis. *Clinical Chemistry, 59,* 180–189. doi:10.1373/clinchem.2012.193342

Le Roux, P.D., Menon, D.K., Citerio, G., Vespa, P., Bader, M.K., Brophy, G.M., ... Taccone, F. (2014). Consensus summary statement of the International Multidisciplinary Consensus Conference on Multimodality Monitoring in Neurocritical Care. *Intensive Care Medicine, 40,* 1189–1209. doi:10.1007/s00134-014-3369-6

Lynam, L.M., Lyons, M.K., Drazkowski, J.F., Sirven, J.I., Noe, K.H., Zimmerman, R.S., & Wilkens, J.A. (2007). Frequency of seizures in patients with newly diagnosed brain tumors: A retrospective review. *Clinical Neurology and Neurosurgery, 109,* 634–638. doi:10.1016/j.clineuro.2007.05.017

Melmed, S. (2011). Pathogenesis of pituitary tumors. *Nature Reviews Endocrinology, 7,* 257–266. doi:10.1038/nrendo.2011.40

Miller, C., & Armonda, R. (2014). Monitoring of cerebral blood flow and ischemia in the critically ill. *Neurocritical Care, 21*(Suppl. 2), 121–128. doi:10.1007/s12028-014-0021-9

Oddo, M., & Bösel, J. (2014). Monitoring of brain and systemic oxygenation in neurocritical care patients. *Neurocritical Care, 21*(Suppl. 2), 103–120. doi:10.1007/s12028-014-0024-6

Olson, D.M., Kofke, W.A., O'Phelan, K., Gupta, P.K., Figueroa, S.A., Smirnakis, S.M., ... Suarez, J.I. (2015). Global monitoring in the neurocritical care unit. *Neurocritical Care, 22,* 337–347. doi:10.1007/s12028-015-0132-y

Olson, D.M., Meek, L.A., & Lynch, J.R. (2004). Accurate patient history contributes to differentiating diabetes insipidus: A case study. *Journal of Neuroscience Nursing, 36,* 228–230. doi:10.1097/01376517-200408000-00011

Olson, D.M., Stutzman, S., Saju, C., Wilson, M., Zhao, W., & Aiyagari, V. (2016). Interrater reliability of pupillary assessments. *Neurocritical Care, 24,* 251–257. doi:10.1007/s12028-015-0182-1

Olson, D.M., Zomorodi, M.G., Britz, G.W., Zomorodi, A.R., Amato, A., & Graffagnino, C. (2013). Continuous cerebral spinal fluid drainage associated with complications in patients admitted with subarachnoid hemorrhage. *Journal of Neurosurgery, 119,* 974–980. doi:10.3171/2013.6.JNS122403

Olson, D.M., Zomorodi, M.G., James, M.L., Cox, C.E., Moretti, E.W., Riemen, K.E., & Graffagnino, C. (2013). Exploring the impact of augmenting sedation assessment with physiologic monitors. *Australian Critical Care, 27,* 145–150. doi:10.1016/j.aucc.2013.09.001

Omuro, A., & DeAngelis, L.M. (2013). Glioblastoma and other malignant gliomas: A clinical review. *JAMA, 310*, 1842–1850. doi:10.1001/jama.2013.280319

Ostrom, Q.T., Bauchet, L., Davis, F.G., Deltour, I., Fisher, J.L., Langer, C.E., … Barnholtz-Sloan, J.S. (2014). The epidemiology of glioma in adults: A "state of the science" review. *Neuro-Oncology, 16*, 896–913. doi:10.1093/neuonc/nou087

Ostrom, Q.T., Gittleman, H., Liao, P., Rouse, C., Chen, Y., Dowling, J., … Barnholtz-Sloan, J.S. (2014). CBTRUS Statistical Report: Primary brain and central nervous system tumors diagnosed in the United States in 2007–2011. *Neuro-Oncology, 16*(Suppl. 4), iv1–iv63. doi:10.1093/neuonc/nou223

Patchell, R.A. (2003). The management of brain metastases. *Cancer Treatment Reviews, 29*, 533–540. doi:10.1016/S0305-7372(03)00105-1

Pedersen, C.L., & Romner, B. (2013). Current treatment of low grade astrocytoma: A review. *Clinical Neurology and Neurosurgery, 115*, 1–8. doi:10.1016/j.clineuro.2012.07.002

Preusser, M., Capper, D., Ilhan-Mutlu, A., Berghoff, A.S., Birner, P., Bartsch, R., … von Deimling, A. (2012). Brain metastases: Pathobiology and emerging targeted therapies. *Acta Neuropathologica, 123*, 205–222. doi:10.1007/s00401-011-0933-9

Raboel, P.H., Bartek, J., Jr., Andresen, M., Bellander, B.M., & Romner, B. (2012). Intracranial pressure monitoring: Invasive versus non-invasive methods—A review. *Critical Care Research and Practice, 2012*, 950393. doi:10.1155/2012/950393

Reddy, G.K., Bollam, P., Caldito, G., Willis, B., Guthikonda, B., & Nanda, A. (2011). Ventriculoperitoneal shunt complications in hydrocephalus patients with intracranial tumors: An analysis of relevant risk factors. *Journal of Neuro-Oncology, 103*, 333–342. doi:10.1007/s11060-010-0393-4

Ridley, A.J., Schwartz, M.A., Burridge, K., Firtel, R.A., Ginsberg, M.H., Borisy, G., … Horwitz, A.R. (2003). Cell migration: Integrating signals from front to back. *Science, 302*, 1704–1709. doi:10.1126/science.1092053

Saloner, D., Uzelac, A., Hetts, S., Martin, A., & Dillon, W. (2010). Modern meningioma imaging techniques. *Journal of Neuro-Oncology, 99*, 333–340. doi:10.1007/s11060-010-0367-6

Scheeren, T.W.L., Schober, P., & Schwarte, L.A. (2012). Monitoring tissue oxygenation by near infrared spectroscopy (NIRS): Background and current applications. *Journal of Clinical Monitoring and Computing, 26*, 279–287. doi:10.1007/s10877-012-9348-y

Schouten, L.J., Rutten, J., Huveneers, H.A.M., & Twijnstra, A. (2002). Incidence of brain metastases in a cohort of patients with carcinoma of the breast, colon, kidney, and lung and melanoma. *Cancer, 94*, 2698–2705. doi:10.1002/cncr.10541

Stupp, R., Brada, M., van den Bent, M., Tonn, J.-C., & Pentheroudakis, G. (2014). High-grade glioma: ESMO clinical practice guidelines for diagnosis, treatment and follow-up. *Annals of Oncology, 25*(Suppl. 3), iii93–iii101. doi:10.1093/annonc/mdu050

Verstappen, C.C.P., Heimans, J.J., Hoekman, K., & Postma, T.J. (2003). Neurotoxic complications of chemotherapy in patients with cancer. *Drugs, 63*, 1549–1563. doi:10.2165/00003495-200363150-00003

Wang, X.-M., Walitt, B., Saligan, L., Tiwari, A.F.Y., Cheung, C.W., & Zhang, Z.-J. (2015). Chemobrain: A critical review and causal hypothesis of link between cytokines and epigenetic reprogramming associated with chemotherapy. *Cytokine, 72*, 86–96. doi:10.1016/j.cyto.2014.12.006

Wilne, S.H., Ferris, R.C., Nathwani, A., & Kennedy, C.R. (2006). The presenting features of brain tumours: A review of 200 cases. *Archives of Disease in Childhood, 91*, 502–506. doi:10.1136/adc.2005.090266

Ziai, W.C., Varelas, P.N., Zeger, S.L., Mirski, M.A., & Ulatowski, J.A. (2003). Neurologic intensive care resource use after brain tumor surgery: An analysis of indications and alternative strategies. *Critical Care Medicine, 31*, 2782–2787. doi:10.1097/01.CCM.0000098860.52812.24

CHAPTER 2

Lung Cancer

Cindy Byrd, DNP, RN, ACNP-BC

Introduction

Lung cancer is the leading cause of cancer death for both men and women in the United States, accounting for an estimated 26% (155,870) of all cancer-related deaths in 2017 (Siegel, Miller, & Jemal, 2017). Currently, more than 400,000 Americans are living with a lung cancer diagnosis, approximately 13% of all newly diagnosed cancers (American Lung Association [ALA], 2016c; Siegel et al., 2017). Lung cancer is the most commonly diagnosed cancer worldwide, accounting for approximately 1.8 million new diagnoses and 1.6 million deaths each year (ALA, 2016c).

The far-reaching effects of lung cancer make it a significant health issue. The National Institutes of Health estimates that lung cancer annually costs the U.S. healthcare system $13.4 billion (ALA, 2016c). This number does not include work-related loss of productivity from patients with lung cancer.

Types of Lung Cancer

Two major types of lung cancer exist: small cell lung cancer (SCLC) and non-small cell lung cancer (NSCLC) (ALA, 2016b). NSCLC accounts for about 80% of all newly diagnosed lung cancers (Burdett, Stewart, & Rydzewska, 2007).

NSCLC can be differentiated into three major types: adenocarcinoma, squamous cell carcinoma, and large cell carcinoma (ALA, 2016b). Adenocarcinoma begins in the cells that line the alveoli where mucus is produced (NCI, 2016). Squamous cell carcinoma originates in tissues formed in the surface of the skin, the passages of the respiratory and digestive tract, and the lining of hollow organs such as the bladder, kidneys, and uterus (NCI, 2016). Large cell carcinoma is named after its origin (in large type cells) and appearance (large cell) under a microscope (National Cancer Institute [NCI], 2016). Less common forms of NSCLC include pleomorphic, carcinoid tumor, salivary gland carcinoma, and unclassified carcinoma. Although different subgroups exist, these types are grouped as NSCLCs because of similar treatment protocols.

SCLC, previously known as oat cell carcinoma, is distinct from other lung cancers because of its clinical and biologic characteristics (NCI, 2016). It is a malignancy that originates from cells in the lung tissue, is very aggressive, and can rapidly metastasize. This cancer is strongly correlated with smoking, exposure to second-hand smoke, a family history of lung cancer, radiation therapy to the breast or chest, asbestos exposure, and radon exposure at home or in the workplace. Prompt identification and staging is required. Often, this type of carcinoma will metastasize early in the disease, with common sites in the mediastinal lymph nodes, liver, bones, adrenal glands, and brain (NCI, 2016). Frequent paraneoplastic syndromes also are prevalent with this type of malignancy, such as syndrome of inappropriate antidiuretic hormone secretion and syndrome of ectopic adrenocorticotropic hormone.

Diagnosis and Treatment

Routine screening is based on risk factors for the development of lung cancer. Patients who qualify for routine screening include those aged 55–80 years, those with a 30 pack-year smoking history, current smokers, or smokers who have quit within the past 15 years (ALA, 2016d). Providers must perform a thorough physical examination and an evaluation of the patient's social history. Table 2-1 outlines testing options used in the diagnosis and staging of lung cancer.

Once the presence of lung cancer is confirmed, the next step is to determine the most appropriate treatment modalities through a comprehensive staging process. This process includes understanding important universal abbreviations. Staging occurs by considering the primary tumor location (T), the regional lymph nodes involved (N), and the distance of metastasis (M). This nomenclature may be reviewed in its entirety on the American Joint Committee on Cancer website (https://cancerstaging.org/pages/default.aspx). Treatment options include surgery, radiation, chemotherapy, or a combination of these therapies.

Radiation Therapy

Radiation therapy is the process of receiving high-energy radiation to decrease tumor size, destroy cancer cells, and alleviate symptoms. This therapy can be used as an adjunct to surgical resection and is often used in conjunction with additional treatment modalities, including surgery and chemotherapy.

Table 2-1. Testing Options Used in the Diagnosis and Staging of Lung Cancer	
Procedure	**Description**
Chest x-ray	No longer recommended as a screening tool; often the first time abnormalities are seen
Sputum cytology	Sputum analyzed under a microscope for abnormal cells
Computed tomography scan	Slices of an area combined by a computer; only proven way to reduce the risk of dying from lung cancer in high-risk populations
Fine needle aspiration	Removal of tissue or fluid using a thin needle under computed tomography scan, ultrasound, or other imaging to identify abnormal tissue
Bronchoscopy	Use of a camera to visualize the trachea and large airways; can be used for direct sampling

Note. Based on information from American Lung Association, 2016a; National Cancer Institute, 2016.

Three radiation sources exist: gamma rays, x-rays, and charged particles. These may be administered to a patient in two ways. The first method is the external delivery of radiation outside the body, termed *external beam therapy. Internal radiation therapy*, or *brachytherapy*, is the second method and the process of inserting or implanting radioactive material into the body.

Radiation therapy for cure is indicated in patients with stage I, II, or III NSCLC with good performance status and whose disease may be covered in radiation therapy without the risk of damaging healthy tissue (National Collaborating Centre for Cancer [NCC-C], 2015). Medically inoperable patients with stage I or II NSCLC should be offered continuous, hyperfractionated, and accelerated radiation therapy as treatment (NCC-C, 2015).

Nursing implications for patients receiving radiation therapy include careful attention to external skin sites, as these areas may become irritated from radiation exposure. Patients should avoid lotions and creams prior to radiation and should bring severe skin burns to the attention of the radiation team.

Chemotherapy Agents and Side Effects

Chemotherapy agents used to treat advanced NSCLC are single third-generation drugs such as docetaxel, gemcitabine, paclitaxel, and vinorelbine plus a platinum drug such as cisplatin or carboplatin (NCC-C, 2015).

Like NSCLC, SCLC has improved survival over supportive care with the use chemotherapy agents that contain platinum, which is the standard of care; however, it is only curative in a minority of patients (Kurup & Hanna, 2004). Because of the small proportion of patients with SCLC (20% of all lung cancers) and the aggressive nature of the disease process, chemotherapy options are limited to platinum-based agents and etoposide.

Platinum-based chemotherapy agents (e.g., cisplatin, carboplatin, oxaliplatin) are the mainstay of cancer therapy, accounting for almost half of all chemotherapy agent use (Johnstone, Park, & Lippard, 2014). Side effects include nephrotoxicity (acute renal failure), ototoxicity (tinnitus), neurotoxicity, hematologic suppression, gastrointestinal distress, hepatic dysfunction, and anaphylaxis (Bristol-Myers Squibb Co., 2011).

In patients with NSCLC in which platinum-based therapy has been unsuccessful or the tumor is unresectable, locally advanced, or untreated, docetaxel is used. Docetaxel's mechanism of action is as an antimitotic agent, meaning it inhibits mitosis, or cell division, to also inhibit cancer growth (Sanofi-Aventis U.S. LLC, 2014). Docetaxel is associated with many serious side effects, including cardiovascular issues such as body fluid retention and vasodilation (Sanofi-Aventis U.S. LLC, 2014). Dermatologic effects include alopecia, disorders of the skin, nail changes, pruritus, rash, and more severe effects such as Stevens-Johnson syndrome and toxic epidermal necrolysis. Gastrointestinal side effects include diarrhea, inflammatory disease of mucous membranes, nausea, stomatitis, vomiting, and more severe side effects such as colitis. Significant hematologic alterations include anemia, leukopenia, and neutropenia. These side effects place patients at significant risk of opportunistic infections, which should always be carefully considered. Docetaxel also can cause significant organ dysfunction, including renal failure, hepatic dysfunction, and anaphylactic reaction.

Gemcitabine is used for patients with inoperable, locally advanced (stage IIIA or IIIB), or metastatic stage IV NSCLC. Gemcitabine's mechanism of action is that of a nucleoside metabolic inhibitor that exhibits antitumor activity by blocking cells from undergoing DNA synthesis (Eli Lilly & Co., 2014). This medication has a similar side effect profile as docetaxel but also has side effects of pulmonary toxicity, including pulmonary edema, pulmonary fibrosis, interstitial pneumonitis, acute respiratory distress syndrome (ARDS), and fatal respiratory failure.

Paclitaxel is an antimicrotubule agent, meaning it attacks the cells during various phases of division as an antimitotic, blocks the progression of mitosis, and prolongs the mitotic checkpoint triggers of apoptosis or reversion of the cell cycle without cell division (Bristol-Myers Squibb Co., 2011). When surgery and/or radiation therapy are not suitable for patients with NSCLC, paclitaxel is used as treatment in combination with cisplatin. It shares a similar side effect profile to other chemotherapy agents, with the most serious being anaphylaxis.

Vinorelbine is a vinca alkaloid with antitumor activity and is indicated as a first-line single agent in combination with cisplatin for treatment of patients with stage III and IV NSCLC. It shares a similar side effect profile with other chemotherapy agents.

Targeted Therapy

Targeted therapy includes either monoclonal antibodies or small-molecule drugs that block the action of certain enzymes and proteins (NCI, 2016). This treatment is indicated for certain cancer types and is used in conjunction with other treatments. A tumor biopsy is needed to determine if targeted therapy is appropriate.

Monoclonal antibodies are drugs that work on the outer surface of cancer cells. They can be used alone or concurrently with other drugs to target defects in cancer cells or make the cells more receptive to the body's immune system. Monoclonal antibodies also can be used as carriers for other drugs or as substrates directly to the cancer (NCI, 2016). For example, ramucirumab can be used in conjunction with docetaxel in stage IV NSCLC with continued tumor growth in addition to a platinum-based therapy (NCI, 2016). Bevacizumab can also be used for the treatment of nonsquamous cell NSCLC and can be given with traditional chemotherapy agents. Small-molecule drugs can enter the cells and inhibit them from normal function, leading to cell death. Examples include erlotinib, afatinib, crizotinib, ceritinib, and cetuximab.

Immunotherapy

Immunotherapy treats lung cancer by stimulating the body's immune response. Nivolumab and pembrolizumab are the two immunotherapy treatments currently approved for lung cancer. Nivolumab is used to treat squamous cell NSCLC that has spread during or after treatment with a platinum-based therapy. It is both a monoclonal antibody and a checkpoint inhibitor that addresses the PD-1 (programmed cell death protein 1) pathway (NCI, 2016). PD-1 binds to PD-L1 (a protein on some normal and cancer cells), allowing an immune response. Nivolumab binds to PD-1 and allows these pathways to be active. Pembrolizumab is used in patients with advanced NSCLC of PD-L1–positive tumor cells.

Surgery

Surgical options are based on tumor size, location, and disease progression (Van Schil et al., 2013). The three typical goals of surgery are cure, tumor debulking, or the symptom palliation. If the procedure's aim is curative, the surgeon's goal is to remove the entire tumor. A debulking procedure removes some of the tumor and may be used if an associated risk of injuring surrounding organs exists (Van Schil et al., 2013). A palliative surgical approach alleviates symptoms associated with the tumor, such as pain or obstruction; this is not a curative measure.

Lung cancer resections can be grouped into three major categories: standard resections, lung parenchymal–sparing procedures, and surgeries that involve the removal of surrounding organs (Van Schil et al., 2013). Standard resections include lobectomy (removal of a lobe of the lung), bilobectomy (removal of two lobes on the right side of the lung), and pneumonectomy (removal of the entire lung) (Burdett et al., 2007). Pneumonectomy was considered the treatment of choice through the 1940s; however, if the lesion can be fully resected, lobectomy currently has a similar survival rate with better patient outcomes (Burdett et al., 2007).

Lung parenchyma is the portion of the lung responsible for gas exchange and includes the alveoli, alveolar ducts, and bronchioles. Lung parenchyma–sparing procedures can be distal or proximal (Van Schil et al., 2013). Distal procedures include segmentectomies and wedge resections. A wedge resection procedure removes a wedge-shaped portion of lung that comprises cancerous cells and some healthy tissue. A segmentectomy is similar but takes out a larger portion of lung tissue without removing the entire lung.

Proximal procedures include bronchoplastic and tracheoplastic operations. The sleeve resection is the most common bronchoplastic procedure performed and is indicated for upper lobe orifice lung cancer. This procedure removes a cancerous lobe of lung and a portion of the bronchus.

A final resection procedure involves lung parenchyma with an adjacent tumor-invaded organ. Common procedures include resection of the chest wall, diaphragm, pericardium, left atrium, superior vena cava, or the apex of the chest (Van Schil et al., 2013). Knowledge of the structures involved during these extended resections is paramount for postoperative management and detection of potential complications.

Medically fit patients with NSCLC should be offered lobectomy for cure. This may be performed as an open thoracic surgery as a first-line choice (NCC-C, 2015); however, debate exists whether this or video-assisted thoracic surgery (VATS) is the optimal technique. Surgical decision should be based on the progression of the patient's condition, the stage of lung cancer, the cell type, and the surgeon's preference.

Patients with borderline fitness and smaller tumors (e.g., T1a/b, N0, M0) should be considered for lung parenchymal–sparing operations if a complete resection cannot be completed. Pneumonectomies, bilobectomies, and bronchial angioplasties should only be performed if needed to obtain clear margins. Patients undergoing surgery with T3 NSCLC with chest wall involvement should receive a complete resection of the tumor with an accompanied extrapleural or en bloc resection (NCC-C, 2015).

Postoperative Care

Thoracic surgery impairs postoperative respiratory function, resulting in a significant amount of postoperative pulmonary complications and leading to morbidity and a high number of deaths. The overall incidence of complications from thoracic surgery varies from 15%–37.5% and is impacted by preoperative comorbidities (Iyer & Yadav, 2013). Complications of both open and VATS procedures include hemorrhage, empyema, air leak, pneumonia, and surgical emphysema. Postoperative care, such as learning pain management techniques, is aimed at reducing the risk for complications.

Pain Management Techniques

Adequate pain management is essential for patients who have undergone thoracic surgery to facilitate active participation in chest physiotherapy and ambulation, which are paramount in reducing postoperative complications. Management includes the use of epidural catheters, paravertebral blocks, systemic analgesia, and intrapleural infusion of local anesthetic (Iyer & Yadav, 2013).

Epidural analgesia is achieved by inserting a catheter at approximately the midpoint of the dermatomal distribution of the skin incision (Iyer & Yadav, 2013). Epidural anesthetics allow for an increased bioavailability of the opioids in the cerebrospinal fluid (Iyer & Yadav, 2013). These anesthetics are often used in combination with medications containing opioid and anesthetic properties (e.g., fentanyl or diamorphine combined with levobupivacaine). The epidural may be delivered at a constant basal rate, by patient-controlled analgesia, or both and is advantageous because of the thoracic segmental effect of minimizing motor and sympathetic blockade. It also reliably increases analgesia with movement and helps to increase respiratory function after thoracotomy (Iyer & Yadav, 2013). Potential disadvantages of an epidural include failure to place properly and hypotension.

An anesthesiologist places paravertebral blocks to provide local pain relief. This is indicated when the afferent pain input is unilateral from the chest or abdomen (Iyer & Yadav, 2013). This type of catheter block is similar to the epidural catheter and can be placed on a continuous infusion of analgesia or by patient demand.

Systemic analgesia, or the use of enteral and parenteral opioids, is still the mainstay of postoperative pain management. Use of patient-controlled analgesia has demonstrated safety and efficacy in pain management in conjunction with enteral opioids (Iyer & Yadav, 2013). Side effects associated with all opioids include nausea, vomiting, ileus, biliary spasms, respiratory depression, and constipation.

Common Postoperative Complications

Postoperative hemorrhage may contribute to surgical bleeding or coagulopathy, with surgical bleeding being more common. Bleeding after thoracic surgery is rare, occurring in 1%–3% of open procedures and less than 2% of VATS procedures (Iyer & Yadav, 2013). Serial drainage from the chest greater than 200 ml/hr and occurring two to four hours after coagulopathy is corrected indicates surgical bleeding and warrants surgical reexploration (Iyer &

Yadav, 2013). Coagulopathies in the presence of hemorrhage should be corrected as quickly as possible with the administration of blood products such as fresh frozen plasma, platelets, and cryoprecipitate as needed based on laboratory findings.

Cardiac complications after thoracic surgery are the most common forms of cardiac arrhythmias, especially atrial fibrillation, which has an incidence of 10%–20% after lobectomy and 40% after pneumonectomy (Asamura et al., 1993). Unstable or hemodynamically compromised patients with atrial fibrillation should immediately undergo electrical cardioversion. A new onset of postoperative atrial fibrillation is often transient and self-limited; rate control should be the first goal of treatment (Iyer & Yadav, 2013). A selective beta 1–blocking agent should be used as a first-line rate control agent in the absence of moderate to severe chronic obstructive pulmonary disease or active bronchospasm. If these conditions are present, diltiazem should be used (Fernando et al., 2011). Amiodarone should not be administered if the patient has severe lung disease or has undergone a pneumonectomy because it increases the risk of ARDS. It was associated with an 11% risk of ARDS formation, as compared to the 1.8% risk for the non-amiodarone group (Iyer & Yadav, 2013).

Pulmonary edema occurs in 5%–14% of thoracic surgery patients (Iyer & Yadav, 2013). Recommendations and statements concerning postoperative fluid administration conclude that no "third space" exists in the thorax (Iyer & Yadav, 2013). Total positive fluid balance in the first 24 hours should not exceed 20 ml/kg, and a urinary output of greater than 0.5 ml/kg is not needed (Iyer & Yadav, 2013). Factors that increase pulmonary venous pressures should be minimized. Hyperinflation of the residual lung and prolonged periods with the residual lung in the dependent position should be avoided (De Decker, Jorens, & Van Schil, 2003). Mindful postoperative fluid resuscitation should be demonstrated in all patients.

Postpneumonectomy syndrome is a bronchial compression resulting from a massive mediastinal shift following pneumonectomy. Postpneumonectomy syndrome is more common after a right pneumonectomy because of the counterclockwise rotation of the mediastinum toward the pneumonectomy space (Iyer & Yadav, 2013), resulting in stretching, distortion, and compression of the left main bronchus between the pulmonary artery anteriorly and the aorta and vertebral column posteriorly (Iyer & Yadav, 2013). Definitive treatment includes surgical repositioning of the mediastinum.

Prolonged air leak is one of the most common postoperative complications. Not all patients have an air leak after resection, but many undergoing a lobectomy, segmentectomy, or complicated wedge resection will leave the operating room with a leak. A prolonged air leak is any leak lasting more than five days and is associated with a greater pulmonary mortality, atelectasis, pneumonia, and empyema and extended hospital stays (Iyer & Yadav, 2013). Treatments include a Heimlich valve, blood patch, chemical pleurodesis, and watchful waiting, as the majority of leaks stop without intervention (Iyer & Yadav, 2013).

Postoperative Respiratory Failure

Postoperative Ventilator Management

Postoperative ventilator management of thoracic surgery can be challenging. Surgical procedures should be considered carefully when choosing ventilator settings. A high-volume, high-pressure ventilation setting has shown to cause diffuse alveolar damage, pulmonary edema, activation of the inflammatory cascade, and barotrauma (Lytle & Brown, 2008). Although no definitive recommendations exist for ventilator settings in this group of patients, accepted guidelines support the use of lower tidal volumes, or 6 ml/kg of predicted body weight (Lytle & Brown, 2008). Because of the risk of a bronchopleural fistula, positive end-expiratory pressure (PEEP) should be minimized or omitted unless atelectasis is significantly impairing oxygenation.

Ventilator Settings

Different ventilator settings use pressure or volume as a basis for breath delivery. As ventilators evolve and become more complex, the line between settings becomes increasingly blurred. It is important to understand traditional ventilator modes and all associated terms, including the following:
- Frequency or respiratory rate—the number of breaths per minute
- Tidal volume—the amount of volume (ml) delivered with each breath
- PEEP—prevents progressive atelectasis by preventing repetitive opening and closing of alveoli and improves compliance and ventilation–perfusion mismatch
- Fraction of inspired oxygen (FiO_2)—percentage of delivered oxygen

Volume Modes

Assist-control ventilation (ACV), also known as continuous mandatory ventilation, is a set volume delivered with each breath. The patient determines the absolute respiratory rate, but a minimum rate is also set (Burnes, 2008). One disadvantage to ACV is that patients breathing rapidly may develop hyperinflation and respiratory alkalosis because of a prolonged inspiratory-to-expiratory time ratio (Burnes, 2008). An advantage is that sedation or paralytics can be increased in extreme cases to totally control a patient's respiratory function.

Synchronized intermittent mandatory ventilation (SIMV) guarantees a certain number of breaths, which are synchronized to coincide with the patient's spontaneous respirations. The patient is partially breathing independently, reducing the risk of respiratory alkalosis and hyperinflation (Burnes, 2008). Disadvantages include increased independent breathing and potentially decreased cardiac output. With few exceptions, provider preference determines ACV or SIMV use. When a patient's respiratory status must be totally controlled, ACV is preferred. If a patient is breathing rapidly on ACV, SIMV is preferred.

Pressure Modes

Pressure-controlled ventilation controls airway pressure and optimizes gas distribution by decelerating flow patterns during inspiration (Burnes, 2008). The decrease in flow patterns reduces peak pressures and improves gas exchange. Parameters include pressure level (inspiratory pressure level), frequency (rate of breath), inspiratory time, FiO_2, PEEP, and sensitivity (pressure or flow triggering). A simple way to remember this mode is that the ventilator is triggered by time, limited by pressure, and only affects inspiration. A disadvantage of pressure-controlled ventilation is its lack of volume guarantee, which may be problematic with changing lung mechanics.

Pressure support ventilation augments spontaneous inspiration with a set amount of pressure support. This mode is patient dependent, with no frequency or volume set, and only affects inspiration. A disadvantage of pressure support ventilation is that a patient may become fatigued and develop respiratory acidosis.

Postoperative noninvasive ventilation (NIV) is the use of noninvasive continuous positive airway pressure (CPAP) and bilevel positive airway pressure (BiPAP) in lung resection patients. CPAP delivers continuous pressure consistently through inspiration and exhalation, which is useful in combating upper airway obstruction (sleep apnea) (MacIntyre, 2003). BiPAP delivers different pressures during inhalation and exhalation, helping to reduce inspiratory muscle load through additional inspiratory pressure (MacIntyre, 2003). BiPAP has shown to be useful during acute chronic obstructive pulmonary disease exacerbations. Both BiPAP and CPAP elevate intrathoracic pressure, which can have a significant effect on cardiac function through both preload and afterload reduction, making NIV a useful tool in acute heart failure by increasing cardiac output and blood pressure (MacIntyre, 2003). Conversely, if a patient is hypovolemic, NIV initiation can have serious cardiovascular implications, including hypotension and decreased cardiac output (MacIntyre, 2003).

Relative contraindications with NIV use exist and need to be evaluated with clinical judgment, including in patients with copious secretions or those at an increased risk of aspiration (Lytle & Brown, 2008). Because the mask is secured to the face, patients with a decreased level of consciousness and inability to remove the mask if needed should not be placed on this type of device. NIV ventilation is often used in patients who have undergone thoracic surgery to avoid prolonged intubation caused by decreased lung function from surgery or other underlying reasons.

Basic Arterial Blood Gas Interpretation and Ventilator Changes

Arterial blood gas (ABG) is the most common laboratory test used to initiate ventilator adjustments. The normal values for test results are acidity (pH) 7.35–7.45, partial pressure of carbon dioxide ($PaCO_2$) 35–45 mm Hg, partial pressure of oxygen (PaO_2) 80–100 mm Hg, bicarbonate (HCO_3) 22–28 mEq/L, base excess –2 to +2, and oxygen saturation (O_2Sat) 97%–100% (Marino, 2014). ABG tests can tell much more than just respiratory function. Many novice interpreters will look at pH first and make a quick assumption based solely on this value; however, a systematic approach is imperative for accurate interpretation.

The first step is to determine if acidosis (pH less than 7.35) or alkalosis (pH greater than 7.45) is present. Next, one must look at $PaCO_2$ and HCO_3 values. If a pH change is associated with an alteration in $PaCO_2$, a respiratory disorder exists. An elevated $PaCO_2$ with a decreased pH is a respiratory acidosis, while a decrease in $PaCO_2$ with an increase in pH is a respiratory alkalosis (Marino, 2014). When a pH change is associated with alterations in HCO_3, a metabolic issue exists. Elevated HCO_3 (greater than 45) is a metabolic alkalosis, while a decrease in HCO_3 (less than 35) is a metabolic acidosis (Marino, 2014).

The third step is to determine if compensation for the primary disturbance is available, meaning the pH is unexpected based on the primary disturbance. Each compensatory change can be calculated using an exact formula (see Table 2-2).

The fourth step is to determine the anion gap (AG) using the following formula: $AG = Na - (Cl + HCO_3)$ (Marino, 2014). A normal AG is 7+4. In critically ill patients, hypoalbuminemia may cause AG interpretation errors. Albumin is a major source of unmeasured anions, resulting in a significant reduction of AG. It may be corrected using the AG obtained from the original equation, or the observed AG, and inserting it into the following equation: adjusted AG = observed AG + 2.5 × [4.5 − measured albumin (g/dl)] (Marino, 2014). The presence or absence of AG in a metabolic acidosis can give insight into the underlying metabolic disturbance.

The primary adjustment for pH is altering $PaCO_2$ and tidal volumes. Adjusting PEEP and FiO_2 affects oxygenation and ventilation. Often, manipulation of one or more of these factors may be limited by surgeon preference or underlying comorbidities. Table 2-3 summarizes basic ventilator adjustments and corresponding responses.

Table 2-2. Acute Changes in Blood Gases

Disorder	Primary Change	Compensatory Change
Respiratory acidosis: Expected pH = 7.40 − [0.08 × (40 − $PaCO_2$)]	Increased $PaCO_2$	Increased HCO_3
Respiratory alkalosis: Expected pH = 7.40 − [0.008 × (40 − $PaCO_2$)]	Decreased $PaCO_2$	Decreased HCO_3
Metabolic acidosis: Expected $PaCO_2$ = (1.5 × HCO_3) + (8 ± 2)	Decreased HCO_3	Decreased $PaCO_2$
Metabolic alkalosis: Expected $PaCO_2$ = (0.7 × HCO_3) + (21 ± 2)	Increased HCO_3	Increased $PaCO_2$

HCO_3—bicarbonate ion; $PaCO_2$—partial pressure of carbon dioxide
Note. Based on information from Marino, 2014.

Table 2-3. Basic Ventilator Adjustments and Corresponding Responses	
Desired Outcome	**Ventilator Changes**
Increased $PaCO_2$	Decreased respiratory rate Decreased Vt
Decreased $PaCO_2$	Increased respiratory rate Increased Vt
Increased oxygenation	Increased FiO_2 Increased PEEP

FiO_2—fraction of inspired oxygen; $PaCO_2$—partial pressure of carbon dioxide; PEEP—positive end-expiratory pressure; Vt—tidal volume

Note. Based on information from Marino, 2014.

Caution and consultation with the surgeon prior to increasing PEEP levels should occur for all postoperative thoracic surgery patients, as intensive communication and collaboration between the critical care team and the surgical team ensures the highest quality care.

Summary

Medical advances over the past 20 years have led to the early diagnosis and aggressive treatment of many malignancies, and lung cancer is no exception (Azoulay & Afessa, 2006). Many intensive care admissions are because of malignancy-related complications or side effects from treatments, such as chemotherapy-related organ toxicities and immunosuppression-related infections (Azoulay & Afessa, 2006). Unit care is aimed at maintaining adequate nutrition, avoiding further toxic agents in already damaged organs, treating infection by removing unnecessary indwelling catheters, avoiding exposure to infections from other intensive care unit patients, and providing overall supportive care (e.g., mechanical ventilation, continuous renal replacement therapy, vasoactive drugs, other life-sustaining treatments).

References

American Lung Association. (2016a). How is lung cancer diagnosed? Retrieved from http://www.lung.org/lung-health-and-diseases/lung-disease-lookup/lung-cancer/learn-about-lung-cancer/how-is-lung-cancer-diagnosed

American Lung Association. (2016b). Lung cancer basics. Retrieved from http://www.lung.org/lung-health-and-diseases/lung-disease-lookup/lung-cancer/learn-about-lung-cancer/what-is-lung-cancer/lung-cancer-basics.html

American Lung Association. (2016c). Lung cancer fact sheet. Retrieved from http://www.lung.org/lung-health-and-diseases/lung-disease-lookup/lung-cancer/resource-library/lung-cancer-fact-sheet.html

American Lung Association. (2016d). Should my patient be screened for lung cancer? Retrieved from http://www.lung.org/lung-health-and-diseases/lung-disease-lookup/lung-cancer/learn-about-lung-cancer/lung-cancer-screening/should-my-patient-be-screened.html

Asamura, H., Naruke, T., Tsuchiya, R., Goya, T., Kondo, H., & Suemasu, K. (1993). What are the risk factors for arrhythmias after thoracic operations? A retrospective multivariate analysis of 267 consecutive thoracic operations. *Journal of Thoracic and Cardiovascular Surgery, 106,* 1104–1110.

Azoulay, E., & Afessa, B. (2006). The intensive care support of patients with malignancy: Do everything that can be done. *Intensive Care Medicine, 32,* 3–5.

Bristol-Myers Squibb Co. (2011). *Taxol® (paclitaxel)* [Package insert]. Princeton, NJ: Author.

Burdett, S., Stewart, L., & Rydzewska, L. (2007). Chemotherapy and surgery versus surgery alone in non-small cell lung cancer. *Cochrane Database of Systematic Reviews, 2007*(3). doi:10.1002/14651858.CD006157.pub2

Burnes, S.M. (2008). Pressure modes of mechanical ventilation: The good, the bad, and the ugly. *AACN Advanced Critical Care, 19,* 399–411. doi:10.4037/15597768-2008-4006

De Decker, K., Jorens, P.G., & Van Schil, P.E. (2003). Cardiac complications after noncardiac thoracic surgery: An evidence-based current review. *Annals of Thoracic Surgery, 75,* 1340–1348. doi:10.1016/S0003-4975(02)04824-5

Eli Lilly & Co. (2014). *Gemzar® (gemcitabine)* [Package insert]. Indianapolis, IN: Author.

Fernando, H.C., Jaklitsch, M.T., Walsh, G.L., Tisdale, J.E., Bridges, C.D., Mitchell, J.D., & Shrager, J.B. (2011). The Society of Thoracic Surgeons practice guideline on the prophylaxis and management of atrial fibrillation associated with general thoracic surgery: Executive summary. *Annals of Thoracic Surgery, 92,* 1144–1152.

Iyer, A., & Yadav, S. (2013). Postoperative care and complications after thoracic surgery. In M.S. Firstenberg (Ed.), *Principles and practice of cardiothoracic surgery* (pp. 33–44). doi:10.5772/55351

Johnstone, T.C., Park, G.Y., & Lippard, S.J. (2014). Understanding and improving platinum anticancer drugs—Phenanthriplatin. *Anticancer Research, 34,* 471–476.

Kurup, A., & Hanna, N.H. (2004). Treatment of small cell lung cancer. *Critical Reviews in Oncology/Hematology, 52,* 117–126.

Lytle, F.T., & Brown, D.R. (2008). Appropriate ventilatory settings for thoracic surgery: Intraoperative and postoperative. *Seminars in Cardiac and Vascular Anesthesia, 12,* 97–108. doi:10.1177/1089253208319869

MacIntyre, N.R. (2003). Mechanical ventilation: Noninvasive strategies in the acute care setting. *Medscape Critical Care.* Retrieved from http://www.medscape.org/viewarticle/450209

Marino, P.L. (2014). *The ICU book* (4th ed.). Philadelphia, PA: Lippincott Williams & Wilkins.

National Cancer Institute. (2016, December 16). Non-small cell lung cancer treatment (PDQ®) [Patient version]. Retrieved from http://www.cancer.gov/types/lung/patient/non-small-cell-lung-treatment-pdq

National Collaborating Centre for Cancer. (2015). *The diagnosis and treatment of lung cancer.* London, England: National Institute for Health and Care Excellence.

Sanofi-Aventis U.S. LLC. (2014). *Taxotere® (docetaxel)* [Package insert]. Bridgewater, NJ: Author.

Siegel, R.L., Miller, K.D., & Jemal, A. (2017). Cancer statistics, 2017. *CA: A Cancer Journal for Clinicians, 67,* 7–30. doi:10.3322/caac.21387

Van Schil, P.E., Balduyck, B., De Waele, M., Hendriks, J.M., Hertoghs, M., & Lauwers, P. (2013). Surgical treatment of early-stage non-small-cell lung cancer. *EJC Supplements, 11,* 110–122. doi:10.1016/j.ejcsup.2013.07.021

CHAPTER 3

Hematologic Malignancies

Brenda K. Shelton, DNP, APRN-CNS, RN, CCRN, AOCN®

Introduction

Patients with hematologic malignancies are among the most complex and difficult to manage in the intensive care unit (ICU). These patients often present with multisystem dysfunction and require immediate antineoplastic therapy, even in the face of critical illness. Although critical illness has historically been associated with poor outcomes in this population, current literature suggests equivalent survival and quality of life compared to other medical patients (Azoulay et al., 2013; McCaughey, Blackwood, Glackin, Brady, & McMullin, 2013; Mokart et al., 2015). Mortality for patients with hematologic malignancy during an ICU stay ranges from 30%–84% (McGrath, Chatterjee, Whiteley, & Ostermann, 2010; Yeo et al., 2012). Variables associated with poorer outcomes in this population include respiratory failure requiring mechanical ventilation, multiorgan failure, refractory sepsis, and shock (Azoulay et al., 2013; Cowan, Altemeier, Johnston, Gernsheimer, & Becker, 2015; Ñamendys-Silva, González-Herrera, García-Guillén, Texcocano-Becerra, & Herrera-Gómez, 2013). This chapter provides an overview of specialized diagnostics, a condensed review of specific hematologic malignancies, and an in-depth discussion of key oncologic emergencies in this population.

Diagnostic Tests

The most common and significant diagnostic tests in patients with hematologic malignancies include complete blood count, coagulation, hemolysis, and bone marrow evaluation (see Table 3-1). Diagnostic tests used for primary disease diagnosis and prognosis are described with specific hematologic malignancies in Table 3-2.

Nurses caring for this patient population should be aware of the value and necessity of less-reported tests, such as red blood cell (RBC) indices, hemolysis, and specialty immunologic evaluations. Many hematologic disorders are genetic in origin; however, specific diagnostic and monitoring tests are not within the scope of this text. Patients with thrombotic thrombocytopenic purpura (TTP) may have a confirmatory diagnosis in the ICU with an ADAMTS13 enzyme level test (Tersteeg et al., 2016), and patients with sickle cell disease may be monitored with hemoglobin variant levels to detect the severity of sickling crisis (Johnston et al., 2016). Unlike critically ill patients without malignancy, inflammation tests (e.g., procalcitonin, C-reactive protein) may be abnormally elevated in those with a malignancy and are not useful for monitoring illness severity (Debiane et al., 2014). Specific tests used in the diagnosis and detection of relapse in patients with hematologic malignancy, such as peripheral circulating blast percentage, flow cytometry, and cytopathology, may be essential in critical care decision making and are directed by oncologists consulting in the care of these patients. Communication and collaboration between oncology and critical care experts is integral to ensure the best quality of care.

Hematologic/Immunologic Therapeutics

Leukapheresis and plasmapheresis are transfusion medicine procedures similar to those used with blood or platelet donation but with the aim to remove excess white blood cells (WBCs) (leukapheresis) or plasma-containing antibodies (plasmapheresis). Pheresis also may be part of the pretransplant preparative regimen, and rarely, patients may require ICU care during this phase of treatment (Schmit-Pokorny, 2013). These procedures require an implanted, large-bore dual-lumen catheter and hemodynamic stability to remove large volumes of blood in a circuit similar to dialysis. Anticoagulation is necessary during the procedure and may place patients at risk for bleeding. The procedure may need to be coordinated or alternated with other essential treatments in the ICU, such as continuous renal replacement therapy or extracorporeal membrane oxygenation.

During these procedures, the nurse should monitor for bleeding, volume deficits, hemodynamic instability, and hypersensitivity reactions. Replacement plasma or blood may be given during the procedure or a reversal of anticoagulation at the end of the procedure. This should be documented in the patient's record. Blood drawn during these procedures may not accurately reflect clinical status. Laboratory diagnostics should be performed after the therapy as well as administration of medications that may be at risk for filtration. Another concern is that the extracorporeal circuit may reduce body temperature and mask fever, requiring other clinical signs and symptoms to drive investigation for infection. Specialty filters designed to remove WBCs or plasma antibodies are used to reduce the risk of clogging.

Table 3-1. Hematologic/Immunologic Diagnostic Tests

Diagnostic Test	Description	Normal Values	Clinical Implications
Red Blood Cell (RBC) Studies			
Hematocrit	Proportion of the volume of RBCs in 100 ml blood	Male: 40%–54% Female: 37%–47% Age > 65 years: 33.1%–50.2%	Increased with dehydration or hemoconcentration Decreased with inadequate RBC production, nutritional deficits, blood loss, anemia of chronic illness, and hemolysis More sensitive to volume changes than hemoglobin
Hemoglobin	Measure of oxygen-carrying pigment that binds with oxygen so that oxygen can be carried to the cells of the microvasculature	Male: 13.5–17.5 g/dl Female: 12–16 g/dl Age > 65 years: 11–16.8 g/dl	Increased with dehydration or hemoconcentration Decreased with inadequate RBC production, nutritional deficits, blood loss, anemia of chronic illness, and hemolysis
Mean corpuscular hemoglobin	Average hemoglobin weight of a single RBC	26–24 pg	Increased macrocytic anemias (e.g., folate deficiency) Decreased microcytic anemias (e.g., iron deficiency) Early indicator of iron deficiency
Mean corpuscular hemoglobin concentration	Average amount of hemoglobin of a single RBC	323–359 g/L	General but useful tool to measure effectiveness of treatment for iron deficiency Described as hypochromic, normochromic, or microchromic
Mean corpuscular volume	Average volume or mass of a single RBC	80–100 fl	Increased macrocytic anemias (e.g., folate deficiency) Decreased microcytic anemias (e.g., iron deficiency)

(Continued on next page)

Table 3-1. Hematologic/Immunologic Diagnostic Tests (Continued)

Diagnostic Test	Description	Normal Values	Clinical Implications
RBC Studies (cont.)			
RBC distribution width (RDW)	Variation in RBC size	12%–15.5%	Differentiates anemia of chronic illness versus iron deficiency
RBC morphology	Variations in size, shape, color, or RBCs caused by disease or toxic exposures	Normal biconcave disc RBC shape; normal RDW and normochromia	Morphologic changes may indicate medical illness, dysfunctional cell production, or damage to the circulating RBCs.
Reticulocyte count	Proportion of immature RBCs in total RBC count	< 2% of total RBC count	Increased when accelerated erythropoiesis occurs Should be increased in response to acute anemia
Iron and Nutrition Studies			
Cobalamin (B_{12}) level	Amount of vitamin B_{12} in the bloodstream	130–950 ng/L	Decreased with nutritional deficiency or hemolytic anemia Increased with solid tumors with and without liver metastases, myeloproliferative disorders, liver disease, and renal failure
Ferritin level	Stores and transports iron; measure of long-term body iron storage	Male: 20–200 ng/ml Female: 15–150 ng/ml	Reflects total iron stores but may be increased with inflammation; usually decreased with iron deficiency
Folic acid/folate level (vitamin B_9)	Amount of folic acid in the bloodstream	3–16 mcg/L	Decreased with nutritional deficiency, hemolytic anemia, or leukemia

(Continued on next page)

Table 3-1. Hematologic/Immunologic Diagnostic Tests *(Continued)*

Diagnostic Test	Description	Normal Values	Clinical Implications
Iron and Nutrition Studies *(cont.)*			
Serum iron	Amount of iron bound to serum proteins	50–150 mcg/dl (9–26.9 mcmol/L)	Levels are nonspecific and vary with time of day and clinical conditions; used in conjunction with other iron tests to detect deficiency or adequate replenishment. Because levels are highest in the morning, the test is usually done in the morning hours.
Soluble transferrin receptor–ferritin ratio	Correlates to the cell surface receptors for transferrin	1.8–4.6 mg/L	Increased values indicate upregulation of transferrin receptors in presence of iron deficiency. More useful than regular transferrin in disorders characterized by inflammation or infection
Total iron-binding capacity (TIBC)	Test of binding of iron on transferrin and amount of unbound transferrin	240–450 mcg/dl	TIBC is low in conditions of iron deficiency.
Transferrin level	Transports iron to cells or back to liver and bone for recycling Indicator of the amount of iron available to support erythropoiesis	Male: 190–360 mg/dl Female: 25–200 mg/dl	More useful for detection of nutritional deficiencies in iron than the serum iron and TIBC Transferrin is also low in liver disease.
Transferrin saturation (TSAT)	Ratio between total iron and TIBC Most reliable indicator of iron availability to produce RBCs in the bone marrow	> 20%	A low TSAT generally indicates iron deficiency.

(Continued on next page)

Table 3-1. Hematologic/Immunologic Diagnostic Tests *(Continued)*

Diagnostic Test	Description	Normal Values	Clinical Implications
Other RBC Studies			
Bilirubin	By-product of pancreatic and hepatic excretion	Total: 0.1–1.3 mg/dl Direct: 0–0.3 mg/dl	Indirect bilirubin increased with hemolysis
Coombs test	Differentiation of immune antibodies Direct Coombs detects antibodies attached to RBCs. Indirect Coombs detects antibodies in serum.	Negative	Used to detect unusual non-ABO blood antibodies that influence blood crossmatching
Erythrocyte sedimentation rate (ESR)	Nonspecific test for inflammation performed by observing the time it takes for RBCs to settle in a column Inflammation alters the cell configuration and impairs this process.	Normal values based on age, with increasing levels with age; higher in females Male: Age ÷ 2 Female: (Age + 10) ÷ 2	Elevated ESR indicates inflammation but is not diagnostic for any specific disease. Used to monitor progress or treatment response in immune and inflammatory diseases
Haptoglobin level	Acute-phase protein that binds with hemoglobin for recycling	Age < 50 years: 0.35–1.90 g/dl Age > 50 years: 0.47–2.10 g/dl	Decreased with hemolysis

(Continued on next page)

Table 3-1. Hematologic/Immunologic Diagnostic Tests *(Continued)*

Diagnostic Test	Description	Normal Values	Clinical Implications
Other RBC Studies *(cont.)*			
Hemoglobin electrophoresis	Blood samples are applied to paper containing an electrical current, and hemoglobins form bands showing the amount of each type of hemoglobin molecule.	The presence of hemoglobin variants HbA and HbA$_2$ is normal, and small amounts of HbF may also be present. Hemoglobin variants HbF, HbS, HbH, and HbM are abnormal findings.	Presence of abnormal hemoglobin variants is diagnostic for specific diseases, such as sickle cell anemia. This can also be used to detect percentages of the variant hemoglobin during treatment and assessment of treatment responses.
Lactate dehydrogenase (LDH)	Measurement of tissue breakdown. Found in many body tissues	140–280 U/L	Increased with malignancy, tumor lysis syndrome, and hemolysis
White Blood Cell (WBC) Studies			
Absolute lymphocyte count	Total number of circulating lymphocytes	Adults: 1,000–4,800/mm^3 Children: 3,000–9,500/mm^3 Approximately 16%–45% of total WBC count	Increased lymphocytes are characteristic of opportunistic and viral infection and hypersensitivity disorders and may also be associated with certain leukemias. Deficient lymphocytes occur with deeply marrow-suppressing treatments, such as those used with hematopoietic stem cell transplant or long-term corticosteroids; these patients are at risk for infection with opportunistic organisms.

(Continued on next page)

Table 3-1. Hematologic/Immunologic Diagnostic Tests *(Continued)*

Diagnostic Test	Description	Normal Values	Clinical Implications
WBC Studies *(cont.)*			
Absolute neutrophil count	Total number of circulating neutrophils (polys or segs) and immature neutrophils (bands)	1,500–8,000/mm³	Reflects the capacity of infection-fighting WBCs Deficiencies occur with cancer treatment, immune suppression, and long-term corticosteroid usage.
WBC count	Total number of WBCs	5,000–10,000/mm³	Elevated WBCs occur in inflammation, infection, and cellular injury/death. Reduced WBCs confer a risk for infection. The specific abnormal WBC provides clues to the precise etiologic disorder.
WBC differential	Description of the WBC distribution across all subtypes Reported as an absolute number and/or the percentage of the total WBC count Cells included are granulocytes (neutrophils), eosinophils, basophils, monocytes, and lymphocytes.	Basophils: 0%–1% Eosinophils: 1%–7% Lymphocytes: 16%–45% Monocytes: 3%–10% Neutrophilic bands: 3%–5% Neutrophils: 45%–74%	Elevations of specific WBCs have unique infectious and inflammation implications. The most important infection-fighting WBC is the neutrophil, so elevations are indicative of systemic bacterial infection, whereas elevated lymphocytes indicate virus, hypersensitivity, and opportunistic infections. Basophils are indicative of delayed hypersensitivity reactions. Eosinophils are elevated in skin and pulmonary disorders as well as some unusual infections, such as spirochetes. Reduced WBCs place individuals at risk for infections related to the specific functions of that cell. Suppression of immune and allergic responses may also reduce specific WBC populations.

(Continued on next page)

Table 3-1. Hematologic/Immunologic Diagnostic Tests *(Continued)*

Diagnostic Test	Description	Normal Values	Clinical Implications
Platelet Studies			
Bleeding time	Measurement of platelet quality The test measures the time required to achieve immediate hemostasis after small vessel injury.	2–9 minutes	Bleeding time abnormalities usually indicate problems with platelet quality caused by medications (aspirin) or diseases (von Willebrand).
Mean platelet volume	Machine-calculated measurement of the average size of platelets in the specimen	7.2–10.4 fl	Large platelets may indicate a myeloproliferative disorder with immature cells or rapid platelet turnover seen in consumptive and hemolytic disorders.
Platelet autoantibody	Tests for self-antibodies against platelets to detect an autoimmune etiology for thrombocytopenia	Negative	Platelet autoantibodies indicate alloimmunization and risk for autoimmune destruction of cells.
Platelet count	Total number of platelets	150,000–350,000/mm^3	Increased with hyperviscosity disorders or increased platelet production High values increase risk of thrombosis. Decreased values increase risk of bleeding.

(Continued on next page)

Table 3-1. Hematologic/Immunologic Diagnostic Tests (Continued)

Diagnostic Test	Description	Normal Values	Clinical Implications
Clotting Studies			
Activated protein C level	An immunosorbent assay test (ELISA) and partial thromboplastin time—based functional protein C assays can detect deficiencies.	65–135 IU/dl	Elevated levels are not clinically significant. Depletion that occurs with some hematologic malignancies and after stem cell transplantation can lead to increased risk of inappropriate clotting.
ADAMTS13	Quantitative serum test for the protease ADAMTS13 to detect deficiencies that lead to hypercoagulation	Immunofluorescence technique used to detect activity level Normal is > 67% activity, although thrombotic thrombocytopenia purpura (TTP) is usually associated with levels < 10%.	A positive ADAMTS13 test shows deficiency of this protease, which is typical of autoimmune TTP, as opposed to aortic valve shearing or hemolytic uremic syndrome. This test is used to guide highly specialized therapy, such as plasmapheresis or eculizumab.
Antithrombin III	Active component of the normal process of thrombolysis on a local vascular level	0.15–0.40 mg/dl	Congenital and acquired antithrombin deficiencies lead to excessive clotting. Common disorders causing acquired deficiency include liver failure, kidney disease, and cancer metastasis.
D-dimer	Measurement of the "D fragment" in clot breakdown	Positive at 1:8 dilutions	Elevated in consumptive clotting disorders where excessive clots are formed and then take part in normal dissolution Elevations reflect the excessive clot formation and may be used to monitor deep vein thrombosis, pulmonary embolism, or stroke resolution.

(Continued on next page)

Table 3-1. Hematologic/Immunologic Diagnostic Tests *(Continued)*

Diagnostic Test	Description	Normal Values	Clinical Implications
Clotting Studies *(cont.)*			
Fibrin degradation products (FDPs)	Measurement of the by-products of fibrin clot break-down	< 10 mcg/ml	FDPs are usually cleared at the same rate they are produced. Excessive clots lead to more FDPs and slower clearance, or accumulation.
Fibrinogen level	Measurement of the amount of the fibrin precursor available for clot production	200–400 mg/dl	Depleted in consumptive disorders with excessive clotting An increase in inflammation and baseline elevation is common in patients with certain malignancies (e.g., acute leukemia, head and neck cancer, Hodgkin).
Hemoglobin stability: isopropanol and heat	Tests for abnormal hemoglobin structure not detectable on hemoglobin electrophoresis testing	Presence of precipitants in the testing blood at 5, 20, or 30 minutes	Abnormal with hemoglobin disorders, such as thalassemia, sickle cell disease, or other uncommon hemoglobinopathies
Partial thromboplastin time	Measurement of the function of the intrinsic pathway of coagulation	18–42 seconds	A prolonged time is present when clotting is impaired through factors in the intrinsic pathway (e.g., heparin's effect of factor VIII) or the final common pathway to a fibrin clot.
Prothrombin time	Measurement of the function of the extrinsic pathway of coagulation	10–13.5 seconds International normalized ratio: 0.9–1.2	Prolonged in absence or inhibition of vitamin K–dependent factors or warfarin

(Continued on next page)

Table 3-1. Hematologic/Immunologic Diagnostic Tests (Continued)

Diagnostic Test	Description	Normal Values	Clinical Implications
Clotting Studies (cont.)			
Thrombin clotting time	Test that adds thrombin to blood specimen, resulting in direct clotting with fibrinogen	11–18 seconds	Prolonged time to achieve clotting with liver disease, abnormal or low fibrinogen levels, and uremia

Note. Based on information from Bonilla & Stiehm, 2017; Erb & Vogel, 2013; Relf & Shelton, 2018; Schrier, 2016; Shelton, 2012, 2018; Zehnder, 2017; Zhu et al., 2010.

Table 3-2. Hematologic Malignancies Overview

Characteristic	Leukemia	Myelodysplastic Syndrome	Lymphoma	Multiple Myeloma
Description	Malignant transformation of white blood cells (WBCs) during maturation process within the bone marrow	Premalignant transformation of WBCs with genetic mutations (primarily JAK2) that create dysfunctional WBC replication and low blood counts of all cell lines within the bone marrow	Malignant transformation of WBCs during maturation process within the lymph node	Malignant transformation of immunoglobulin-producing lymphocyte WBCs, creating malignant immunoglobulin
Classifications	Major groupings are by acuity and cell line (e.g., acute lymphocytic, acute myelocytic, chronic myelocytic, chronic lymphocytic), but cytogenetic classifications are an emerging trend.	Classification is based on the cell line affected, dysplastic characteristics, and the degree of immature cells (e.g., refractory anemia with multilineage dysplasia, refractory anemia with excess blasts). Some overlap syndromes may also be present between myelodysplastic syndrome (MDS) and some chronic leukemias, such as chronic myelomonocytic leukemia.	Major groupings are Hodgkin lymphoma and non-Hodgkin lymphoma. Under each of these subheadings are a variety of disorders named by cellular characteristics.	Myeloma and smoldering myeloma are the classifications of multiple myeloma. Another variation of abnormal immunoglobulin, called monoclonal gammopathy of undetermined significance (MGUS), is further subdivided into non-IgM MGUS and light-chain MGUS. Solitary plasmacytoma is another plasma cell disorder in this family.

(Continued on next page)

Table 3-2. Hematologic Malignancies Overview (Continued)

Characteristic	Leukemia	Myelodysplastic Syndrome	Lymphoma	Multiple Myeloma
Pertinent cytogenetics	Poor: Complex karyotypes, biphenotypic leukemia, hypodiploidy, t(9;22), (q34;q11.2), t(4;11), and (q21;q23) in acute lymphoblastic leukemia (ALL), often occurring with secondary leukemia Favorable: NPM1 in young adults, t(8;21), and inv(16)/t(16;16) in acute myeloid leukemia (AML); hyperdiploidy, t(10;14), abn(9p), and normal karyotype in ALL; Philadelphia chromosome and BCR-ABL in chronic myeloid leukemia (CML) Unclear: Secondary aberrations	Poor: High-percentage blasts in bone marrow, number of cytopenias, multiple chromosomal abnormalities, 7q/monosomy, transfusion dependence Favorable: Del(5q) as only anomaly, del(20q) as only anomaly, loss of Y chromosome Unclear: Trisomy 8, del1(2p), abnormal 17p, 11q23, chromosome 3	Poor: High percentage of cells with abnormal metaphases, > 6 chromosomal breaks, aberrations involving 1p21–22, 6q23–26, or short arm of chromosome 17 Favorable: A t(2;5)(p23;q35) fusion protein and response to anaplastic lymphoma kinase (ALK) proteins in large cell lymphoma Unclear: Uncertain if cytogenetics are important in adult T-cell lymphoma or Hodgkin lymphoma	Poor: t(14;16), t(4;14), del(17p), chromosome 1 aberrations del(1p), amplification 1q21 Favorable: Hyperdiploidy Unclear: Chromosome 13 aberrations, t(11;14)

(Continued on next page)

Table 3-2. Hematologic Malignancies Overview *(Continued)*

Characteristic	Leukemia	Myelodysplastic Syndrome	Lymphoma	Multiple Myeloma
Prognosis	Widely variable and dependent on subtype Chronic leukemias generally have a better prognosis, but even these depend on cytogenetics. With chronic leukemias having good cytogenetic markers (e.g., Philadelphia chromosome in CML, *BCR-ABL* mutation in CML), survival may be years when given long-term continuous therapy. Acute leukemia is associated with an average survival of 2–5 years, but this is dependent on many factors.	Generally poor prognosis and high conversion rate to acute leukemia Part of prognostic implications related to subtypes and specific genetic markers	It is widely variable, but more highly proliferative subtypes respond quickly to treatment, and long-term disease-free survival is possible with intense chemotherapy followed by transplant. More indolent forms are chronic but more refractory to treatment. It may take years for these diseases to become life threatening. In general, Hodgkin lymphoma is thought to have a better prognosis than non-Hodgkin lymphoma.	Considered a chronic disease Early MGUS disease may be present for years without progression. It has many available treatment options, but disease recurrence is common. Even single hematopoietic stem cell transplant limits disease-free survival, so some centers perform tandem transplants.

(Continued on next page)

Table 3-2. Hematologic Malignancies Overview (Continued)

Characteristic	Leukemia	Myelodysplastic Syndrome	Lymphoma	Multiple Myeloma
Demographics	Acute leukemia has bimodal distribution, with some occurring in patients aged 20–35 years and others aged 50–60 years. Chronic leukemia is dependent on whether it is myeloid (CML) or lymphocytic (CLL) in origin. CML occurs in patients aged 30–40 years. It recurs in patients' 50s or 60s. CLL is more common in adults older than 70 years, but variants may occur in younger adults. Leukemia is slightly more prevalent in men than women.	Demographics vary by etiology. In patients with specific single chromosomal abnormalities, the disease may manifest earlier. In patients having therapy-related MDS, it occurs within 5 years after treatment with antineoplastic agents and shows no gender prevalence. In general, it is more common in men than women and in Whites and non-Hispanics.	Hodgkin lymphoma has historically been associated with young adults, but bimodal distribution exists, with a second prevalence being in the fifth or sixth decade of age. Its association to Epstein-Barr virus may lead to incidences at any time. In the United States, Hodgkin lymphoma is more prevalent in men and Whites. Non-Hodgkin lymphoma has a more even distribution across age, gender, and ethnicity.	This disease is more common in the older population, with a higher incidence in men than women and with more than twice the incidence among African Americans than Whites. It may have increased incidence within families.

(Continued on next page)

Table 3-2. Hematologic Malignancies Overview (Continued)

Characteristic	Leukemia	Myelodysplastic Syndrome	Lymphoma	Multiple Myeloma
Diagnosis	Complete blood count (CBC) provides clinical cues about blood cell production problems. The presence of peripheral blasts exceeding 15% is indicative of abnormal production and possible leukemia. A definitive diagnosis is by bone marrow aspirate and a biopsy with flow cytometry for key genetic mutations.	CBC provides clinical cues about diminished blood cell production. A definitive diagnosis is by bone marrow aspirate and a biopsy with flow cytometry for key genetic mutations.	CBC provides clinical cues about blood cell production problems, but it may only be abnormal if the lymphoma has infiltrated the bone marrow. A lymph node biopsy with flow cytometry helps differentiate specific types of lymphomas.	Serum and urinary immunoglobulin proteins are used to detect abnormal M proteins indicative of multiple myeloma. Clonal plasma cells and cytogenetics are evaluated by plasmacytoma biopsy or bone marrow biopsy.
Additional clinical evaluation	Acute inflammation is common at diagnosis but should become less apparent when in remission. Inflammatory markers, such as C-reactive protein or fibrinogen level, are elevated in acute disease.	None	Lactate dehydrogenase (LDH) levels are useful to monitor the amount of tumor burden. Positron-emission tomography (PET) scans are used when it is difficult to differentiate scar tissue from previous masses and lymphadenopathy, as opposed to active disease. Increased metabolic uptake indicates active disease. This technique is most common with Hodgkin lymphoma assessment.	Skeletal survey, including spine, pelvis, skull, humeri, and femora A fluorodeoxyglucose-PET scan can differentiate MGUS from infection or another malignancy.

(Continued on next page)

	Table 3-2. Hematologic Malignancies Overview *(Continued)*			
Characteristic	**Leukemia**	**Myelodysplastic Syndrome**	**Lymphoma**	**Multiple Myeloma**
Key signs and symptoms	Infection is a significant problem because of dysfunctional WBCs at the onset of disease and profound marrow suppression after treatment. Refractoriness to platelets may also lead to bleeding concerns. Other common signs/symptoms include fatigue, anemia, and constitutional symptoms.	Most common presenting signs and symptoms are chronic fatigue, easy bruising, and low-grade, nonhealing infections. Symptoms relate to the specific cytopenia experienced by the patient. Effects may include chronic infection, bleeding, and anemia.	Most common presenting symptom is a nonpainful enlarged lymph node or mass near a lymph node. Significant lymphadenopathy can cause organ dysfunction, respiratory distress, or neurologic impairment. Infiltration into organs, such as the bowel, lungs, and heart, may also lead to symptoms such as airway obstruction, cardiac tamponade, or bowel obstruction.	Fatigue, weakness, bone pain, reduced urine output Thrombotic complications can lead to deep vein thrombosis, pulmonary embolism, and their associated signs and symptoms.
Usual treatment	Treatment is determined by whether disease is acute or chronic; myelocytic cell line or lymphocytic cell line. Chronic leukemia rarely may be observed without immediate treatment. Systemic chemotherapy with or without hematopoietic stem cell transplant is almost	Early and minimally dysplastic forms of MDS may only require observation. As cytopenia becomes more chronic or severe, transfusions and targeted therapy (often agents targeting the JAK2 mutation) are indicated.	Treatment is based on the stage of the disease and location of involved lymph nodes. For isolated disease above the diaphragm and involving one lymph node group, targeted radiation may be the only therapy needed. Cytogenetics may dictate the	MGUS may be observed until more significant mutations and immunoglobulin production becomes a problem. Isolated plasmacytoma may be treated with radiation therapy. Patients with high immunoglobulin levels and

(Continued on next page)

Table 3-2. Hematologic Malignancies Overview (Continued)

Characteristic	Leukemia	Myelodysplastic Syndrome	Lymphoma	Multiple Myeloma
Usual treatment *(cont.)*	always indicated, but the urgency of its administration depends on the type of leukemia, cell proliferation rates, and clinical findings. Active agents for treatment of AML often include antitumor antibiotics and antimetabolites. ALL is treated with a combination of agents from several categories, including L-asparaginase and vinca alkaloids. BCR-ABL tyrosine kinase inhibitors are the mainstay for treatment of CML. CLL may be treated with antimetabolites, monoclonal antibodies, and other novel agents.	In severe and refractory disease, the treatment of choice is hematopoietic stem cell transplant. The most common agents used to treat MDS are JAK2 inhibitors.	need to add antineoplastic therapy in patients having high risk for relapse. In more advanced disease, antineoplastic therapy with or without hematopoietic stem cell transplant is indicated. Many lymphomas are characterized by a CD20 marker that can be targeted with immune therapy/monoclonal antibodies. Most treatment regimens include an alkylating agent, antitumor antibiotic, and the anti-CD20 antibody rituximab. Other new and novel agents are emerging.	hyperviscosity may be acutely managed with plasmapheresis for removal of excessive M-protein levels. Usual treatment includes systemic antineoplastic therapy with or without hematopoietic stem cell transplant. Antineoplastic agents commonly used for treatment include antiangiogenesis agents, proteasome inhibitors, histone deacetylase inhibitors, immune modulating agents, dexamethasone, and monoclonal antibodies. Because of the risk for bone demineralization, bisphosphonates are often routinely administered.

(Continued on next page)

Table 3-2. Hematologic Malignancies Overview (Continued)

Characteristic	Leukemia	Myelodysplastic Syndrome	Lymphoma	Multiple Myeloma
Complications	Primary complications are infection, bleeding, and anemia. High WBC counts (> 100,000/mm³ in AML; > 400,000/mm³ in ALL) or high blast percentage with high proliferation rates lead to a high risk for leukostasis, a disorder of organ thromboses from high blood counts and hyperviscosity. Most commonly affected organs are the brain, lungs, and kidneys. High proliferation rates and responsiveness to therapy leads to high incidence of tumor lysis syndrome, especially if associated with high blast percentage and acute leukemia at the time of new diagnosis or disease relapse. Specific leukemia subtypes exhibit unique complications, such as disseminated intravascular coagulation with acute granulocytic leukemia.	Refractoriness to transfusions with alloimmunization is common in this population. Transformation to acute leukemia occurs in a significant number of patients.	Lymphoma produces large lymph nodes and masses that interfere with body functions and normal fluid distribution. Common clinical problems include edema, increased intracranial pressure, pericardial and pleural effusions, superior vena cava syndrome, tracheobronchial obstruction, and venous thrombosis. Less common manifestations of obstruction from masses include bowel obstruction, hydronephrosis, and spinal cord compression. High proliferation rates and responsiveness to therapy leads to high incidence of tumor lysis syndrome, especially if associated with large bulky disease and high LDH levels.	Most common problems relate to hyperviscosity from immunoglobulin, including thromboses, stroke, and myocardial infarction. Anemia is common. Immunoglobulin destruction of the kidneys often produces renal impairment that can progress to renal failure. Hypercalcemia or pathologic fractures occur because of renal failure and bone demineralization.

Note. Based on information from Byar, 2013; Devine, 2013; Faiman & Bilotti, 2013; Goodrich et al., 2013; Handy et al., 2013; Olsen, 2013; Peterson et al., 2013; Relf & Shelton, 2018; Rogers, 2013; Shelton, 2012; Viele, 2013; Zitella, 2013.

Hematologic/Immunologic System Cancers

Hematologic malignancies comprise the cancers of blood-forming cell lines and specifically result in WBC malignancies. The major differences between malignancies—leukemia, myelodysplastic syndrome, lymphoma, and multiple myeloma—are determined in the origin of the malignant cell line (Olsen, 2013). Leukemia includes cancers that originate in the early cell precursors or in the cells that remain in the bone marrow. Myelodysplastic syndrome is a premalignant transformation of WBCs with genetic mutations that cause dysfunctional WBC replication and low blood counts of all cell lines in the bone marrow. Lymphomas are lymphocytes that migrate to the lymph nodes then become malignant. Multiple myeloma is a malignancy that begins within the plasma cell (differentiated lymphocyte).

Hematologic malignancies primarily grow rapidly and are highly invasive, although specific subtypes may be more chronic in nature. Knowing the natural history of a defined malignant diagnosis is essential to understanding typical critical illness patterns for these patients. Prognostic indicators, such as a cytogenetics, help the clinician to appreciate treatment decisions and the expected trajectory for patients after recovery from critical illness. Each malignancy has unique clinical characteristics and management strategies. A brief overview of these disorders is summarized in Table 3-2.

Historically, these hematologic malignancies have almost exclusively been treated with high-dose antineoplastic therapy with or without a follow-up hematopoietic stem cell transplantation to replace the impaired immune system with new hematopoietic stem cells. In addition to myelosuppression with infection and bleeding, unique complications have been identified in this population, such as sinusoidal obstruction syndrome and atypical hemolytic uremic syndrome (Anderson-Reitz & Clancy, 2013; Nayer & Asif, 2016; Relf & Shelton, 2018). These chemotherapy agents also may cause toxicities not typical of other critical care medications, such as differentiation syndrome or hemorrhagic cystitis (Sanz & Montesinos, 2014; Shelton, 2012). Newer therapies targeting specific genetic mutations (e.g., *BCR-ABL* in chronic myeloid leukemia) have introduced different toxicities that are less familiar to oncology specialists, such as reversible cardiomyopathy and dysrhythmias, autoimmune colitis, and pancreatitis (Polovich, Olsen, & LeFebvre, 2014). Nonrespiratory oncologic emergencies that may occur in patients with hematologic malignancies and disorders are briefly described in Table 3-3.

Nonmalignant Hematologic/Immunologic Disorders

Benign Hematologic Disorders

Concomitant hematologic or immunologic disease that may require acute and critical care management is common with malignant disease. Additionally,

Table 3-3. Nonrespiratory Oncologic Emergencies in Patients With Hematologic Malignancies and Disorders

Oncologic Emergency	Description	Risk Groups
Acalculous cholecystitis	Disorder of gallbladder or biliary tree inflammation and reduced flow of bile Presents with right upper quadrant abdominal pain, fatty or clay-colored stools, fever, tachycardia, and possible hypotension. Abdominal ultrasound shows dilated or thickened wall of the gallbladder without stones. May require a hepatobiliary iminodiacetic acid or computed tomography scan with contrast for definitive diagnosis	Abdominal surgery Chronic hypoperfusion (shock) Disseminated sepsis Total parenteral nutrition
Disseminated intravascular coagulation (DIC)	Excessive microvascular clotting in DIC leads to depletion of clotting factors and combined thrombosis and hemorrhage with multiorgan failure. Coagulation test abnormalities include thrombocytopenia, decreased fibrinogen, prolonged prothrombin time or partial thromboplastin time, and elevated D-dimer levels. In patients with hematologic malignancies, who are often already thrombocytopenic, reduced fibrinogen is more commonly followed to assess and manage disease. Treatment first requires treatment of reversible etiologies. Reactive transfusion with platelets and clotting factors may be necessary. Defibrotide is used for primary thrombotic DIC. Heparin at low doses may be used in DIC related to progranulocytic leukemia.	Progranulocytic leukemia at diagnosis or during initial therapy Sepsis at diagnosis or during therapy Severe leukostasis

(Continued on next page)

Table 3-3. Nonrespiratory Oncologic Emergencies in Patients With Hematologic Malignancies and Disorders *(Continued)*

Oncologic Emergency	Description	Risk Groups
Engraftment syndrome	This syndrome of cytokine release occurs as the lymphocytes recover after myeloablative therapy. It is difficult to distinguish from sepsis because lymphocytes engraft before neutrophils. It is characterized by fever, erythema, rash, fluid retention, respiratory distress, renal dysfunction, hematuria, and transaminase elevations. The syndrome may require aggressive organ failure support, but it will resolve when neutrophil recovery occurs.	After hematopoietic stem cell transplantation (HSCT), particularly with mismatched donors or umbilical cord transplant After treatment with immunomodulatory agents, such as bortezomib and lenalidomide, or when HSCT has been employed for autoimmune disorders or solid tumors More common in women Patients with acute leukemia, particularly lymphocytic subtype
Hemolytic uremic syndrome (HUS), atypical subtype	This syndrome of microangiopathic hemolytic anemia, thrombocytopenia, and renal failure has two forms: typical and atypical. This is based on the triggering mechanism of the microangiopathy. Although similar to thrombotic thrombocytopenia purpura, it does not have the usual neurologic symptoms associated with that disorder. Atypical HUS is triggered by microvascular endothelial damage to the kidney and abnormal complement pathways. Plasma exchange remains a common treatment, but recent use of the C5 (complement) antibody eculizumab has been highly successful at limiting long-term renal failure.	Most common with graft-versus-host disease after transplant Exposure to specific medications (e.g., calcineurin inhibitors)

(Continued on next page)

Table 3-3. Nonrespiratory Oncologic Emergencies in Patients With Hematologic Malignancies and Disorders *(Continued)*

Oncologic Emergency	Description	Risk Groups
Hemorrhagic cystitis	Bladder mucosal injury when the metabolite acrolein is retained. Erosion of the bladder mucosa with hemorrhage from small vessels produces significant bleeding within the bladder. It usually occurs within 2–7 days of medication administration, but it may be as late as two weeks after administration. May be abrogated by high-flow IV hydration during medication administration. Continuous bladder irrigation during bleeding reduces risk of retained clots. Concomitant precisely dosed mesna to counteract the toxic effects of acrolein. Experimental therapies have included prostaglandin and alum bladder irrigation or hyperbaric oxygen. Exact mechanism of viral-induced hemorrhagic cystitis is not known. Antiviral therapies have been used with moderate success. Ganciclovir alone or combined with acyclovir may be effective against cytomegalovirus. Cidofovir has been used with some success for viral-related hemorrhagic cystitis.	Alkylating chemotherapy agents used to treat hematologic malignancies (e.g., busulfan, cyclophosphamide, ifosfamide, thiotepa) Post-transplant viruses (e.g., cytomegalovirus, BK virus, JC virus)

(Continued on next page)

Table 3-3. Nonrespiratory Oncologic Emergencies in Patients With Hematologic Malignancies and Disorders (Continued)

Oncologic Emergency	Description	Risk Groups
Hypercalcemia	May occur from several mechanisms. Lymphoma may cause this complication through increased absorption of calcitriol and reduced renal clearance of calcium. T-cell lymphoma may also create ectopic parathyroid hormone or activate receptor activator of nuclear factor kappa-B ligand (RANKL) expression. The complication is more common in patients with multiple myeloma caused by osteoclastic activity and RANKL expression by tumor cells. Risk can be increased in patients with renal dysfunction. It may be prevented or minimized with monthly bisphosphonate therapy in at-risk patients. IV hydration with normal saline enhances calcium excretion. Emergent rapid-acting bisphosphonates (e.g., zoledronate) may also effectively lower calcium. Other less often used medications that can lower calcium include mithramycin and calcitonin.	Most common with multiple myeloma May occur in patients with lymphoma having bone marrow involvement
Idiopathic hyperammonemia syndrome	A syndrome of elevated ammonia without concurrent rises in transaminases Proposed to be an unusual outcome of profound neutropenia and altered metabolic pathways Management is supportive and may involve respiratory support, airway protection, lactulose, acetate infusion, or renal replacement therapy.	During neutropenia after highly immunosuppressive chemotherapy; most cases have been reported with treatment of acute leukemia.

(Continued on next page)

Table 3-3. Nonrespiratory Oncologic Emergencies in Patients With Hematologic Malignancies and Disorders *(Continued)*

Oncologic Emergency	Description	Risk Groups
Leukostasis	Excess number and size of immature cells found in acute leukemia cause vascular obstruction and organ failure. For unclear reasons, the brain, lungs, and kidneys are most prone to injury with this disorder, resulting in respiratory and renal failure and strokes. Immediate antineoplastic therapy is indicated. Rapid-acting chemotherapy agents, such as cyclophosphamide or hydroxyurea, are usually the preferred initial treatment until the patient's clinical condition is stabilized. Most clinicians recommend leukapheresis to remove a large portion of the white blood cells (WBCs) from circulation prior to antineoplastic chemotherapy. This is thought to reduce the risk for severe tumor lysis syndrome and its consequences.	Most common with acute myeloid leukemia (monocytic subtype) where cells are large and easily clumping, a WBC count > 100,000/mm^3, or high proliferation rate and blast percentage May occur with chronic leukemia or acute lymphocytic leukemia with WBC counts > 300,000–400,000/mm^3 Occurs with Burkitt lymphoma or other high-grade lymphomas with rapid proliferation rates Associated with differentiating agents, such as bortezomib, lenalidomide, and rituximab

(Continued on next page)

Table 3-3. Nonrespiratory Oncologic Emergencies in Patients With Hematologic Malignancies and Disorders *(Continued)*

Oncologic Emergency	Description	Risk Groups
Pericardial effusion	Excess fluid accumulation in the pericardial space, impeding normal venous return and filling of the heart Leads to edema, hepatic congestions and other signs and symptoms of right heart failure and reduced cardiac output leading to end-organ dysfunction, and hypotension Primary diagnosis with echocardiogram that shows both pericardial fluid and right ventricular collapse from high pericardial pressure. Excess pericardial fluid may be evident on chest x-ray or computed tomography scan, but the degree of impaired cardiac output may not be defined. Emergent treatment may include large-volume fluid administration, but draining the fluid from the pericardial sac is the definitive treatment. Cancer-related pericardial effusions may be slow to develop, causing subtle symptoms and resulting in large volume of fluid at removal. Malignant infiltration of the pericardium may alter the fluid appearance, making it cloudy, chylous, or bloody.	Cancers: Acute lymphocytic leukemia, primary effusion lymphoma Therapy: Alemtuzumab, cytosine arabinoside

(Continued on next page)

Table 3-3. Nonrespiratory Oncologic Emergencies in Patients With Hematologic Malignancies and Disorders *(Continued)*

Oncologic Emergency	Description	Risk Groups
Posterior reversible encephalopathy syndrome	Also termed *posterior reversible leukoencephalopathy syndrome*, it is a rare neurologic disorder linked to hypertension. It is unclear whether the same trigger mechanism for hypertension is the pathology or whether the high blood pressure is a consequence of the neurovascular injury and inflammation. Characterized by headaches, altered mental status, and visual disturbances that may progress to seizures. Tinnitus and vertigo have also been reported. Classic computed tomography and magnetic resonance imaging features exist, including bilateral attenuation abnormalities, vasogenic edema, and increased signal intensity in the posterior brain, which may involve parietal, temporal, and/or occipital lobes. The syndrome is managed with symptomatic support, such as mechanical ventilation, anticonvulsants, and antihypertensive medications. Corticosteroids have been used with some success to reverse neurologic symptoms.	Calcineurin inhibitors (e.g., cyclosporine, tacrolimus) Angiogenesis inhibitors (e.g., bevacizumab, mTOR inhibitors)

(Continued on next page)

Table 3-3. Nonrespiratory Oncologic Emergencies in Patients With Hematologic Malignancies and Disorders *(Continued)*

Oncologic Emergency	Description	Risk Groups
Sinusoidal obstruction syndrome/hepatic veno-occlusive disease	Inflammatory stimulation of venous endothelial layers of the veins and sinusoids of the liver Progresses to fibrotic changes and occlusion of the hepatic venous vessels and portal hypertension and tendency for thromboses Early symptoms include abdominal pain, fluid retention, elevated direct bilirubin, and other signs and symptoms of obstructive liver disease. Onset of symptoms begins 8–20 days after start of therapy, and progression occurs over 1–3 weeks with a plateau after that time. Presence of painful ascites, thrombocytopenia, prolonged clotting times, hyperammonemia, metabolic alkalosis, and increased vagal tone signals more severe hepatic destruction. May appear symptomatically similar to graft-versus-host disease, but sonography can differentiate the two disorders. Abdominal ultrasonography will reveal hepatomegaly, and Doppler technology confirms venous wall stiffness and estimated portal pressures. Treatment is supportive with fluid restriction, clotting factors, and renal replacement therapy. Defibrotide has antithrombotic properties thought to reduce hepatic thromboses with permanent and irreversible liver damage.	High-dose radiation therapy involving abdomen (e.g., total body irradiation in transplant) High-dose alkylating agents (e.g., busulfan, cyclophosphamide, thiotepa) Monoclonal antibodies (e.g., alemtuzumab) Calcineurin inhibitors (e.g., sirolimus) Azole antifungal agents Hypersensitivity induced (e.g., dacarbazine, methotrexate) Herbal remedies (e.g., *Gynura segetum*, Tusangi; tea containing pyrrolizidine alkaloids) Pretreatment older age, previous history of hepatitis, heavily pretreated with alkylating agents, increased bilirubin or increased ferritin

(Continued on next page)

Table 3-3. Nonrespiratory Oncologic Emergencies in Patients With Hematologic Malignancies and Disorders (Continued)

Oncologic Emergency	Description	Risk Groups
Spinal cord compression	Paravertebral tumor can obstruct blood supply, directly compress the spinal cord, or most commonly invade the vertebral body from the anterior surface. Vertebral collapse and compression fractures can then cause cord compression. Cord compression symptoms correlate to the location of injury. Early cord compression presents as pain and sensory changes, usually in the lower extremities. Motor changes, such as weakness or diminished reflexes, occur later. Total paralysis and loss of autonomic function (incontinent bladder or bowel) are late findings. Diagnosis can be confirmed by magnetic resonance imaging. Emergent treatment with corticosteroids may provide temporary relief of cord injury, but it must be followed by definitive treatment of the etiology. Antineoplastic therapy is indicated, such as chemotherapy/immunotherapy and targeted radiation therapy in radiosensitive tumors.	Lymphoma, especially with abdominal involvement Multiple myeloma, especially with plasmacytoma
Syndrome of inappropriate antidiuretic hormone secretion	Excess production of antidiuretic hormone incongruent with normal feedback mechanisms leads to fluid retention and hyponatremia. It is often linked to the presence and severity of disease. Fluid restrictions and treatment of the cancer are often the only interventions required, but refractory disease may require hypertonic saline administration.	Ectopic antidiuretic hormone production occurs with lymphoma with high tumor burden (often represented by high lactate dehydrogenase or leukocytosis). May be more prevalent in primary central nervous system lymphoma and HIV-related lymphoma

(Continued on next page)

Table 3-3. Nonrespiratory Oncologic Emergencies in Patients With Hematologic Malignancies and Disorders (Continued)

Oncologic Emergency	Description	Risk Groups
Tumor lysis syndrome	Rapid lysis of neoplastic cells that exceeds the clearance capacity of the kidneys Internal cell components are released into the systemic circulation, leading to hyperkalemia, hyperuricemia, and hyperphosphatemia. Calcium is pushed back into the bones in the presence of high phosphorus, leading to hypocalcemia. May be present even before treatment in patients with malignancies having high proliferation rate Leukemias with high blast percentages may increase risk of lysis prior to treatment. Self-lysis is characterized by more severe hyperuricemia, and treatment-related lysis is more likely to produce hyperphosphatemia. The syndrome usually occurs within the first 48 hours, but it may develop as late as 3–5 days and rarely lasts longer than 7 days. Treatment usually includes phosphate-binding agents and allopurinol to prevent uric acid production. If the uric acid is initially high, rasburicase can lower uric acid levels. Initial hydration with high-volume normal saline prevents calcium phosphate precipitants and reduces the risk for acute kidney injury.	Rapidly proliferating malignancies (e.g., acute leukemia, Burkitt lymphoma) Large tumor burden of at-risk malignancies indicated by high WBC counts (leukemia, lymphoma) or high LDH Renal impairment that slows clearance Administration of differentiating agents (e.g., bortezomib, rituximab)

(Continued on next page)

Table 3-3. Nonrespiratory Oncologic Emergencies in Patients With Hematologic Malignancies and Disorders (Continued)

Oncologic Emergency	Description	Risk Groups
Typhlitis/neutropenic enterocolitis	A gastrointestinal complication of poor perfusion to a segment of bowel in the presence of gastrointestinal microbes. The distal small bowel (ileum) and area of the appendix are at particular risk due to poor perfusion, tortuosity, and potential for gram-negative bacteria to translocate across the ileocecal valve. Bacteria proliferate and translocate across the inflamed bowel lumen, causing gram-negative bacteremia. Gases produced by bacteria may also cause pneumatosis intestinalis. It is most common with prolonged neutropenia and the presence of gram-negative bacteria in the gut. Prophylactic oral antimicrobials and growth factors have reduced the incidence and severity of this disorder, but it remains problematic among patients with hematologic malignancies, particularly those with refractory disease and poor count recovery. It presents as dull or acute abdominal pain focused in the right abdomen, abdominal distension, diarrhea or gastrointestinal bleeding, and sepsis-related symptoms such as fever, tachypnea, tachycardia, hypotension, and acidosis. Diagnosis can be made by abdominal computed tomography scan. It is managed like other instances of abdominal sepsis with fluids, broad-spectrum antimicrobials, and gut rest; although, the option of intestinal resection is a high risk in this population.	Prolonged neutropenia from refractory disease Failure to engraft after therapy or HSCT Specific agents associated with higher risk (e.g., cytosine arabinoside, daunomycin, docetaxel, doxorubicin, idarubicin, methotrexate, pegylated asparaginase, rituximab, topotecan, vincristine) Failure to comply with oral antimicrobial prophylaxis regimens Intact appendix, prior bowel surgery, or prior *Clostridium difficile* infection

Note. Based on information from Anderson-Reitz & Clancy, 2013; S. Chen et al., 2015; Y.-H. Chen et al., 2010; Cope, 2016; Davies, 2016; Franchini, 2015; Granata et al., 2015; Kaplan, 2016; Picard et al., 2015; Relf & Shelton 2018; Schmidt et al., 2016.

patients with nonmalignant hematologic/immunologic disorders often are man-aged by oncologists and have similar clinical problems to patients with hemato-logic malignancies. The most common of these disorders include autoimmune diseases, myelodysplastic syndrome, myelofibrosis, hemophagocytic syndrome, immune and thrombotic thrombocytopenia, and RBC problems (e.g., hemo-lytic anemia, polycythemia vera, sickle cell disease) (Deadmond & Smith-Gagen, 2015; Shelton, 2012). At times, these disorders are independent of malignancy, although many have been associated with increased development of hematopoi-etic malignancy and may present as concomitant illnesses.

The specific association of malignant conditions with complications such as hemolytic anemia and immune thrombocytopenic purpura (ITP) is well known (Izzedine & Perazella, 2015). The malignancies most likely associated with hemo-lytic anemia are colon cancer, chronic lymphocytic leukemia, and lymphoma (Izzedine & Perazella, 2015). Hemolytic anemia also has been associated with specific antineoplastic agents, such as mitomycin, gemcitabine, and anti–vascular endothelial growth factor (Izzedine & Perazella, 2015; Polovich et al., 2014). Vari-ant or atypical hemolytic uremic syndrome (HUS) has been identified in patients after hematopoietic stem cell transplantation (HSCT) and chemotherapy for some hematologic malignancies (Nayer & Asif, 2016). It is often difficult to clin-ically differentiate from the typical hematologic disorder of HUS or TTP (Kap-pler, Ronan-Bentle, & Graham, 2014). TTP has been strongly linked to breast cancer and lymphoma (Liebman, 2014). Additionally, many of these hematologic patients receive similar therapies to patients with cancer (e.g., antineoplastic med-ications, blood component transfusions, infection prevention strategies). Com-mon clinical issues include bleeding, infection, and perfusion deficit from anemia. The variety of these disorders is beyond the scope of this book, but key patient care implications are noted in Table 3-4.

Bleeding

When hematologic disorders require critical care intervention, special con-siderations exist regarding bleeding and thrombosis risk. Medication review for agents that worsen thrombocytopenia, alter coagulation, or enhance thrombo-sis can minimize bleeding or clotting risk and may identify confounding risks for hematologic complications.

Bleeding occurs in approximately 10% of patients with cancer. Those with a hematologic malignancy experience this complication more often than those with solid tumors (Federici et al., 2014). Transfusion thresholds in patients with hema-tologic disorders or hematologic malignancies may be considerably different than usual cases in the intensive care unit. Studies have shown that patients can toler-ate platelet counts as low as $10,000/mm^3$ when injury risk is limited (Erb & Vogel, 2013; Kreuger, Middelburg, Zwaginga, van der Bom, & Kerkhoffs, 2015). When invasive procedures are required, concomitant products may be infused, but the risk of bleeding is exacerbated, and it may not be possible to achieve optimal plate-

Table 3-4. Key Features of Nonmalignant Hematologic/Immunologic Disorders

Disorder	Description	Key Critical Care Implications
Antiphospholipid syndrome	An autoimmune hypercoagulable state caused by antiphospholipid antibodies. Thromboses occur in both arteries and veins and can lead to pregnancy complications such as miscarriage and stillbirth. It is diagnosed by a presence of lupus anticoagulant, anti–beta-2 glycoprotein, or anticardiolipin antibodies. It may occur as a primary disorder or be associated with autoimmune diseases such as systemic lupus erythematosus.	Excessive clotting may be refractory to traditional anticoagulation methods and require intermediate or critical care for management of life-threatening clots or thrombolytic therapy. Newer interventional management of clots with thrombectomy and catheter-directed thrombolytics may require a higher level of care and monitoring.
Aplastic anemia	This disorder destroys the stem cell population within the bone marrow, leading to inadequate production of red blood cells (RBCs), white blood cells (WBCs), and platelets. The clinical consequences are anemia, infection, and bleeding. Acute aplastic anemia may resolve with removal of the etiologic factor, but nonresponse to this strategy may require a fast track to bone marrow transplantation. Delays with excessive blood product transfusions may result in transfusion refractoriness and marrow rejection.	These patients have no compensatory mechanisms and are at high risk for hematologic complications that are only temporarily responsive to supportive therapy. Bone marrow transplant for these patients may be essential but also fraught with complications unless a complete human leukocyte antigen match is available.
Hemolytic anemia	This anemia is an IV lysis of RBCs with subsequent circulating RBC fragments. It may be immune related or genetically induced (e.g., sickle cell disease). Primary clinical effects include severe anemia, microvascular occlusion with organ ischemia, and renal failure.	Reduced-functioning RBCs can lead to ischemic complications, such as myocardial infarction, pulmonary infarction, and bowel infarction. Hemolysis and circulating cell fragments also lead to organ failure. In critically ill patients, hemolysis and anemia exacerbate ischemic conditions and complicate treatment. Removal of the etiologic factor is the most effective treatment.

(Continued on next page)

Table 3-4. Key Features of Nonmalignant Hematologic/Immunologic Disorders *(Continued)*

Disorder	Description	Key Critical Care Implications
Hemophagocytic lymphohistiocytosis (HLH)	HLH is an overstimulated immune system response with self-phagocytosis of WBCs. Symptoms mimic infection but with more dramatic clinical findings. The disease is confirmed by hematology tests, liver function tests, and markers of inflammation (e.g., ferritin, interleukin-2 receptor levels). Bone marrow examination shows hemophagocytosis and specific genetic mutations by flow cytometry. The disease may occur independently or as a precursor to the diagnosis of lymphoma.	The treatment of choice is immune suppression with corticosteroids with chemotherapy (usually etoposide) or antithymocyte globulin.
Hemophilia	This group of hereditary genetic impairment of clotting factors (e.g., hemophilia A [factor VIII], hemophilia B [factor IX], hemophilia C [factor XI]) leads to bleeding with minimal injury.	Bleeding, particularly in the joints or deep muscles, is the most common complication of this disorder. Patients require hospitalization and transfusion with clotting factor or after injury with risk for bleeding or prior to invasive procedures. The most common cause of serious consequences and death is intracranial hemorrhage, which may require critical care support.

(Continued on next page)

Table 3-4. Key Features of Nonmalignant Hematologic/Immunologic Disorders (Continued)

Disorder	Description	Key Critical Care Implications
Myelofibrosis	Myelofibrosis is disrupted normal production of blood cells with scarring of the bone marrow. Resulting complications include anemia with enlarged spleen or liver. It is now considered a form of chronic leukemia with a specific mutation called JAK2 mutation, but it often leads to acute myeloid leukemia over time. Myelofibrosis may also be linked to polycythemia vera and exposure to industrial chemicals or radiation. Other common outcomes include portal hypertension, hypersplenism, painful bones and joints, and hyperuricemia with gout.	An enlarged spleen is painful, and splenic infarction or rupture is a high-risk complication that may require emergent surgical intervention or critical care. Coexisting portal hypertension and risk for bleeding complicate patient management. Thrombocytopenia is common late in the disease course and increases the risk for injury related to bleeding. Sudden withdrawal of medications used to treat this disorder (JAK2 inhibitors) can lead to a sudden and severe cytokine storm that mimics sepsis. Patients may also be at risk for infection, making it difficult to differentiate unless an accurate medication adherence history is obtained.
Myelodysplastic syndrome (MDS)	MDS occurs with the ineffective production of all blood cells and may initially present with anemia. MDS can eventually cause cytopenia and convert to acute myeloid leukemia.	MDS with long-term cytopenia and need for chronic transfusions is related to chronic transfusion reactions and refractoriness to transfusion response. This complicates the ability to provide transfusion support for invasive interventions and critical care support. Patients may also have a long-term history of chronic and refractory infections, making infection with unusual microbes (e.g., fungi) or drug-resistant organisms a common concern for this population. Patients with initial MDS that converts to acute leukemia are known to have a more refractory disease and require more aggressive chemotherapy with a high incidence of adverse reactions.

(Continued on next page)

Table 3-4. Key Features of Nonmalignant Hematologic/Immunologic Disorders *(Continued)*

Disorder	Description	Key Critical Care Implications
Polycythemia vera	Polycythemia vera is a Philadelphia chromosome–negative myeloproliferative neoplasm leading to high RBC counts. This results in increased risk of thrombosis and often evolves into MDS or acute leukemia.	This disorder has many neoplastic features and is often managed by oncologists. Thrombotic complications may also lead to thrombohemorrhagic events. Because transformation to MDS and acute leukemia is common, leukocytosis and thrombocytopenia are also common. The same JAK2 mutation found in some patients with MDS can be present with polycythemia vera, so treatment may be similar.
Porphyria	Porphyria is a usually inherited metabolic derangement of porphyrins required to create heme and carry oxygen to the tissues, leading to liver, nerve, and skin abnormalities. Symptoms may include mental status changes, seizures, restlessness, insomnia, pain, tingling, weakness, or paralysis. Abdominal pain, vomiting, and diarrhea may also be present. Cutaneous symptoms may include sun-related changes, such as painful skin redness, fragile skin, increased hair growth, or brown urine.	Complications may include dehydration, anemia, muscle weakness with decreased respiratory effort, hyponatremia, hypertension, renal insufficiency, or hepatic failure. Multiorgan support may be required during acute exacerbation episodes. Treatment is supportive or may involve injections of hemin.

(Continued on next page)

Table 3-4. Key Features of Nonmalignant Hematologic/Immunologic Disorders (Continued)

Disorder	Description	Key Critical Care Implications
Sickle cell disease	Sickle cell disease is a genetic disorder of hemoglobin S where the red blood cell becomes disfigured (sickle shaped) in the presence of hypoxia. Sickled cells and intravascular cell lysis causes all the features of hemolytic anemia. Sickle cells occlude the microvasculature, causing tissue ischemia and injury with pain. Infection risk is also increased due to a damaged spleen.	Hemolysis and subsequent anemia with ischemia and injury or renal failure may require critical care intervention. Careful balance of oxygen supply and demand to minimize hemolysis may require fluid administration and oxygen support. Care must be taken with fluids, as many patients have developed long-term pulmonary hypertension and heart failure from increased workload on the heart during sickling episodes. Organ ischemia and injury can lead to complications such as myocardial infarction, bowel infarction, splenic rupture, or renal insufficiency. Blood viscosity can lead to intracranial infarction and hemorrhage, venous thrombosis, and pulmonary infarction. Iron overload may occur when frequent transfusions are required to replenish lysed cells. Tissue occlusion can also cause pain, and management may be complex and difficult to resolve.
Thalassemia	Thalassemia is an inherited autosomal recessive anemia that results in abnormal oxygen transport and self-hemolysis. The most common results of this disorder are from hyperviscosity and microvascular occlusion. Hypersplenism, heart failure, and iron overload often occur. Infection risk is also increased due to a damaged spleen.	Implications are similar to hemolytic anemia or sickle cell anemia.

Note. Based on information from Rogers, 2013; Rosselet, 2013; Shelton, 2012.

let levels of 50,000/mm³ (Erb & Vogel, 2013; O'Leary & Mack, 2013; Tong, Tadros, & Vaziri, 2015). These patients may be resistant to platelet transfusion (alloimmunization) or require specially processed products, although no strong evidence supports this practice (Riedijk et al., 2015). Nurses can anticipate that platelet products may be single-donor, multi-unit products, and patients can have a history of febrile or allergic reactions requiring premedications. The usual hemoglobin goal for patients with hematologic disorders is 7–8 mg/dl, although many patients are stable at even lower levels (Carson et al., 2012; Chen, 2015). Given normal low RBC counts, transfusions may be administered based on symptoms rather than threshold values.

Despite low thresholds for transfusion, many patients receive large volumes of blood products throughout critical illness because of blood losses and metabolic destruction of hematopoietic cells. In such patients, ongoing risk exists for complications of transfusion, such as transfusion-related lung injury, transfusion-related graft-versus-host disease, and rare viral illnesses (Federici et al., 2014). Critical care nurses must be alert to acute changes in respiratory status, such as increased respiratory rate, cough, coarse breath sounds, or the occurrence of new pulmonary infiltrates within six hours of transfusion (Kim & Na, 2015; Vande Vusse et al., 2015; Vlaar et al., 2010; Vlaar & Juffermans, 2013). Assessment for symptoms in high-risk patients receiving large-volume transfusions or with a history of transfusion reactions permits aggressive, immediate management. Cold agglutinin reactions requiring blood warming are also more prevalent in patients with hematologic/immunologic disorders and hematologic malignancies compared to other medical-surgical diseases (Berentsen & Tjønnfjord, 2012).

Expertise in management of excessive bleeding is a required skill when caring for patients with hematologic disorders. Because patients may marginally respond or have contraindications to transfusions, local and topical antibleeding strategies are essential. Extended manual pressure on puncture sites and topical hemostatics, such as Gelfoam®, oxidized cellulose, and topical thrombin, may be useful adjuncts (Shelton, 2012). Blood conservation strategies, such as blood waste reinfusion and chest tube drainage reinfusion, are also helpful supportive therapies that minimize the blood lost through laboratory testing or from drains.

Thrombosis

Some hematologic disorders have increased risk of thrombosis instead of bleeding. Thrombosis is triggered by vascular injury, tissue injury, inflammation, and hyperviscosity. Many hematologic/immunologic disorders are characterized by high levels of inflammation. Usual thrombosis prevention interventions are employed, although the presence of thrombocytopenia may require use of less effective mechanical compression devices rather than anticoagulants (Erb & Vogel, 2013). Other proactive thrombosis prevention may include increased in-bed exercises, adequate hydration, and avoidance of large multilumen venous catheters when possible (Erb & Vogel, 2013). Nursing care for patients with thrombosis may include assessment of viscosity tests or assistance with phlebotomy and pheresis. Daily assessment for the need of thrombosis prevention and for the escalation of prophylaxis measures when anticoagulation contraindications resolve should be priorities for the interprofessional team.

Infection

Patients with immunologic disorders are inherently at risk for infection, but the clinical profile of infection types and severity of illness may vary considerably. In patients with hematologic malignancy, infection caused by dysfunctional or depleted WBCs is common. Patients may receive targeted immunosuppressive medications or corticosteroids to treat their autoimmune disorder, making them highly susceptible to infection; however, they are likely to demonstrate few signs or symptoms. Given long-term suppression of WBC function, typical bacteria seen in critically ill patients may not be the only consideration when infection is suspected (Shelton, 2018). Patients should be screened and tested for atypical bacteria, as well as fungal and viral pathogens, at the first sign of infection. Many patients also receive essential prophylactic antimicrobials against these unusual infection sources. These must be maintained even during critical illness. Oral antimicrobial prophylaxis against gastrointestinal bacteria, *Pneumocystis jirovecii* fungi, and viruses should not be omitted from care and may require conversion to IV alternatives if the patient has a nonfunctioning gut (Melichar & Zezulová, 2011; National Comprehensive Cancer Network® [NCCN®], 2017).

Patients with immunologic disorders and/or hematologic malignancy are at risk for and experience complex and frequent infections. Constant exposure to antimicrobial agents magnifies the risk for infection with secondary pathogens, such as *Clostridium difficile* and *Candida* species (Surawicz et al., 2013). Uncommon locations and infection sources must be evaluated, requiring an array of diagnostic tests, such as multisite cultures, lumbar puncture, pan-computed tomography scan, and ultrasound. Unusual complications occur in this population, such as typhlitis/neutropenic enterocolitis and acalculous cholecystitis (Shafi & Bresalier, 2010; Song & Marcon, 2017).

Unlike in critically ill patients, who are considered febrile and potentially infected at a temperature of 38.3°C (100.4°F), the threshold for potential infection in this population is a temperature of 38.0°C recorded twice within an hour (NCCN, 2017). This lower threshold for fever requires that critical care nurses alter fever evaluation protocols. The risk for unusual infections may also necessitate fungal and viral cultures less frequently prescribed in the ICU setting. Special tests for fungus, such as beta-D-glucan and galactomannan, may be ordered and sent to outside laboratories, and special viral culture media may need to be obtained (Shelton, 2018; Zitella, 2011).

Critical care nurses need to understand viral polymerase chain reaction (PCR) tests, tests defining viral load, and the importance of these tests to patient management. Antiviral prophylaxis medications are dosed differently than when used for therapeutic management of disease, and nurses play an integral role in helping to prescribe the appropriate drugs and dosage for viral illness. Viral copies may also drive implementation of multidrug regimens to adequately suppress common opportunistic viruses, such as cytomegalovirus (Sansoni et al., 2014).

Additionally, patients experiencing frequent infections are often treated with different frontline, broad-spectrum antimicrobial therapy. Third- or fourth-generation cephalosporins are seldom used, and beta-lactam/beta-lactamase inhibitors or carbapenems are the preferred fever agents (NCCN, 2017). In cases of severe and refractory infection during bone marrow aplasia, granulocyte transfusions may be administered to boost the patient's ability to combat the infection until WBC count recovery (Estcourt et al., 2015; Nesher & Rolston, 2013; Öztürkmen, Altuntas, & Olcay, 2013; Safdar, Rodriguez, Zuniga, Al Akhrass, & Pande, 2014). For patients with chronic lymphocyte suppression, especially with sinus or pulmonary infections, immunoglobulin levels may be assessed and supported with IV immunoglobulin infusions (McCormack, 2013; Raanani et al., 2009).

Patients with an infection may be transferred to the intensive care unit when they develop severe infectious complications, such as refractory infection or septic shock. Management principles for these patients mirror other standard management strategies for critically ill individuals and are addressed in other critical care references (Dellinger et al., 2013). The underlying care priority is to ascertain the source of infection and aggressively manage it while maintaining adequate tissue perfusion. Special considerations exist for management of sepsis in these patients beyond the scope of this chapter; however, they may be accessed through specialty references (Mokart et al., 2015; Torres et al., 2015). Usual sepsis screening criteria may be overly sensitive for this population, fluid therapy may result in greater risk for capillary permeability disorders, and the history of immune compromise and antimicrobial exposure may complicate typical therapy choices.

Respiratory Complications

The most common cause of critical illness in patients with hematologic malignancies and nonmalignant hematologic/immunologic disorders is respiratory failure (Vadde & Pastores, 2015). The etiologies for this complication may be tumor related, treatment related, or infectious in nature. Diagnostic evaluation includes assessment of risks associated with specific malignancy diagnoses, tumor in the lungs or pleura, cardiogenic pulmonary edema, and a medication review for potential toxicities.

Minimally invasive tests, such as arterial blood gases, will aid in identifying whether hypoxia or hypercarbia characterizes the disorder. Chest x-rays are nonspecific but useful when a structural defect is suspected. Computed tomography scans with contrast are helpful in differentiating disorders of the pleura, parenchyma, and vascular structures in the lungs (Wielpütz, Heußel, Herth, & Kauczor, 2014). Many of the unusual disorders seen in this patient population will require bronchoscopy with lavage, brush, or biopsy, or, alternatively, an open-lung biopsy. Despite relative contraindications to these procedures, such as severe and refractory thrombocytopenia, expert proceduralists have performed bronchoscopy in patients with active bleeding or high-risk individuals without significant morbidity (Nandagopal, Veeraputhiran, Jain, Soubani, & Schiffer, 2016). Research suggests that bronchoscopy with lavage can be safely performed in patients with very low platelet counts (Nandagopal et al., 2016).

Disease-related respiratory failure may be related to tumor-induced tracheobronchial airway obstruction, pulmonary alveolar proteinosis, and pleural effusions. Treatment-related pulmonary toxicities occur with variable frequency, such as diffuse alveolar hemorrhage, differentiation syndrome, interstitial pneumonitis, or radiation pneumonitis (Polovich et al., 2014). Differentiation of these disorders is important for intensive care clinicians to understand because survival is highly dependent on prompt, appropriate therapy. Respiratory distress is more commonly related to pulmonary infections than other etiologies and is the most common clinical problem causing respiratory failure. Given the broad spectrum of possible respiratory pathogens, early bronchoscopy has been advocated for diagnostic evaluation in this patient population (Chellapandian et al., 2015; Kim & Na, 2015). When a patient's respiratory status declines without a definitive diagnosis, the risks and benefits of open lung biopsy may be considered (Chellapandian et al., 2015). A thorough review of the specific features of respiratory pathogens is beyond the scope of this text but is available in specialty references (Shelton, 2018). A summary of the causes of respiratory failure and their key features is included in Table 3-5.

Early targeted intervention for respiratory complications has been associated with improved outcomes (Vadde & Pastores, 2015). Noninvasive ventilation with continuous positive airway pressure or bilevel positive airway pressure in carefully selected patients can provide temporary support while the etiology of respiratory compromise is addressed (Saillard, Mokart, Lemiale, & Azoulay, 2014; Vadde & Pastores, 2015). High-flow nasal cannula is another innovative therapy that can deliver hyperconcentrated oxygen (Lee, Rhee, & Lee, 2015), and heliox (combined helium and oxygen) may be implemented to deliver oxygen despite airway obstruction (Beurskens, Wösten-van Asperen, Preckel, & Juffermans, 2015). Despite an armamentarium of supportive care options, aggressive assessment for the etiology of respiratory distress is the preferred management strategy (Saillard et al., 2014).

Table 3-5. Respiratory Complications of Hematologic Malignancies and Nonmalignant Hematologic Disorders

Disorder	Description	High-Risk Factors	Assessment/Diagnosis	Treatment
Bronchiolitis obliterans organizing pneumonia	Also known as cryptogenic organizing pneumonia Granulation tissue within the small airways and extending into the alveolus	Typically occurs > 100 days after transplant Most common after allogeneic transplant, especially with unrelated donors or concomitant graft-versus-host disease	Dyspnea, late inspiratory crackles Pulmonary function tests show decreased vital capacity, normal flow rate, and decreased diffusing capacity. A chest x-ray shows bilateral patchy consolidation that may be migratory with serial x-rays. Computed tomography (CT) scan findings include bilateral air space consolidation and ground-glass opacities. Consolidation is usually subpleural, or peribronchial ground-glass opacities have no specific pattern of distribution. Nodules with smooth and distinct margins may be observed but have no specific pattern of distribution.	Corticosteroids are the treatment of choice but are also associated with inconsistent results.

(Continued on next page)

Table 3-5. Respiratory Complications of Hematologic Malignancies and Nonmalignant Hematologic Disorders *(Continued)*

Disorder	Description	High-Risk Factors	Assessment/Diagnosis	Treatment
Differentiation syndrome	Antineoplastic agents that enhance malignant cell differentiation for purposes of more effective targeted apoptosis can also trigger inflammation, or differentiation syndrome. Widespread inflammation occurs because of the release of cytokines during engraftment or cell proliferation. Although a normal process, the inflammatory outcome may produce significant adverse signs and symptoms.	Most common in acute progranulocytic leukemia receiving arsenic trioxide, or all-trans-retinoic acid Has also been reported with proteasome inhibitors (e.g., bortezomib) or agents that target a tumor marker, such as CD20 receptors (e.g., rituximab)	Clinical signs/symptoms of respiratory compromise as white blood cells release cytokines (e.g., crackles, cough, hypoxemia, increased work of breathing) Fever Diffuse skin rash Timing of this syndrome is usually 7–20 days after start of treatment. Chest x-ray and CT scan show diffuse, bilateral pulmonary infiltrates, and general haziness associated with increased lung water.	Fluid restriction may decrease risk of developing. Chemotherapy may be held while corticosteroids are administered. Treatment is resumed after stabilization while receiving steroids.

(Continued on next page)

Table 3-5. Respiratory Complications of Hematologic Malignancies and Nonmalignant Hematologic Disorders (Continued)

Disorder	Description	High-Risk Factors	Assessment/Diagnosis	Treatment
Diffuse alveolar hemorrhage	Microvascular bleeding into alveoli in setting of inflammation and endothelial injury Usually reversible when detected early and managed aggressively	Newly diagnosed leukemia, especially with leukostasis Postmyeloablative hematopoietic stem cell transplantation (usually within the first two weeks) and a toxicity of the preparative regimen Strong association with cyclophosphamide in doses > 100 mg/kg, thalidomide (rare) Graft-versus-host disease Viral illness (e.g., adenovirus, cytomegalovirus, influenza, respiratory syncytial virus, rhinovirus, parainfluenza)	Sudden and profound dyspnea, air hunger, tachypnea, moderate to severe hypoxemia, cough, and/or chest discomfort Mild to moderate hemoptysis (rare) Increased static and peak airway pressures Chest x-rays (diffuse bilateral infiltrates); it may be difficult to differentiate from pneumonia without follow-up CT scan or bronchoscopy. Bronchoscopy with lavage is the most definitive test, as it quickly reveals hemosiderin-laden macrophages.	Oxygen therapy: Positive-pressure ventilation (noninvasively or invasively) Transfusion with platelets and coagulation products Corticosteroids

(Continued on next page)

Table 3-5. Respiratory Complications of Hematologic Malignancies and Nonmalignant Hematologic Disorders *(Continued)*

Disorder	Description	High-Risk Factors	Assessment/Diagnosis	Treatment
Hypersensitivity pulmonary edema or bronchospasm	Acute inflammatory reaction to direct exposure to offending agent triggers cytokine release, capillary permeability, and a syndrome similar to noncardiogenic pulmonary edema or acute respiratory distress syndrome. Bronchospasm may be an alternate clinical presentation. The degree of injury and unidentified host variables dictate whether it is a reversible process or progresses to pulmonary fibrosis.	Hypersensitivity reactions with acute noncardiogenic pulmonary edema or acute respiratory distress syndrome that occur from direct injury with drugs: • Alemtuzumab • Bortezomib • Cytarabine, especially with doses > 5 g/m²; usually occurs 6–12 hours after the dose • Fludarabine • Gemtuzumab • Lenalidomide • Methotrexate • Mitoxantrone • Rituximab • Vinorelbine between 3–8 days after administration Etoposide has only been associated with bronchospasm. Concomitant administration of growth factors may worsen symptoms.	Respiratory effort, such as dyspnea and tachypnea, may be first indicator of toxicity. Breath sounds are coarse and wet, with diffuse crackles or gurgles. Hypoxemia is prevalent. Food intake is usually greater than exercise output, leading to weight gain. Chest x-ray or chest CT shows bilateral patchy infiltrates. Sputum cultures or bronchoscopic specimens are negative for infectious etiologies. A component of alveolar hemorrhage is suspected but not consistent or proven to be part of the syndrome.	Fluid restrictions and prophylactic diuresis with weight gain may be used as a prevention. Offending chemotherapy will be stopped until the complication resolves. Diuresis may help oxygenation. Oxygen therapy is provided as needed to maintain an oxygen saturation above 88%–90%. Noninvasive positive pressure support through bilevel pressure support or high-flow nasal cannula has been helpful. Corticosteroids administered early may abrogate symptoms.

(Continued on next page)

Table 3-5. Respiratory Complications of Hematologic Malignancies and Nonmalignant Hematologic Disorders *(Continued)*

Disorder	Description	High-Risk Factors	Assessment/Diagnosis	Treatment
Interstitial pneumonitis with pulmonary fibrosis	Alveolar damage leading to inflammation, followed by fibrosis of the lung parenchyma Damage is thought to occur because of endothelial injury and activation of fibroblasts. Stiff and noncompliant lungs are the end result, and pulmonary hypertension may also occur.	Metabolism with accumulation of toxic metabolites that cause injury may occur with cyclophosphamide, ifosfamide, carmustine, and busulfan at doses > 500 mg. Mixed pathologic mechanisms have been associated with bleomycin lung toxicity. Cumulative dose effects are known for this drug, and lifetime maximum dose should not exceed 450–500 units. Busulfan recommended lifetime dose is < 500 mg. Multikinase inhibitors inhibit tyrosine kinase pathways in pneumocytes, causing fibrosis. Increased incidence occurs with patients over age 70	Dyspnea with slow to moderate progression of associated symptoms, such as fatigue, tachypnea, and increased work of breathing Late effects include hypoxemia and hypercarbia. Rarely includes fever Onset may occur 15 weeks to 6 or more years after exposure. Pulmonary function tests with assessment of diffusing lung capacity for carbon monoxide have been helpful in detecting early cyclophosphamide toxicity, but these have not been studied in other disorders. Arterial blood gases may show hypoxemia. Chest x-ray will initially be normal at onset of symptoms, but bilateral ground-glass opacities in the acute phase may be first visible on chest CT scan. Ground-glass infiltrates convert to	Initial treatment is to eliminate the offending agent if possible. Oxygen is used conservatively to avoid exacerbating toxicity with overlapping oxygen toxicity. Corticosteroids may be helpful.

(Continued on next page)

Table 3-5. Respiratory Complications of Hematologic Malignancies and Nonmalignant Hematologic Disorders (Continued)

Disorder	Description	High-Risk Factors	Assessment/Diagnosis	Treatment
Interstitial pneumonitis with pulmonary fibrosis (cont.)		years, a history of smoking, prior lung and autoimmune disease, chest irradiation, declining creatinine clearance, and exposure to oxygen at > 50% inspired oxygen.	fibrotic airways with honeycombing pattern after fibrosis.	
Leukostasis (pulmonary)	Hyperviscosity from a high number and large size of white blood cells (WBCs) causes pulmonary vascular occlusion with WBCs, leading to inflammation with increased capillary permeability. Hypoxemia and increased pulmonary congestion are characteristic of this complication.	High WBC counts (> 100,000/mm^3), high rate of rise, or high blast percentage in acute leukemia. Monocytic subtype is the highest risk due to level of immaturity and large size of cells. If present with chronic leukemia or acute lymphocytic leukemia, counts may be as high as 300,000–400,000/mm^3.	Dyspnea, tachypnea, and increased work of breathing. Breath sounds are coarse with gurgles and wet breath sounds. Acute hypoxemia is primary respiratory impairment. Typical chest x-ray and CT findings of leukostasis include bilateral patchy infiltrates that look similar to other pneumonic processes but often occur more acutely.	Treat malignancy with rapid-acting chemotherapy (e.g., cyclophosphamide), or hydroxyurea until definitive chemotherapy can be safely administered. Leukapheresis to remove excess WBCs may be helpful to reduce symptoms.

(Continued on next page)

Table 3-5. Respiratory Complications of Hematologic Malignancies and Nonmalignant Hematologic Disorders *(Continued)*

Disorder	Description	High-Risk Factors	Assessment/Diagnosis	Treatment
Radiation pneumonitis	Radiation injury causing damage to type I pneumocytes, resulting in interstitial and alveolar edema	Chest radiation is more common with lymphoma or lymphoblastic leukemia.	Dyspnea, low-grade fever, cough, and chest discomfort Occurs 4–12 weeks after completion of radiation course or as early as one week after end of therapy Especially common in patients receiving a high total dose of radiation or concomitant chemotherapy Chest x-ray shows the nonspecific ground-glass opacities and air space consolidation primarily in the radiation port. Pleural effusion (ipsilateral) or atelectasis may also occur. A fluorodeoxyglucose positron-emission tomography scan shows increased metabolic activity in area of injury.	Symptoms may be mild and resolve spontaneously. Corticosteroids are the treatment of choice. Regardless of treatment responsiveness, it may progress to radiation lung fibrosis.
Pleural effusions	Excess fluid accumulation between the visceral and parietal pleura Fluid increases thoracic pressure and impedes lung expansion.	Large chest masses disrupt normal pleural fluid dynamics and circulation, leading to trapped fluid. Malignancy invasion into the pleural fluid increases permeability and fluid production.	Dyspnea and increased work of breathing precede altered gas exchange. Hypercarbia may result if chest wall movement is greatly impaired. Hypoxemia occurs late. Breath sounds and chest excursion are diminished on affected side.	Some effusions may be observed, particularly if treatment of malignancy is thought to improve the effusion. Fluid restrictions have not been proven effective at reducing severity.

(Continued on next page)

Table 3-5. Respiratory Complications of Hematologic Malignancies and Nonmalignant Hematologic Disorders (Continued)

Disorder	Description	High-Risk Factors	Assessment/Diagnosis	Treatment
Pleural effusions (cont.)		Primary effusion lymphoma and specific subtypes of acute lymphocytic leukemia may have increased risk. Concomitant disorders, such as heart failure and hypothyroidism, may increase risk. Treatment with certain antineoplastic agents, such as cytosine arabinoside and dasatinib, may increase risk.	Pleural rub may be present, but it is often position dependent. Affected lung dull to percussion Deviated trachea away from affected side Chest x-ray shows fluid meniscus and blunting of diaphragmatic dome. Fluid tracking up side of the lung may also be visible. The x-ray should be performed upright to avoid fluid tracking the length of the lung and underestimation of effusion. A chest CT differentiates pneumonia and other parenchymal disease from effusion when multiple pulmonary disorders are present. Diagnostic thoracentesis with fluid sent for chemistry (exudative versus transudative), cytopathology (malignant cells), or flow cytometry (more sensitive for malignant cells in hematologic malignancies)	Therapeutic thoracentesis to remove significant fluid may be performed up to three times a week. With frequent and rapid recurrence, more permanent drainage methods are indicated. Short-term catheter drainage via chest tube with pleurodesis may be helpful, but this method has fallen out of favor. Video-assisted thoracoscopic surgery with talc pleurodesis or pleuroperitoneal shunt may have long-term effectiveness. Tunneled silastic pleural catheter for intermittent home drainage is popular, easy to manage, and safe.

(Continued on next page)

Table 3-5. Respiratory Complications of Hematologic Malignancies and Nonmalignant Hematologic Disorders (Continued)

Disorder	Description	High-Risk Factors	Assessment/Diagnosis	Treatment
Pulmonary alveolar proteinosis	Disrupted surfactant homeostasis with accumulation of phospholipid proteinaceous material inside the alveoli Associated with antibodies to granulocyte macrophage–colony-stimulating factor (GM-CSF)	Hematologic malignancies, especially chronic myeloid leukemia Exposure to inorganic toxins, such as silicone Adverse effect of immunosuppressive drugs on occasion More prevalent in men aged 30–50 years and smokers	Dyspnea Cough Nail clubbing Bronchoalveolar lavage is evidence of proteinaceous fluid. Immunohistochemical tests show GM-CSF antibodies. A CT scan of the lung shows patchy ground-glass opacities and interlobar thickening producing a "crazy-paving pattern" characteristic of the disease. Bronchoscopic lavage shows alveolar macrophages and eosinophils and myelin-like lamellar bodies. Open lung biopsy is likely to be periodic acid–Schiff stain-positive.	Oxygen and mechanical ventilation Pulmonary hygiene GM-CSF (replacement subcutaneous or inhalation) Plasmapheresis may be helpful. Whole lung lavage, including segments or entire lung, is the treatment of choice in refractory disease. Extracorporeal membrane circulation or cardiopulmonary bypass may be required with bilateral lung lavage; saline is usually the lavage fluid of choice. A double-lumen endotracheal tube may be required. Hyperbaric oxygen and liquid oxygen ventilation have been used experimentally.

(Continued on next page)

Table 3-5. Respiratory Complications of Hematologic Malignancies and Nonmalignant Hematologic Disorders *(Continued)*

Disorder	Description	High-Risk Factors	Assessment/Diagnosis	Treatment
Tracheobron-chial obstruction	Masses in the chest, particularly when they are high or anterior in location, occlude the upper airways (trachea or mainstem bronchi) Obstruction may be compressive or invasive into the airways or blood vessels.	High or anterior chest masses Usually lymphoma, but occasionally myeloma-related plasmacytoma or mass-producing acute lymphocytic leukemia	Dyspnea, tachypnea, air hunger Increased work of breathing Stridor or wheezes Hypoxemia Obstruction of high airways leads to reduced or absent aeration of lower airways, causing reduced breath sounds, abnormal chest excursion, or development of trapped secretions below the area of obstruction and pneumonia. Chest x-rays show the location of the mass. A chest CT angiogram with contrast differentiates the precise location and degree of invasion into the airway, lung parenchyma, and vasculature. Bronchoscopy allows visualization of airway occlusion and option for direct intervention.	Temporary airway opening may be accomplished with stenting, laser, and photodynamic therapy. Hematologic malignancies usually rapidly respond to chemotherapy, although radiation therapy may also shrink the tumor. Additional interventions to temporize airway are to use extra long or bifurcated endotracheal tubes or suture tubes in place to avoid displacement, particularly if tube placement must pass by obstruction. Prone positioning may offer benefit in airway management if the mass is located anterior to airways.

(Continued on next page)

Table 3-5. Respiratory Complications of Hematologic Malignancies and Nonmalignant Hematologic Disorders *(Continued)*

Disorder	Description	High-Risk Factors	Assessment/Diagnosis	Treatment
Veno-occlusive disease (pulmonary)	Endothelial wall damage with fibrotic tissue within the pulmonary venous circulation. Engorgement of alveolar capillaries and dilated lymphatics leads to interstitial edema and venous fibrosis. The clinical result is right-sided heart failure and pulmonary hypertension.	High risk: matched, unrelated donor transplant with graft-versus-host disease; treatment with high-dose alkylating agents (e.g., busulfan) Additional risks: dasatinib, mitomycin, familial pulmonary hypertension, preexisting lung disease, viral illness during post-transplant period Peak incidence is 40–60 days after transplant.	Dyspnea Fatigue Right heart failure symptoms: elevated jugular venous pulsations, hepatomegaly, edema Late findings may include left heart failure. Echocardiogram may show increased right heart pressures. CT scan shows patchy ground-glass or nodular opacities and central vascular engorgement in the perihilar region.	Treatment of reversible causes, such as viral illness Symptomatic management of heart failure Usual treatments for pulmonary hypertension (e.g., calcium channel blockers, prostacyclins) are contraindicated because they may cause pulmonary edema. Nitric oxide, prostanoids, phosphodiesterase inhibitors, and endothelin receptor antagonists have shown limited benefit. Corticosteroids or other graft-versus-host disease treatment may be helpful. Anticoagulant and antithrombotic agents may be useful.

Note. Based on information from Abdelmalak et al., 2015; Davies, 2016; Lee et al., 2015; Polovich et al., 2014; Saillard et al., 2014; Stephens, 2013; Vymazal & Krecmerova, 2015.

Hematologic/Immunologic Disorders Related to Cancer Treatment

Oncologic treatment is aimed at eradicating the greatest number of malignant cells while preserving normal cell function as much as possible. Despite attempts to minimize life-threatening adverse effects of therapy, myelosuppression occurs in approximately half of all patients with cancer (Shelton, 2016). Specific hematologic/immunologic effects of therapy involve RBCs, WBCs, and platelets. Coagulation protein abnormalities are also hematologic in nature. The primary clinical effects are anemia, infection, and bleeding. These effects are intensified in the patient with hematologic malignancy because the prescribed antineoplastic therapy must eradicate all bone marrow cells to be effective against the malignancy.

Medication-Induced Hematologic/Immunologic Toxicity

Antineoplastic and immunosuppressive medications are most known for their suppressive effects on the hematologic and immunologic systems. The degree, timing, and features of these functional deficits vary with agent, dose, and administration schedule. The time from therapy to return of normal blood may range from 21 days with nonmyeloablative transplant to more than 60 days with some leukemia therapies (Polovich et al., 2014). Some newer targeted therapies directed toward specific mutations may not cause significant myelosuppression. Nurses caring for these patients should consult with oncologic experts to predict and plan for these details. Critical care interventions that may be influenced by this knowledge include the removal or insertion of venous catheters, the timing of invasive interventions (e.g., surgery), the threshold for therapeutic interventions (e.g., transfusion therapy, antimicrobials), and the addition of supportive care (e.g., growth factors). In critical care practice, other medical-surgical medications may exacerbate the myelosuppressive effects of antineoplastic therapy and should be considered as alternate etiologies or exacerbating factors. Examples of critical care medications with concomitant hematologic/immunologic and myelosuppressive effects are included in Table 3-6.

A small group of antineoplastic therapies also exist that can cause inflammatory vasculitis, leading to capillary permeability, hypotension, and generalized organ dysfunction. Although most often associated with interleukin-2, this syndrome exists in some patients receiving high-dose cytarabine (Polovich et al., 2014). The recent exploration of immune activation to enhance self-antitumor effects with immune checkpoint inhibitors (e.g., PD-1, PD-L1, CTLA-4) or chimeric antigen receptor–directed T lymphocytes (e.g., CAR T cells) has produced similar clinical findings (Costa et al., 2016; Holzinger, Barden, & Abken, 2016). Although these adverse effects may be addressed in sources related to fluid or electrolyte imbalance, their inflammatory etiology should not be ignored. Treatment with corticosteroids

Table 3-6. Critical Care and Oncologic Medications Associated With Hematologic/Immunologic Disorders

Hematologic/ Immunologic Effects	Medication Class/Specific Medication
Anemia	Anticonvulsants (e.g., phenobarbital, phenytoin, primidone, valproic acid) Antimicrobials (e.g., pentamidine, sulfasalazine, sulfamethoxazole, trimethoprim) Calcineurin inhibitors (e.g., cyclosporine, tacrolimus, sirolimus) Cephalosporins Cholestyramine Choline magnesium salicylate, choline salicylate Citalopram Cloxacillin Colchicine Demeclocycline hydrochloride Escitalopram Flutamide Gastric acid blocking agents (block absorption of vitamin B_{12}) (e.g., proton pump inhibitors, histamine-2 blockers) Isosorbide nitrate Loop diuretics (e.g., bumetanide, furosemide) Meperidine Metformin Neomycin sulfate Nitrous oxide Opiates (e.g., codeine, fentanyl) Oseltamivir Phenazopyridine Phenothiazines Reverse transcriptase inhibitors (e.g., lamivudine, stavudine, zidovudine) Rosiglitazone maleate Zinc
Hemolytic anemia	Cyclophosphamide Cyclosporine Dapsone Levodopa Levofloxacin Methyldopa Nitrofurantoin Penicillin and its derivatives Quinidine Rasburicase Rituximab

(Continued on next page)

Table 3-6. Critical Care and Oncologic Medications Associated With Hematologic/Immunologic Disorders *(Continued)*

Hematologic/ Immunologic Effects	Medication Class/Specific Medication
Leukopenia	Analgesics (e.g., acetaminophen, nonsteroidal anti-inflammatory agents, COX inhibitors, naproxen, phenylbutazone) Antiepileptics (e.g., carbamazepine, phenytoin, trimethadione, valproic acid) Antihistamines (e.g., cimetidine) Antimicrobials (e.g., acyclovir, carbapenems, cephalosporins, chloramphenicol, flucytosine, gentamycin, isoniazid, levamisole, linezolid, macrolides, metronidazole, minocycline, nitrofurantoin, norfloxacin, penicillin, rifampicin, streptomycin, trimethoprim-sulfamethoxazole, vancomycin, antiretrovirals) Antiplatelet drugs/glycoprotein IIb/IIIa inhibitors (e.g., aspirin, clopidogrel, dipyridamole) Antithyroid medications (e.g., carbimazole, methimazole, propylthiouracil) Calcineurin inhibitors (e.g., cyclosporine, sirolimus, tacrolimus) Cardiovascular medications (e.g., amiodarone, captopril, digoxin, lisinopril, methyldopa, nifedipine, procainamide, propranolol, ticlopidine) Dicoumarol anticoagulants Diuretics (e.g., furosemide, hydralazine, hydrochlorothiazide, spironolactone) Glucocorticoids (e.g., dexamethasone, methylprednisolone) Miscellaneous drugs (e.g., acetazolamide, allopurinol, arsenic, colchicine, flutamide, levodopa) Motility agents (e.g., macrolides, metoclopramide) Oral hypoglycemic agents (e.g., glimepiride, metformin) Proton pump inhibitors (e.g., famotidine, omeprazole) Psychiatric agents (e.g., amoxapine, clomipramine, chlorpromazine, clozapine, desipramine, diazepam, doxepin, fluoxetine, haloperidol, imipramine, olanzapine, phenothiazine, risperidone) Reverse transcriptase inhibitors (e.g., lamivudine, stavudine, zidovudine)
Lymphopenia	Calcineurin inhibitors (e.g., cyclosporine, sirolimus, tacrolimus) Glucocorticoids (e.g., dexamethasone, methylprednisolone) Reverse transcriptase inhibitors (e.g., lamivudine, stavudine, zidovudine)

(Continued on next page)

Table 3-6. Critical Care and Oncologic Medications Associated With Hematologic/Immunologic Disorders *(Continued)*	
Hematologic/ Immunologic Effects	**Medication Class/Specific Medication**
Thrombocytopenia	Aminoglycosides Catecholamines (e.g., dopamine, epinephrine, norepinephrine) Dextran Heparin and heparinoids Loop diuretics Nonsteroidal anti-inflammatory agents Penicillin (e.g., carbenicillin, ticarcillin) Phenothiazines Salicylates Sulfonamides Thiazide diuretics Tricyclic antidepressants Trimethoprim-sulfamethoxazole Vitamin E

Note. Based on information from Erb & Vogel, 2013; O'Leary & Mack, 2013; Polovich et al., 2014; Shelton, 2012.

or the antitumor necrosis factor agent tocilizumab exemplify the immune source of these reactions (Holzinger et al., 2016; Salama & Moschos, 2017).

Immunosuppressive medications may be given to control disease or prevent rejection after HSCT. Patients who require critical care interventions while receiving immunosuppressive medications may need additional specialized care. These individuals usually receive prophylactic antimicrobial therapy against common organisms that may need to be maintained by changing to the IV form. Additionally, these medications achieve their action by steady state blood levels, which can be altered by renal and hepatic impairment; therefore, careful monitoring of blood levels with frequent dose adjustments should be attended to during critical illness. References for optimal immunosuppressive blood levels must be readily available for critical care clinicians. Other concerning adverse effects of immunosuppressive agents include unusual infections, hypomagnesemia, renal impairment, hypertension, and encephalopathy syndrome (Mitchell, 2013). Posterior reversible encephalopathy syndrome is a disorder that occurs in patients receiving certain chemotherapy agents (e.g., tyrosine kinase inhibitors) or calcineurin inhibitor immunosuppressive agents (e.g., tacrolimus). It is recognized by a constellation of new-onset neurologic symptoms, such as acute mental status changes, seizures, hypertension, and impaired airway protection in the absence of hyperammonemia (Schmidt et al., 2016). Corticosteroids also have immunosuppressive effects and are frequently included in regimens to treat lymphoma or multiple myeloma.

Radiation-Induced Hematologic/Immunologic Toxicity

Radiation therapy to the axial skeleton and long bones may cause myelosuppression. Patients who have received radiation to the hip and spine, such as with isolated bone lesions in multiple myeloma, are at a particularly high risk for this complication. The onset of myelosuppression begins with leukopenia at about two to five weeks after the start of therapy, with usual peak effects during week 3. Bone marrow recovery usually occurs three to seven weeks after the end of therapy. With current intensity-modulated and conformal radiation techniques that more precisely target the tumor without surrounding tissue exposure, the risk for radiation-induced bone marrow suppression in nonbone radiation regimens is greatly reduced. Recognition of this risk and implementation of monitoring and supportive measures can abrogate this adverse effect.

Selected Hematologic/Immunologic Disorders

Disseminated Intravascular Coagulation

Disseminated intravascular coagulation (DIC) is a disorder of excessive and unmitigated clotting. Excessive clotting stimulus from vessel injury, inflammation, tissue injury, or a foreign body in the bloodstream can initiate a cascade of unchecked microvascular clotting. In patients with cancer, this clotting may be related to the presence of inflammation, large tumor burden, or the consequence of specific cancer procoagulants (Levi, 2014). Although it is possible to have DIC with any cancer, the risk is considerably higher in hematologic malignancy and hepatocellular cancer (Yamashita et al., 2014). Progranulocytic leukemia is notable for causing this complication in as much as 79% of patients presenting with new or refractory disease. The promyelocyte membrane directly secretes the procoagulant tissue factor into the bloodstream and may be present in the case of tumor self-lysis but is more common during antineoplastic therapy (Rashidi & Fisher, 2013).

The key to optimal DIC care is recognition of the risk and identification of the disorder during its thrombotic phase rather than after clotting components are depleted in the hemorrhagic phase. Platelets are the first clotting component used; therefore, decreases in platelet count might be the most sensitive early indicator of DIC. In patients with leukemia who have chronic thrombocytopenia, fibrinogen level is monitored, and although baseline is often elevated, decreases in fibrinogen may be indicative of DIC and warrant administration of low-dose heparin (Kaplan, 2013).

Engraftment Syndrome

Peri-engraftment syndrome, also known as cytokine release syndrome, is a disorder of bone marrow response to the return growth or engraftment of WBCs after myelosuppressive therapy. The syndrome is triggered by the release of cytokines from the lymphocytes as they repopulate the bone marrow. These cytokines produce vasodilation and capillary leaking strikingly similar to sepsis from microorganism invasion. Because lymphocytes engraft prior to granulocytes, the patient may still appear to have leukopenia and demonstrate signs and symptoms functionally indistinguishable from sepsis.

Individuals most at risk for development of engraftment syndrome are women; patients with acute leukemia, particularly the lymphocytic subtype; and patients who have undergone HSCT, particularly with mismatched donors or umbilical cord transplant (Relf & Shelton, 2018). More recently, this syndrome has been noted after treatment with immunomodulatory agents, such as bortezomib and lenalidomide, or when HSCT has been employed for autoimmune disorders or solid tumors (Cornell et al., 2013).

Patients at risk are assessed for signs and symptoms of inflammation and infection. Given that symptoms often precede evidence of granulocyte recovery, management usually includes antimicrobial therapy for potential infection. Early signs and symptoms of engraftment include fever, total body erythema, rash, fluid retention, respiratory distress, and mental status changes (Spitzer, 2015; Thoele, 2014). Renal impairment with rising creatinine may follow, but the addition of hematuria is relatively unique to engraftment syndrome (Thoele, 2014). Individuals often experience a rise in transaminases or demonstrate gastrointestinal bleeding (Thoele, 2014). The Spitzer (2015) criteria include all three major criteria (temperature, rash, pulmonary infiltrates) or two major criteria and one or more minor criteria (hepatic dysfunction, renal dysfunction, weight gain, transient encephalopathy). Symptoms are usually rapid in onset and begin to resolve once WBC count reaches 2,500–3,000/mm^3 (Hong et al., 2013). No defining diagnostic test has emerged to diagnose this disorder, although some suggest a rise in C-reactive protein may be indicative of engraftment (Hong et al., 2013). Negative cultures will be present in engraftment syndrome, although just more than half of immunocompromised patients with presumed infection do not have a confirmed source; this alone cannot be used to differentiate the two disorders (Nazer, Al-Shaer, & Hawari, 2013; Samonis et al., 2013).

Management of engraftment syndrome is supportive and directed toward specific clinical complications. While clinicians are determining whether the signs and symptoms relate to engraftment, broad-spectrum antibacterial therapy will be instituted. Nursing care involves continuous monitoring for possible infection, frequent vital signs, and hemodynamic support for hypotension. It also includes oxygen therapy, evaluation for medication toxicity, and complication prevention.

Leukostasis

Leukostasis is a complication of new-onset or relapsed hematologic malignancies in which a high number of circulating immature WBCs cause hyperviscosity and microvascular occlusion (Schiffer, 2016). For unclear reasons, the microvascular damage occurs primarily in the brain, lungs, and kidneys (Röllig & Ehninger, 2015; Schiffer, 2016). Because it is a disorder caused by excess WBCs, leukostasis is almost exclusively associated with leukemia. Interestingly, not all leukemias with high WBC counts seem to cause this disorder. It is primarily associated with acute myeloid leukemias with monocyte subtypes and WBC counts greater than $100,000/mm^3$, with a rapid rate of rise, or with a large percentage of blasts (Pham & Schwartz, 2015; Schiffer, 2016). These specific leukemia subtypes and genetic mutations are thought to have more adhesion molecules that damage the endothelial lining of microvessels (DiNardo et al., 2015). Rapidly proliferating lymphomas have also been linked to this syndrome, such as Burkitt and lymphoblastic lymphoma, lymphocytic leukemia with WBC counts greater than $300,000/mm^3$, and plasma cell leukemia (multiple myeloma variant) (Pham & Schwartz, 2015; Röllig & Ehninger, 2015).

Patients experiencing leukostasis often have an acute onset of symptoms occurring over hours to days. Patients may appear to be asymptomatic and suddenly develop mental status changes, respiratory distress, and renal failure. Other organ failure may follow with the onset of significant tumor- and hypoperfusion-induced acidosis. Early mortality may be as high as 40% within the first few days of this complication (Van de Louw, Schneider, Desai, & Claxton, 2016). Confirmation of leukostasis is primarily based on risk factors and clinical symptomatology, although classic lung computed tomography findings have been identified, and microhemorrhages in the cerebrum may also support the diagnosis (Schiffer, 2016).

Management of leukostasis requires emergent antineoplastic therapy directed at rapid tumor reduction or the removal of a portion of cells via leukapheresis (Pastore, Pastore, Wittmann, Hiddemann, & Spiekermann, 2014; Pham & Schwartz, 2015; Röllig & Ehninger, 2015; Schiffer, 2016). Antineoplastic therapy must be implemented with rapid-acting agents to quickly reduce the burden of tumor within 24 hours. Standard chemotherapy may take days to achieve this objective, so hydroxyurea or cyclophosphamide are often the immediate treatment given. It is unclear whether dialysis removes cyclophosphamide; therefore, continuous renal replacement therapy may be stopped during cyclophosphamide infusion and for approximately eight hours afterward in critically ill patients with leukostasis and concomitant tumor lysis syndrome. Hydroxyurea may be contraindicated when dialysis is also required. Leukapheresis presents the same clinical dilemma, necessitating alternating dialysis and pheresis. A single leukapheresis treatment usually reduces WBC counts by $20,000–40,000/mm^3$. Treatments occur once or twice daily until WBC count is less than $30,000–40,000/mm^3$ (Aqui & O'Doherty, 2014). When immediate leukapheresis is not available, high-volume hydration or exchange transfusions may be necessary (Schiffer, 2016). It is common for patients receiving treatment for leukostasis to have rapid lysis of cells and to develop tumor lysis syndrome and renal failure. Patients with leukostasis have complex care issues and often require frequent vital signs and neurologic assessment, respiratory support, antineoplastic therapy, and dialysis. Nurses will often have competing clinical demands and challenges in maintaining adequate IV access for the many required medications and therapies.

Summary

Patients with hematologic cancer often present with multisystem dysfunction and require immediate antineoplastic therapy, even in the face of critical illness. Bleeding, infections, and respiratory failure in patients with hematologic malignancies often require intensive care nursing. These patients are best supported in the ICU by critical care oncology nurses. Variables in the hematologic cancer population associated with poorer outcomes include respiratory failure requiring mechanical ventilation, multiorgan failure, refractory sepsis, and shock.

References

Abdelmalak, B.B., Khanna, A.K., Culver, D.A., & Popovich, M.J. (2015). Therapeutic whole-lung lavage for pulmonary alveolar proteinosis. A procedural update. *Journal of Bronchology and Interventional Pulmonology, 22,* 251–258. doi:10.1097/LBR.0000000000000180

Anderson-Reitz, L., & Clancy, C. (2013). Hepatorenal complications. In S.A. Ezzone (Ed.), *Hematopoietic stem cell transplantation: A manual for nursing practice* (2nd ed., pp. 191–199). Pittsburgh, PA: Oncology Nursing Society.

Aqui, N., & O'Doherty, U. (2014). Leukocytapheresis for the treatment of hyperleukocytosis secondary to acute leukemia. *Hematology: American Society of Hematology Education Program Book, 2014, 457*–460. doi:10.1182/asheducation-2014.1.457

Azoulay, E., Mokart, D., Pène, F., Lambert, J., Kouatchet, A., Mayaux, J., … Lemiale, V. (2013). Outcomes of critically ill patients with hematologic malignancies: Prospective multicenter data from France and Belgium—A Groupe de Recherche Respiratoire en Réanimation Onco-Hématologique study. *Journal of Clinical Oncology, 31,* 2810–2818. doi:10.1200/JCO.2012.47.2365

Berentsen, S., & Tjønnfjord, G.E. (2012). Diagnosis and treatment of cold agglutinin mediated autoimmune hemolytic anemia. *Blood Reviews, 26,* 107–115. doi:10.1016/j.blre.2012.01.002

Beurskens, C.J.P., Wösten-van Asperen, R.M., Preckel, B., & Juffermans, N.P. (2015). The potential of heliox as a therapy for acute respiratory distress syndrome in adults and children: A descriptive review. *Respiration, 89,* 166–174. doi:10.1159/000369472

Bonilla, F.A., & Stiehm, E.R. (2017, January 23). Laboratory evaluation of the immune system [Literature review current through August 2017]. Retrieved from http://www.uptodate.com/contents/laboratory-evaluation-of-the-immune-system

Byar, K. (2013). Mature T-cell and NK-cell neoplasms. In M. Olsen & L.J. Zitella (Eds.), *Hematologic malignancies in adults* (pp. 411–444). Pittsburgh, PA: Oncology Nursing Society.

Carson, J.L., Grossman, B.J., Kleinman, S., Tinmouth, A.T., Marques, M.B., Fung, M.K., … Clinical Transfusion Medicine Committee of the AABB. (2012). Red blood cell transfusion: A clinical practice guideline from the AABB. *Annals of Internal Medicine, 157,* 49–58. doi:10.7326/0003-4819-157-1-201206190-00429

Chellapandian, D., Lehrnbecher, T., Phillips, B., Fisher, B.T., Zaoutis, T.E., Steinbach, W.J., … Sung, L. (2015). Bronchoalveolar lavage and lung biopsy in patients with cancer and hematopoietic stem-cell transplantation recipients: A systematic review and meta-analysis. *Journal of Clinical Oncology, 33,* 501–509. doi:10.1200/JCO.2014.58.0480

Chen, L. (2015). A study in scarlet: Restrictive red blood cell transfusion strategy. *Critical Care Nursing Quarterly, 38,* 217–219. doi:10.1097/CNQ.00000000000065

Chen, S., Hu, J., Xu, L., Brandon, D., Yu, J., & Zhang, J. (2015). Posterior reversible encephalopathy syndrome after transplantation: A review. *Molecular Neurobiology, 53,* 6897–6909.

Chen, Y.-H., Chiou, T.-J., Hsu, Y.-N., & Liu, C.-Y. (2010). Idiopathic hyperammonemia after chemotherapy with vinorelbine, topotecan, and cisplatin in a patient with acute lymphocytic leukemia. *Hematology/Oncology and Stem Cell Therapy, 3,* 199–202. doi:10.5144/1658-3876.2010.199

Cope, D.G. (2016). Metabolic emergencies. In B. Gobel, S. Triest-Robertson, & W.H. Vogel (Eds.), *Advanced oncology nursing certification review and resource manual* (2nd ed., pp. 643–692). Pittsburgh, PA: Oncology Nursing Society.

Cornell, R.F., Hari, P., Zhang, M.-J., Zhong, X., Thompson, J., Fenske, T.S., … Drobyski, W.R. (2013). Divergent effects of novel immunomodulatory agents and cyclophosphamide on the risk of engraftment syndrome after autologous peripheral blood stem cell transplantation for multiple myeloma. *Biology of Blood and Marrow Transplantation, 19,* 1368–1373. doi:10.1016/j.bbmt.2013.06.017

Costa, R., Carneiro, B.A., Agulnik, M., Rademaker, A.W., Pai, S.G., Villaflor, V.M., … Giles, F.J. (2016). Toxicity profile of approved anti-PD-1 monoclonal antibodies in solid tumors: A systematic review and meta-analysis of randomized clinical trials. *Oncotarget, 8,* 8910–8920. doi:10.18632/oncotarget.13315

Cowan, A.J., Altemeier, W.A., Johnston, C., Gernsheimer, T., & Becker, P.S. (2015). Management of acute myeloid leukemia in the intensive care setting. *Journal of Intensive Care Medicine, 30,* 375–384. doi:10.1177/0885066614530959

Davies, M.J. (2016). Cardiac and pulmonary toxicities. In B. Gobel, S. Triest-Robertson, & W.H. Vogel (Eds.), *Advanced oncology nursing certification review and resource manual* (2nd ed., pp. 491–524). Pittsburgh, PA: Oncology Nursing Society.

Deadmond, M.A., & Smith-Gagen, J.A. (2015). Changing incidence of myeloproliferative neoplasms: Trends and subgroup risk profiles in the USA, 1973–2011. *Journal of Cancer Research and Clinical Oncology, 141,* 2131–2138. doi:10.1007/s00432-015-1983-5

Debiane, L., Hachem, R.Y., Al Wohoush, I., Shomali, W., Bahu, R.R., Jiang, Y., … Raad, I. (2014). The utility of proadrenomedullin and procalcitonin in comparison to C-reactive protein as predictors of sepsis and bloodstream infections in critically ill patients with cancer. *Critical Care Medicine, 42,* 2500–2507. doi:10.1097/CCM.00000000000526

Dellinger, R.P., Levy, M.M., Rhodes, A., Annane, D., Gerlach, H., Opal, S.M., … Surviving Sepsis Campaign Guidelines Committee including the Pediatric Subgroup. (2013). Surviving Sepsis Campaign: International guidelines for management of severe sepsis and septic shock, 2012. *Intensive Care Medicine, 39,* 165–228. doi:10.1007/s00134-012-2769-8

Devine, H. (2013). Myelodysplastic syndromes. In S.A. Ezzone (Ed.), *Hematopoietic stem cell transplantation: A manual for nursing practice* (2nd ed., pp. 23–46). Pittsburgh, PA: Oncology Nursing Society.

DiNardo, C.D., Tang, G., Pemmaraju, N., Wang, S.A., Pike, A., Garcia-Manero, G., … Kantarjian, H.M. (2015). Acute myeloid leukemia with t(10;11): A pathological entity with distinct clinical presentation. *Clinical Lymphoma, Myeloma and Leukemia, 15,* 47–51. doi:10.1016/j.clml.2014.06.022

Erb, C.H., & Vogel, W.H. (2013). Management of the complications of hematologic malignancy and treatment. In M. Olsen & L.J. Zitella (Eds.), *Hematologic malignancies in adults* (pp. 537–648). Pittsburgh, PA: Oncology Nursing Society.

Estcourt, L.J., Stanworth, S.J., Doree, C., Blanco, P., Hopewell, S., Trivella, M., & Massey, E. (2015). Granulocyte transfusions for preventing infections in patients with neutropenia or neutrophil dysfunction. *Cochrane Database of Systematic Reviews, 2015*(6). doi:10.1002/14651858.CD005341.pub3

Faiman, B., & Bilotti, E. (2013). Multiple myeloma. In M. Olsen & L.J. Zitella (Eds.), *Hematologic malignancies in adults* (pp. 445–498). Pittsburgh, PA: Oncology Nursing Society.

Federici, A.B., Intini, D., Lattuada, A., Vanelli, C., Arrigoni, L., Sacchi, E., & Russo, U. (2014). Supportive transfusion therapy in cancer patients with acquired defects of hemostasis. *Thrombosis Research, 133*(Suppl. 2), S56–S62. doi:10.1016/S0049-3848(14)50010-2

Franchini, M. (2015). Atypical hemolytic uremic syndrome: From diagnosis to treatment. *Clinical Chemistry and Laboratory Medicine, 53*, 1679–1688. doi:10.1515/cclm-2015-0024

Goodrich, A., McNally, G.A., Ridgeway, J., & Zitella, L.J. (2013). Mature B-cell neoplasms. In M. Olsen & L.J. Zitella (Eds.), *Hematologic malignancies in adults* (pp. 201–362). Pittsburgh, PA: Oncology Nursing Society.

Granata, G., Greco, A., Iannella, G., Granata, M., Manno, A., Savastano, E., & Magliulo, G. (2015). Posterior reversible encephalopathy syndrome—Insight into pathogenesis, clinical variants and treatment approaches. *Autoimmunity Reviews, 14*, 830–836. doi:10.1016/j.autrev.2015.05.006

Handy, C.M., Olsen, M., & Zitella, L.J. (2013). Precursor lymphoid neoplasms. In M. Olsen & L.J. Zitella (Eds.), *Hematologic malignancies in adults* (pp. 157–200). Pittsburgh, PA: Oncology Nursing Society.

Holzinger, A., Barden, M., & Abken, H. (2016). The growing world of CAR T cell trials: A systematic review. *Cancer Immunology, Immunotherapy, 65*, 1433–1450. doi:10.1007/s00262-016-1895-5

Hong, K.T., Kang, H.J., Kim, N.H., Kim, M.S., Lee, J.W., Kim, H., … Ahn, H.S. (2013). Peri-engraftment syndrome in allogeneic hematopoietic SCT. *Bone Marrow Transplantation, 48*, 523–528. doi:10.1038/bmt.2012.171

Izzedine, H., & Perazella, M.A. (2015). Thrombotic microangiopathy, cancer, and cancer drugs. *American Journal of Kidney Diseases, 66*, 857–868. doi:10.1053/j.ajkd.2015.02.340

Johnston, D.J., Scott, A.V., Barodka, V.M., Park, S., Wasey, J.O., Ness, P.M., … Frank, S.M. (2016). Morbidity and mortality after high-dose transfusion. *Anesthesiology, 124*, 387–395. doi:10.1097/ALN.0000000000000945

Kaplan, M. (2013). Disseminated intravascular coagulation. In M. Kaplan (Ed.), *Understanding and managing oncologic emergencies: A resource for nurses* (2nd ed., pp. 69–102). Pittsburgh, PA: Oncology Nursing Society.

Kaplan, M. (2016). Structural emergencies. In B. Gobel, S. Triest-Robertson, & W.H. Vogel (Eds.), *Advanced oncology nursing certification review and resource manual* (2nd ed., pp. 693–736). Pittsburgh, PA: Oncology Nursing Society.

Kappler, S., Ronan-Bentle, S., & Graham, A. (2014). Thrombotic microangiopathies (TTP, HUS, HELLP). *Emergency Medicine Clinics of North America, 32*, 649–671. doi:10.1016/j.emc.2014.04.008

Kim, J., & Na, S. (2015). Transfusion-related acute lung injury: Clinical perspectives. *Korean Journal of Anesthesiology, 68*, 101–105. doi:10.4097/kjae.2015.68.2.101

Kreuger, A.L., Middelburg, R.A., Zwaginga, J.J., van der Bom, J.G., & Kerkhoffs, J.-L.H. (2015). Clinical practice of platelet transfusions in haemato-oncology. *Vox Sanguinis, 109*, 91–94. doi:10.1111/vox.12254

Lee, H.Y., Rhee, C.K., & Lee, J.W. (2015). Feasibility of high-flow nasal cannula oxygen therapy for acute respiratory failure in patients with hematologic malignancy: A retrospective single-center study. *Journal of Critical Care, 30*, 773–774. doi:10.1016/j.jcrc.2015.03.014

Levi, M. (2014). Cancer-related coagulopathies. *Thrombosis Research, 133*(Suppl. 2), S70–S75. doi:10.1016/S0049-3848(14)50012-6

Liebman, H.A. (2014). Thrombocytopenia in cancer patients. *Thrombosis Research, 133*(Suppl. 2), S63–S69. doi:10.1016/S0049-3848(14)50011-4

McCaughey, C., Blackwood, B., Glackin, M., Brady, M., & McMullin, M.F. (2013). Characteristics and outcomes of haematology patients admitted to the intensive care unit. *Nursing in Critical Care, 18*, 193–199. doi:10.1111/nicc.12005

McCormack, P.L. (2013). Immune globulin (human) 10% liquid: A review of its use in primary immunodeficiency disorders. *BioDrugs, 27*, 393–400. doi:10.1007/s40259-013-0044-3

McGrath, S., Chatterjee, F., Whiteley, C., & Ostermann, M. (2010). ICU and 6-month outcome of oncology patients in the intensive care unit. *QJM, 103,* 397–403. doi:10.1093/qjmed/hcq032

Melichar, B., & Zezulová, M. (2011). The significance of altered gastrointestinal permeability in cancer patients. *Current Opinion in Supportive and Palliative Care, 5,* 47–54. doi:10.1097/SPC.0b013e328343a043

Mitchell, S.A. (2013). Acute and chronic graft-versus-host disease. In S.A. Ezzone (Ed.), *Hematopoietic stem cell transplantation: A manual for nursing practice* (2nd ed., pp. 103–154). Pittsburgh, PA: Oncology Nursing Society.

Mokart, D., Darmon, M., Resche-Rigon, M., Lemiale, V., Pène, F., Mayaux, J., ... Azoulay, E. (2015). Prognosis of neutropenic patients admitted to the intensive care unit. *Intensive Care Medicine, 41,* 296–303. doi:10.1007/s00134-014-3615-y

Ñamendys-Silva, S.A., González-Herrera, M.O., García-Guillén, F.J., Texcocano-Becerra, J., & Herrera-Gómez, A. (2013). Outcome of critically ill patients with hematological malignancies. *Annals of Hematology, 92,* 699–705. doi:10.1007/s00277-013-1675-7

Nandagopal, L., Veeraputhiran, M., Jain, T., Soubani, A.O., & Schiffer, C.A. (2016). Bronchoscopy can be done safely in patients with thrombocytopenia. *Transfusion, 56,* 344–348. doi:10.1111/trf.13348

National Comprehensive Cancer Network. (2017). *NCCN Clinical Practice Guidelines in Oncology (NCCN Guidelines®): Prevention and treatment of cancer-related infections* [v.2.2017]. Retrieved from https://www.nccn.org/professionals/physician_gls/PDF/infections.pdf

Nayer, A., & Asif, A. (2016). Atypical hemolytic-uremic syndrome: A clinical review. *American Journal of Therapeutics, 23,* e151–e158. doi:10.1097/MJT.0b013e31829b59dc

Nazer, L., Al-Shaer, M., & Hawari, F. (2013). Drug utilization pattern and cost for the treatment of severe sepsis and septic shock in critically ill cancer patients. *International Journal of Clinical Pharmacy, 35,* 1245–1250. doi:10.1007/s11096-013-9860-2

Nesher, L., & Rolston, K.V.I. (2013). Neutropenic enterocolitis: A growing concern in the era of widespread use of aggressive chemotherapy. *Clinical Infectious Diseases, 56,* 711–717. doi:10.1093/cid/cis998

O'Leary, C., & Mack, L. (2013). Bleeding and thrombosis. In M. Kaplan (Ed.), *Understanding and managing oncologic emergencies: A resource for nurses* (2nd ed., pp. 1–42). Pittsburgh, PA: Oncology Nursing Society.

Olsen, M. (2013). Overview of hematologic malignancies. In M. Olsen & L.J. Zitella (Eds.), *Hematologic malignancies in adults* (pp. 1–17). Pittsburgh, PA: Oncology Nursing Society.

Öztürkmen, S., Altuntas, F., & Olcay, L. (2013). Granulocyte transfusion therapy in paediatric patients with severe neutropenic infection. *Transfusion and Apheresis Science, 48,* 381–385. doi:10.1016/j.transci.2013.04.022

Pastore, F., Pastore, A., Wittmann, G., Hiddemann, W., & Spiekermann, K. (2014). The role of therapeutic leukapheresis in hyperleukocytotic AML. *PLOS ONE, 9,* e95062. doi:10.1371/journal.pone.0095062

Peterson, G.J., Trautman, K., Hoffner, B., & Zakrocki, J. (2013). Acute myeloid leukemia and acute leukemias of ambiguous lineage. In M. Olsen & L.J. Zitella (Eds.), *Hematologic malignancies in adults* (pp. 101–156). Pittsburgh, PA: Oncology Nursing Society.

Pham, H.P., & Schwartz, J. (2015). How we approach a patient with symptoms of leukostasis requiring emergent leukocytapheresis. *Transfusion, 55,* 2306–2311. doi:10.1111/trf.13210

Picard, C., Burtey, S., Bornet, C., Curti, C., Montana, M., & Vanelle, P. (2015). Pathophysiology and treatment of typical and atypical hemolytic uremic syndrome. *Pathologie Biologie, 63,* 136–143. doi:10.1016/j.patbio.2015.03.001

Polovich, M., Olsen, M., & LeFebvre, K.B. (Eds.). (2014). *Chemotherapy and biotherapy guidelines and recommendations for practice* (4th ed.). Pittsburgh, PA: Oncology Nursing Society.

Raanani, P., Gafter-Gvili, A., Paul, M., Ben-Bassat, I., Leibovici, L., & Shpilberg, O. (2009). Immunoglobulin prophylaxis in hematopoietic stem cell transplantation: Systematic review and meta-analysis. *Journal of Clinical Oncology, 27,* 770–781. doi:10.1200/JCO.2008.16.8450

Rashidi, A., & Fisher, S.I. (2013). Therapy-related acute promyelocytic leukemia: A systematic review. *Medical Oncology, 30,* 625–635. doi:10.1007/s12032-013-0625-5

Relf, M.V., & Shelton, B.K. (2018). Common immunologic disorders. In P.G. Morton & D.K. Fontaine (Eds.), *Critical care nursing: A holistic approach* (11th ed., pp. 948–981). Philadelphia, PA: Wolters Kluwer.

Riedijk, M., van den Bergh, W.M., van Vliet, M., Kusadasi, N., Span, L.R., Tuinman, P.R., ... HEMA-ICU Study Group. (2015). Characteristics and outcomes of patients with a haematological malignancy admitted to the intensive care unit for a neurological event. *Critical Care and Resuscitation, 17,* 268–273.

Rogers, B.B. (2013). Myelodysplastic/myeloproliferative neoplasms. In M. Olsen & L.J. Zitella (Eds.), *Hematologic malignancies in adults* (pp. 79–100). Pittsburgh, PA: Oncology Nursing Society.

Röllig, C., & Ehninger, G. (2015). How I treat hyperleukocytosis in acute myeloid leukemia. *Blood, 125,* 3246–3252. doi:10.1182/blood-2014-10-551507

Rosselet, R.M. (2013). Hematologic effects. In S.A. Ezzone (Ed.), *Hematopoietic stem cell transplantation: A manual for nursing practice* (2nd ed., pp. 155–172). Pittsburgh, PA: Oncology Nursing Society.

Safdar, A., Rodriguez, G., Zuniga, J., Al Akhrass, F., & Pande, A. (2014). Use of healthy-donor granulocyte transfusions to treat infections in neutropenic patients with myeloid or lymphoid neoplasms: Experience in 74 patients treated with 373 granulocyte transfusions. *Acta Haematologica, 131,* 50–58. doi:10.1159/000351174

Saillard, C., Mokart, D., Lemiale, V., & Azoulay, E. (2014). Mechanical ventilation in cancer patients. *Minerva Anestesiologica, 80,* 712–725.

Salama, A.K., & Moschos, S.J. (2017). Next steps in immuno-oncology: Enhancing antitumor effects through appropriate patient selection and rationally designed combination strategies. *Annals of Oncology, 28,* 57–74. doi:10.1093/annonc/mdw534

Samonis, G., Vardakas, K.Z., Maraki, S., Tansarli, G.S., Dimopoulou, D., Kofteridis, D.P., ... Falagas, M.E. (2013). A prospective study of characteristics and outcomes of bacteremia in patients with solid organ or hematologic malignancies. *Supportive Care in Cancer, 21,* 2521–2526. doi:10.1007/s00520-013-1816-5

Sansoni, P., Vescovini, R., Fagnoni, F.F., Akbar, A., Arens, R., Chiu, Y.-L., ... Nikolich-Zugich, J. (2014). New advances in CMV and immunosenescence. *Experimental Gerontology, 55,* 54–62. doi:10.1016/j.exger.2014.03.020

Sanz, M.A., & Montesinos, P. (2014). How we prevent and treat differentiation syndrome in patients with acute promyelocytic leukemia. *Blood, 123,* 2777–2782. doi:10.1182/blood-2013-10-512640

Schiffer, C.A. (2016). Hyperleukocytosis and leukostasis in hematologic malignancies [Literature review current through August 2017]. Retrieved from https://www.uptodate.com/contents/hyperleukocytosis-and-leukostasis-in-hematologic-malignancies

Schmidt, V., Prell, T., Treschl, A., Klink, A., Hochhaus, A., & Sayer, H.G. (2016). Clinical management of posterior reversible encephalopathy syndrome after allogeneic hematopoietic stem cell transplantation: A case series and review of the literature. *Acta Haematologica, 135,* 1–10. doi:10.1159/000430489

Schmit-Pokorny, K. (2013). Stem cell collection. In S.A. Ezzone (Ed.), *Hematopoietic stem cell transplantation: A manual for nursing practice* (2nd ed., pp. 23–46). Pittsburgh, PA: Oncology Nursing Society.

Schrier, S.L. (2016). Approach to the adult patient with anemia [Literature review current through August 2017]. Retrieved from https://www.uptodate.com/contents/approach-to-the-adult-patient-with-anemia

Shafi, M.A., & Bresalier, R.S. (2010). The gastrointestinal complications of oncologic therapy. *Gastroenterology Clinics of North America, 39,* 629–647. doi:10.1016/j.gtc.2010.08.004

Shelton, B.K. (2012). Hematology and oncology problems. In J.G.W. Foster & S.S. Prevost (Eds.), *Advanced practice nursing of adults in acute care* (pp. 591–651). Philadelphia, PA: F.A. Davis.

Shelton, B.K. (2016). Myelosuppression and second malignancies. In B. Gobel, S. Triest-Robertson, & W.H. Vogel (Eds.), *Advanced oncology nursing certification review and resource manual* (2nd ed., pp. 451–490). Pittsburgh, PA: Oncology Nursing Society.

Shelton, B.K. (2018). Infections. In C.H. Yarbro, D. Wujcik, & B.H. Gobel (Eds.), *Cancer nursing: Principles and practice* (8th ed., pp. 818–850). Burlington, MA: Jones & Bartlett Learning.

Song, L.-M.W.K., & Marcon, N.E. (2017). Neutropenic enterocolitis (typhlitis) [Literature review current through August 2017]. Retrieved from https://www.uptodate.com/contents/neutropenic-enterocolitis-typhlitis

Spitzer, T.R. (2015). Engraftment syndrome: Double-edged sword of hematopoietic cell transplants. *Bone Marrow Transplantation, 50,* 469–475. doi:10.1038/bmt.2014.296

Stephens, J. (2013). Cardiopulmonary complications. In S.A. Ezzone (Ed.), *Hematopoietic stem cell transplantation: A manual for nursing practice* (2nd ed., pp. 201–229). Pittsburgh, PA: Oncology Nursing Society.

Surawicz, C.M., Brandt, L.J., Binion, D.G., Ananthakrishnan, A.N., Curry, S.R., Gilligan, P.H., ... Zuckerbraun, B.S. (2013). Guidelines for diagnosis, treatment, and prevention of *Clostridium difficile* infections. *American Journal of Gastroenterology, 108,* 478–498. doi:10.1038/ajg.2013.4

Tersteeg, C., Verhenne, S., Roose, E., Schelpe, A.-S., Deckmyn, H., De Meyer, S.F., & Vanhoorelbeke, K. (2016). ADAMTS13 and anti-ADAMTS13 autoantibodies in thrombotic thrombocytopenic purpura: Current perspectives and new treatment strategies. *Expert Review of Hematology, 9,* 209–221. doi:10.1586/17474086.2016.1122515

Thoele, K. (2014). Engraftment syndrome in hematopoietic stem cell transplantations. *Clinical Journal of Oncology Nursing, 18,* 349–354. doi:10.1188/14.CJON.349-354

Tong, M.C., Tadros, M., & Vaziri, H. (2015). Endoscopy in neutropenic and/or thrombocytopenic patients. *World Journal of Gastroenterology, 21,* 13166–13176. doi:10.3748/wjg.v21.i46.13166

Torres, V.B.L., Azevedo, L.C.P., Silva, U.V.A., Caruso, P., Torelly, A.P., Silva, E., ... Soares, M. (2015). Sepsis-associated outcomes in critically ill patients with malignancies. *Annals of the American Thoracic Society, 12,* 1185–1192. doi:10.1513/AnnalsATS.201501-046OC

Vadde, R., & Pastores, S.M. (2015). Management of acute respiratory failure in patients with hematological malignancy. *Journal of Intensive Care Medicine.* Advance online publication. doi:10.1177/0885066615601046

Van de Louw, A., Schneider, C.W., Desai, R.J., & Claxton, D.F. (2016). Initial respiratory status in hyperleukocytic acute myeloid leukemia: Prognostic significance and effect of leukapheresis. *Leukemia and Lymphoma, 57,* 1319–1326. doi:10.3109/10428194.2015.1094695

Vande Vusse, L.K., Caldwell, E., Tran, E., Hogl, L., Dinwiddie, S., López, J.A., ... Watkins, T.R. (2015). The epidemiology of transfusion-related acute lung injury varies according to the applied definition of lung injury onset time. *Annals of the American Thoracic Society, 12,* 1328–1335. doi:10.1513/AnnalsATS.201504-246OC

Viele, C.S. (2013). Myeloproliferative neoplasms (Ph–) and chronic myeloid leukemias. In M. Olsen & L.J. Zitella (Eds.), *Hematologic malignancies in adults* (pp. 19–50). Pittsburgh, PA: Oncology Nursing Society.

Vlaar, A.P.J., Binnekade, J.M., Prins, D., van Stein, D., Hofstra, J.J., Schultz, M.J., & Juffermans, N.P. (2010). Risk factors and outcomes of transfusion-related acute lung injury in the critically ill: A nested casecontrol study. *Critical Care Medicine, 38,* 771–778. doi:10.1097/CCM.0b013e3181cc4d4b

Vlaar, A.P.J., & Juffermans, N.P. (2013). Transfusion-related acute lung injury: A clinical review. *Lancet, 382,* 984–994. doi:10.1016/S0140-6736(12)62197-7

Vymazal, T., & Krecmerova, M. (2015). Respiratory strategies and airway management in patients with pulmonary alveolar proteinosis: A review. *BioMed Research International, 2015,* 639543. doi:10.1155/2015/639543

Wielpütz, M.O., Heußel, C.P., Herth, F.J.F., & Kauczor, H. (2014). Radiological diagnosis in lung disease: Factoring treatment options into the choice of diagnostic modality. *Deutsches Ärzteblatt International, 111,* 181–187. doi:10.3238/arztebl.2014.0181

Yamashita, Y., Wada, H., Nomura, H., Mizuno, T., Saito, K., Yamada, N., ... Katayama, N. (2014). Elevated fibrin-related markers in patients with malignant diseases frequently associated with disseminated intravascular coagulation and venous thromboembolism. *Internal Medicine, 53,* 413–419. doi:10.2169/internalmedicine.53.1102

Yeo, C.D., Kim, J.W., Kim, S.C., Kim, Y.K., Kim, K.H., Kim, H.J., … Rhee, C.K. (2012). Prognostic factors in critically ill patients with hematologic malignancies admitted to the intensive care unit. *Journal of Critical Care, 27,* 739 e1–739.e6. doi:10.1016/j.jcrc.2012.07.014

Zehnder, J.L. (2017). Clinical use of coagulation tests [Literature review current through August 2017]. Retrieved from http://www.uptodate.com/contents/clinical-use-of-coagulation-tests

Zhu, A., Kaneshiro, M., & Kaunitz, J.D. (2010). Evaluation and treatment of iron deficiency anemia: A gastroenterological perspective. *Digestive Diseases and Sciences, 55,* 548–559. doi:10.1007/s10620-009-1108-6

Zitella, L. (2011). Invasive aspergillosis in an allogeneic hematopoietic cell transplant patient. *Oncology, 25*(Suppl. 7), 15–20.

Zitella, L.J. (2013). Hodgkin lymphoma. In M. Olsen & L.J. Zitella (Eds.), *Hematologic malignancies in adults* (pp. 363–410). Pittsburgh, PA: Oncology Nursing Society.

CHAPTER 4

Hepatic, Pancreatic, and Biliary Cancers

Lisa Parks, MS, ANP-BC

Introduction

The treatment of hepatic, pancreatic, and biliary cancers often leads to life-threatening situations requiring intensive care. For example, hepatectomy or transarterial chemoembolization can cause liver failure, which is best treated in the intensive care unit. Surgery or endoscopic retrograde cholangiopancreatography (ERCP) can lead to pancreatitis and cause septic shock, and ERCP in cholangiocarcinoma may result in cholangitis and septic shock. This chapter will discuss critical care interventions of these and similar side effects of hepatic, pancreatic, and biliary cancer treatments.

Hepatocellular Carcinoma

Hepatocellular carcinoma (HCC) is the sixth most prevalent cancer worldwide and the third leading cause of cancer death (Salgia & Singal, 2014). Cirrhosis and the hepatitis C virus (HCV) are the greatest risk factors of HCC development (Bernal & Wendon, 2013). HCV and nonalcoholic steatohepatitis are prominent risk factors in the United States and Europe (Galuppo, Ramaiah, Ponte, & Gedaly, 2014), while the hepatitis B virus is predominantly seen worldwide. Other risk factors include older age, male gender, obesity, diabetes, and alcohol and tobacco abuse (Salgia & Singal, 2014). Treatment for HCC includes resection, locoregional therapies, and chemotherapy (Chung,

2015; Page, Cosgrove, Philosophe, & Pawlik, 2014). Hepatectomy performed in patients of advanced age and with multiple comorbidities increases surgical risk (e.g., extended resections, repeat hepatectomies) (Russell, 2015). Liver failure is a complication after liver resection, and its only treatment is supportive care, which includes treatment to the body systems affected by the failure.

Liver Failure

Postoperative hepatic insufficiency has many surgical and patient risk factors. Prolonged operating room time, excessive blood loss during surgery, extent of resection with a small liver remnant, ischemia, and infection are considered surgical risk factors (Russell, 2015). Patient risk factors include older age, steatosis, fibrosis, cirrhosis, and chemotherapy-induced liver damage (Russell, 2015). Liver insufficiency is defined on postoperative day 3 as a bilirubin level greater than 3 mg/dl. Numerous proposed definitions exist for the criteria of liver failure. An elevated international normalized ratio (INR) and elevated bilirubin on or after postoperative day 5 are widely accepted indicators of liver failure (Russell, 2015).

Neurologic Complications

Hepatic encephalopathy results from portosystemic shunting and hepatocellular dysfunction. Patients with hepatic encephalopathy are at an increased risk of respiratory failure because of ventilation–perfusion mismatch, pulmonary aspiration, acute lung injury, acute respiratory distress syndrome (ARDS), sepsis, pleural effusion, atelectasis, and noncardiogenic pulmonary edema (Al-Khafaji & Huang, 2011; Sargent, 2010). As treatment, lactulose is administered orally or rectally to increase bowel movements (Hansen, Sasaki, & Zucker, 2010). Lactulose acidifies bowel content and slows ammonia absorption, which decreases blood ammonia levels. The goal is to adjust the lactulose to four to five daily bowel movements (Fullwood & Sargent, 2014).

Cardiovascular Complications

Patients with HCC have a dilated vasculature because of splanchnic and peripheral vasodilation, which presents as low blood pressure and high cardiac output (Panackel, Thomas, Sebastian, & Mathai, 2015). Cirrhotic cardiomyopathy is a type of cardiac dysfunction that has impaired contractile responsiveness to stress or altered diastolic relaxation, which prolongs the QT interval. Cirrhotic cardiomyopathy can cause heart failure, renal failure, and ultimately cardiovascular collapse. Once heart failure is present, heart failure management principles are followed as supportive treatment (Al-Khafaji & Huang, 2011).

Impaired sympathetic response causes impaired cardiac contractility with orthostasis and reduced response to vasoconstrictors, requiring careful titration of inotropes and vasopressors. Patients are likely to develop adrenal insufficiency because of high levels of inflammatory cytokines (Møller & Bendtsen, 2015). IV corticosteroids may be considered when hypotension responds poorly to fluid resuscitation (e.g., isotonic crystalloid and colloid solutions) and vasopressors (Bernal & Wendon, 2013).

Pulmonary Complications

Hepatopulmonary syndrome is the presence of hypoxia caused by ventilation–perfusion mismatch, intrapulmonary shunting, and pulmonary capillary vasodilation (Al-Khafaji & Huang, 2011; Sargent, 2010) and is treated with supplemental oxygen. Patients can develop ARDS from inflammatory cytokines and pulmonary dysfunction. Therapy is supportive, and possible interventions include low tidal volume and high positive end-expiratory pressure (PEEP) (Al-Khafaji & Huang, 2011).

Gastrointestinal Complications

Gastrointestinal bleeding may be a complication of portal hypertension and liver failure. Bleeding can be from gastric and esophageal varices and requires volume resuscitation, blood transfusions, vasoconstrictors, prophylactic antibiotics, and endoscopy. Vitamin K may also be administered (Al-Khafaji & Huang, 2011). Patients with gastrointestinal bleeding are usually intubated to minimize aspiration risk. The aim of variceal bleeding management is to decrease portal pressure with vasopressin and octreotide. Antibiotic prophylaxis for seven days decreases the occurrence of spontaneous bacterial peritonitis (SBP), sepsis, recurrent bleeding, hospital length of stay, and mortality (Al-Khafaji & Huang, 2011).

Hepatorenal Syndrome

Hepatorenal syndrome is an acute kidney injury in patients with liver failure and ascites in the absence of a cause of renal failure. Treatment includes avoidance of nephrotoxins, volume resuscitation, vasoconstrictors, and paracentesis. Albumin may be administered for volume expansion (Al-Khafaji & Huang, 2011). Continuous renal replacement therapy improves the stability of cardiovascular and intracranial function. Bicarbonate-buffered replacement fluid is often used, as the liver is unable to use lactate or acetate to make bicarbonate (Sargent, 2010).

Infection

SBP is the most common infection in patients with liver failure. It can present with no or vague symptoms and can accelerate liver failure. If SBP is suspected, paracentesis should be performed and blood cultures sent (Sargent, 2010). Antibiotic coverage should be directed at gram-negative bacteria, such as *Escherichia coli (E. coli)* and *Klebsiella pneumonia*, and gram-positive cocci, such as *Streptococcus* and *Enterococcus*. Third-generation cephalosporins are commonly prescribed. A lack of clinical improvement should prompt repeat abdominal imaging and paracentesis (Al-Khafaji & Huang, 2011).

Hyperlactatemia

Lactate production is the result of poor tissue perfusion and anaerobic metabolism. Hyperlactatemia may occur because of poor systemic microcirculation and failure of the liver to clear lactate, leading to hemodynamic instability. High levels of lactate are a predictor of mortality (Sargent, 2010). Treatment of hyperlactatemia should be aggressive and includes appropriate antibiotic use to treat sepsis, adequate systemic oxygen delivery, fluid resuscitation, and avoidance of adrenergic agonists (Suetrong & Walley, 2015).

Hypoglycemia

A high plasma insulin level leads to reduced hepatic uptake and glucogenesis. Glucose infusions are often used to maintain normal blood glucose (Bernal & Wendon, 2013). Daily phosphate, magnesium, and potassium supplementation may be required (Sargent, 2010).

Coagulopathy

Increased consumption of fibrinolytic proteins, anticoagulant proteins, and procoagulant factors with decreased synthesis occurs in liver failure, leading to a prolonged prothrombin time and INR (Sargent, 2010). Stress ulcer prophylaxis with a histamine-2 receptor blocker or a proton pump inhibitor should be implemented to decrease the risk of gastrointestinal bleeding. Fresh frozen plasma should be given for active bleeding for an INR greater than 1.5 for invasive procedures. In patients with a platelet count below 10,000/mm^3, thrombocytopenia is corrected with platelet administration for active bleeding or in invasive procedures (Al-Khafaji & Huang, 2011).

Chemotherapy Side Effects

Sorafenib is the only approved therapy for advanced HCC. It is a multikinase inhibitor with antiprolific and antiangiogenic effects (Galuppo et al., 2014). Side effects typically include hand-foot syndrome and diarrhea (Colagrande, Regini, Taliani, Nardi, & Inghilesi, 2015).

Radiation Side Effects

Radiation-induced liver disease (RILD) creates a venoocclusive disease after conventional radiation therapy (Kimura et al., 2015). Recent advances in radiation techniques provide high radiation doses to focal HCC. Focal radiation therapy has shown injury on imaging to normal and cirrhotic tissue. Stereotactic body radiation therapy and particle therapy have shown no contribution to RILD.

Nursing Implications

Nurses should be aware that hepatic dysfunction can affect the bioavailability of enterally administered drugs through the reduction of the first-pass effect, which involves cytochrome P450. A reduction in the first-pass effect results in a larger amount of the drug reaching the systemic circulation. Common critical care drugs, such as labetalol, metoprolol, midazolam, morphine, nifedipine, and propranolol administered enterally, exhibit increased bioavailability (Lin & Smith, 2010). Delayed gastric emptying may lead to prolonged time for absorption of medications from the small intestine. Diarrhea may limit medication absorption as intestinal transit time increases. The use of vasopressors reduces blood flow to the intestinal tract and absorption of medications (Hansen et al., 2010).

The liver produces albumin, making a low serum albumin level common in patients with liver disease. Medications bound to albumin can result in a high amount of circulating free drug in patients with liver failure, leading to excessive side effects. In the critical care setting, lower doses of medications should be considered, and drug levels should be monitored (Lin & Smith, 2010).

Cholangiocarcinoma

Cholangiocarcinoma is a cancer of the epithelial cells of the biliary tree. The World Health Organization defines two categories of cholangiocarcinoma: intrahepatic (ICC) and extrahepatic (ECC). ECC is further defined as hilar and distal, with hilar accounting for 60%–70% of all cholangiocarcinomas (Kogut, Bastawrous, Padia, & Bhargava, 2013). Surgery is the only potential curative therapy. Biliary obstruction may be a result of tumor progression and requires decompression through stenting of the bile ducts. Decompression of the biliary tree is done via ERCP with stenting. Percutaneous transhepatic cholangiography (PTC) drainage is the treatment for biliary obstruction (Brown, Parmar, & Geller, 2014).

Cholangitis

Acute cholangitis is an infection of the biliary tree. Bile duct obstruction raises the intrabiliary pressure and increases ductal permeability, allowing bacteria into the vascular system and resulting in bacteremia (Butte, Hameed, & Ball, 2015; Weber et al., 2013). Patients may present with a wide range of symptoms, including severe infection and shock. The Tokyo Guidelines include signs of systemic inflammation (fever), cholestasis, and findings on imaging to define the grade of acute cholangitis (Nishino et al., 2014). Grade I is mild and a diagnosis of exclusion. Grade II is systemic inflammation without organ dysfunction. Grade III is concurrent dysfunction of at least one organ system (Butte et al., 2015).

If acute cholangitis is suspected, the patient should be admitted to the intensive care unit. Typically, crystalloid fluid is given for fluid resuscitation and albumin is given to increase intracellular fluid volume. If mean arterial pressure is less than 65 mm Hg, vasopressive therapy can be initiated. The first therapy choice is norepinephrine with the addition of epinephrine and/or vasopressin. Inotropic therapy with dobutamine can also be used if myocardial dysfunction is noted or in the case of hypoperfusion. Corticosteroids such as hydrocortisone are recommended after fluid resuscitation if vasopressor therapy is unsuccessful (Lee et al., 2013; Lehman & Thiessen, 2015).

E. coli is the normal pathogen in patients with acute cholangitis, but *Enterococcus* and *Klebsiella* species may also be present (Weber et al., 2013). Broad-spectrum penicillin/beta-lactamase inhibitors, such as ampicillin/sulbactam and piperacillin/tazobactam, and third- or fourth-generation cephalosporins are recommended in acute cholangitis (Kogure et al., 2011). Hospital-acquired cholangitis is often caused by multiple resistant organisms, such as vancomycin-resistant enterococci, methicillin-resistant *Staphylococcus aureus*, and *Pseudomonas* (Mosler, 2011). The type and duration of antibiotic therapy should be based on disease severity. Mild cases should be treated for two to three days, and moderate to severe cases should be treated for at least five to seven days. Ultimately, the patient's clinical picture determines therapy length. Biliary and blood cultures may be used to broaden or narrow the spectrum of antibiotics (Mosler, 2011).

For patients requiring mechanical ventilation with ARDS, a tidal volume of 6 ml/kg of predicted body weight should be targeted with PEEP (Lehman & Thiessen, 2015). Sedation should be minimized, with the patient weaned off as soon as possible.

Overall prognosis of malignancy-causing biliary obstruction is poor. Malignant biliary strictures are managed endoscopically or via percutaneous drainage (Kogut et al., 2013). Patients who have undergone previous endoscopes, have a preexisting sphincterotomy, or have a biliary bypass are at high risk for a superimposed infection. The presence of biliary dilatation or hyperbilirubinemia alone does not indicate that drainage is necessary; however, it may be required to lower bilirubin, enabling the patient to receive chemotherapy.

Chemotherapy Side Effects

Gemcitabine and cisplatin in combination is the standard of care in patients with cholangiocarcinoma (Avan et al., 2015; Lafaro et al., 2015). Sorafenib, erlotinib, lapatinib, panitumumab, cetuximab, sunitinib, and bevacizumab are the targets of the vascular endothelial growth factor involved in angiogenesis and the epidermal growth factor involved in cell proliferation. These have been studied alone or in combination with gemcitabine with no increase in overall survival (Lafaro et al., 2015). Gemcitabine has the potential for pulmonary toxicity with ARDS (Tutar, Buyukoglan, Gülmez, Oymak, & Demir, 2012).

Radiation Side Effects

The role of external beam radiation therapy is controversial in the adjuvant setting and for inoperable ICC (Lafaro et al., 2015). Several small studies have shown improvement in one- and two-year survival with doses greater than or equal to 75 Gy. No radiation side effects have been documented.

Nursing Implications

Biliary drain care is important in preventing recurrent biliary obstruction. Drains should be flushed at least every eight hours or more often if sludge or sediment is present. A change in drainage output or color should be reported to the medical team. The nurse should expect a decrease in total bilirubin with a functioning stent or PTC. The patient should be instructed that the stent will need to be exchanged every six weeks, or sooner if symptoms develop. Symptoms include an inability to flush the drain, fevers, chills, or jaundice, and patients should contact their provider if any of these are present. A patient with PTC drains is usually discharged on antibiotics to prevent recurrent cholangitis. If PTC drains are unable to be internalized because of tumor, the patient should be instructed to maintain hydration above drain output.

Pancreatic Cancer

Pancreatitis

Acute pancreatitis (AP) is an inflammatory disease of the pancreas caused by alcohol, gallstones, hypertriglyceridemia, hypocalcemia, drugs, or after biliary tree manipulation by ERCP (Bolado et al., 2015). Serum lipase and computed tomography of the abdomen and pelvis are recommended to diagnose AP (Yokoe et al., 2015). Magnetic resonance imaging is useful in diagnosing hemorrhagic necrotizing pancreatitis. Tumors causing obstruction of the ampulla, including intraductal papillary mucinous neoplasm, neuroendocrine carcinoma, pancreatic adenocarcinoma, or metastases from other malignancies, have also been associated with AP (Bolado et al., 2015; Yadav & Lowenfels, 2013). AP results in microcirculation disturbances in the pancreatic parenchyma, which can lead to tissue ischemia and cell death (Howard, 2013). This presents as pancreatic and peripancreatic necrosis on imaging. Infected pancreatic necrosis can lead to sepsis and death. Close clinical monitoring with aggressive fluid resuscitation and supplemental oxygenation is the basis of supportive care.

AP is divided into two phases. Within the first week of onset, cytokines through the systematic inflammatory response assist in reversible organ failure. A rise in temperature is caused by the autodigestion of the pancreas by pancreatic enzymes. As the patient's condition deteriorates, toxins released by the necrosing pancreas maintain the elevated temperature. Destruction of the capillaries leads to fluid leaking into the abdominal cavity and hypovolemic shock. If the patient is in shock, short-time rapid fluid resuscitation may be used. Permeability of the vessel walls allows bacterial debris to pass to organs, leading to organ failure. Pulmonary edema can occur as fluid shifts across the alveolar–capillary membrane. The focus of treatment for this phase is volume resuscitation with an extracellular solution: Ringer's lactate. Enteral nutrition and treatment of sources of active infection are also part of the treatment plan. Pain is severe and persistent and requires consistent narcotics administration for relief. Death in this phase is attributed to multisystem organ failure (Upchurch, 2014).

The second phase of AP occurs two to four weeks following initial onset. The patient develops systemic sepsis and persistent or new-onset multisystem organ failure. Pancreatic necrosis peaks two to four weeks after onset and is the cause of secondary pancreatic infection with bacterial or fungal organisms (Thandassery et al., 2015). The most commonly found organisms are gram-negative (e.g., *E. coli, Klebsiella, Enterobacter*) and gram-positive (e.g., *Staphylococcus, Streptococcus, Candida*). Targeted antimicrobial therapy is essential. Secondary fungal infection with *Candida* is associated with increased hospital mortality.

Hemodynamic Resuscitation

Cardiovascular and microcirculatory failure in the early stages of AP determines patient outcome. Systemic vasodilation and myocardial dysfunction are also factors contributing to hypotension. Patients may exhibit tachycardia, tachyarrhythmia, weak pulses, cold and mottled skin, and low urine output. Arterial hypotension will develop as a late symptom. The extent of hypovolemia is underestimated, making repeated physical examination and urine output monitoring essential for volume replacement.

Respiratory Treatment

Two time frames exist for the development of pulmonary complications due to AP. On admission, 15% of patients will demonstrate lung injury (Hasibeder, Torgersen, Rieger, & Dünser, 2009). After five days, up to 70% of patients will exhibit acute lung injury (Hasibeder et al., 2009). Acute lung injury is caused by inflammatory changes with leukocyte plugging of capillaries, the formation of pulmonary edema, atelectasis, and reduced chest wall compliance caused by increased intra-abdominal pressure. Symptoms include respiratory distress, diaphoresis, and anxiety. Mechanical ventilation for lung protection includes PEEP and tidal volumes of 6 ml/kg of ideal body weight. Lung complications in the later phase of AP are associated with pulmonary or extrapulmonary infections.

Intra-Abdominal Hypertension

Body organ edema with ascites formation and distension of intestinal loops increases abdominal pressure and results in vascular compression, reduced venous return, decreased cardiac output, increased arteriolar resistance, and impaired organ blood flow. Tissue hypoxia is aggravated by arterial hypoxia, which results from impaired respirations. Abdominal distension, oliguria, and increased ventricular filling pressures are the first clinical symptoms of intra-abdominal hypertension. Treatment involves gastric decompression, postural changes, sedation, neuromuscular relaxation, and negative fluid balance if possible.

Nutrition

Enteral nutrition within 72 hours of AP reduces infectious complications. Enteral nutrition maintains the integrity of the intestinal barrier, while total parenteral nutrition is associated with a proinflammatory response. Patients with severe shock are likely to develop paralytic ileus and compromised mucosal perfusion. Jejunal enteral feeding into an atonic bowel can cause the intraluminal pressure to exceed the mucosal perfusion pressure, causing ischemia.

Summary

Cancers of the upper gastrointestinal tract and their treatments have the potential to cause life-threatening illnesses, requiring the knowledge and skill of oncology and critical care nurses. Sepsis management is the foundation of care for these critical conditions, including liver failure, acute pancreatitis, and cholangitis. Surviving Sepsis Campaign's 2016 guidelines for managing severe sepsis and septic shock can be viewed at www.survivingsepsis.org/guidelines/pages/default.aspx.

References

Al-Khafaji, A., & Huang, D.T. (2011). Critical care management of patients with end-stage liver disease. *Critical Care Medicine, 36,* 1157–1166. doi:10.1097/CCM.0b013e318211fdc4

Avan, A., Postma, T.J., Ceresa, C., Avan, A., Cavaletti, G., Giovannetti, E., & Peters, G.J. (2015). Platinum-induced neurotoxicity and preventive strategies: Past, present, and future. *Oncologist, 20,* 411–432. doi:10.1634/theoncologist.2014-0044

Bernal, W., & Wendon, J. (2013). Acute liver failure. *New England Journal of Medicine, 369,* 2525–2534. doi:10.1056/NEJMra1208937

Bolado, F., Tarifa, A., Zazpe, C., Urman, J.M., Herrera, J., & Vila, J.J. (2015). Acute recurrent pancreatitis secondary to hepatocellular carcinoma invading the biliary tree. *Pancreatology, 15,* 191–193. doi:10.1016/j.pan.2015.01.007

Brown, K.M., Parmar, A.D., & Geller, D.A. (2014). Intrahepatic cholangiocarcinoma. *Surgical Oncology Clinics of North America, 23,* 231–246. doi:10.1016/j.soc.2013.10.004

Butte, J.M., Hameed, M., & Ball, C.G. (2015). Hepato-pancreato-biliary emergencies for the acute care surgeon: Etiology, diagnosis and treatment. *World Journal of Emergency Surgery, 10,* 1–10. doi:10.1186/s13017-015-00001-y

Chung, V. (2015). Systemic therapy for hepatocellular carcinoma and cholangiocarcinoma. *Surgical Oncology Clinics of North America, 24,* 187–198. doi:10.1016/j.soc.2014.09.009

Colagrande, S., Regini, F., Taliani, G.G., Nardi, C., & Inghilesi, A.L. (2015). Advanced hepatocellular carcinoma and sorafenib: Diagnosis, indications, clinical and radiological follow-up. *World Journal of Hepatology, 7,* 1041–1053. doi:10.4254/wjh.v7.i8.1041

Fullwood, D., & Sargent, S. (2014). Complications in acute liver failure: Managing hepatic encephalopathy and cerebral edema. *Gastrointestinal Nursing, 12*(3), 27–34. doi:10.12968/gasn.2014.12.3.27

Galuppo, R., Ramaiah, D., Ponte, O.M., & Gedaly, R. (2014). Molecular therapies in hepatocellular carcinoma: What can we target? *Digestive Diseases and Sciences, 59,* 1688–1697. doi:10.1007/s10620-014-3058-x

Hansen, L., Sasaki, A., & Zucker, B. (2010). End-stage liver disease: Challenges and practice implications. *Nursing Clinics of North America, 45,* 411–426. doi:10.1016/j.cnur.2010.03.005

Hasibeder, W.R., Torgersen, C., Rieger, M., & Dünser, M. (2009). Critical care of the patient with acute pancreatitis. *Anesthesiology and Intensive Care, 37,* 190–206.

Howard, T.J. (2013). The role of antimicrobial therapy in severe acute pancreatitis. *Surgical Clinics of North America, 93,* 585–593. doi:10.1016/j.suc.2013.02.006

Kimura, T., Takahashi, S., Takahashi, I., Nishibuchi, I., Doi, Y., Kenjo, M., … Nagata, Y. (2015). The time course of dynamic computed tomographic appearance of radiation injury to the cirrhotic liver following stereotactic body radiation therapy for hepatocellular carcinoma. *PLOS ONE, 10,* e0125231. doi:10.1371/journal.pone.0125231

Kogure, H., Tsujino, T., Yamamoto, K., Mizuno, S., Yashima, Y., Yagioka, H., … Koike, K. (2011). Fever-based antibiotic therapy for acute cholangitis following successful endoscopic biliary drainage. *Journal of Gastroenterology, 46,* 1411–1417. doi:10.1007/s00535-011-0451-5

Kogut, M., Bastawrous, S., Padia, S., & Bhargava, P. (2013). Hepatobiliary oncologic emergencies: Imaging appearances and therapeutic options. *Current Problems in Diagnostic Radiology, 42,* 113–126. doi:10.1067/j.cpradiol.2012.08.003

Lafaro, K.J., Cosgrove, D., Geschwind, J.-F.H., Kamel, I., Herman, J.M., & Pawlik, T.M. (2015). Multidisciplinary care of patients with intrahepatic cholangiocarcinoma: Updates in management. *Gastroenterology Research and Practice, 2015,* 860861. doi:10.1155/2015/860861

Lee, B.S., Hwang, J.-H., Lee, S.H., Jang, S.E., Jang, E.S., Jo, H.J., … Ahn, S. (2013). Risk factors of organ failure in patients with bacteremic cholangitis. *Digestive Diseases and Sciences, 58,* 1091–1099. doi:10.1007/s10620-012-2478-8

Lehman, K., & Thiessen, K. (2015). Sepsis guidelines: Clinical practice implications. *Nurse Practitioner, 40,* 1–6. doi:10.1097/01.NPR.0000465120.42654.86

Lin, S., & Smith, B.S. (2010). Drug dosing considerations for the critically ill patient with liver disease. *Clinical Care Nursing Clinics of North America, 22,* 335–340. doi:10.1016/j.ccel.2010.04.006

Møller, S., & Bendtsen, F. (2015). Cirrhotic multiorgan syndrome. *Digestive Diseases and Sciences, 66,* 3209–3225. doi:10.1007/s10620-015-3752-3

Mosler, P. (2011). Management of acute cholangitis. *Current Gastroenterology Reports, 13,* 166–172. doi:10.1007/s11894-010-0171-7

Nishino, T., Hamano, T., Mitsunaga, Y., Shirato, I., Shirato, M., Tagata, T., ... Mitsunaga, A. (2014). Clinical evaluation of the Tokyo Guidelines 2013 for severity assessment of acute cholangitis. *Journal of Hepato-Biliary-Pancreatic Sciences, 21,* 841–849. doi:10.1002/jhbp.189

Page, A., Cosgrove, D., Philosophe, B., & Pawlik, T.M. (2014). Hepatocellular carcinoma: Diagnosis, management, and prognosis. *Surgical Oncology Clinics of North America, 23,* 289–311. doi:10.1016/j.soc.2013.10.006

Panackel, C., Thomas, R., Sebastian, B., & Mathai, S.K. (2015). Recent advances in management of acute liver failure. *Indian Journal of Critical Care Medicine, 19,* 27–33. doi:10.4103/0972-5229 .148636.

Russell, M.C. (2015). Complications following hepatectomy. *Surgical Oncology Clinics of North America, 24,* 73–96. doi:10.1016/j.soc.2014.09.008

Salgia, R., & Singal, A.G. (2014). Hepatocellular carcinoma and other liver lesions. *Medical Clinics of North America, 98,* 103–118. doi:10.1016/j.mcna.2013.09.003

Sargent, S. (2010). An overview of acute liver failure: Managing rapid deterioration. *Gastrointestinal Nursing, 8*(9), 36–42. doi:10.12968/gasn.2010.8.9.79852

Suetrong, B., & Walley, K.R. (2015). Lactic acidosis in sepsis: It's not all anaerobic: Implications for diagnosis and management. *Chest, 149,* 252–261. doi:10.1378/chest.15-1703

Thandassery, R.B., Yadav, T.D., Dutta, U., Appasani, S., Singh, K., & Kochhar, R. (2015). Hypotension in the first week of acute pancreatitis and APACHE II score predict development of infected pancreatic necrosis. *Digestive Diseases and Sciences, 60,* 537–542. doi:10.1007/s10620-014-3081-y

Tutar, N., Buyukoglan, H., Gülmez, I., Oymak, F.S., & Demir, R. (2012). Gemcitabine induced pulmonary toxicity with late onset [Abstract]. *European Journal of General Medicine, 9,* 208–210.

Upchurch, E. (2014). Local complications of acute pancreatitis. *British Journal of Hospital Medicine, 75,* 698–702. doi:10.12968/hmed.2014.75.12.698

Weber, A., Schneider, J., Wagenpfeil, S., Winkle, P., Riedel, J., Wantia, N., ... Huber, W. (2013). Spectrum of pathogens in acute cholangitis in patients with and without biliary endoprosthesis. *Journal of Infection, 67,* 111–121. doi:10.1016/j.jinf.2013.04.008

Yadav, D., & Lowenfels, A.B. (2013). The epidemiology of pancreatitis and pancreatic cancer. *Gastroenterology, 144,* 1252–1261. doi:10.1053/j.gastro.2013.01.068

Yokoe, M., Takada, T., Mayumi, T., Yoshida, M., Isaji, S., Wada, K., ... Hirata, K. (2015). Japanese guidelines for the management of acute pancreatitis: Japanese Guidelines 2015. *Journal of Hepato-Biliary-Pancreatic Sciences, 22,* 405–432. doi:10.1002/jhbp.259

CHAPTER 5

Gynecologic Cancers

Catherine Hydzik, MS, CNS, AOCN®, and
Karen M. Perialis, MSN, RN, ANP-BC, OCN®

Introduction

Patients treated for a gynecologic (GYN) malignancy may also have a life-threatening illness, making it essential to recognize early symptoms, promptly diagnose, and begin treatment. Patients may experience symptoms and side effects ranging from within normal limits to severe toxicities, and on a continuum from well to critically ill. It may be helpful to use an objective scale to assess and measure toxicities, such as the National Cancer Institute's (NCI's) Common Terminology Criteria for Adverse Events (see Table 5-1). This tool provides a consistent method to document side effects and toxicities. This chapter presents an overview of GYN malignancies and the potential critical events for women undergoing treatment.

Overview of Gynecologic Cancers

GYN cancers are caused by the uncontrolled growth and spread of abnormal cells originating in female reproductive organs, including the cervix, ovaries, fallopian tubes, uterus, endometrium, vagina, and vulva. Gestational trophoblastic disease is a rare type of GYN malignancy caused by the uncontrolled growth of a human trophoblast, which is a product of conception. Multiple factors are associated with GYN cancers, including oncogenes and tumor suppressor genes, which can promote cancer growth (Cancer.Net, 2015). The abnormal functioning of these genes can be caused by several factors, including environmental exposures, aging, smoking, diet, viruses, hormones, lifetime number of menstrual cycles,

Table 5-1. Common Terminology Criteria for Adverse Events Grading

Adverse Event	Grade				
	1	2	3	4	5
Allergic reaction	Transient flushing or rash, drug fever < 38°C (< 100.4°F); intervention not indicated	Intervention or infusion interruption indicated; responds promptly to symptomatic treatment (e.g., antihistamines, nonsteroidal anti-inflammatory drugs, narcotics); prophylactic medications indicated for ≤ 24 hours	Prolonged (e.g., not rapidly responsive to symptomatic medication and/or brief interruption of infusion); recurrence of symptoms following initial improvement; hospitalization indicated for clinical sequelae (e.g., renal impairment, pulmonary infiltrates)	Life-threatening consequences; urgent intervention indicated	Death
Anaphylaxis	—	—	Symptomatic bronchospasm, with or without urticaria; parenteral intervention indicated; allergy-related edema/angioedema; hypotension	Life-threatening consequences; urgent intervention indicated	Death
Anorexia	Loss of appetite without alteration in eating habits	Oral intake altered without significant weight loss or malnutrition; oral nutritional supplements indicated	Associated with significant weight loss or malnutrition (e.g., inadequate oral caloric and/or fluid intake); tube feeding or total parenteral nutrition (TPN) indicated	Life-threatening consequences; urgent intervention indicated	Death

(Continued on next page)

Table 5-1. Common Terminology Criteria for Adverse Events Grading *(Continued)*

Adverse Event	Grade				
	1	2	3	4	5
Constipation	Occasional or intermittent symptoms; occasional use of stool softeners, laxatives, dietary modification, or enema	Persistent symptoms with regular use of laxatives or enemas; limiting instrumental activities of daily living (ADL)	Obstipation with manual evacuation indicated; limiting self-care ADL	Life-threatening consequences; urgent intervention indicated	Death
Cough	Mild symptoms; nonprescription intervention indicated	Moderate symptoms; medical intervention indicated; limiting instrumental ADL	Severe symptoms; limiting self-care ADL	—	—
Dehydration	Increased oral fluids indicated; dry mucous membranes; diminished skin turgor	IV fluids indicated < 24 hours	IV fluids or hospitalization indicated	Life-threatening consequences; urgent intervention indicated	Death
Dermatitis radiation	Faint erythema or dry desquamation	Moderate to brisk erythema; patchy moist desquamation, mostly confined to skinfolds and creases; moderate edema	Moist desquamation in areas other than skinfolds and creases; bleeding induced by minor trauma or abrasion	Life-threatening consequences; skin necrosis or ulceration of full thickness dermis; spontaneous bleeding from involved site; skin graft indicated	Death

(Continued on next page)

Table 5-1. Common Terminology Criteria for Adverse Events Grading (Continued)

Adverse Event	Grade				
	1	2	3	4	5
Diarrhea	Increase of < 4 stools per day over baseline; mild increase in ostomy output compared to baseline	Increase of 4–6 stools per day over baseline; moderate increase in ostomy output compared to baseline	Increase of ≥ 7 stools per day over baseline; incontinence; hospitalization indicated; severe increase in ostomy output compared to baseline; limiting self-care ADL	Life-threatening consequences; urgent intervention indicated	Death
Dry mouth	Symptomatic (e.g., dry or thick saliva) without significant dietary alteration; unstimulated saliva flow > 0.2 ml/min	Moderate symptoms; oral intake alterations (e.g., copious water, other lubricants, diet limited to purees and/or soft, moist foods); unstimulated saliva 0.1–0.2 ml/min	Inability to adequately aliment orally; tube feeding or TPN indicated; unstimulated saliva < 0.1 ml/min	—	—
Dyspnea	Shortness of breath with moderate exertion	Shortness of breath with minimal exertion; limiting instrumental ADL	Shortness of breath at rest; limiting self-care ADL	Life-threatening consequences; urgent intervention indicated	Death
Esophagitis	Asymptomatic; clinical or diagnostic observations only; intervention not indicated	Symptomatic; altered eating/swallowing; oral supplements indicated	Severely altered eating/swallowing; tube feeding, TPN, or hospitalization indicated	Life-threatening consequences; urgent operative intervention indicated	Death

(Continued on next page)

Table 5-1. Common Terminology Criteria for Adverse Events Grading (Continued)

Adverse Event	Grade				
	1	2	3	4	5
Fatigue	Fatigue relieved by rest	Fatigue not relieved by rest; limiting instrumental ADL	Fatigue not relieved by rest, limiting self-care ADL	—	—
Febrile neutropenia	—	—	Absolute neutrophil count (ANC) < 1,000/mm^3 with a single temperature of > 38.3°C (101°F) or a sustained temperature ≥ 38°C (100.4°F) for more than 1 hour	ANC < 1,000/mm^3 with a single temperature of > 38.3°C (101°F) or a sustained temperature of ≥ 38°C (100.4°F) for more than 1 hour	Death
Fever	38.0°–39.0°C (100.4°–102.2°F)	> 39.0°–40.0°C (102.3°–104.0°F)	> 40.0°C (> 104.0°F) for ≤ 24 hours	>40.0°C (> 104.0°F) for > 24 hours	Death
Headache	Mild pain	Moderate pain; limiting instrumental ADL	Severe pain; limiting self-care ADL	—	—
Hepatic failure	—	—	Asterixis; mild encephalopathy; limiting self-care ADL	Moderate to severe encephalopathy; coma; life-threatening consequences	Death

(Continued on next page)

Adverse Event	Grade				
	1	2	3	4	5
Infusion-related reaction	Mild transient reaction; infusion interruption not indicated; intervention not indicated	Therapy or infusion interruption indicated but responds promptly to symptomatic treatment (e.g., antihistamines, nonsteroidal anti-inflammatory drugs, narcotics, IV fluids); prophylactic medications indicated for ≤ 24 hours	Prolonged (e.g., not rapidly responsive to symptomatic medication and/or brief interruption of infusion); recurrence of symptoms following initial improvement; hospitalization indicated for clinical sequelae	Life-threatening consequences; urgent intervention indicated	Death
Mucositis, oral	Asymptomatic or mild symptoms; intervention not indicated	Moderate pain; not interfering with oral intake; modified diet indicated	Severe pain; interfering with oral intake	Life-threatening consequences; urgent intervention indicated	Death
Multiorgan failure	—	—	Shock with azotemia and acid–base disturbances; significant coagulation abnormalities	Life-threatening consequences (e.g., vasopressor dependent and oliguric or anuric or ischemic colitis or lactic acidosis)	Death
Nausea	Loss of appetite without alteration in eating habits	Oral intake decreased without significant weight loss, dehydration, or malnutrition	Inadequate oral caloric or fluid intake; tube feeding, TPN, or hospitalization indicated	—	—

Table 5-1. Common Terminology Criteria for Adverse Events Grading (Continued)

(Continued on next page)

Table 5-1. Common Terminology Criteria for Adverse Events Grading *(Continued)*

Adverse Event	Grade				
	1	2	3	4	5
Pain	Mild pain	Moderate pain; limiting instrumental ADL	Severe pain; limiting self-care ADL	—	—
Proctitis	Rectal discomfort, intervention not indicated	Symptoms (e.g., rectal discomfort, passing blood or mucus); medical intervention indicated; limiting instrumental ADL	Severe symptoms; fecal urgency or stool incontinence; limiting self-care ADL	Life-threatening consequences; urgent intervention indicated	Death
Pruritus	Mild or localized; topical intervention indicated	Intense or widespread; intermittent; skin changes from scratching (e.g., edema, papulation, excoriations, lichenification, oozing/crusts); oral intervention indicated; limiting instrumental ADL	Intense or widespread; constant; limiting self-care ADL or sleep; oral corticosteroid or immunosuppressive therapy indicated	—	—
Seizure	Brief partial seizure; no loss of consciousness	Brief generalized seizure	Multiple seizures despite medical intervention	Life-threatening; prolonged repetitive seizures	Death
Sepsis	—	—	—	Life-threatening consequences; urgent intervention indicated	Death

(Continued on next page)

Table 5-1. Common Terminology Criteria for Adverse Events Grading (Continued)

Adverse Event	Grade				
	1	2	3	4	5
Urinary frequency	Present	Limiting instrumental ADL; medical management indicated	—	—	—
Vaginal discharge	Mild vaginal discharge (greater than baseline for patient)	Moderate to heavy vaginal discharge; use of perineal pad or tampon indicated	—	—	—
Vomiting	1–2 episodes (separated by 5 minutes) in 24 hours	3–5 episodes (separated by 5 minutes) in 24 hours	≥ 6 episodes (separated by 5 minutes) in 24 hours; tube feeding, TPN, or hospitalization indicated	Life-threatening consequences; urgent intervention indicated	Death
Wound infection	—	Localized; local intervention indicated (e.g., topical antibiotic, antifungal, or antiviral)	IV antibiotic, antifungal, or antiviral intervention indicated; radiologic or operative intervention indicated	Life-threatening consequences; urgent intervention indicated	Death

Note. From *Common Terminology Criteria for Adverse Events* [v.4.03], by National Cancer Institute Cancer Therapy Evaluation Program, 2010. Retrieved from https://evs.nci.nih.gov/ftp1/CTCAE/CTCAE_4.03_2010-06-14_QuickReference_5x7.pdf.

and genetic influences (Foundation for Women's Cancer, n.d.). GYN cancers are associated with an advanced age (older than 40 years), obesity, genetic predisposition, and possibly the use of fertility drugs for more than a year. Cervical cancers are associated with women younger than 40 years of age (Benard, Watson, Castle, & Saraiya, 2012). The use of hormonal birth control agents, multiple pregnancies, and tubal ligations are associated with a lower risk of some GYN cancers.

Multiple genes are associated with GYN cancers, such as *BRCA1*, *BRCA2*, *MSH1*, *MLH1*, *MSH6*, *PMS2*, *EPCAM*, *BRIP1*, *RAD51D*, *RAD51C*, and many others (Lancaster, Powell, Chen, & Richardson, 2015). High-risk forms of the human papillomavirus, such as 16 and 18, are responsible for 70% of all cases of cervical cancer (NCI, 2015a). An estimated 98,000 women will be diagnosed with a GYN malignancy in 2017, and approximately 30,000 will die from the disease (American Cancer Society [ACS], 2017a) (see Table 5-2).

Symptoms vary by both the location and stage of the tumor. Diagnosis begins with vague symptoms, a computed tomography scan or magnetic resonance imaging, and a surgically obtained pathology. Current treatment modalities include surgical debulking, chemotherapy, biotherapy, and radiation therapy (RT). Because of the nature of these treatment modalities and the location of the tumors in the lower abdomen (see Figure 5-1), commonly associated disease-specific complications exist that require critical nursing interventions.

As previously mentioned, women diagnosed with a GYN malignancy may be treated with one or a combination of treatment modalities. The physician decides the treatment plan based on diagnosis, stage, grade (pathology), and medical history, as well as patient input and performance status. Table 5-3 provides an overview of treatment options for women with GYN cancers based on disease location.

Table 5-2. Estimated Number of New Cancer Cases and Deaths, United States, 2017		
Cancer	Estimated New Cases (Female)	Estimated Deaths (Female)
Uterine cervix	12,820	4,210
Uterine corpus	61,380	10,920
Ovary	22,440	14,080
Vulva	6,020	1,150
Vagina and other genital	4,810	1,240

Note. From *Cancer Facts and Figures 2017* (p. 3), by American Cancer Society, 2017. Retrieved from https://www.cancer.org/content/dam/cancer-org/research/cancer-facts-and-statistics/annual-cancer-facts-and-figures/2017/cancer-facts-and-figures-2017.pdf. Copyright 2017 by American Cancer Society. Adapted with permission.

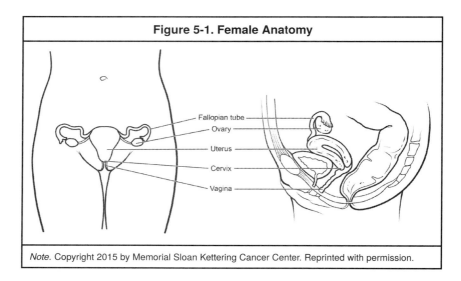

Figure 5-1. Female Anatomy

Fallopian tube
Ovary
Uterus
Cervix
Vagina

Note. Copyright 2015 by Memorial Sloan Kettering Cancer Center. Reprinted with permission.

Caring for a patient with a GYN malignancy is challenging and requires comprehensive nursing assessment, patient and caregiver education, and interventions tailored to the patient's specific needs throughout the trajectory of treatment. At initial diagnosis, the nurse must focus on assessment and patient/caregiver education regarding the disease, the immediate treatment plan/goal of therapy, and the evaluation of coping strategies. Patients and caregivers need information about treatment modalities and potential side effects, which should be verbally discussed. Written instructions also should be given to the patient for reference. The nurse plays a pivotal role in assessing the patient's anxiety level and providing educational information to facilitate coping and lessen anxiety. Anxiety and chronic fatigue are most commonly experienced by patients throughout the disease course.

Treatment Modalities

Three options exist when treating patients with GYN cancers: surgery, chemotherapy, and RT.

Surgery

Surgery type is dependent on the stage of the disease and the patient's health characteristics. Debulking surgery is often performed initially to remove the bulk of the cancer as safely as possible. Potential problems for patients who have undergone GYN surgery are changes in body image and sexuality and risk of

Table 5-3. Treatment Options for Gynecologic Cancers Based on Disease Site

Site	Surgery	Chemotherapy	Radiation Oncology
Cervical	• Simple/extra-fascial • Hysterectomy • Modified radical hysterectomy • Pelvic exenteration • Simple/radical trachelectomy	• Cisplatin/paclitaxel/bevacizumab • Carboplatin • Carboplatin/paclitaxel • Topotecan/paclitaxel • Cisplatin/gemcitabine • Cisplatin/topotecan • Cisplatin concurrently with radiation • Paclitaxel • Vinorelbine • Multiple second-line therapies available	• External beam radiation therapy (EBRT) • Brachytherapy
Ovarian	• Laparotomy/total hysterectomy and bilateral salpingo-oophorectomy with comprehensive staging • Fertility-sparing surgery can be considered in patients who wish to preserve fertility. • Palliative surgical procedures • Paracentesis/indwelling peritoneal catheter • Thoracentesis/indwelling pleural catheter • Ureteral stents/nephrostomy • Gastrostomy tube/intestinal stents/relief of intestinal obstruction	• Paclitaxel IV/cisplatin intraperitoneal (IP)/paclitaxel IP • Paclitaxel/carboplatin + bevacizumab • Docetaxel/carboplatin • Carboplatin • Carboplatin/gemcitabine + bevacizumab • Carboplatin/liposomal doxorubicin • Cisplatin • Cisplatin/gemcitabine • Docetaxel • Gemcitabine • Liposomal doxorubicin + bevacizumab • Paclitaxel • Topotecan + bevacizumab • Mutiple second-line therapies available; please see guidelines at www.nccn.org	• Palliative localized radiation therapy (RT) for symptom control in patients with recurrent disease

(Continued on next page)

Table 5-3. Treatment Options for Gynecologic Cancers Based on Disease Site *(Continued)*

Site	Surgery	Chemotherapy	Radiation Oncology

Uterine and endometrial	• Total hysterectomy and bilateral salpingo-oophorectomy and surgical staging
	• Radical hysterectomy
	• Fertility-sparing surgery can be considered in patients with early-stage disease and/or good-risk tumors who wish to preserve fertility.
		• Carboplatin/paclitaxel
		• Cisplatin/paclitaxel
		• Cisplatin/doxorubicin + paclitaxel
		• Carboplatin/docetaxel
		• Ifosfamide/paclitaxel
		• Cisplatin/ifosfamide
		• Cisplatin
		• Carboplatin
		• Doxorubicin
		• Liposomal doxorubicin
		• Paclitaxel
		• Topotecan
		• Bevacizumab
		• Temsirolimus
		• Docetaxel
		• Ifosfamide
		• Hormonal therapy
		  − Megestrol/tamoxifen (alternating)
		  − Progestational agents
		  − Aromatase inhibitors
		  − Tamoxifen
			• Observation
			• EBRT
			• Pelvic radiation + vaginal brachytherapy + chemotherapy

Vulvovaginal	• Local excision or radical surgery (vaginectomy/radical hysterectomy/pelvic exenteration), often replaced with RT • Radical vulvectomy	• 5-Fluorouracil and/or cisplatin	• Brachytherapy • Intravaginal therapy (intracavitary) • Interstitial therapy • EBRT
Gestational trophoblastic disease/germ cell tumors	• Suction curettage • Hysterectomy without oophorectomy may be considered.	• Methotrexate • Dactinomycin • EMA/CO (dactinomycin, etoposide, methotrexate and leucovorin/vincristine and cyclophosphamide) • EP/EMA (etoposide and cisplatin with dactinomycin, etoposide, and methotrexate)	• The role of concurrent intrathecal therapy and cranial RT is controversial for patients with brain metastases.

(Continued on next page)

Table 5-3. Treatment Options for Gynecologic Cancers Based on Disease Site *(Continued)*			
Site	Surgery	Chemotherapy	Radiation Oncology
Gestational trophoblastic disease/germ cell tumors *(cont.)*		• The role of intrathecal therapy is controversial for patients with brain metastases. • Germ cell tumors • Bleomycin/etoposide/cisplatin • Etoposide/cisplatin	

Note. Based on information from Berkowitz et al., 2016, 2017; Karam et al., 2015; National Comprehensive Cancer Network, 2016, 2017a, 2017b, 2017c.

infection, bleeding, pulmonary embolism, pain, changes in urinary and bowel habits, and lymphedema. Table 5-4 highlights potential side effects related to surgery.

Chemotherapy

Chemotherapy agents for GYN cancers are administered by various routes, including oral, IV, intraoperative, or intraperitoneal (IP), depending on the stage and the size of the residual disease. Side effects are drug specific. The most common side effects are myelosuppression, fatigue, mucositis, constipation, diarrhea, nausea and vomiting, alopecia, alteration in electrolytes, potential for hypersensitivity reactions, cardiotoxicity, and fluid retention. The incidence and severity of these side effects are largely dependent on the patient's characteristics, such as diagnosis, stage, performance status, comorbidities, and individual treatment regimen (e.g., agent, dosage, schedule). These women often are treated in the outpatient setting. Patients and caregivers should be educated on the specific agents, potential acute side effects, and side effect management. Patients must know when to call the healthcare provider to discuss a side effect (e.g., fever, nausea and vomiting). The potential acute side effects of chemotherapy are summarized by agent in Table 5-5.

IP chemotherapy may be administered via an IP port or catheter. The unique management for patients receiving IP chemotherapy is outlined in Table 5-6.

Radiation Therapy

RT for patients with GYN cancer is usually administered in the outpatient setting. RT may consist of external beam RT, low- or high-dose brachytherapy, or a combination of both. Brachytherapy is a form of radiation therapy in which a radiation source is placed into a body cavity (intracavitary) or into tissue (interstitial).

Advanced technology in RT and the imaging field has allowed more targeted radiation treatment with less adverse toxicities and side effects. Side effects may vary by type and site of radiation and by combined modalities. Because of the proximity of the urethra, bladder, and rectum, these structures may be predisposed to injury from radiation. The major side effects of external beam RT to the pelvis include diarrhea, cystitis, alterations in vaginal mucous membranes, and fatigue. It is important that patients and caregivers are educated about RT

Table 5-4. Nursing Care for the Patient Undergoing Gynecologic Surgery		
Potential Problems/Side Effects	Intervention and Rationale	Patient Education and Instruction
Risk for pulmonary embolism	Assess who is at risk (i.e., patients with a prior history of pulmonary embolism). Monitor vital signs. Auscultate breath sounds. Assess for shortness of breath and color. Assess for leg pain and signs of thrombophlebitis. Apply antiembolic compression or devices to both lower extremities. Perform active range-of-motion exercises to prevent embolism. Ambulate as soon as possible. Administer anticoagulants as ordered.	Instruct patient regarding: • Potential risk of pulmonary embolism • Importance of wearing the antiembolic compression or devices • Rationale for performing range-of-motion exercises • When to call the healthcare professional
Wound infection/ breakdown/fistulas	Identify patients at high risk for infections, skin breakdown, and possible rectovaginal fistula formation. Assess wound and monitor changes. Monitor vital signs.	Instruct patient regarding: • Reporting signs and symptoms of infection • Monitoring temperature • Reporting abnormal vaginal discharge or change in bowel habits • Reporting redness or skin breakdown

(Continued on next page)

Table 5-4. Nursing Care for the Patient Undergoing Gynecologic Surgery *(Continued)*		
Potential Problems/Side Effects	**Intervention and Rationale**	**Patient Education and Instruction**

Lower-extremity lymphedema	Identify patients at risk (treatment: radiation therapy and lymph node dissection). Lower-extremity lymphedema occurs in up to 80% of those who had lymph node dissection in the groin or those who have compression of pelvic or inguinal lymph nodes. Monitor weight and offer weight reduction strategies (diet and exercise). Refer to lymphedema specialist. Perform complete decongestive therapy, including manual lymph drainage, compression techniques, exercise, and self-care training. Evaluate for compression hosiery.	Instruct patient regarding:
		• Maintaining ideal body weight
		• Prevention of infection
		• Skin care
		  – Inspect skin for changes and signs and symptoms of infection: cuts, scrapes, abrasions, redness, swelling, warmth, and insect bites.
		  – Use a mild soap and apply cream; avoid scented products.
		  – Keep skinfolds clean and dry.
		  – Use sunscreen (SPF > 30).
		  – Protect skin.
		    * Wear loose clothing and properly fitted, closed-toe shoes.
		    * Assess fit of jewelry (e.g., toe ring).
		    * Avoid extreme temperature changes.
		• Activity/mobility/exercise
		  – Encourage ambulation, emphasize importance of changing position, and avoid crossing legs or sitting at a 90° angle.
		  – Elevate legs when sitting for a long period.
		• Air travel
		  – Consider wearing compression hosiery.
		  – Ambulate as often as possible.
		  – Request a seat with enough leg room.

(Continued on next page)

Table 5-4. Nursing Care for the Patient Undergoing Gynecologic Surgery *(Continued)*

Potential Problems/Side Effects	Intervention and Rationale	Patient Education and Instruction
Changes in body image and sexuality	Encourage patient to express feelings. Acknowledge that patient may see body differently. Discuss patient concerns about sexuality and plan ways to manage the problem. Review potential side effects (e.g., hormonal changes, vaginal changes, dyspareunia, decreased sexual interest, arousal, and satisfaction).	Instruct patient regarding: • Referrals to pelvic floor physical therapist and women's health sexual therapist • Exploring other methods of expression (hand-holding and hugs) See information under radiation.

Note. Based on information from Almadrones-Cassidy, 2010; Armer et al., 2017; Mann, 2017.

and how to manage its side effects. Nursing management for patients who receive either external beam RT or brachytherapy to the pelvis is outlined in Table 5-7.

Common Complications in Gynecologic Cancers

The common potential complications that patients with GYN cancers may experience are based on the disease and treatment.

Infection

Women with GYN cancers are susceptible to infections for a multitude of reasons. The tumor may cause pressure on or invade the structures of adjacent organs, including the peritoneal space, intestines, and bladder or rectovaginal walls. Surgical excision, lymph node removal, urinary- or bowel-diversion techniques, or the use of indwelling devices can increase the susceptibility to infection. The use of antineoplastic therapies and combination biologic therapies can affect the immune system's ability to detect and respond to infections. Drug-induced mucositis and skin breakdown related to chemotherapy or RT can also increase the susceptibility to infections. The female genital tract is rich in anaerobic microflora and normal vaginal bacteria that can become problematic in

Table 5-5. Potential Side Effects for Chemotherapy and Biologic Therapy Agents

Drug Class	Agent	Side Effects
Alkylating agents	Carboplatin (Paraplatin®)	Hypersensitivity reactions Less renal toxicity than cisplatin Myelosuppression Nausea and vomiting (moderate)
	Cisplatin (Platinol®)	Hypersensitivity reactions Hypomagnesemia Hypocalcemia Hypokalemia Myelosuppression Nausea and vomiting (high) Nephrotoxicity Neurotoxicity Ototoxicity
	Cyclophosphamide (Cytoxan®)	Alopecia Anorexia Hemorrhagic cystitis Myelosuppression Nausea and vomiting (high/moderate; dose dependent) Ovarian failure Secondary malignancy
	Ifosfamide (Ifex®)	Alopecia Hemorrhagic cystitis (to prevent, administer mesna) Methylene blue used to treat ifosfamide-induced encephalopathy Myelosuppression Nausea and vomiting (moderate) Neurotoxicity
Antibiotic agents	Bleomycin (Blenoxane®)	Fever and chills Hypersensitivity reactions Mucositis Nausea and vomiting (minimal) Photosensitivity Pulmonary, renal, and hepatic toxicity
	Dactinomycin (actinomycin D, Cosmegen®)	Alopecia Diarrhea Hepatic and renal toxicity Mucositis Myelosuppression Nausea and vomiting (moderate) Ovarian suppression Radiation recall

(Continued on next page)

Table 5-5. Potential Side Effects for Chemotherapy and Biologic Therapy Agents *(Continued)*

Drug Class	Agent	Side Effects
Antibiotic agents *(cont.)*	Doxorubicin (Adriamycin®)	Alopecia Cardiotoxicity Hepatotoxicity Mucositis Myelosuppression Nausea and vomiting (high/moderate; dose dependent) Photosensitivity Radiation recall Red urine
	Liposomal doxorubicin (Doxil®)	Alopecia Cardiotoxicity Electrolyte changes Mucositis Myelosuppression Nausea and vomiting (low) Palmar-plantar erythrodysesthesia Photosensitivity Radiation recall Red urine
	Mitomycin (Mutamycin®)	Alopecia Anorexia Congestive heart failure (doses > 30 mg/m^2) Fatigue Mucositis Myelosuppression Nausea and vomiting (low) Pulmonary and renal toxicity
Antimetabolite agents	5-Fluorouracil (Adrucil®)	Alopecia Anorexia Darkening of veins Diarrhea Mucositis Myelosuppression Nausea and vomiting (low) Ocular toxicity Photosensitivity

(Continued on next page)

Table 5-5. Potential Side Effects for Chemotherapy and Biologic Therapy Agents *(Continued)*

Drug Class	Agent	Side Effects
Antimetabolite agents *(cont.)*	Gemcitabine (Gemzar®)	Flu-like symptoms Myelosuppression Nausea and vomiting (low) Mucositis Rash Peripheral edema Pulmonary toxicity; infused longer than 30 minutes can increase pulmonary toxicity
	Methotrexate (Mexate®)	Avoid multivitamins with folic acid. For high dose, monitor methotrexate level and hydrate. Mucositis Myelosuppression Nausea and vomiting (minimal: ≤ 50 mg/m^2, low: > 50 to < 250 mg/m^2; moderate: ≥ 250 mg/m^2) Photosensitivity Renal, hepatic, and neurologic toxicity
Camptothecins	Irinotecan (Camptosar®)	Alopecia Diarrhea Fever Increased bilirubin Mucositis Myelosuppression Nausea and vomiting (moderate) Weakness
	Topotecan (Hycamtin®)	Alopecia Fatigue Headache Interstitial lung disease Myelosuppression Nausea and vomiting (low)
Plant alkaloids (vinca alkaloids)	Docetaxel (Taxotere®)	Alopecia Fluid retention Hypersensitivity reactions Mucositis Myelosuppression Nausea and vomiting (low) Skin/nail changes

(Continued on next page)

Table 5-5. Potential Side Effects for Chemotherapy and Biologic Therapy Agents *(Continued)*

Drug Class	Agent	Side Effects
Plant alkaloids (vinca alkaloids) *(cont.)*	Etoposide (VP-16, Toposar®)	Alopecia Anorexia Myelosuppression Nausea and vomiting (low) Hypotension
	Paclitaxel (Taxol®)	Alopecia Cardiotoxicity Diarrhea Facial flushing Fatigue Hypersensitivity reactions Mucositis Myalgia Myelosuppression Nausea and vomiting (low) Peripheral neuropathy
	Vinorelbine (Navelbine®)	Alopecia Constipation Myelosuppression Nausea and vomiting (minimal) Neurologic and hepatic toxicities
Monoclonal antibodies	Bevacizumab (Avastin®)	Congestive heart failure Diarrhea Hemorrhage Hypertension Hyponatremia Leukopenia Nausea and vomiting (minimal) Proteinuria Thromboembolism
Hormonal therapy	Tamoxifen (Nolvadex®)	Hot flashes Hypercalcemia Menstrual irregularity Nausea and vomiting Vaginal discharge/bleeding

(Continued on next page)

Table 5-5. Potential Side Effects for Chemotherapy and Biologic Therapy Agents *(Continued)*		
Drug Class	**Agent**	**Side Effects**
Small-molecule kinase inhibitor	Temsirolimus (Torisel®)	Anorexia Asthenia Bowel perforations Edema Elevated alkaline phosphate, aspartate aminotransferase Elevated creatinine Hyperglycemia Hyperlipidemia Hypersensitivity reactions Hypertriglyceridemia Hypophosphatemia Interstitial lung disease Lymphopenia Mucositis Myelosuppression Nausea and vomiting (minimal) Opportunistic infections Rash

Note. Based on information from National Comprehensive Cancer Network, 2017a; Polovich et al., 2014.

those with GYN malignancies who are undergoing treatment. The nurse's ability to detect early signs and symptoms of infections is imperative in helping prevent sepsis. Infection leading to sepsis is a common reason for patient admission to the intensive care unit.

Tumor-Related Infections

Dependent on the anatomic location and the extent of the tumor, infections can arise at local tumor sites or in the deep pelvic structures. Some infections can present as ovarian or pelvic abscesses and endometritis. Other infections associated with tumor effect on adjacent structures include pyelonephritis, renal abscesses, or peritonitis. Life-threatening infections, such as pneumonia, peritonitis, and septicemia, hold the highest mortality rate for all cancer types. Because of faster detection of infections and the use of broad-spectrum antibiotics, the overall mortality rate has steadily declined in the last two decades; however, the spread of multidrug-resistant organisms may mitigate these advances (Safdar, Rolston, Bennett, Press, & Armstrong, 2013).

Surgery-Related Infections

Some patients undergo advanced surgeries, such as pelvic exenteration and tumor debulking, in which infection can be a serious complication. Women can

Table 5-6. Unique Nursing Considerations for Intraperitoneal Chemotherapy

Rationale for Intraperitoneal (IP) Chemotherapy: IP chemotherapy delivers a higher concentration and a longer half-life of the chemotherapy in the peritoneal space compared with IV therapy. Clinical trials have documented a survival benefit over IV chemotherapy alone in select patients with ovarian cancer.

Potential Problems/ Side Effects	Intervention and Rationale	Patient Education and Instruction
Abdominal distension/ pain	Assess abdomen prior to therapy. Assess for pain using the 0–10 scale. • If pain occurs during infusion, slow the infusion until discomfort stops. • Administer pain medications as needed/ordered.	Eat a light meal. Wear comfortable, loose-fitting clothes. Turn side-to-side post-therapy. Increase ambulation.
Dyspnea	Assess pretreatment respiratory status. Provide emotional support and help patient understand that this is a temporary side effect.	Report difficulty breathing. Use measures to relieve shortness of breath. • Elevate head of bed. • Sit upright. Increase ambulation.
Electrolyte imbalance	Monitor electrolytes (e.g., magnesium, potassium, calcium) and administer replacement electrolytes as ordered. Assess for signs and symptoms of hypomagnesemia, hypokalemia, and hypocalcemia.	Instruct patient about diet and supplements.
Frequent urination	Monitor voiding pattern.	Inform patient of this side effect. • Void prior to treatment. • Call if normal urination pattern does not return within 48 hours.
Infection	Assess port site. Monitor vital signs.	Report signs and symptoms of infection.

Note. Based on information from Anastasia, 2012; Huffman et al., 2015; Hydzik, 2007; Marin et al., 2007; National Cancer Institute, 2006; National Comprehensive Cancer Network, 2017a, 2017b, 2017c; Polovich et al., 2014; Potter & Held-Warmkessel, 2008.

Table 5-7. Nursing Care for the Patient Receiving External Beam Radiation Therapy

Potential Problems/ Side Effects	Intervention and Rationale	Patient Education and Instruction
Radiation dermatitis	Assess for risk factors (patient/treatment). Assess skin at least weekly or if patient reports symptoms. Assess for erythema, folliculitis (inflammation of hair follicles, presenting as itchy, raised, red rash), hyperpigmentation, dry desquamation (dryness and itching), moist desquamation (loss of epidermis, exposed dermis, serous exudate, pain), and discomfort; a grading scale is helpful (see National Cancer Institute Cancer Therapy Evaluation Program, 2010). Assess for signs or symptoms of infection. Culture the wound if the possibility of an infection is suspected. Based on skin assessment, institute skin management plan.	Instruct patient regarding: • Adequate nutritional intake • Skin care • Gentle washing of skin with tepid water and mild perfume-free soap, using soft washcloth • Wearing loose-fitting, soft cotton clothing • Using skin-care products without perfume or lanolin • Avoiding scratching skin • Protecting skin from extreme temperatures (hot/cold) • Not using adhesive tape or bandages in the treatment field • Swimming, as it is OK for intact skin • Using sunscreen (SPF 30 or higher) • Caring for skin reactions • Calling healthcare professionals when necessary
Change in urinary symptoms: Cystitis	Assess patient's bladder function, patterns of urinary elimination (e.g., symptoms of urgency, frequency, dysuria, nocturia), and history of urinary tract infections. Assess labs. Assess for fever. Obtain urine for a urinalysis and urine culture and sensitivity. Administer anti-inflammatory agent, antibiotic therapy, antispasmodics, or anticholinergic drugs if indicated and ordered.	Instruct patient regarding: • Signs and symptoms will subside gradually within 2–8 weeks following completion of radiation • Maintaining adequate amount of fluid intake (1–2 L/day) • Avoiding foods that irritate the bladder mucosa (e.g., caffeine [coffee, tea], spicy foods, alcohol, chocolate) • Monitoring urinary output • Reporting signs and symptoms of bladder irritation, dysuria, urgency with decreased urine volume, and signs of hematuria • When to notify healthcare professionals

(Continued on next page)

Table 5-7. Nursing Care for the Patient Receiving External Beam Radiation Therapy *(Continued)*

Potential Problems/ Side Effects	Intervention and Rationale	Patient Education and Instruction
Change in bowel: Diarrhea	Assess patient's bowel pattern. Assess frequency and amount of diarrhea using a scale (see National Cancer Institute Cancer Therapy Evaluation Program, 2010). Administer antidiarrheal medication as ordered. Assess for signs and symptoms of dehydration. Monitor weight and chemistries. Assess patient's nutrition status and refer to a nutritionist as needed. Administer IV hydration as ordered. Obtain stool culture as ordered.	Instruct patient regarding: • Encouraging oral intake • Dietary changes – Low-residue diet – Avoidance of caffeine products, sweets, highly seasoned or greasy foods, and extreme temperature changes – Small, frequent meals • Medications (psyllium, antidiarrheal, anti-inflammatory, or antispasmodic) • Care of perianal skin (i.e., sitz bath [clean after each bowel movement and apply a barrier cream]) • When to notify healthcare professionals
Change in vaginal mucous membranes: • Atrophy • Dryness • Shortening • Stenosis	Assess for vaginal discharge. Assess for pruritus. Assess for dyspareunia. Assess the potential for estrogen depletion. Assess the impact on sexual activity and satisfaction.	Instruct patient regarding: • Preparing patient/partner of possible side effect • Importance of cleansing vaginal area with warm water and mild soap, and patting skin with towel to dry • Sitz bath as needed • Keeping skin free from moisture • Wearing loose-fitting, soft cotton clothing • Applying corticosteroid and/or antibiotic if indicated and as ordered • Using vaginal moisturizers several times a week to improve tissue quality and comfort, thus improving vaginal health • Using vaginal lubricants during intercourse to minimize dryness, pain, irritation, or mucosal tears

(Continued on next page)

Table 5-7. Nursing Care for the Patient Receiving External Beam Radiation Therapy *(Continued)*		
Potential Problems/ Side Effects	Intervention and Rationale	Patient Education and Instruction
Change in vaginal mucous membranes *(cont.)*		• Use of vaginal and estrogen therapy as indicated • Pelvic floor exercises • Use of vaginal dilators (4–6 weeks after radiation therapy) • When to notify healthcare professionals

Note. Based on information from Gosselin et al., 2017; Iwamoto et al., 2012; McQuestion, 2011; Thorpe et al., 2017; Wong et al., 2013.

experience wound infections with dehiscence, urinary fistulas with urinary tract infections, and pelvic abscesses. With postradical vulvar resections and inguinal lymph node dissections, a high rate of site-related cellulitis with or without lymphedema exists. Intra-abdominal and pelvic abscesses can also be caused by tumor necrosis, surgical instrumentation, reconstruction, or prosthetic devices. Identifying the symptoms of infection early and obtaining blood cultures and site-specific cultures are critical. Prompt initiation of antibiotics that target organisms that commonly originate in the intestinal or cutaneous areas is key to eradicating the infection.

Chemotherapy- and Radiation-Related Infections

Patients who receive chemotherapy have an increased risk of infection, most commonly because of neutropenia. Neutropenia for less than one week in the GYN oncology population is associated with infections caused by *Staphylococcus aureus*, *Pseudomonas*, *Escherichia coli*, and coliform bacterium. Patients with neutropenia that lasts for longer than five to seven days are at an additional risk for infections of fungal origin, such as the *Candida* species (Safdar et al., 2013). Patients with severe neutropenia are at high risk for severe morbidity and mortality unless IV antibiotics are initiated at the first evidence of clinical signs or fever. Implantable devices, such as centrally located infusion catheters and peritoneal infusion ports, are possible sites for infections. The most common organism to infect implanted venous catheters is gram-negative bacteria. In patients with oral mucositis, streptococcal infections are common. Radiation can cause microvascular damage to the tissues, which can lead to further difficulties in treating these infections (Safdar et al., 2013). Growth factor use has been a monumental reason for decreased chemotherapy-associated infections over the past decade. Additional common infections include urinary tract, wound sites, cellulitis, peritonitis, and fasciitis.

Nursing Implications

Nursing plays a critical role in assessing early and late signs and symptoms of infection. Nurses should be familiar with monitoring for redness, swelling, drainage, pain, bleeding, and temperature changes. Monitoring vital signs for tachycardia, hypotension, changes in respiratory rate, and temperature increase or decrease is crucial for the detection of possible sepsis. Laboratory values, such as complete blood counts with a differential count, should be routinely done, as well as notifying the provider of abnormal laboratory values. Drawing blood cultures and cultures of other relevant possible infection sites as ordered should be done promptly so that antimicrobial therapy administration can be initiated. Please refer to Chapter 12 for further information regarding sepsis management.

Stroke and Cardiac Complications

It is estimated that the incidence of stroke is less than 1% following GYN oncology surgery (Obermair, Ibeanu, Janial, Armstrong, & Bristow, 2013). General risk factors for stroke, such as a history of prior strokes, transient ischemic attacks, atherosclerosis, hypertension, diabetes, and the administration of some biotherapy agents, apply to the oncology population as well (Ng, Chan, & Gelb, 2011). Cardiac complications during and following GYN surgery are estimated to be between 0.5% and 3% (Obermair et al., 2013). The administration of cardiac protective medications, prevention of hypotension, maintenance of normothermia, and postoperative troponin blood levels are commonly used in practice for cardiac protection and detection of cardiac status. Chemotherapy drugs used for GYN malignancies (e.g., anthracyclines such as doxorubicin) can cause cardiotoxicity over time. Increased toxicity that can lead to chronic heart failure is usually seen after a lifetime cumulative dose of doxorubicin greater than 550 mg/m^2 (Mutch, Yashar, Markman, & Rubin, 2005). Cardioprotective agents, such as dexrazoxane, are often started at a lifetime cumulative dose of 300 mg/m^2 (Mutch et al., 2005). A chemotherapy/biotherapy hypersensitivity reaction can cause cardiac strain, and patients should be monitored for cardiac events.

Nursing plays a critical role in assessing for neurologic and cardiac changes. Neurologic and cardiac assessments are critical after surgery. Mental status changes, signs of stroke, and cardiac changes should be immediately discussed with the healthcare provider. Nurses should be educated regarding the increased use of some biotherapy treatment options associated with stroke, cardiac events, or bleeding.

Hemorrhage

Intraoperative hemorrhage is defined as a blood loss of greater than 1,000 ml or if an intraoperative blood transfusion is necessary (Vergote et al., 2010).

Patients undergoing surgery for GYN malignancies, such as ovarian cancer, have a 4%–7.5% chance of hemorrhage (Vergote et al., 2010). The use of bevacizumab may contribute to the increased chance of bowel perforation or hemorrhage and may need to be discontinued 28 days prior to any invasive procedures.

Patients need to be assessed for bleeding around the tumor sites within the abdomen and the wound sites and have vital signs monitored. Chemotherapy can reduce platelets, which can lead to bleeding. Complete blood counts are monitored for thrombocytopenia.

Bowel Obstruction and Perforation

Patients with GYN cancers are at risk for small and large bowel obstructions throughout their disease course. Postoperative small bowel obstructions can be from a mechanical block, adhesions, and tumors on the bowel or intussusceptions. Prompt recognition and management of small bowel obstructions are imperative to prevent bowel ischemia and necrosis. Because of the location of GYN tumors in the abdomen, pressure on any area of the bowel can cause the bowel to crimp or obstruct. It is estimated that as many as half of all women with ovarian cancer develop intermittent or actual bowel obstructions during the disease course. A bowel obstruction may be the first sign that disease has recurred. In most cases, the cause of the bowel obstruction is from the progressive growth of the tumor near or on the outer lining of the bowel. The presence of peritoneal carcinomatosis throughout the abdomen may increase the risk of bowel perforations in this population. Interventions may include bowel rest with nasogastric suction or surgical interventions. Bowel perforation is one of the top indicators that critical care management is needed.

Presenting symptoms often include nausea and vomiting, abdominal pain, cramping, distension, diarrhea, constipation, and obstipation. Bowel sounds may be high pitched or absent, and the healthcare provider should be notified. An abdominal x-ray, upright and flat plate, or computed tomography scan will be ordered for diagnosis. If the bowel is obstructed, the radiographic films will show multiple dilated loops of bowel and the appearance of air fluid levels. The patient should be given nothing by mouth, and once asymptomatic, the patient can often resume eating with clear liquids and should be assessed for tolerability. Slow advancement to full liquids and solid foods can occur if obstruction does not return. If hospitalized, the patient should be given nothing by mouth, and a bowel decompression should be instituted by placement of a nasogastric tube to suction. IV hydration and nutrition must be provided. If these actions do not help resolve the obstruction, a surgical intervention may be required (e.g., a resection of adhesions, a colostomy, the placing of a percutaneous endoscopic gastrostomy tube).

Pulmonary Toxicity

Multiple chemotherapy agents used for GYN malignancies can cause pulmonary fibrosis. Some of the agents, such as bleomycin (germ cell tumors) and gemcitabine (ovarian tumors), are known to cause pulmonary toxicity. Prior to the administration of bleomycin, a pulmonary function test, including carbon monoxide diffusing capacity testing, should be completed. These tests should be repeated if the patient develops any symptoms, such as cough, dyspnea, crackles on lung examination, or abnormal test imaging. The mainstay of pulmonary fibrosis treatment is corticosteroids; however, these have little to no effect on established fibrotic lesions (Obermair et al., 2013). Pleural effusions can be the initial symptom that leads a female patient to an ovarian cancer diagnosis and can occur later in the disease course. Approximately 25%–30% of patients with ovarian cancer will develop a pleural effusion (Eriksson & Frazier, 2000). When fluid builds rapidly in the pleural space, the patient can become symptomatic and rapidly advance to respiratory failure. Symptoms include shortness of breath, hypoxia, cough, and pleuritic chest pain. A diagnosis is made from markedly decreased breath sounds and confirmation via x-ray with anteroposterior and lateral views. Patients may commonly require a thoracentesis or the placement of a chest tube to prevent respiratory compromise. For recurring pleural effusions, sclerosing agents may be used to help prevent further accumulation, although it is estimated that fluid tends to rebuild quickly without cancer treatment. A pulmonary embolism can be a minor or fatal event in patients with cancer. A new onset of pulmonary symptoms, including acute chest pain or pleuritic chest pain, warrants immediate evaluation and diagnostics for a possible pulmonary embolism. Patient oxygen saturations may be low, requiring oxygen or advanced ventilation.

Knowledge of a patient's history of pulmonary embolisms or deep vein thrombosis is helpful. Change in the patient's respiratory status, color, breath sounds, and vital signs should be reported immediately (Safdar et al., 2013). Patients with complaints of pleuritic chest pain or lower-extremity pain should be tested for the presence of a thrombosis. Preventive measures, such as ambulation, range-of-motion exercise, venodynes, and anticoagulants, are helpful in thrombosis prevention.

Malnutrition

Many patients with cancer suffer from malnourishment at some time throughout the disease or treatment course. Up to 85% of patients experience weight loss or malnutrition during the cancer journey (Sauer & Voss, 2012). Because rapid tumor growth increases metabolic demands, the body uses accelerated methods to provide energy. These changes can lead to protein loss, nitrogen imbalances, and altered insulin use. GYN cancers can cause mechanical types of cachexia because of abdominal distension by ascites or tumor compression of the bowel. Chemotherapy and RT can cause nausea and appetite suppression, leading to decreased oral intake. IP chemotherapy can temporarily compete for space in the abdomen and may cause a decreased appetite around the time of administration. The psychological effects of cancer are associated with anxiety, depression, and the feeling of loss of control. These can lead to a sustained loss of appetite or anorexia.

Anorexia can cause chronic muscle wasting, hypoalbuminemia, and potential drug metabolism issues. The use of dietary supplements, appetite stimulants, and total parenteral nutrition may support nutritional needs.

Patients should be assessed for signs and symptoms of malnutrition. Referrals to dietitians may be indicated for nutrition advice. Signs and symptoms of malnutrition include dry, flaky skin that bruises easily; hair changes; bleeding gums; dull or dark sunken eyes; muscle wasting; and confusion. Blood albumin levels should be routinely drawn to assess for hypoalbuminemia. Patients with chemotherapy-induced nausea and vomiting are at high risk of malnutrition, requiring early referrals to dietitians (Davidson et al., 2012). Nursing interventions include providing the patient with some dietary advice, such as consuming small, frequent, high-protein meals.

Gastrointestinal Toxicity

GYN cancers are treated with multiagent chemotherapies and are associated with some degree of gastrointestinal toxicity, such as nausea and vomiting and anorexia. Chemotherapy-induced nausea and vomiting is one of the most distressing acute side effects of cancer treatment, occurring in up to 80% of patients (NCI, 2015b). Nausea is classified into three categories: anticipatory, acute onset, and delayed (ACS, 2017b). Anticipatory nausea occurs prior to the actual chemotherapy administration and should be treated with antiemetic medications prior to the patient's entrance into the chemotherapy area. Acute nausea begins within one hour of chemotherapy administration, and delayed nausea occurs more than 24 hours after chemotherapy administration (ACS, 2017b). The aggressive uses of antiemetics are tailored to the emetic potential of the treatment. Because GYN cancers are commonly treated with moderate or high emetogenic chemotherapy regimens, multiple antiemetics are indicated. Despite antiemetics, some patients may still experience nausea and vomiting, leading to dehydration and electrolyte imbalances. Dehydration is a common acute complication in these patients. Additional gastrointestinal toxicities caused by chemotherapy and RT include oral mucositis, esophagitis, gastroenteritis, diarrhea, and constipation. Nurses are familiar with assessing and intervening in common complaints of bowel changes. Diarrhea should be graded, and aggressive use of antidiarrheal agents should be implemented. Constipation can occur because of the use of antiemetics, pain medications, and mechanical obstructions. Stool softeners and laxatives are often clinically indicated to treat constipation.

Oral cavity assessment and nausea and vomiting and diarrhea grading should be completed prior to chemotherapy or RT administration (Safdar et al., 2013). Any concerns should be brought to the healthcare provider for intervention. Chemotherapy, biotherapy, or RT may need to be reduced or held, dependent on the extent of toxicity. Behavioral modifications, antiemetic drugs, bowel medications, and oral protective agents should be administered as ordered to help prevent further advancement of gastrointestinal toxicities. Dietary education should be provided for both diarrhea and constipation management. Hydration and electrolyte repletion is often indicated in patients treated for GYN malignancies.

Ascites

Ascites commonly develops in the presence of advanced ovarian malignancies and occurs because of tumor implants blocking or impeding normal peritoneal lymph flow and the increased fluid production in the abdomen. For women with ovarian cancer, ascites can cause continual pressure, pain, and diminished pulmonary capacity, which can significantly affect activities of daily living (Obermair et al., 2013). These patients often experience symptoms of early satiety or anorexia.

Assessment for ascites includes a review of the patient's symptoms, measurement of abdominal girth, percussion of the abdomen, and detection of the fluid wave. In the presence of ascites, dullness is heard in the flanks and tympany resonates in the middle abdomen. Fluid shifts may be seen with as little as 500 ml of ascites fluid buildup when the patient repositions from side to side. Preparation for paracentesis may include prothrombin time/international normalized ratio, complete blood count, and ultrasound marking. In addition, possible insertion of a permanent drainage catheter may be needed for those who require frequent removal of ascites or for comfort measures.

Hepatotoxicity and Renal Toxicity

During the disease course, multiple chemotherapy agents are used for treatment. Many of these agents can strain the liver and kidneys. Routine serum laboratory testing for liver function tests, such as bilirubin, aspartate aminotransferase, alanine aminotransferase, and alkaline phosphatase, should be drawn prior to the administration of hepatotoxic chemotherapy agents. Doses of chemotherapy agents may have to be reduced or not given if liver function tests are elevated. Platinum chemotherapy agents, such as carboplatin and cisplatin, are a mainstay of therapy for many GYN cancers and can be highly renal toxic. Serum creatinine levels and glomerular filtration rate are used both for dosing the agents and in deciding whether the agent should be administered.

Nurses should be familiar with assessing for signs and symptoms of liver abnormalities, such as jaundice, bleeding, abdominal swelling, disorientation, and sleepiness. Drawing liver function tests as ordered and notifying the healthcare provider of abnormalities are nursing assessments.

Nurses should also be comfortable assessing for signs and symptoms of renal abnormalities, such as swelling, vomiting, decreased urinary output, and weakness. Drawing kidney tests, such as blood urea nitrogen and creatinine, as ordered, and notifying the healthcare provider of abnormalities is expected. Patients who decompensate into renal failure may need access to an intensive care unit that can provide dialysis.

Neurotoxicity

Taxanes, platinum analogs, and vinca alkaloids are treatment mainstays for many GYN cancers. Some of the drugs, such as paclitaxel, docetaxel, carboplatin, cisplatin, vincristine, and etoposide, are given as standard treatment and can cause peripheral neuropathy (PN). Chemotherapy-induced PN is often a dose-limiting toxicity of cisplatin and paclitaxel. PN may warrant pharmacologic interventions with medications such as alpha 2-adrenergic agonists, anticonvulsants, antidepressants, corticosteroids, or anesthetic medications.

Nurses should obtain a patient's subjective report of symptoms, pain, and influence on activities of daily living as well as a complete neurologic physical assessment. Abnormal findings should be communicated to the healthcare provider prior to chemotherapy administration. Safety should be addressed and education should be provided to the patient regarding fall prevention and adaptive environmental changes that can be implemented in the home.

Pain

Two of the most complex problems in patients with advanced GYN disease are the fear and management of pain. It is estimated that 75% of patients with cancer will have unrelieved pain at some point with advanced disease (Thapa, Rastogi, & Ahuja, 2011). Some causes of pain in this population include cancer infiltrating the bone, nerve infiltration, PN, adhesions, radiation fibrosis, surgery, tumor pressure, abdominal distension, swelling, and bowel, vaginal, or ureter fistula development.

Assessing the patient's pain and advocating for pain management are essential responsibilities. Successful cancer pain management can be achieved with nonpharmacologic and pharmacologic interventions. Cancer pain and its management has been extensively studied over the past 10 years. A nurse's role in pain medication selection and follow-up pain-relief assessments, including balancing side effects, is critical. Patient education should consist of treatment scheduling, common side effects, and strategies to promote adherence. Nonpharmacologic pain management can include massage, deep breathing, alternating heat and cold, biofeedback, music or art therapy, and acupuncture. The use of short- or long-acting, transdermal, and continuous-infusion pain medications can help successfully relieve continuous pain.

Hypersensitivity Reactions

The risk of severe hypersensitivity reactions and related negative health effects remains a valid concern. Patients with GYN cancer receive chemotherapy agents such as carboplatin, cisplatin, paclitaxel, docetaxel, and etoposide, all of which are associated with a high risk of hypersensitivity reactions. The frequency of hypersensitivity reactions to drugs has risen over the last 10 years because of increased exposure and the use of better and more allergenic medications to help manage them (Castells Guitart, 2014). This population will be premedicated with the use of antihistamines, leukotriene blockers, and corticosteroids prior to high-risk chemotherapy administration. Although these medications are used to prevent hypersensitivity reactions, they still occur frequently. Some of the common platinum hypersensitivity reaction symptoms include diffuse erythroderma, tachycardia, chest tightness, wheezing, facial swelling, dyspnea, hypertension, or hypotension (Markman et al., 1999). The use of desensitization or graded infusion regimens for platinum agents is becoming an increasingly common practice, and conversion to an extended infusion schedule is often done prophylactically (O'Cearbhaill et al., 2010).

Nurses need to be aware of the common agents associated with hypersensitivity reactions and implement close monitoring for signs and symptoms, such as facial flushing, palmar/plantar redness, shortness of breath, tachycardia, hypertension, hypotension, hives, nausea and vomiting, or a feeling of impending doom. On recognition of the symptoms, the nurse needs to immediately stop the causative agent, notify the healthcare provider, administer rescue medications, monitor vital signs, and reassure the patient. Hypersensitivity reactions can be mild to fatal and should always be taken seriously and treated aggressively. Because these agents are some of the most effective treatments for GYN malignancies, patients may be rechallenged or a desensitization or graded infusion may be used.

Suggested Reading

Markman, M., & Walker, J.L. (2006). Intraperitoneal chemotherapy of ovarian cancer: A review, with a focus on practical aspects of treatment. *Journal of Clinical Oncology, 24,* 988–994.

Robinson, J.B., Singh, D., Bodurka-Bevers, D.C., Wharton, J.T., Gershenson, D.M., & Wolf, J.K. (2001). Hypersensitivity reactions and the utility of oral and intravenous desensitization in patients with gynecologic malignancies. *Gynecologic Oncology, 82,* 550–558. doi:10.1006/gyno .2001.6331

Society of Gynecologic Oncology. (n.d.). SGO genetics toolkit. Retrieved from http://www.sgo.org /genetics

Spriggs, D.R. (2012). Drug development for chronic cancers: Time to think differently? *Journal of Clinical Oncology, 30,* 3779–3780. doi:10.1200/JCO.2012.42.3269

Summary

GYN malignancy remains a considerable risk for the U.S. female population. These patients need recognition of their vague symptoms, prompt diagnosis, and a treatment plan within a reasonable time frame. Many critical issues are specific to this patient population and need to be managed effectively. Nurses remain the frontline critical component in caring for these patients and making a difference in each patient's cancer journey. Nurses play an essential role in improving the quality of care for women with GYN cancers—whatever the type of treatment. Healthcare providers and patients can be directed to Internet sites that will provide additional information related to their cancers, the treatment, and possible clinical trials for which they may be eligible (see Figure 5-2).

Figure 5-2. Resources Related to Women With Gynecologic Cancer

- American Society for Radiation Oncology: www.astro.org
- American Society of Clinical Oncology: www.asco.org
- Gynecologic Cancer Foundation: www.thegcf.org
- Gynecologic Oncology Group: www.gog.org
- National Cancer Institute: www.cancer.gov
- National Comprehensive Cancer Network®: www.nccn.org
- National Lymphedema Network: www.lymphnet.org/le-faqs/nln-position-papers
- Oncology Nursing Society: www.ons.org
- Ovarian Cancer Research Fund Alliance: https://ocrfa.org
- Society of Gynecologic Nurse Oncologists: www.sgno.org
- Society of Gynecologic Oncology: www.sgo.org

Funding for this work comes from the Memorial Sloan Kettering Cancer Center Support Grant/Core Grant (P30 CA008748).

References

Almadrones-Cassidy, L. (Ed.). (2010). *Site-specific cancer series: Gynecologic cancers.* Pittsburgh, PA: Oncology Nursing Society.

American Cancer Society. (2017a). *Cancer facts and figures 2017.* Retrieved from https://www.cancer.org/content/dam/cancer-org/research/cancer-facts-and-statistics/annual-cancer-facts-and-figures/2017/cancer-facts-and-figures-2017.pdf

American Cancer Society. (2017b). Chemotherapy-related nausea and vomiting. Retrieved from https://www.cancer.org/treatment/treatments-and-side-effects/physical-side-effects/nausea-and-vomiting/chemo-and-nausea-vomiting.html

Anastasia, P. (2012). Intraperitoneal chemotherapy for ovarian cancer. *Oncology Nursing Forum, 39,* 346–349. doi:10.1188/12.ONF.346-349

Armer, J.M., Beck, M., Burns, B.R., Deng, J., Fu, M.R., Lockwood, S., … Poage, E.G. (2017, January 13). ONS putting evidence into practice: Lymphedema. Retrieved from https://www.ons.org/practice-resources/pep/lymphedema

Benard, V.B., Watson, M., Castle, P.E., & Saraiya, M. (2012). Cervical carcinoma rates among young females in the United States. *Obstetrics and Gynecology, 120,* 1117–1123.

Berkowitz, R.S., Goldstein, D.P., & Horowitz, N.S. (2016, September 12). Initial management of low-risk gestational trophoblastic neoplasia [Literature review current through August 2017]. Retrieved from https://www.uptodate.com/contents/initial-management-of-low-risk-gestational-trophoblastic-neoplasia

Berkowitz, R.S., Goldstein, D.P., & Horowitz, N.S. (2017, April 19). Gestational trophoblastic neoplasia: Epidemiology, clinical features, diagnosis, staging, and risk stratification [Literature review current through August 2017]. Retrieved from http://www.uptodate.com/contents/gestational-trophoblastic-neoplasia-epidemiology-clinical-features-diagnosis-staging-and-risk-stratification

Cancer.Net. (2015). The genetics of cancer: About genes. Retrieved from http://www.cancer.net/navigating-cancer-care/cancer-basics/genetics/genetics-cancer

Castells Guitart, M.C. (2014). Rapid drug desensitization for hypersensitivity reactions to chemotherapy and monoclonal antibodies in the 21st century. *Journal of Investigational Allergology and Clinical Immunology, 24*, 72–79.

Davidson, W., Teleni, L., Muller, J., Ferguson, M., McCarthy, A.L., Vick, J., & Isenring, E. (2012). Malnutrition and chemotherapy-induced nausea and vomiting: Implications for practice [Online exclusive]. *Oncology Nursing Forum, 39*, E340–E345. doi:10.1188/12.ONF.E340-E345

Eriksson, J.H., & Frazier, S.R. (2000). Epithelial cancers of the ovary and fallopian tube. In G.J. Moore-Higgs (Ed.), *Women and cancer: A gynecologic oncology nursing perspective* (2nd ed., pp. 186–234). Burlington, MA: Jones & Bartlett Learning.

Foundation for Women's Cancer. (n.d.). About gynecologic cancers. Retrieved from http://www.foundationforwomenscancer.org/about-gynecologic-cancers

Gosselin, T., Beamer, L., Ciccolini, K., Merritt, C., Omabegho, M., Shaftic, A., & Lucas, A.S. (2017, May 10). ONS putting evidence into practice: Radiodermatitis. Retrieved from https://www.ons.org/practice-resources/pep/radiodermatitis

Huffman, L.B., Hartenbach, E.M., Carter, J., Rash, J.K., & Kushner, D.M. (2015). Maintaining sexual health throughout gynecologic cancer survivorship: A comprehensive review and clinical guide. *Gynecologic Oncology, 140*, 359–368. doi:10.1016/j.ygyno.2015.11.010

Hydzik, C. (2007). Implementation of intraperitoneal chemotherapy for the treatment of ovarian cancer. *Clinical Journal of Oncology Nursing, 11*, 221–225. doi:10.1188/07.CJON.221-225

Iwamoto, R.R., Haas, M.L., & Gosselin, T. (Eds.). (2012). *Manual for radiation oncology nursing practice and education* (4th ed.). Pittsburgh, PA: Oncology Nursing Society.

Karam, A., Berek, J.S., & Kidd, E.A. (2015, July 6). Vaginal cancer [Literature review current through August 2017]. Retrieved from http://www.uptodate.com/contents/vaginal-cancer

Karam, A., Berek, J.S., & Russo, A.L. (2016, September 6). Squamous cell carcinoma of the vulva: Staging and surgical treatment [Literature review current through August 2017]. Retrieved from http://www.uptodate.com/contents/squamous-cell-carcinoma-of-the-vulva-staging-and-surgical-treatment

Lancaster, J.M., Powell, C.B., Chen, L.-M., & Richardson, D.L. (2015). Society of Gynecologic Oncology statement on risk assessment for inherited gynecologic cancer predispositions. *Gynecologic Oncology, 136*, 3–7. doi:10.1016/j.ygyno.2014.09.009

Mann, J., Jr. (2017, April 27). Complications of gynecologic surgery [Literature review current through August 2017]. Retrieved from http://www.uptodate.com/contents/complications-of-gynecologic-surgery

Marin, K., Oleszewski, K., & Muehlbauer, P. (2007). Intraperitoneal chemotherapy: Implications beyond ovarian cancer. *Clinical Journal of Oncology Nursing, 11*, 881–889. doi:10.1188/CJON.07.881-889

Markman, M., Kennedy, A., Webster, K., Elson, P., Peterson, G., Kulp, B., & Belinson, J. (1999). Clinical features of hypersensitivity reactions to carboplatin. *Journal of Clinical Oncology, 17*, 1141.

McQuestion, M. (2011). Evidence-based skin care management in radiation therapy: Clinical update. *Seminars in Oncology Nursing, 27*, e1–e17. doi:10.1016/j.soncn.2011.02.009

Mutch, D.G., Yashar, C., Markman, M., & Rubin, S.C. (2005). Management of late effects of gynecologic cancer treatment. In W.J. Hoskins, C.A. Perez, R.C. Young, R. Barakat, M. Markman, & M. Randall (Eds.), *Principles and practice of gynecologic oncology* (4th ed., pp. 1132–1147). Philadelphia, PA: Wolters Kluwer Health/Lippincott Williams & Wilkins.

National Cancer Institute. (2006). *NCI clinical announcement: Intraperitoneal chemotherapy for ovarian cancer.* Retrieved from https://ctep.cancer.gov/highlights/docs/clin_annc_010506.pdf

National Cancer Institute. (2015a). HPV and cancer. Retrieved from https://www.cancer.gov/about-cancer/causes-prevention/risk/infectious-agents/hpv-fact-sheet

National Cancer Institute. (2015b). Nausea and vomiting (PDQ®) [Patient version]. Retrieved from https://www.cancer.gov/about-cancer/treatment/side-effects/nausea/nausea-pdq

National Cancer Institute Cancer Therapy Evaluation Program. (2010). *Common terminology criteria for adverse events* [v.4.03]. Retrieved from http://evs.nci.nih.gov/ftp1/CTCAE/About.html

National Comprehensive Cancer Network. (2016). *NCCN Clinical Practice Guidelines in Oncology (NCCN Guidelines®): Cervical cancer* [v.1.2017]. Retrieved from https://www.nccn.org/professionals/physician_gls/PDF/cervical.pdf

National Comprehensive Cancer Network. (2017a). *NCCN Clinical Practice Guidelines in Oncology (NCCN Guidelines®): Antiemesis* [v.2.2017]. Retrieved from http://www.nccn.org/professionals/physician_gls/pdf/antiemesis.pdf

National Comprehensive Cancer Network. (2017b). *NCCN Clinical Practice Guidelines in Oncology (NCCN Guidelines®): Ovarian cancer, including fallopian tube cancer and primary peritoneal cancer* [v.1.2017]. Retrieved from https://www.nccn.org/professionals/physician_gls/PDF/ovarian.pdf

National Comprehensive Cancer Network. (2017c). *NCCN Clinical Practice Guidelines in Oncology (NCCN Guidelines®): Uterine neoplasms* [v.2.2017]. Retrieved from https://www.nccn.org/professionals/physician_gls/pdf/uterine.pdf

Ng, J.L.W., Chan, M.T.V., & Gelb, A.W. (2011). Perioperative stroke in noncardiac, nonneurosurgical surgery. *Anesthesiology, 115,* 879–890. doi:10.1097/ALN.0b013e31822e9499

Obermair, A., Ibeanu, O.A., Janial, D.D., Armstrong, D.K., & Bristow, R.E. (2013). Management of acute and chronic complications of gynecological cancer treatment. In R.R. Barakat, A. Berchuck, M. Markman, & E. Randall (Eds.), *Principles and practice of gynecologic oncology* (6th ed., pp. 988–1002). Philadelphia, PA: Wolters Kluwer Health/Lippincott Williams & Wilkins.

O'Cearbhaill, R., Zhou, Q., Iasonos, A., Hensley, M.L., Tew, W.P., Aghajanian, C., ... Sabbatini, P.J. (2010). The prophylactic conversion to an extended infusion schedule and use of premedication to prevent hypersensitivity reactions in ovarian cancer patients during carboplatin retreatment. *Gynecologic Oncology, 116,* 326–331. doi:10.1016/j.ygyno.2009.10.070

Polovich, M., Olsen, M., & LeFebvre, K.B. (Eds.). (2014). *Chemotherapy and biotherapy guidelines and recommendations for practice* (4th ed.). Pittsburgh, PA: Oncology Nursing Society.

Potter, K.L., & Held-Warmkessel, J. (2008). Intraperitoneal chemotherapy for women with ovarian cancer: Nursing care and considerations. *Clinical Journal of Oncology Nursing, 12,* 265–271. doi:10.1188/08.CJON.265-271

Safdar, A., Rolston, K., Bennett, G.L., Press, R., & Armstrong, D. (2013). Management of infections in patients with gynecologic malignancy. In R.R. Barakat, A. Berchuck, M. Markman, & E. Randall (Eds.), *Principles and practice of gynecologic oncology* (6th ed., pp. 967–988). Philadelphia, PA: Wolters Kluwer Health/Lippincott Williams & Wilkins.

Sauer, A.C., & Voss, A.C. (2012). *Improving outcomes with nutrition in patients with cancer* [White paper]. Retrieved from https://pdfs.semanticscholar.org/0ec5/7525627045d98b134a4d9b65d5a664073250.pdf

Thapa, D., Rastogi, V., & Ahuja, V. (2011). Cancer pain management: Current status. *Journal of Anaesthesiology and Clinical Pharmacology, 27,* 162–168. doi:10.4103/0970-9185.81820

Thorpe, D.M., Byar, K.L., Conley, S., Drapek, L., Held-Warmkessel, J., Ramsdell, M.J., ... Wolles, B. (2017, February 27). ONS putting evidence into practice: Diarrhea. Retrieved from https://www.ons.org/practice-resources/pep/diarrhea

Vergote, I., Tropé, C.G., Amant, F., Kristensen, G.B., Ehlen, T., Johnson, N., ... Reed, N.S. (2010). Neoadjuvant chemotherapy or primary surgery in stage IIIC or IV ovarian cancer. *New England Journal of Medicine, 363,* 943–953. doi:10.1056/NEJMoa0908806

Wong, R.S., Bensadoum, R.-J., Boers-Doets, C.B., Bryce, J., Chan, A., Epstein, J.B., ... Lacouture, M.E. (2013). Clinical practice guidelines for the prevention and treatment of acute and late radiation reactions from the MASCC Skin Toxicity Study Group. *Supportive Care in Cancer, 21,* 2933–2948. doi:10.1007/s00520-013-1896-2

CHAPTER 6

Gastrointestinal Cancers

Lisa Parks, MS, ANP-BC

Introduction

Colorectal cancer is the fourth most common cancer, with the second highest mortality rate in the United States (Porpiglia & Sigurdson, 2015). Despite its commonness, its incidence has decreased over time because of advancements in screening and prevention with colonoscopy and flexible sigmoidoscopy. About 40% of patients with colorectal cancer will have local disease on presentation (Porpiglia & Sigurdson, 2015). These patients have a five-year survival rate of 66.5% (Porpiglia & Sigurdson, 2015).

Surgery is the recommended treatment for patients with nonmetastatic colon cancer. The standard of care is a colectomy with en bloc resection of regional lymph nodes. The goal of resection is 5 cm margins, both proximally and distally, with at least a sampling of 12 lymph nodes for cancer staging (Porpiglia & Sigurdson, 2015). Recently, laparoscopic and robotic surgery have been used for less invasive resection and quicker recovery.

Adjuvant chemotherapy is the standard of care for patients with high-risk stage II or stage III colon cancer after curative resection (Kumar et al., 2015). Side effects include nausea and vomiting, diarrhea, mucositis, hemorrhage, and gastrointestinal (GI) perforation. Stereotactic body radiation therapy (SBRT) toxicity is a concern when the tumor is near GI organs. GI ulceration and perforation can be seen with high-dose chemotherapy. With SBRT and anti–vascular endothelial growth factor agents, potential exists for late luminal GI side effects (e.g., perforation) (Pollom et al., 2015). The mechanism of late effects of radiation is generally considered to be related to fibrosis and endothelial abnormality. The intestine after radiation has decreased motility and is more prone to mechanical friction and damage.

Common Complications in Gastrointestinal Cancers

Anastomotic Leak and Sepsis

Anastomotic leak rates in colorectal surgery are 1%–21% with a mortality of 3%–22% (Landmann, 2014). An anastomotic leak is defined by postoperative timing (early vs. late), extent of anastomotic dehiscence, location (intraperitoneal vs. extraperitoneal), patient presentation, and degree of sepsis (uncontrolled leak vs. contained abscess). Patients who develop an anastomotic leak within the first week of surgery will have an atypical abdominal examination that will often include peritoneal signs. They may also experience increased abdominal pain, fever, decreased urinary output, leukocytosis, and tachycardia. A computed tomography (CT) scan may be performed to confirm the leak, but surgical reexploration may be the best treatment for patients with peritoneal symptoms. Reexploration is preferred within the first seven days after initial surgery because of less fibrinopurulent exudate and easier tissue dissection for operative field visualization (Sneider & Davids, 2014). Late anastomotic leak or an intraperitoneal abscess may develop in patients seven days after surgery. These patients will present with vague abdominal complaints, low-grade fever, an inability to tolerate an oral diet, and decreased urination. These leaks show on a CT scan as a contained abscess, which can be managed with drainage by radiology via aspiration or by the placement of an abscess drain and antibiotic administration. Drainage is recommended for abscesses greater than 4 cm in size with or without antibiotics (Sneider & Davids, 2014).

In the presence of hypotension or sepsis, an ileostomy is indicated to divert the source of fecal contamination. In an early anastomotic leak, repair of the primary anastomosis with ostomy diversion or a Hartmann procedure with exteriorization of both anastomotic endo or a redo anastomosis with proximal diversion is performed (Sneider & Davids, 2014).

Bevacizumab is a humanized monoclonal antibody that targets vascular endothelial growth factor A. This class of drugs restricts the neoangiogenesis necessary for tumor growth. Bevacizumab is associated with an increased incidence of postoperative complications, including impaired wound healing and anastomotic leak. It is also associated with late anastomotic complications (Sneider & Davids, 2014).

Sepsis is the systematic inflammatory response to infection associated with hypoperfusion and tissue injury. Prolonged hypotension and microvascular ischemia are predisposing factors for tissue ischemia and anastomotic failure. Rapid progression to septic shock is caused by inhibition of the sympathetic nervous system and the loss of baroreceptor reflex control of arterial blood pressure (Choudhuri & Uppal, 2013). Early initiation of broad-spectrum antibiotics is essential for sepsis treatment (Sartelli et al., 2013). Cultures should be taken to assess for fungi and atypical organisms. *Pseudomonas*, *Enterococci*, and *Staphylococci* infections are difficult to treat because of antibiotic resistance and carry a high mortality in patients with sepsis (Weledji & Ngowe, 2013).

Fluid resuscitation in the first six hours of septic shock may use blood products instead of crystalloids to expand extravascular volume. Colloid resuscitation requires less fluid to achieve the same results but is more expensive and may have restricted use in some settings. Serial lactate measurements are an excellent determination of the response and adequacy of fluid resuscitation. A decreased lactate is associated with decreased mortality (Ahmed & Oropello, 2010). If lactate level does not decrease with adequate resuscitation and cardiac function, an intra-abdominal source (e.g., mesenteric ischemia) should be considered. Inotropic agents may be used to maintain adequate blood pressure and preserve perfusion pressure. Norepinephrine and dopamine are first-line vasopressor agents used to correct hypotension (Sartelli et al., 2013). Epinephrine increases mean blood pressure but may decrease regional blood flow to the splanchnic circulation.

Sepsis potentiates the catabolic response in the critically ill patient. Exaggerated muscle protein breakdown caused by catabolic hormones, insulin resistance, and the release of cytokines contributes to the catabolic response. Supplemental glucose via total parenteral nutrition (TPN) or enteral nutrition leads to increased respiratory effort from carbon dioxide production. At least 50% of energy requirements should be administered as a lipid, which reduces the volume required for administration (Choudhuri & Uppal, 2013). If possible, enteral feeding is the optimal method for meeting the patient's nutritional requirements. TPN is used if the enteral route is unavailable because of surgical healing. The goal of feeding the critically ill patient is to halve net protein catabolism.

Respiratory Complications

Patients are usually extubated within 24 hours postoperatively, but some fail extubation because of respiratory failure, usually presenting as a noncardiogenic pulmonary edema from subacute lung injury (ALI) or acute respiratory distress syndrome (ARDS). ALI causes infiltrates and results from a systemic inflammatory response to tissue injury and trauma during the surgical procedure. It may also be caused by sepsis, hemorrhage, and blood transfusion and exacerbated by perioperative fluid resuscitation in hemodynamically unstable patients. Respiratory failure is attributed to pneumonia in postsurgical patients who have a fever and infiltrates on chest x-ray. Aspiration is another important cause of pneumonia and ALI and may occur in patients with encephalopathy and GI dysfunction. These patients have had a nasogastric tube removed and are unable to protect their airway. Aspiration pneumonia may occur with vomiting and should be noted during tracheal suctioning.

Preexisting lung disease, such as asthma and chronic obstructive lung disease, may increase respiratory complications. The effects of chemotherapy and radiation therapy may cause pneumonitis, pleurisy, interstitial fibrosis, and pulmonary hemorrhage and may prolong the need for ventilator support. Patients who undergo diaphragmatic stripping of tumor or diaphragm resection may develop pneumothorax, pleural effusions, or hemothorax requiring chest tubes. These patients are predisposed to extrapulmonary failure from diaphragm dysfunction. Patients who are not weaned from the ventilator and unlikely to be extubated after 7–10 days should undergo a tracheostomy (Ahmed & Oropello, 2010).

Complications After Complete Cytoreduction With Heated Intraperitoneal Chemotherapy

Cytoreductive surgery with heated intraperitoneal chemotherapy (HIPEC) is a treatment option for advanced, locally metastatic or peritoneal carcinomatosis. Tumor debulking, GI anastomoses, and heated chemotherapy contribute to extensive peritoneal inflammation and a systemic inflammatory response. All major surgeries produce transient postoperative impaired immunity. This excessive inflammatory response leads to the suppression of cell-mediated immunity and predisposes the patient to postoperative peritonitis (Honoré et al., 2013). HIPEC induces fluid losses, and volume resuscitation and blood product transfusion can cause platelet and coagulation factor dilution. The most common complications with HIPEC are anastomotic leaks, intestinal perforation, abscesses, and intra-abdominal bleeding. Intestinal perforations may be from inadvertent surgical injury during debulking. Prior radiation exposure, chemotherapy, steroids, and malnutrition predispose the patient to leaks or tissue perforation caused by tissue friability (Sneider & Davids, 2014). Intraperitoneal chemotherapy and hyperthermia lead to bowel edema, and perforations can occur at the site of surgical anastomoses. Intra-abdominal contamination can present as peritonitis, wound infection, and intra-abdominal abscess.

Intravascular volume losses from the peritoneal surface and intraoperative blood loss can be substantial. An inflammatory response causes development of third-space fluid distribution. It is important to monitor intra-abdominal drain output and note any high-output drains with ascites. These drains are sometimes emptied on delay to slow the production of ascites. Postoperative fluid loss greater than 5 L/day is possible after HIPEC and will require close monitoring of intake, output, and fluid replacement (Ahmed & Oropello, 2010).

Gastrointestinal Bleeding

The most common presentation of an upper GI (UGI) hemorrhage is hematemesis or melena, while the symptom of a lower GI (LGI) hemorrhage is bright red blood per rectum (Feinman & Haut, 2014a, 2014b). Comorbidities, such as congestive heart failure, renal disease, liver disease, or vascular disease, increase the overall mortality risk with GI bleeding. Patients with liver disease may have esophageal and gastric varices as well as coagulopathies that predispose the patient to UGI bleeding. Medications such as steroids, nonsteroidal anti-inflammatory drugs, and anticoagulants also increase the risk of bleeding (Meltzer & Klein, 2014).

UGI bleeding assessment begins with the ABCs: airway, breathing, and circulation (Meltzer & Klein, 2014). Airway control is important because aspiration of vomited blood is associated with significant morbidity and mortality (Meltzer & Klein, 2014). Intubation to protect the airway may be indicated in cases of profuse vomiting or altered mental status. Breathing is assessed with pulse oximetry. Sedating agents, such as propofol in hypovolemic shock, should be reduced by 90% because changing distribution volume and drug clearance could lead to respiratory depression (Kiliç, Konan, & Kaynaroğlu, 2011). Oxygen saturation below 90% requires further evaluation with arterial blood gases and chest x-ray. Supplemental oxygen or intubation with ventilation may be required. Patients in shock may not be able to maintain vital organ perfusion, even with compensatory mechanisms. Respiratory compensation may lead to increased respiratory effort and systemic oxygen use, requiring mechanical ventilation. Hemodynamic status is assessed with blood pressure, heart rate, and signs of end-organ perfusion with altered mental status, decreased urine output, and increased lactate. Older adult patients and those on antihypertensives may not become tachycardic; other assessment criteria should be used.

Heavy sustained bleeding may cause hypovolemic shock, leading to cardiopulmonary compromise. Initial fluid replacement should be crystalloid or colloid. A hemoglobin of 7–9 g/dl is the target range, except in coronary artery disease, tissue hypoperfusion, or active hemorrhage (Kiliç et al., 2011). In these cases, a blood transfusion may be given with a hemoglobin greater than 9 g/dl based on the patient's clinical symptoms, such as tachycardia. Packed red blood cells should be administered when more than 30% of the circulating volume has been lost (Mitra, Marrow, & Nayer, 2012). Platelet transfusion should be considered in patients who are actively bleeding with a platelet count less than 50 × 10^9/L (Mitra et al., 2012). To maintain an international normalized ratio of 1.5 or less, fresh frozen plasma should be considered in bleeding patients with a fibrogen count less than 1 g/L or a prothrombin time greater than 1.5 times the upper limit of normal (Mitra et al., 2012). Coagulopathy may be seen in patients with liver failure or in those who are anticoagulated. Coagulopathy correction should not delay urgent endoscopy. These products may be simultaneously administered.

Although management of a bleeding lesion requires endoscopic or surgical intervention, preendoscopic pharmacologic therapy may assist in achieving hemostasis. Reducing acid secretion may stabilize a UGI bleed. An IV drip of a proton pump inhibitor (PPI) should be started and infused for 72 hours (Mitra et al., 2012). The patient can then be converted to high-dose oral therapy. Use of vasoactive medications, such as somatostatin and vasopressin, is well established for control of variceal sources of bleeding. Vasoactive medications cause splanchnic vasoconstriction, reducing blood flow to the viscera and decreasing portal pressure (Feinman & Haut, 2014a, 2014b).

Endoscopy is the standard for UGI bleeding and is recommended within 24 hours of presentation. This therapy includes injection with vasoconstrictors, thermal coagulation, and mechanical clipping and is recommended for active arterial bleeding, nonbleeding visible vessels, and ulcers with adherent clot. Esophageal varices are treated with variceal band ligation using elastic rubber bands. If banding cannot be achieved, sclerotherapy may be used. For gastric variceal hemorrhage, cyanoacrylate is the preferred treatment. In severe refractory variceal bleeding, a transjugular intrahepatic portosystemic shunt can be performed by an interventional radiologist. This procedure reduces the pressure in the varices by creating an artificial shunt between the portal venous system and the hepatic veins. A second endoscopy should be performed within 24 hours in patients likely to have rebleeding or if initial scope visualization was suboptimal (Gerson, Fidler, Cave, & Leighton, 2015). After endoscopic evaluation with active bleeding, an angiography and embolization may be completed.

Antibiotic prophylaxis is recommended in all patients with variceal bleeding, as studies have shown it to reduce mortality (Mitra et al., 2012). Beta-blocker prophylaxis should be used long term to prevent variceal bleeding. If a peptic ulcer is found, the patient should be tested for *Helicobacter pylori*. If the bacterium is found, a seven-day course of a PPI with metronidazole and clarithromycin or amoxicillin and clarithromycin should be prescribed.

LGI bleeding originates below the duodenojejunal junction at the ligament of Treitz. This includes the small intestine, colon, rectum, and anus (Feinman & Haut, 2014a, 2014b). The severity of LGI bleeding is less than that of UGI bleeding, with 80% of cases spontaneously resolving. Anywhere from 60%–80% of LGI bleeding occurs in the colon and rectum and is caused by diverticular bleeding, ischemic colitis, tumors and polyps, radiation proctitis, and colitis (Marion et al., 2014). Diverticular bleeding accounts for 20%–50% of LGI bleeding and is caused by erosion of the small arteries in the wall of the diverticulum. This bleeding usually resolves 85% of the time with medical management (Marion et al., 2014). Ischemic colitis includes secondary erosive lesions from arterial or venous hypoxia of the colon or rectum (Porpiglia & Sigurdson, 2015). A colonoscopy is the standard treatment for LGI bleeding but should be avoided emergently because of poor visualization without a bowel prep (Pfeifer, 2011). Colonoscopy is both diagnostic and therapeutic. Hemostatic modalities include monopolar or bipolar electrocoagulation, argon plasma coagulation, submucosal injection of epinephrine solution, or occlusion of a visible vessel by hemostatic clips.

In an emergent situation, angiography is the most important examination for both UGI and LGI bleeding. Angiography localizes the source of bleeding and allows embolization of the bleeding source. Hemodynamic stabilization with IV fluids and blood products are standard medical management for both UGI and LGI bleeding. Severe bleeding is the loss of more than 1,500 ml in a 24-hour period. Clotting factors should be assessed and corrected (Pfeifer, 2011).

Small Bowel Perforation

Closed-loop small bowel obstruction and tumor are the most common causes of small bowel perforation (Hines, Rosenblat, Duncan, Friedman, & Katz, 2013). Medications, including nonsteroidal anti-inflammatory drugs and potassium chloride, have been implicated in small bowel perforation. Free air on CT scan may be present in about 50% of cases. Other CT findings include mural thickening, abnormal mural enhancement, and mesenteric fat stranding. The small intestine is the most frequently injured bowel during laparoscopic surgery. Radiation injury may also lead to small bowel perforation. Lymphoma accounts for 18%–38% of small bowel malignancies and is the most common small bowel tumor to present with perforation (Hines et al., 2013). The risk of perforation in lymphoma is increased in patients treated with systemic chemotherapy and steroids (Hines et al., 2013).

Intra-Abdominal Hypertension

Intra-abdominal hypertension (IAH) is a sustained elevation of intra-abdominal pressure (IAP) of 12 mm Hg or greater, and abdominal compartment syndrome (ACS) is a sustained IAP greater than 20 mm Hg with new organ dysfunction or failure (Björck & Wanhainen, 2014). IAH can lead to multisystem organ failure and death. ACS can be attributed to postoperative bleeding, mechanical intestinal obstruction, postoperative closure of the abdomen under tension, severe intra-abdominal infection, large-volume fluid replacement, ascites, ileus, sepsis, and morbid obesity (Lee, 2012).

The effect of IAH on the splanchnic organs causes diminished gut perfusion, leading to ischemia, acidosis of the mucosal bed, capillary leak, intestinal edema, and translocation of gut bacteria. As IAP increases, pressure is placed on the arteries, capillaries, and veins in the abdominal cavity, decreasing arterial flow to the abdominal organs and causing poor venous drainage. The decreased oxygenation to the gut leads to intramucosal acidosis (Delgado, 2013). The ischemic intestine loses its protective mucosal barrier, which increases permeability to intestinal contents. Edema develops in the intestinal wall, increasing IAP. Intestinal flora translocates via the villi into the lymph and vascular systems. This is the beginning of sepsis. The loss of the mucosal barrier predisposes patients with IAH to stress ulcers. IAH exerts pressure on the blood vessels, leading to edema and ischemia. This decreased blood flow causes poor wound healing and dehiscence of abdominal surgical wounds (Lee, 2012).

Liver

Hepatic perfusion and liver function are impaired by low blood flow, leading to decreased blood glucose metabolism, mitochondrial malfunction, and decreased lactate clearance, which causes lactic acidosis (Lee, 2012).

Renal

IAH leads to impaired renal function. The compression on the renal system results in decreased renal perfusion, arterial pulse pressure, and cardiac output and increased systemic vascular resistance (Delgado, 2013). An elevated serum creatinine may not appear for two to three days after IAH (Lee, 2012). This elevated creatinine is termed *acute kidney injury*. IV fluids may be used to improve renal perfusion.

Pulmonary

As the abdomen distends, the diaphragm is impinged. Pulmonary dysfunction may be one of the first signs of ACS. Tidal volume is reduced, leading to hypoxemia, and carbon dioxide is retained, causing hypercarbia and respiratory acidosis (Delgado, 2013). Compression atelectasis decreases the ratio of partial pressure of oxygen in arterial blood to fraction of inspired oxygen, and hospital-acquired pneumonia may develop (Lee, 2012). IAH can cause elevated peak airway and plateau pressures on ventilated patients and lead to ALI, requiring low tidal volumes. When ALI is not present with ACS, low tidal volumes will not improve pulmonary dysfunction.

Cardiovascular

Increased intrathoracic pressure compresses the heart and vessels, resembling tamponade. Central venous and pulmonary artery wedge pressure are elevated and may falsely convince clinicians that the patient is volume overloaded (Lee, 2012). Compression of the inferior vena cava decreases venous return, which also decreases preload and cardiac output. The elevated intrathoracic pressure increases pulmonary vascular resistance and right ventricular afterload. IAH also causes pressure of the femoral veins, increasing venous stasis and the development of deep vein thrombosis, which raises the risk of pulmonary emboli development (Lee, 2012).

Neurologic

Increased intrathoracic pressure puts pressure on the jugular veins, decreasing drainage of the cerebrospinal fluid and blood and leading to increased intracranial pressure. This can result in a reduction of cerebral perfusion pressure, causing an altered level of consciousness and ischemia (Delgado, 2013).

Nursing Implications

The standard of measuring IAP is via a urinary catheter. A transducer or manometer technique can be used. Once IAH is detected, the goal is to decrease IAP to 15 mm Hg or less. CT with angiography is the best radiology test to determine ACS. Intraluminal contents should be monitored for daily bowel movement and a bowel program implemented to avoid constipation. A nasogastric tube is inserted to decompress the stomach. To improve abdominal wall compliance, positioning in the prone position is avoided and the head of the bed should be elevated more than 20°. Neuromuscular blockade may be administered to decrease abdominal muscle pressure. If the patient is fluid overloaded, diuresis and dialysis can be used to decrease volume. Patients with severe lactic acidosis may require a sodium bicarbonate drip. A morphine or fentanyl drip is often used to treat the pain. A sedative may be used to treat anxiety and tachypnea. Early enteral nutrition will help to maintain the integrity of the mucosal barrier and stimulate bowel movements (Björck & Wanhainen, 2014).

The most common surgical treatment is a decompressive laparotomy. An open abdomen is at serious risk of infection, sepsis, and fluid loss. The goal is to close the abdomen as soon as possible.

Summary

GI cancer and its treatments can lead to other abdominal emergencies. Complications can occur after surgery, including GI bleeding, anastomotic leaks, bowel perforation, and ACS. Chemotherapy may also cause bowel perforation and GI bleeding. It is important for the critical care nurse to be knowledgeable regarding complications of the cancer and its treatments.

References

Ahmed, S., & Oropello, J.M. (2010). Critical care issues in oncology surgery patients. *Critical Care Clinics, 26,* 93–106. doi:10.1016/j.ccc.2009.10.004

Björck, M., & Wanhainen, A. (2014). Management of abdominal compartment syndrome and the open abdomen. *European Journal of Vascular and Endovascular Surgery, 47,* 279–287. doi:10.1016 /j.ejvs.2013.12.014

Choudhuri, A., & Uppal, R. (2013). Predictors of septic shock following anastomotic leak after major gastrointestinal surgery: An audit from a tertiary care institute. *Indian Journal of Critical Care Medicine, 17,* 298–303. doi:10.4103/0972-5229.120322

Delgado, L.A. (2013). Abdominal compartment syndrome: A guide for the gastrointestinal nurse. *Gastrointestinal Nursing, 11*(5), 42–48. doi:10.12968/gasn.2013.11.5.42

Feinman, M., & Haut, E.R. (2014a). Lower gastrointestinal bleeding. *Surgical Clinics of North America, 94,* 55–63. doi:10.1016/j.suc.2013.10.005

Feinman, M., & Haut, E.R. (2014b). Upper gastrointestinal bleeding. *Surgical Clinics of North America, 94,* 43–53. doi:10.1016/j.suc.2013.10.004

Gerson, L.B., Fidler, J.L., Cave, D.R., & Leighton, J.A. (2015). ACG clinical guideline: Diagnosis and management of small bowel bleeding. *American Journal of Gastroenterology, 110,* 1265–1287. doi:10.1038/ajg.2015.246

Hines, J., Rosenblat, J., Duncan, D.R., Friedman, B., & Katz, D.S. (2013). Perforation of the mesenteric small bowel: Etiologies and CT findings. *Emergency Radiology, 20,* 155–161. doi:10.1007 /s10140-012-1095-3

Honoré, C., Sourrouille, I., Suria, S., Chalumeau-Lemoine, L., Dumont, F., Goéré, D., & Elias, D. (2013). Postoperative peritonitis without an underlying digestive fistula after complete cytoreductive surgery plus HIPEC. *Saudi Journal of Gastroenterology, 19,* 271–277. doi:10.4103/1319 -3767-121033

Kiliç, Y.A., Konan, A., & Kaynaroğlu, V. (2011). Resuscitation and monitoring in gastrointestinal bleeding. *European Journal of Trauma and Emergency Surgery, 37,* 329–337. doi:10.1007/s00068 -011-0113-6

Kumar, A., Kennecke, H.F., Renouf, D.J., Lim, H.J., Gill, S., Woods, R., … Cheung, W.Y. (2015). Adjuvant chemotherapy use and outcomes of patients with high-risk versus low-risk stage II colon cancer. *Cancer, 121,* 527–534. doi:10.1002/cncr.29072

Landmann, R.G. (2014). Surgical management of anastomotic leak following colorectal surgery. *Seminars in Colon and Rectal Surgery, 6,* 58–66. doi:10.1053/j.scrs.2014.05.001

Lee, R.K. (2012). Intra-abdominal hypertension and abdominal compartment syndrome: A comprehensive overview. *Critical Care Nurse, 32,* 19–31. doi:10.4037/ccn2012662

Marion, Y., Lebreton, G., Le Pennec, V., Hourna, E., Viennot, S., & Alves, A. (2014). The management of lower gastrointestinal bleeding. *Journal of Visceral Surgery, 151,* 191–201. doi:10.1016 /j.jviscsurg.2014.03.008

Meltzer, A.C., & Klein, J.C. (2014). Upper gastrointestinal bleeding: Patient presentation, risk stratification, and early management. *Gastroenterology Clinics of North America, 43,* 665–675. doi:10 .1016/j.gtc.2014.08.002

Mitra, V., Marrow, B., & Nayar, M. (2012). Management of acute upper gastrointestinal bleeding. *Gastrointestinal Nursing, 10*(7), 34–41. doi:10.12968/gasn.2012.10.7.34

Pfeifer, J. (2011). Surgical management of lower gastrointestinal bleeding. *European Journal of Trauma and Emergency Surgery, 37,* 365–372. doi:10.1007/s00068-011-0122-5

Pollom, E.L., Deng, L., Pai, R.K., Brown, J.M., Giaccia, A., Loo, B.W., Jr., … Chang, D.T. (2015). Gastrointestinal toxicities with combined antiangiogenic and stereotactic body radiation therapy. *International Journal of Radiation Oncology, Biology, Physics, 92,* 568–576. doi:10.1016/j.ijrobp.2015.02.016

Porpiglia, A.S., & Sigurdson, E.R. (2015). Surgical options in the treatment of lower gastrointestinal tract cancers. *Current Treatment Options in Oncology, 16,* 46. doi:10.1007/s11864-015-0363-3

Sartelli, M., Catena, F., Ansaloni, L., Moore, E., Malangoni, M., Velmahos, G., … Ishii, W. (2013). Complicated intra-abdominal infections in a worldwide context: An observational prospective study (CIAOW Study). *World Journal of Emergency Surgery, 8,* 1. doi:10.1186/1749-7922-8-1

Sneider, E.B., & Davids, J.S. (2014). Effect of chemotherapy, radiation, or immunosuppression on the integrity of the intestinal anastomosis. *Seminars in Colon and Rectal Surgery, 25,* 105–109. doi:10.1053/j.scrs.2014.04.008

Weledji, E.P., & Ngowe, M. (2013). The challenge of intra-abdominal sepsis. *International Journal of Surgery, 11,* 290–295. doi:10.1016/j.ijsu.2013.02.021

CHAPTER 7

Bone and Soft Tissue Sarcomas

Laetitia Simeral, RN, MSN, CRNP

Introduction

Sarcoma is a diverse group of solid tumors in tissues of mesenchymal origin (e.g., bone, cartilage, muscle, fat, nerve, blood vessels) (Skubitz & D'Adamo, 2007). This rare malignancy will account for an estimated 12,390 cases of soft tissue sarcoma and 3,260 cases of bone sarcomas in 2017 (Siegel, Miller, & Jemal, 2017). Sarcoma is broadly divided into bone and soft tissue types. Bone sarcomas comprise three main categories: osteosarcoma, Ewing sarcoma, and chondrosarcoma. More than 50 different subtypes of soft tissue sarcomas exist, with leiomyosarcoma and liposarcoma being the most common. This chapter will discuss the pathophysiology, treatment, side effects, and complications related to bone and soft tissue sarcomas.

Pathophysiology

Sarcoma can affect individuals of all ages, from infants to older adults. These tumors may develop anywhere in the body but typically present as a gradually growing, painless mass, which may become quite large before causing pain from tumor compression of adjoining structures (i.e., edema or paresthesia) (Goldblum, Weiss, & Folpe, 2013). They may also present as cutaneous nodules (i.e., angiosarcoma) or areas of necrosis. Imaging techniques most commonly used for staging purposes are computed tomography scans and magnetic resonance imaging. These techniques assess the primary tumor size, location, and any evidence of metastasis. A biopsy (core needle or fine needle aspiration) is needed to confirm a diagnosis and should be performed by a radiologist or surgeon with experience in sarcoma at a major cancer center; biopsy technique and location are critical to the success of any future surgical resection (Skubitz & D'Adamo, 2007). Pathology also needs to be reviewed by an experienced sarcoma pathologist, as determining subtype is critical in choosing the appropriate treatment modality (Skubitz & D'Adamo, 2007).

Treatment

Treatment of bone and soft tissue sarcomas involves an interprofessional approach. Surgery, chemotherapy, and radiation therapy are often combined and used with neoadjuvant, adjuvant, or palliative intent. Soft tissue sarcoma is predominantly a surgical disease, but radiation therapy and chemotherapy may be used to improve local and distant disease control.

Some soft tissue sarcomas are more sensitive to chemotherapy than others (i.e., synovial and myxoid/round cell liposarcoma), placing added emphasis on determining subtype. Neoadjuvant chemotherapy in soft tissue sarcomas may be used for tumor cytoreduction, immediate treatment of micrometastases, and as an early indicator of chemotherapy/radiation therapy (necrosis) effectiveness. It is usually used in large (greater than 10 cm) or recurrent high-grade tumors to increase the chance of limb-salvage resection (DeLaney et al., 2003); however, no clear evidence exists that neoadjuvant chemotherapy is beneficial, making this therapy institution dependent and not a standard of care (Grobmyer et al., 2004).

The most common chemotherapy agents used in the treatment of soft tissue sarcomas are anthracyclines, ifosfamide, gemcitabine, and taxanes. Recent clinical trials focusing specifically on sarcoma subtypes have led to the approval of some reasonable treatment options, such as pazopanib for the treatment of metastatic nonadipocytic soft tissue sarcoma and trabectedin for the treatment of leiomyosarcoma and liposarcoma (van der Graaf et al., 2012).

Treatment of Ewing sarcoma and osteosarcoma consists of neoadjuvant chemotherapy, followed by surgery or radiation therapy, and then completion of the chemotherapy in an adjuvant setting (Anninga et al., 2011; Grier et al., 2003).

First-line chemotherapy for Ewing sarcoma comprises a multidrug regimen of cyclophosphamide, doxorubicin, and vincristine alternating with ifosfamide and etoposide, while first-line chemotherapy for osteosarcoma comprises neoadjuvant treatment with high-dose methotrexate, doxorubicin, and high-dose cisplatin, followed by surgical resection (wide excision or amputation), and then completion of chemotherapy in an adjuvant setting (Eilber & Rosen, 1989). Treatment for both takes about a year.

The primary goal of surgery in bone sarcomas is to control the tumor, and the secondary goal is to preserve function. The feasibility of limb-salvage surgery for bone sarcomas depends on clinical presentation, stage of disease, local extent of the tumor, and tumor response to chemotherapy.

Chemotherapy Side Effects

Most chemotherapy drugs used to treat bone and soft tissue sarcomas can cause serious and sometimes life-threatening complications if not recognized early and aggressively managed. These drugs are often given at higher than usual doses, causing more pronounced and severe side effects.

Patients with metastatic disease often have already received several lines of chemotherapy and may be at risk for developing more significant toxicities (e.g., compromised bone marrow). For this reason, patients with sarcoma should be treated in major sarcoma centers staffed with experienced medical professionals who can immediately recognize and aggressively manage any complications. These side effects highlight the need for close and frequent communication between patients and healthcare providers. Unplanned patient visits to the clinic and unexpected hospital admissions can be common. Established protocols for handling these potentially life-threatening emergencies promote patient safety and timely intervention.

Neutropenia

Chemotherapy for bone and soft tissue sarcomas typically leads to profound neutropenia during the nadir period (7–10 days after treatment) (Kurtin, 2012). White blood cell and absolute neutrophil counts can drop well below 1,000/mm^3 during this time (Crawford, Dale, & Lyman, 2004). This occurs despite the widespread use of growth factors (filgrastim and pegfilgrastim). Febrile neutropenia is a serious complication of the chemotherapy regimens used for sarcomas and can lead to septic shock and death if not properly and aggressively managed. Patients need to be educated on the signs and symptoms of possible infection during the nadir period. Open communication between patients and medical providers is essential in providing necessary interventions.

Anemia

Anemia is another likely side effect of chemotherapy for bone and soft tissue sarcomas. It is common for patients to require blood transfusions during the treatment course.

Thrombocytopenia

Thrombocytopenia also occurs frequently and may lead to bleeding, as platelets will often fall below 10,000/mm^3 during the nadir period (Kurtin,

2012). This is especially true in heavily pretreated patients with metastatic disease. Platelet transfusions are common, especially in the later stages of treatment.

Nausea and Vomiting

Despite the use of neurokinin-1 receptor antagonists and serotonin antiemetics, nausea and vomiting may still be prevalent in this patient population. If not controlled, nausea and vomiting can lead to significant dehydration and electrolyte imbalances, sometimes requiring hospitalization for aggressive fluid and electrolyte resuscitation. This can also contribute to poor quality of life and lead to added distress for patients and their caregivers. High-dose cisplatin use in the treatment of osteosarcoma can result in delayed nausea and vomiting. This may lead to hospitalization and require around-the-clock IV hydration and electrolyte repletion, as patients are unable to tolerate any oral intake.

Mucositis

Mucositis is another potential chemotherapy complication in this population and occurs because of the extensive use of anthracyclines and the potential for delayed excretion of high-dose methotrexate in the treatment of osteosarcoma. It typically is seen in the oral cavity and esophagus. Mucositis can be as mild as having a sore mouth and gums or as severe as having disseminated oral ulcers or thrush and not being able to tolerate any oral intake. Although milder cases can be managed with supportive care at home, severe cases usually require hospitalization to manage dehydration, electrolyte imbalances, and pain. Though rare, diarrhea and constipation may occur at any time during these long treatment periods. These side effects are usually managed at home but may sometimes require more aggressive measures, especially in a profound myelosuppression setting.

Ifosfamide-Related Encephalopathy

Ifosfamide-related encephalopathy is a rare complication stemming from the use of ifosfamide and the delayed excretion of chloroacetaldehyde. Patients may develop mild confusion and remain fully functional, or they may become severely disoriented, agitated, and unable to take care of themselves. This state usually resolves with discontinuation of the drug, continuous and aggressive IV hydration, and the use of IV methylene blue (Pelgrims et al., 2000).

Nephrotoxicity

Extensive use of alkylating agents (cyclophosphamide and ifosfamide) and high-dose cisplatin and methotrexate can result in significant nephrotoxicity in patients treated for bone and soft tissue sarcomas (Perazella & Moeckel, 2010). Close monitoring of renal function throughout treatment and for years after is critical for the early detection and prevention of this potentially serious complication. IV hydration with proper alkalization of the urine must be administered throughout the chemotherapy infusion and for several days after. Electrolytes, particularly potassium and magnesium, also must be checked often and supplemented daily.

Hemorrhagic Cystitis

Hemorrhagic cystitis is another potential complication of chemotherapy with ifosfamide but can be prevented with the appropriate use of mesna during ifosfamide administration.

Cardiomyopathy

Cardiomyopathy is a well-known complication of using anthracycline-based chemotherapy. As anthracyclines are standard in the treatment of bone and soft tissue sarcomas, this complication must be carefully monitored during treatment and for years after.

Judicious use of echocardiography and dexrazoxane, a cardioprotective agent, are essential when treating patients with regimens that include anthracyclines (Shakir & Rasul, 2009). Access to cardiologists experienced in treating cardiomyopathy from exposure to anthracyclines is critical.

Radiation Side Effects

As with chemotherapy, radiation therapy can be neoadjuvant, adjuvant, or palliative in the treatment of bone and soft tissue sarcomas. Side effects from radiation tend to be more localized and better tolerated than chemotherapy; however, bone marrow suppression and mucositis can occur depending on the anatomic site being radiated.

Bone marrow suppression can be a side effect of radiation to the pelvis and can be exacerbated if the patient is receiving concurrent myelosuppressive chemotherapy with radiation therapy.

Similarly, patients with head and neck sarcomas receiving concurrent radiation therapy and chemotherapy have the potential to experience significant worsening of oral and esophageal mucositis. A collaborative relationship between healthcare providers in medical and radiation oncology will ensure that patients with cancer are receiving timely and appropriate interventions, such as IV hydration and palliative radiation for severe tumor-related pain.

Nursing Implications

Oncology nurses and advanced practice oncology nurses play a significant role in educating patients and their families about a diagnosis of bone or soft tissue sarcoma and navigating them through an often-complicated treatment plan.

As patients begin chemotherapy treatment, nurses will need to rely on their oncology expertise and experiences treating sarcomas and their side effects.

Patient care relies heavily on the involvement of other disciplines, such as social work, palliative care, physical therapy, and nutrition. As the ages of patients diagnosed with sarcoma are broad, healthcare professionals must be well versed on the different age-related needs of this population.

Summary

Bone and soft tissue sarcomas are very rare tumors that can affect any part of the body and occur at any age. Given their rarity and the need for an interprofessional team approach, care should take place at a dedicated sarcoma center.

The use of chemotherapy to treat bone or soft tissue sarcomas can lead to significant toxicities, including myelosuppression, cardiotoxicity, nephrotoxicity, and dehydration. Management of these toxicities can be done in the outpatient setting, but hospitalization is often required; therefore, oncology nurses play an integral part in recognizing and managing these complications and must be educated on the intricacies of caring for patients with soft tissue and bone sarcomas.

References

Anninga, J.K., Gelderblom, H., Fiocco, M., Kroep, J.R., Taminiau, A.H.M., Hogendoorn, P.C.W., & Egeler, R.M. (2011). Chemotherapeutic adjuvant treatment for osteosarcoma: Where do we stand? *European Journal of Cancer, 47,* 2431–2445. doi:10.1016/j.ejca.2011.05.030

Crawford, J., Dale, D.C., & Lyman, G.H. (2004). Chemotherapy-induced neutropenia. *Cancer, 100,* 228–237. doi:10.1002/cncr.11882

DeLaney, T.F., Spiro, I.J., Suit, H.D., Gebhardt, M.C., Hornicek, F.J., Mankin, H.J., ... Harmon, D.C. (2003). Neoadjuvant chemotherapy and radiotherapy for large extremity soft-tissue sarcomas. *International Journal of Radiation Oncology, Biology, Physics, 56,* 1117–1127. doi:10.1016/S0360-3016(03)00186-X

Eilber, F.R., & Rosen, G. (1989). Adjuvant chemotherapy for osteosarcoma. *Seminars in Oncology, 16,* 312–322.

Goldblum, J.R., Weiss, S.W., & Folpe, A.L. (Eds.). (2013). *Enzinger and Weiss's soft tissue tumors: Expert consult* (6th ed.). Philadelphia, PA: Elsevier Saunders.

Grier, H.E., Krailo, M.D., Tarbell, N.J., Link, M.P., Fryer, C.J.H., Pritchard, D.J., ... Miser, J.S. (2003). Addition of ifosfamide and etoposide to standard chemotherapy for Ewing's sarcoma and primitive neuroectodermal tumor of bone. *New England Journal of Medicine, 348,* 694–701. doi:10.1056/nejmoa020890

Grobmyer, S.R., Maki, R.G., Demetri, G.D., Mazumdar, M., Riedel, E., Brennan, M.F., & Singer, S. (2004). Neo-adjuvant chemotherapy for primary high-grade extremity soft tissue sarcoma. *Annals of Oncology, 15,* 1667–1672. doi:10.1093/annonc/mdh431

Kurtin, S. (2012). Myeloid toxicity of cancer treatment. *Journal of the Advanced Practitioner in Oncology, 3,* 209–224.

Pelgrims, J., De Vos, F., Van den Brande, J., Schrijvers, D., Prové, A., & Vermorken, J.B. (2000). Methylene blue in the treatment and prevention of ifosfamide-induced encephalopathy: Report of 12 cases and a review of the literature. *British Journal of Cancer, 82,* 291–294. doi:10.1054/bjoc.1999.0917

Perazella, M.A., & Moeckel, G.W. (2010). Nephrotoxicity from chemotherapeutic agents: Clinical manifestations, pathobiology and prevention/therapy. *Seminars in Nephrology, 30,* 570–581. doi:10.1016/j.semnephrol.2010.09.005

Shakir, D.K., & Rasul, K.I. (2009). Chemotherapy induced cardiomyopathy: Pathogenesis, monitoring and management. *Journal of Clinical Medicine Research, 1,* 8–12. doi:10.4021/jocmr2009.02.1225

Siegel, R.L., Miller, K.D., & Jemal, A. (2017). Cancer statistics, 2017. *CA: A Cancer Journal for Clinicians, 67,* 7–30. doi:10.3322/caac.21387

Skubitz, K.M., & D'Adamo, D.R. (2007). Sarcoma. *Mayo Clinic Proceedings, 82,* 1409–1432. doi:10.4065/82.11.1409

van der Graaf, W.T.A., Blay, J.-Y., Chawla, S.P., Kim, D.-W., Nguyen, B.B., Casali, P.G., ... Hohenberger, P. (2012). Pazopanib for metastatic soft tissue sarcoma (PALETTE): A randomised, double-blind, placebo-controlled phase 3 trial. *Lancet, 379,* 1879–1886. doi:10.1016/S0140-6736(12)60651-5

CHAPTER 8

Renal Failure and Obstructive Uropathy

Ladan Golestaneh, MD, MS, Yelena Drexler, MD,
and Neelja Kumar, MD

Introduction

Renal disease is a common and frequently underdiagnosed condition in patients with malignancy. Certain cancers are associated with especially high rates of acute kidney injury (AKI), including kidney cancers (44% risk of AKI at one year), multiple myeloma (33%), and other hematologic cancers (up to 36%) (Campbell, Hu, & Okusa, 2014). Because of recent standardization and updates to diagnostic criteria for AKI, the term *acute renal failure* has been replaced by *acute kidney injury*. With this updated terminology, the pool of patients with AKI has expanded, as has diagnostic precision (Bagshaw, George, & Bellomo, 2008). AKI refers to the development of impaired renal function over the course of hours to days and has been associated with poor outcomes and iatrogenic complications. Renal damage is best characterized by measuring the increase in serum creatinine and the duration and degree of oliguria (Lin & Chen, 2012); however, using serum creatinine or urine output measurements alone can underestimate the degree of kidney disease, especially in patients with cancer. Furthermore, creatinine-based estimations of glomerular filtration rate frequently lead to inaccurate medication dosing in this population (Buemi et al., 2009; Humphreys, Soiffer, & Magee, 2005; Launay-Vacher et al., 2007). Adaptation of frequently used medications and oncologic therapies in response to AKI is complex and requires interprofessional efforts by a dedicated team. The implications of AKI occurrence over the course of hospitalization are far-reaching and have been shown to cause both short-term and long-term morbidity and mortality (Hsu et al., 2016).

In critically ill patients with cancer, AKI is associated with longer duration of ventilator support, severe impairment in functional status, and delays in administration of lifesaving chemotherapeutic agents (Lameire, Flombaum, Moreau, & Ronco, 2005). Multiorgan dysfunction syndrome (MODS) is a consequence of sepsis and some treatment strategies in this vulnerable patient population. Acute tubular necrosis (ATN), as a component of MODS, is the most common cause of AKI in the intensive care unit (ICU) setting and connotes a poor prognosis (Humphreys et al., 2005; Lameire, Van Biesen, & Vanholder, 2008; Soares et al., 2006); however, of those who survive critical illness, rates of kidney recovery are high (Soares et al., 2006). The overall prognosis of AKI is dependent on many factors, including cancer type (solid vs. hematologic), disease severity, the presence of critical illness, and the oncology therapy (Rosolem et al., 2012; Soares et al., 2006). Mortality with AKI is up to 81% but varies in the ICU, as it depends on precise etiology and the need for renal replacement therapy (RRT). RRT use for AKI is higher in ICU patients with cancer as compared to other ICU patients. This provision of RRT is increasing because of rising ICU admissions of patients with cancer (Maccariello et al., 2011; Rosolem et al., 2012). Furthermore, formal guidelines are not available for dosing of chemotherapeutics in AKI or dialysis-dependent AKI. Thus, the presence of kidney disease may preclude the use of aggressive cancer therapy (Maccariello et al., 2011; Rosolem et al., 2012).

Types of Renal Disease

The cause of AKI is usually multifactorial in patients with malignancy, and hypovolemia, sepsis, and exposure to nephrotoxic agents are the most common etiologies (Kapoor & Chan, 2001; Lam & Humphreys, 2012; Launay-Vacher et al., 2007; Salahudeen & Bonventre, 2013). The cancer itself, or its treatment, also may be the cause. Tumor lysis syndrome (TLS) and myeloma cast nephropathy are common primary cancer-related causes of AKI with an abrupt onset and severe course. Paraneoplastic glomerular disease, infiltrative diseases, thrombotic microangiopathy (TMA), and other forms of chemotherapy-associated kidney disease are more indolent (Lameire et al., 2005). MODS is commonly seen in critically ill patients with cancer and is associated with septic ATN as well as concomitant cardiac and liver failure, which can lead to cardiorenal or hepatorenal syndromes, respectively. Ischemic ATN and contrast-induced nephropathy are also commonly encountered causes of AKI in this group of patients (Finkel & Foringer, 2007; Humphreys et al., 2005). Different AKI types and their associated treatments will be discussed in subsequent sections.

Hemodynamic Acute Kidney Injury

Systemic manifestations of cancer or its treatment can result in volume depletion (Benoit & Hoste, 2010; Lameire, Van Biesen, & Vanholder, 2010).

Prerenal azotemia results from vomiting, decreased oral intake, diarrhea, and high insensible losses. The nephron is not perfused because of volume depletion and compensates by vasoconstriction of the renal arterial bed at the cost of worsening azotemia. Treatment comprises volume repletion with isotonic fluids and restoration of circulatory volume (Bagshaw et al., 2008; Benoit & Hoste, 2010; Buemi et al., 2009; Lameire et al., 2010). Cardiorenal syndrome is a kidney dysfunction in response to heart failure and involves a complex set of hemodynamic and hormonal changes, which are upregulated because of decreased effective arterial pressure (Ronco, Haapio, House, Anavekar, & Bellomo, 2008). Although renal pathophysiology in cardiorenal cases is similar to prerenal azotemia, treatment is different and centered on improving cardiac output and effective arterial blood volume. Malignant pericardial tamponade is an extreme case of cardiorenal syndrome commonly encountered with malignant effusions, wherein the decrease in renal perfusion is abrupt and severe because of ventricular compression. Treatment includes decompression via percutaneous drainage (pericardiocentesis) or a pericardial window (Lameire et al., 2008, 2010). Hepatorenal syndrome involves splanchnic vasodilation and the release of vasoactive peptides that dilate systemic vessels, resulting in decreased perfusion pressure to vital organs such as the kidneys (Ginès & Schrier, 2009). It commonly occurs in veno-occlusive disease after hematopoietic stem cell transplantation (HSCT) and in cancers complicated by liver metastases or direct occupation of the liver parenchyma by tumor (Bower, Robinson, & Cox, 2015; Soares et al., 2006). Although the renal pathophysiology is similar to prerenal azotemia, treatment and implications are quite different, and mortality can reach up to 100% at 40 days (Ginès & Schrier, 2009). Vasoconstrictor drugs, such as midodrine, vasopressin, and terlipressin (a vasopressin analog), have been used to increase mean arterial pressure and thus improve renal perfusion (Epstein, 1992). Finally, capillary leak syndrome from interleukin-2 administration in certain malignancies results in massive third-spacing and decreased effective arterial pressure, which leads to neurohormonal reflexes, renal vasoconstriction, and azotemia.

Renal artery obstruction is caused by thrombosis (procoagulant state), compression (tumor), or embolism, where renal perfusion is impeded and the kidneys respond in a similar manner to prerenal azotemia (Bower et al., 2015; Rosner & Dalkin, 2012). Certain medications may also lead to renal vasoconstriction and reduced perfusion pressure (the hallmark of hemodynamic renal disease), including nonsteroidal anti-inflammatory drugs (NSAIDs), angiotensin-converting enzyme (ACE) inhibitors, and calcineurin inhibitors (Finkel & Foringer, 2007; Kapoor & Chan, 2001; Salahudeen & Bonventre, 2013). Novel biomarkers may help differentiate hemodynamic kidney injury from intrinsic causes such as ATN (Lameire, 2007). What these renal disorders share is a decrease in renal perfusion, and treatment of hemodynamic AKI ultimately rests on the restoration of renal perfusion with goal-directed therapy targeted at the underlying cause of decreased perfusion.

Intrinsic Renal Disease

Intrinsic renal disease comprises all disease states that cause parenchymal damage in the kidney and is classified based on the components of the nephron: arteriole, glomerulus, tubule, and the interstitium. Unlike hemodynamic renal disease, parenchymal renal disease is not as readily reversible, and the pathophysiology of these disorders involves renal tissue inflammation or damage.

Pathologic processes specific to malignancy that affect the vascular system (arteriole) include hypercoagulable states, which most commonly occur in patients with hematologic cancers and can lead to renal infarction. Renal vein thrombosis may occur because of external compression or the hyperviscosity syndrome associated with some cancers but should not cause clinically significant AKI unless it is bilateral (Buemi et al., 2009; Parikh & Coca, 2006). Leukostasis, a consequence of hyperleukocytosis most commonly seen in patients with leukemia, can cause AKI and presents similarly to hyperviscosity syndrome (e.g., headache, dizziness, seizure, impaired consciousness, blurry vision, papilledema). It is treated with leukoreduction (leukapheresis) (Buemi et al., 2009; Lameire et al., 2008). Hemophagocytic lymphohistiocytosis is a rare condition that can cause cytokine release syndrome. AKI develops in up to 16% of these cases because of severe endothelial dysfunction (Lam & Humphreys, 2012; Salahudeen & Bonventre, 2013). TMA is a diagnosis that affects the renal arteriole and is specific to malignant conditions.

Thrombotic Microangiopathy

TMA is a common complication in patients with cancer and is an overlooked cause of AKI. It is caused by endothelial injury and microvascular thrombosis and manifests clinically with microangiopathic hemolytic anemia, thrombocytopenia, and organ damage. The kidney is most frequently affected (George & Nester, 2014). Classic TMA syndromes include thrombotic thrombocytopenic purpura (TTP), diarrhea-associated hemolytic uremic syndrome, and atypical hemolytic uremic syndrome. In patients with malignancy, TMA can result from the cancer itself, chemotherapeutic agents, or because of HSCT. Most cases of cancer-related TMA (90%) occur in patients with metastatic disease, and mucin-producing adenocarcinomas are the most common type of malignancy (Izzedine & Perazella, 2015). Many chemotherapeutic agents have been associated with TMA, including mitomycin C, gemcitabine, and anti–vascular endothelial growth factor therapy (e.g., bevacizumab) (see Table 8-1) (Al-Nouri, Reese, Terrell, Vesely, & George, 2015; Perazella, 2012). TMA is also a common cause of AKI in patients who have received HSCT and may be triggered by infections, graft-versus-host disease (GVHD), calcineurin inhibitor use for GVHD prophylaxis, or total body irradiation (Parikh & Coca, 2006). TMA is more frequent after allogeneic HSCT (15%) than with autologous HSCT (less than 1%) and is more common with myeloablative versus reduced-intensity conditioning regimens (Riedl et al., 2014).

Supportive care for TMA includes drug discontinuation, blood pressure control, volume management, dialysis (if necessary), and treatment of any condi-

Table 8-1. Common Nephrotoxic Agents Encountered in Patients With Malignancy		
Nephrotoxic Effect	**Agents**	**Comments**
Hemodynamic	Angiotensin-converting enzyme inhibitors	Cause efferent vasodilation and reduce filtration fraction
	Nonsteroidal anti-inflammatory drugs (NSAIDs)	Cause prostaglandin-mediated vasoconstriction Risk factors include volume depletion, concomitant hypercalcemia, chronic kidney disease, and older age.
Glomerular	Bisphosphonates • Pamidronate • Zoledronate	Associated with collapsing focal segmental glomerulosclerosis Toxicity is dose and infusion-time dependent. Zoledronate: incidence of 9%–24% (Perazella & Markowitz, 2008)
	NSAIDs	Associated with membranous nephropathy and minimal change disease
Thrombotic microangiopathy (TMA)	Mitomycin C	Alkylating agent used to treat gastric, pancreatic, and rectal cancers Development related to cumulative dose Kidney damage is usually irreversible, and the prognosis is poor, with one-third of patients requiring dialysis and overall mortality of up to 75% at four months (Zakarija & Bennett, 2005).
	Gemcitabine	Used to treat lymphoma and pancreatic, lung, bladder, and breast cancer TMA incidence is low, but overall mortality is high (40%–90%). Development of acute kidney injury, worsening hypertension, and hematologic manifestations are common, and kidney injury is usually irreversible despite drug discontinuation (Izzedine & Perazella, 2015).
	Vascular endothelial growth factor inhibitors • Bevacizumab • Tyrosine kinase inhibitors	Antiangiogenesis therapy used to treat a variety of solid tumors Approximately 21%–64% of patients on bevacizumab therapy develop proteinuria, and 3%–36% develop hypertension (Eremina et al., 2008).

(Continued on next page)

Table 8-1. Common Nephrotoxic Agents Encountered in Patients With Malignancy *(Continued)*

Nephrotoxic Effect	Agents	Comments
TMA *(cont.)*	Calcineurin inhibitors • Cyclosporine • Tacrolimus	Used after hematopoietic stem cell transplantation for prophylaxis against graft-versus-host disease (GVHD) Cause endothelial cell injury If sirolimus is used for GVHD prophylaxis in combination with a calcineurin inhibitor, TMA incidence may increase (Laskin et al., 2011).
Direct tubular toxicity	Contrast dye	Risk factors include volume depletion, concomitant use of nephrotoxic agents, and chronic kidney disease. Prevention involves correction of hypovolemia, use of iso-osmolar contrast media, and limiting volume of the contrast load.
	Amphotericin B	Used for treatment of fungal infections Creates cell membrane pores in tubular cells
	Vancomycin	Frequently used to treat bacterial infections Acute tubular necrosis development is dose dependent.
	Aminoglycoside antibiotics • Amikacin • Gentamicin • Tobramycin	Risk factors include chronic kidney disease, prolonged duration of therapy, frequent dosing, and elevated plasma levels. Cause mitochondrial dysfunction
	Streptozotocin	Antineoplastic agent used for pancreatic cancer Toxicity is dose related and cumulative.
	Ifosfamide	Antineoplastic agent used in multiple cancers Causes direct proximal tubular toxicity by depleting glutathione
	Cisplatin	Frequently used antineoplastic agent Causes direct cell death and vasoconstriction with selective injury of proximal tubule cells Can also cause Fanconi-like syndrome and hypomagnesemia Combination therapy with ifosfamide increases the risk of nephrotoxicity (Berns & Ford, 1997).

(Continued on next page)

Table 8-1. Common Nephrotoxic Agents Encountered in Patients With Malignancy *(Continued)*		
Nephrotoxic Effect	**Agents**	**Comments**
Direct tubular toxicity *(cont.)*	Tyrosine kinase inhibitors • Dasatinib • Imatinib	Direct toxicity to tubules (Gafter-Gvili et al., 2009)
Acute interstitial nephritis	Antibiotics • Penicillins • Cephalospo-rins	The classic triad of symptoms (fever, rash, eosinophilia) is more common than with other agents.
	NSAIDs	Prevalence is increasing, especially among older patients.
Urologic	Cyclophospha-mide Ifosfamide	Can cause hemorrhagic cystitis Preventive treatments include mesna, normal saline, and continuous bladder irrigation.

tions that may have triggered the episode (e.g., infections, GVHD) (Izzedine & Perazella, 2015). The first step in managing suspected chemotherapy-related or calcineurin inhibitor–associated TMA should be immediate discontinuation of the offending drug. Blood pressure should ideally be controlled with ACE inhibitors or angiotensin receptor blockers. Volume overload should be managed with diuretics. Worsening kidney function might necessitate dialysis, and patients should be monitored closely for development of any acute dialysis indications, such as electrolyte abnormalities or volume overload that is unable to be medically managed. If TMA is severe or no clinical improvement occurs after withdrawal of the offending drug, additional specific treatments can be considered; however, quality evidence is lacking. Potential additional treatments for chemotherapy-associated and HSCT-associated TMA include therapeutic plasma exchange, rituximab, and eculizumab (Laskin, Goebel, Davies, & Jodele, 2011). The median response rate to therapeutic plasma exchange ranges from 27%–80%; however, mortality rates can be very high (greater than 80%), and the procedure itself carries risks, including placement of central venous access and patient exposure to additional blood products (Laskin et al., 2011). In the absence of controlled studies, therapeutic plasma exchange is currently not the standard of care but can be considered in select patients. Rituximab, an anti-CD20 monoclonal antibody, is used in recurrent TTP, and eculizumab, a terminal complement inhibitor, is used in atypical hemolytic uremic syndrome. The number of successful treatments is growing with these agents; however, their benefits have yet to be studied in prospective, controlled trials (Izzedine & Perazella, 2015; Laskin et al., 2011).

Glomerular Disease

Glomerular diseases that affect patients with cancer include membranous nephropathy, membranoproliferative glomerulonephritis, and minimal change disease (Buemi et al., 2009; Ganguli, Sawinski, & Berns, 2015; Maesaka, Mittal, & Fishbane, 1997). Up to 11% of membranous nephropathy cases are associated with solid tumors. Membranoproliferative glomerulonephritis (cryoglobulinemic and primary) and minimal change disease are commonly seen with hematologic malignancies (Buemi et al., 2009; Ganguli et al., 2015). Focal segmental glomerulosclerosis is also seen with lymphoma and some solid tumors. Crescentic glomerulonephritis associated with antineutrophil cytoplasmic antibodies has sometimes been tied to lymphomas and rarely with solid tumors (Pamuk et al., 2007). The treatment for these disorders is tailored to the underlying malignancy with no established therapies for the kidney disease itself.

Tubular Disease and Acute Tubular Necrosis

Sepsis is the most common cause of ATN in patients with tubular disease. Nephrotoxic drugs are the second most common (Benoit & Hoste, 2010; Campbell et al., 2014; Li Cavoli et al., 2015). Neutropenia and chemotherapeutic agents increase the risk of infections, and severe sepsis and septic shock are common, especially in patients with hematologic cancer (Benoit & Hoste, 2010; Campbell et al., 2014; Humphreys et al., 2005; Rosolem et al., 2012). The pathophysiology of septic ATN involves vasodilation, hemodynamic failure with decreased effective circulatory volume, inflammation, and endothelial damage (Bagshaw et al., 2008; Lameire et al., 2005; Salahudeen & Bonventre, 2013). The most common infective organisms are bacterial, but fungal and other opportunistic infections are also prevalent (Rosolem et al., 2012; Salahudeen & Bonventre, 2013). Early goal-directed therapy with aggressive volume resuscitation, vasopressor medications, and early administration of antibiotics is essential for septic shock (Rosolem et al., 2012; Salahudeen & Bonventre, 2013). Activated protein C may be useful in severe sepsis (Lameire et al., 2008). If renal failure worsens and conservative measures fail, RRT may be offered.

Other causes of ATN include ischemia caused by hypotension and tubular toxicity caused by a variety of medications (see Table 8-1). Direct tubular toxicity and crystal precipitation in response to certain offending agents are the most common mechanisms for medication-induced AKI. IV contrast is also a frequent culprit. Contrast-induced nephropathy following computed tomography scans and angiography is mediated by intense vasoconstriction and direct osmotic toxicity to the renal tubular cells, and patients with malignancies are especially prone to receiving contrast studies during their illness.

Interstitial Disease

Acute interstitial nephritis (AIN) is another common cause of AKI. The infiltration of the interstitial space in the nephron with lymphocytes, in the case of aggressive lymphomas, and eosinophils, in response to a systemic allergen, represents the pathophysiology of AIN (Li Cavoli et al., 2015). Renal failure can be subacute or abrupt. Several medications have been implicated in AIN, especially antibiotics (e.g., penicillin, cephalosporin) and NSAIDs (Praga & González, 2010). Aggressive cellular infiltration of the nephron's interstitial space can also occur in hematologic cancers and some solid tumors. Metastases to the renal parenchyma from extrarenal primary malignancies, such as lung, gastric, and breast cancers, can rarely (less than 1%) cause AKI (Kapoor & Chan, 2001). Lymphomatous infiltration is an interstitial infiltration of malignant cells reported in patients with non-Hodgkin lymphoma. It can rarely cause AKI and presents as large, echogenic kidneys on imaging (Kapoor & Chan, 2001; Maesaka et al., 1997). Symptoms include flank pain, hematuria, abdominal distension, and hypertension. Renal parenchymal infiltration is responsive to steroids and chemotherapy for the underlying malignancy (Buemi et al., 2009; Kapoor & Chan, 2001).

Obstructive Renal Disease

Obstructive renal disease comprises disorders that affect urologic organs (e.g., ureters, bladder, urethra) and the flow of urine. Infiltration, external compression, and obstruction of the urinary collecting system can cause obstructive uropathy, leading to the development of hydronephrosis and renal failure. Urinary tract obstruction is more common in patients with cancer than the general population (Campbell et al., 2014; Kapoor & Chan, 2001). Patients with ovarian, uterine, cervical, prostate, or bladder malignancies, as well as those with metastatic disease affecting the pelvis, are particularly prone to obstructive kidney disease. Extensive lymph node enlargement and radiation-induced or sarcomatous retroperitoneal fibrosis present in a similar manner and can cause extensive compression of the urinary tract (Finkel & Foringer, 2007; Kapoor & Chan, 2001). The development of obstructive renal disease is a poor prognostic sign, as it often signifies an advanced cancer stage (Kapoor & Chan, 2001). Percutaneous nephrostomy and placement of ureteral stents are the mainstays of therapy for obstructive renal disease. In patients with bladder cancer requiring cystectomy, the creation of ileal conduits or continent diversions (e.g., orthotopic neobladder) may be complicated by obstruction at the ureteral anastomosis or the conduit/reservoir outflow (Campbell et al., 2014; Finkel & Foringer, 2007). This may be treated with percutaneous drainage or with placement of a Foley or suprapubic catheter (Kapoor & Chan, 2001). Bladder outlet obstruction can also occur in patients with gross hematuria, leading to the passage of blood clots (Berns & Ford, 1997; Humphreys et al., 2005). Potential causes include bladder tumors and hemorrhagic cystitis. Hemorrhagic cystitis can be caused by radiation injury, chemotherapeutic agents (e.g., cyclophosphamide), and viral infections (e.g., BK virus, post-HSCT adenovirus) (Buemi et al., 2009; Ganguli et al., 2015).

Some etiologies for renal and urologic disease in patients with malignancy deserve their own categories because they are specific to malignant conditions and have specific diagnostic and prognostic implications.

Tumor Lysis Syndrome

TLS is the most common malignancy-related emergency and classically occurs after the initiation of chemotherapy (Wilson & Berns, 2012). The highest risk occurs in highly metabolic malignancies, such as acute lymphoblastic leukemia, acute myeloid leukemia, and Burkitt lymphoma, with an incidence of 6%–26.4% (Wilson & Berns, 2012). Solid tumors that are highly responsive to chemotherapy are also commonly associated with this syndrome (Darmon, Malak, Guichard, & Schlemmer, 2008). TLS has recently been reported after treatment with steroids, bortezomib, thalidomide, rituximab, and radiation therapy (Mirrakhimov, Voore, Khan, & Ali, 2015). The pathophysiology underlying this syndrome is the massive lysis of cells and the release of intracellular components. This can lead to hyperkalemia, hyperuricemia, hyperphosphatemia, or secondary hypocalcemia, resulting in cardiac arrhythmias, seizures, MODS, or death. AKI has been found to be independently associated with mortality in these patients (Darmon, Guichard, Vincent, Schlemmer, & Azoulay, 2010). The release of intracellular purine nucleic acids, specifically adenosine and guanine, results in elevated uric acid levels, which cause tubular toxicity and deposition of both uric acid and calcium phosphate crystals within the renal parenchyma (Mato et al., 2006; Wilson & Berns, 2012). Risk assessment in patients with a malignancy is important to determine preventive measures. Risk stratification involves factors such as type of malignancy, white blood cell count, and chemotherapy treatment (see Figure 8-1).

Hydration remains a critical aspect of TLS treatment. Supportive measures, at times requiring dialysis modalities, are implemented once TLS has developed. The metabolic derangements associated with this syndrome can be life threatening, and their presence must be addressed and prevented if possible. It is recommended that hydration with crystalloid fluids begins 24–48 hours prior to administration of chemotherapy and continues for up to 72 hours after completion. The goal is to increase urine output to a target of about 100 ml/hr to enhance clearance of phosphate, potassium, and uric acid (Howard, Jones, & Pui, 2011). Patients at intermediate risk for developing TLS should receive allopurinol with hydration. Low-risk patients should be carefully monitored but conservatively managed with fluids (Cairo & Bishop, 2004; Coiffier, Altman, Pui, Younes, & Cairo, 2008). Allopurinol, a competitive inhibitor of xanthine oxidase that prevents production of uric acid, can be administered for 24 hours prior to the initiation of chemotherapy to prevent TLS development. The dose is usually 100 mg/m^2 every eight hours, but patients with renal failure require

---

Figure 8-1. Risk Stratification for Tumor Lysis Syndrome

High Risk
- Advanced Burkitt lymphoma/leukemia or early stage with elevated lactate dehydrogenase (LDH)
- Acute lymphoblastic leukemia (ALL) with white blood cell (WBC) count > 100,000/mm³ or less if LDH is > twice the upper limit of normal (ULN)
- Acute myeloid leukemia (AML) with WBC > 100,000/mm³
- Diffuse large B-cell lymphoma (DLBCL) and LDH > twice ULN and bulky disease

Intermediate Risk
- ALL with WBC count < 100,000/mm³ and LDH < twice ULN
- AML with WBC count 25,000–100,000/mm³
- DLBCL with LDH > twice ULN but not bulky disease

Low Risk
- Indolent lymphomas, chronic lymphocytic leukemia, chronic phase of chronic myeloid leukemia, multiple myeloma, solid tumors
- AML with WBC count < 25,000/mm³ and LDH < twice ULN

Note. Based on information from Coiffier et al., 2008.

---

a significant dose reduction (Cairo & Bishop, 2004). Potential adverse effects include rash, Stevens-Johnson syndrome, toxic epidermal necrolysis, hypersensitivity, hepatitis, eosinophilia, and myelosuppression (Arrambide & Toto, 1993; Wilson & Berns, 2012). Other purine analogs, including 6-mercaptopurine and azathioprine, are metabolized by xanthine oxidase; thus, their metabolism will be decreased by allopurinol. Concomitant use should be avoided, or the dose should be significantly reduced. In contrast to allopurinol, rasburicase is a medication that can decrease uric acid levels, as it is a recombinant urate oxidase. Uric acid is converted into a water-soluble compound called allantoin, which is easily excreted. The dose used is 0.15–0.20 mg/kg IV in 50 ml of normal saline infused over 30 minutes for up to five days (Cairo & Bishop, 2004; Rampello, Fricia, & Malaguarnera, 2006). Clinically, it is often only administered once or twice, as it is very effective in rapidly decreasing serum uric acid levels, but can be repeated if levels remain elevated. This medication should not be used in patients with glucose-6-phosphate-dehydrogenase deficiency (Rampello et al., 2006). No studies have evaluated morbidity or mortality outcomes with the use of this medication.

Multiple Myeloma

Multiple myeloma is unique among malignancies, as it is frequently associated with renal disease and presents with a wide array of renal manifestations (Ganguli et al., 2015; Kleeberg et al., 2009). Myeloma accounted for 58% of all AKI episodes in patients with cancer in one series. It has been reported that 50% of patients with myeloma experience renal failure, and 10% of those cases require dialysis (Ganguli et al., 2015). Myeloma cast nephropathy, light-chain deposition disease, amyloidosis, cryoglobulinemia, and hyperviscosity are some renal manifestations of myeloma. Cast nephropathy is the most common cause of AKI in association with myeloma and involves the precipitation of filtered light chains at high concentrations that are bound to the Tamm-Horsfall protein in the loop of Henle and distal tubule (Kleeberg et al., 2009). Severe ATN ensues and causes interstitial damage and a high rate of irreversible kidney failure. Hypovolemia and concomitant exposure to nephrotoxic agents further contribute to the severity of cast nephropathy. Therapeutic plasma exchange is the traditional therapy used to remove free light chains from the plasma and reduce the filtered load to the kidney, thereby reducing the amount of protein and opportunity for precipitation. Its use, though intuitive, is controversial. Studies to illustrate definitive proof of benefit have been inconsistent (Kleeberg et al., 2009). Newer continuous renal replacement therapy (CRRT) techniques with high-flux filters have also been examined with some success in the treatment of cast nephropathy. These techniques use hemofiltration as their mode of light-chain clearance (Berghmans, Meert, Markiewicz, & Sculier, 2004). If early chemotherapy or stem cell transplantation are being considered, these treatments may be beneficial. With timely myeloma treatment, cast nephropathy and other causes of myeloma kidney disease may stabilize but seldom recover to baseline. Renal failure should not be considered a contraindication to intensive treatment with chemotherapy, and an aggressive course of treatment should be pursued with the renal disease component as a significant consideration (Kleeberg et al., 2009). Newer anti–vascular endothelial growth factor therapy agents, such as bevacizumab, show promise in the treatment of myeloma-associated renal failure (Rosolem et al., 2012; Soares et al., 2006).

Common Electrolyte Derangements

Severe electrolyte derangements (e.g., hyperkalemia, hyponatremia, hypercalcemia) and acid–base disturbances are common findings in patients with cancer and are categorized under kidney disease considerations. The consequences of these derangements can be life threatening.

Metabolic Acidosis

Metabolic acidosis is a complication of certain forms of malignancy and chemotherapy treatment (Lameire et al., 2010; Schlondorff, Mendez, Rennke, & Magee, 2007). Hyperchloremic metabolic acidosis can occur in the setting of severe diarrhea, as well as different types of renal tubular acidosis (RTA). Type 2 (proximal) RTA is seen with multiple myeloma (light-chain excretion causes proximal tubular toxicity) and medications (e.g., cisplatin, ifosfamide) (Berns &

Ford, 1997; Bower et al., 2015; Lameire et al., 2010). Patients may present with an isolated proximal RTA or with Fanconi syndrome, which is characterized by renal wasting of phosphorus, glucose, and amino acids. Type 1 (distal) RTA can be seen with amphotericin B use (Lameire, 2007; Lameire et al., 2010). Voltage-dependent RTA occurs with subacute urinary obstruction and is frequently accompanied by hyperkalemia (Benoit & Hoste, 2010). Anion gap metabolic acidosis occurs with sepsis and MODS, as seen in other etiologies of shock.

Lactic acidosis most commonly occurs because of hypoperfusion, such as in MODS and hypotension. It can also less commonly occur because of disruption of aerobic pathways in high cell turnover states or mitochondrial dysfunction. In patients with hematologic cancer, lactic acidosis is caused by the apoptosis of malignant cells with a high rate of lactic acid production or from tumor ischemia from impaired neovascularization. Another form of lactic acidosis, D-lactic acidosis, can occur after intestinal surgery and ostomy creation and particularly in patients with short bowel (Bower et al., 2015). In these patients, intestinal bacteria metabolize glucose and starch into D-lactic acid, which is then systemically absorbed. Renal failure can also cause both hyperchloremic and anion gap metabolic acidosis. In turn, acidic urine promotes precipitation of uric acid crystals and can cause intratubular obstruction and tubular damage. The immediate treatment of severe acidosis is sodium bicarbonate administration, which allows blood pH to approach a level more conducive to proper heart and vascular function (usually greater than 7.1) (Benoit & Hoste, 2010). RRT should be considered an emergent intervention for cases of refractory metabolic acidosis (Benoit & Hoste, 2010).

Hyponatremia

Hyponatremia occurs in up to 5% of hospitalized patients with malignancy (Lameire et al., 2010). In one study, 11% of hospitalized hyponatremic patients had a concomitant cancer diagnosis (Finkel & Foringer, 2007; Kapoor & Chan, 2001). Syndrome of inappropriate antidiuretic hormone secretion (SIADH) is a common etiology, and potential causes include nausea, pain, central nervous system and pulmonary processes, stress, and ectopic antidiuretic hormone production by tumor (Kapoor & Chan, 2001; Schlondorff et al., 2007). In patients diagnosed with hyponatremia, two-thirds can be explained by volume depletion and SIADH (Schlondorff et al., 2007). The presence of hyponatremia also imparts a higher mortality in this population. Chemotherapeutic agents such as vincristine, vinblastine, and cyclophosphamide can cause hyponatremia (Berns & Ford, 1997; Bower et al., 2015; Lameire et al., 2010). Renal disease and decreased oral intake also increase hyponatremia risk (Kapoor & Chan, 2001). Depending on the degree of hyponatremia and whether the patient is symptomatic, treatment can be conservative (e.g., fluid restriction, sodium chloride [salt] tablets, loop diuretics) or aggressive (e.g., hypertonic saline solutions, ICU-level care). Care must be taken to avoid rapid overcorrection of severe hyponatremia, as central pontine myelinolysis is a devastating consequence. Treatment can include vasopressin receptor antagonists, including IV conivaptan or oral tolvaptan; however, no improvement in survival has been demonstrated (Kapoor & Chan, 2001; Lameire et al., 2010; Schlondorff et al., 2007).

Hypernatremia

Hypernatremia can occur with aggressive hypertonic saline, bicarbonate infusion, or impaired free-water intake in the setting of high water losses from the skin, gastrointestinal (GI) tract, or in the urine (Bower et al., 2015; Schlondorff et al., 2007). Tumor infiltration of the thirst center can disrupt osmoreceptors, leading to decreased antidiuretic hormone secretion and the development of central diabetes insipidus (DI) (Lameire et al., 2010). Medications (e.g., ifosfamide, amphotericin, foscarnet), chronic obstruction, and hypercalcemia can cause resistance to the effect of antidiuretic hormone secretion in the kidneys and the development of nephrogenic DI (Benoit & Hoste, 2010; Lameire et al., 2008). With either form of DI, excretion of dilute urine will contribute to hypernatremia. Severe hypernatremia can cause altered mentation and organ dysfunction. Treatment includes careful free-water repletion and the removal of the offending agent, if possible.

Hyperkalemia

Hyperkalemia is one of the most dreaded electrolyte disturbances in clinical medicine. Severe hyperkalemia can cause myocardial dysfunction and cardiac arrest. Potassium is an intracellular ion and handled almost exclusively by the kidneys (with some contribution from the GI tract). The causes of hyperkalemia are numerous, but common etiologies in patients with cancer involve renal failure and rapid cell turnover. In TLS, ongoing cell turnover perpetuates persistent hyperkalemia, increasing the risk of cardiac events. Through the same mechanism, phosphate levels also remain elevated as cells continue to lyse (Arrambide & Toto, 1993; Howard et al., 2011; Wilson & Berns, 2012). An electrocardiogram is recommended in patients with hyperkalemia and includes evaluation of peaked T waves, prolongation of the PR interval, widening of the QRS interval, and ultimately, a sine wave. Medical management of hyperkalemia should be initiated immediately and includes short-acting regular insulin (0.1 U/kg IV), dextrose (2 ml/kg), high-dose beta-2 agonist nebulizer (albuterol 10–20 mg in 4 ml of normal saline inhaled over 10 minutes), sodium bicarbonate (1–2 mEq/kg IV), sodium polystyrene sulfonate (1 g/kg with 50% sorbitol orally), and calcium gluconate (100–200 mg/kg/dose, only if electrocardiographic changes are noted) (Maxwell, Linden, O'Donnell, Hamilton, & McVeigh, 2013; Rampello et al., 2006). In the immediate setting, hemodialysis can rapidly correct hyperkalemia; however, CRRT with high dialysate or replacement flow rates of 3–4 L/hr is often used in ongoing electrolyte abnormalities (Lameire et al., 2008, 2010).

Hypophosphatemia, Hypokalemia, and Hypomagnesemia

Though distinct entities, hypophosphatemia, hypokalemia, and hypomagnesemia frequently occur concomitantly in malignancy because of excess GI losses, poor oral intake, and rapid uptake from high cell turnover in rapidly growing tumors (Halfdanarson, Hogan, & Moynihan, 2006; Kapoor & Chan, 2001). These electrolyte derangements can also occur with Fanconi syndrome in multiple myeloma and with agents such as ifosfamide and cisplatin. A refeeding syndrome, which can occur in acutely ill malnourished patients who are given glucose or enteral nutrition, also manifests with hypophosphatemia, hypokalemia, and hypomagnesemia and is secondary to cellular uptake of these electrolytes. Vomiting (such as from chemotherapy), severe diarrhea, and malabsorption can cause phosphate, magnesium, and potassium depletion via GI losses. Phosphate-depleting cytokines are known to exist in certain cancers (Halfdanarson et al., 2006; Lameire et al., 2010).

Intracellular shifts, catecholamine surges, hyperalimentation, metabolic alkalosis, decreased GI absorption, increased GI and renal losses, and renal tubular damage may contribute to hypophosphatemia. Tumor-induced osteomalacia with mesenchymal tumors is well described and involves elevated urinary phosphate excretion.

Hypokalemia can result from increased GI or urinary losses or from a shift of potassium into cells. Shifts occur in those with leukocytosis, in response to granulocyte macrophage–colony-stimulating factor, or when metabolic alkalosis induces kaliuresis (Lameire et al., 2010). Diuretics and steroids can also contribute to these shifts. Fluids administered to these patients should be without dextrose, and drugs such as amiloride and spironolactone have been used as treatment.

Hypomagnesemia can also occur with certain therapeutic agents, including amphotericin, foscarnet, aminoglycosides, cisplatin, and calcineurin inhibitors. Both IV and oral electrolyte repletion are therapy mainstays (Bower et al., 2015; Lameire et al., 2010).

Hypercalcemia

Hypercalcemia is a common metabolic derangement found in patients with malignancy and has various clinical presentations. Cancers often associated with this condition include breast, lung, and multiple myeloma (Carroll & Schade, 2003; Seccareccia, 2010). Hypercalcemia may be mild (serum calcium 10.5–11.9 mg/dl), moderate (12–13.9 mg/dl), or severe (greater than 14 mg/dl). The severity of symptoms typically correlates with the degree of hypercalcemia. The prevalence of hypercalcemia in this patient population ranges from 20%–30% and is associated with high mortality. The median duration of survival is two to six months after diagnosis (Carroll & Schade, 2003; Seccareccia, 2010).

The mechanism of hypercalcemia development is often hormonal. Certain tumors secrete parathyroid hormone–related peptide (PTHrP), which stimulates osteoclast activity, bone resorption, and intestinal and renal tubular cal-cium reabsorption (Carroll & Schade, 2003; Lumachi, Brunello, Roma, & Basso, 2009). Compared to parathyroid hormone (PTH), which stimulates both bone resorption and formation, PTHrP only stimulates osteoclast activity and bone resorption and has minimal effect on bone formation (Carroll & Schade, 2003; Rosner & Dalkin, 2012). Another mechanism of hypercalcemia is a local increase in osteoclast activity surrounding the tumor within the bone marrow. Patients with hypercalcemia often present with fatigue, decreased appetite, nausea, consti-pation, weight loss, bone pain, dehydration, and intermittent confusion.

Other presenting features include polyuria and polydipsia caused by the develop-ment of nephrogenic DI, muscle aches, and more severe symptoms, including con-fusion, seizures, and coma. As calcium in the body is both in a free ionized state and bound to albumin, measurement of total calcium levels, especially in patients with malignancy, is often inaccurate, as it is affected by albumin levels as well as immu-noglobulins in certain cancers (Rosner & Dalkin, 2012; Seccareccia, 2010; Stewart, 2005). Using a correction factor (i.e., adding 0.8 mg/dl to the total calcium level for every 1 g/dl that the albumin level is below 4) is often inaccurate, and it is recom-mended that an ionized calcium level be measured in these patients.

Evaluation of hypercalcemia should include measurements of serum PTH, PTHrP, 25-hydroxyvitamin D, 1,25-dihydroxyvitamin, and creatinine levels. Dehydration and subsequent decline in glomerular filtration rate are major con-cerns. Treatment includes aggressive volume expansion with normal saline at 250–500 ml/hr with a goal urine output of 75–100 ml/hr.

Renal failure is often a concurrent finding, as hypercalcemia also results in vasoconstriction, natriuresis, and impaired concentration, leading to excessive fluid loss (Stewart, 2005). Careful monitoring for hypernatremia during volume repletion is recommended. Although no sufficient clinical data exist to support the use of loop diuretics, which enhances calcium excretion within the loop of Henle, it is often required in patients with hypercalcemia who become volume overloaded (LeGrand, Leskuski, & Zama, 2008).

IV bisphosphonates, which inhibit osteoclast activity, are often used in the treatment of hypercalcemia and have been extremely effective in patients with malignancy (Rogers, 2003). Their use may also provide symptomatic relief of malignant bone pain. Pamidronate and zoledronate are approved for treatment of malignancy-associated hypercalcemia (Rogers, 2003).

Unless its underlying cause is addressed and mitigated, hypercalcemia will recur, and the patient will likely need repeated courses of the bisphosphonate. Though previously considered to be an integral part of hypercalcemia treatment, cortico-steroids have been used less frequently and instead are more often used in certain 1,25-dihydroxyvitamin D–secreting tumors, such as Hodgkin and non-Hodgkin lymphomas. Steroids inhibit alpha-1-hydroxylase activity, decreasing the presence of activated vitamin D and calcium levels. Calcitonin inhibits osteoclast activity and increases urinary excretion of calcium, and though it is a treatment that works rapidly, its effects are short lived, as the patient develops a downregulation of calcitonin receptors, resulting in tachyphylaxis (Solimando, 2001). It is often used in patients with very severe hypercalcemia with dramatic presentations to achieve rapid correction while bisphosphonates become effective, but its efficacy is limited to the first 48 hours. Dialysis is indicated in patients with severe hypercalcemia and AKI with oliguria. In this subset of patients, volume resuscitation is limited, and dialysis with a low calcium dialysate bath is a feasible alternative.

Hypocalcemia

Hypocalcemia often presents with renal failure, TLS, metastatic cancer, and bisphosphonate therapy (Stewart, 2005). Manifestations of acute hypocalcemia include tetany (perioral and acral paresthesias and muscle spasms), blood pressure variation, and seizures. At extremes, hypocalcemia can cause QT interval prolongation and eventual dysrhythmias. Treatment must involve correction of hypomagnesemia, followed by calcium repletion with calcium gluconate and calcium chloride. Hyperphosphatemia can be treated with phosphate binders; however, calcium acetate should be avoided, as the calcium load can cause potential harm. Severely elevated phosphate levels can be treated with a short course (one to two days) of aluminum hydroxide 50–150 mg/kg per day orally every six hours (Carroll & Schade, 2003; Rosner & Dalkin, 2012).

Renal Replacement Therapy

Several types of RRT exist, including intermittent hemodialysis (IHD), CRRT (e.g., continuous venovenous hemofiltration, continuous venovenous hemodialysis, continuous venovenous hemodiafiltration), sustained low-efficiency dialysis (SLED), and peritoneal dialysis. Among ICU patients with cancer, 13%–42% have AKI and 8%–59.6% receive RRT (Berghmans & Sculier, 2004; Rosolem et al., 2012; Soares et al., 2006). In one series, up to 55% of patients with hematologic malignancies received RRT (compared to 5.7% who did not) (Darmon & Azoulay, 2009; Darmon et al., 2007). This is partially explained by higher susceptibility to infection and nephrotoxic antibiotic use in this subset of patients. The incidence of RRT needs is highest in patients with myeloma and with septic shock (Darmon et al., 2007).

When making decisions regarding the timing of dialysis initiation in this patient population, classic indications are used (e.g., fluid overload, refractory hyperkalemia, refractory acidosis, uremic symptoms). RRT is typically initiated in those with hyperkalemia, severe acidosis, severe pulmonary edema, and with severe renal failure. When deciding to start RRT in critically ill patients with cancer, it is important to consider whether their ability to receive lifesaving therapeutics would be altered (Darmon & Azoulay, 2009). TLS is a particularly important indication for dialysis because of the severity of the electrolyte disturbances. Most commonly, RRT is used in patients with sepsis and myeloma. Characteristics of the illness other than cancer often have more bearing on prognosis than the cancer itself (Berghmans et al., 2004). Of those who survive their ICU course, renal prognosis is good. Survival rates have improved in hematologic cancers because of new chemotherapy and biologics as well as stem cell transplantation, but this is at the cost of new opportunities for nephrotoxicity (Humphreys et al., 2005; Launay-Vacher et al., 2007). Dialysis dependence is associated with up to 85% mortality. A study conducted by Soares et al. (2006) evaluated six-month survival in a cohort of patients with cancer and renal failure at the time of ICU admission and was based on Acute Kidney Injury Network criteria. The malignancies represented included non-Hodgkin lymphoma, leukemia, and GI, urogenital, head and neck, lung, breast, and brain cancers (Humphreys et al., 2005; Launay-Vacher et al., 2007). The most common causes of ICU admission other than AKI were sepsis, respiratory failure, cardiovascular shock, cardiac arrest, and GI bleed. RRT was used in 32% of patients, including IHD in 9%, SLED in 65%, and CRRT in 26% (Benoit & Hoste, 2010; Maccariello et al., 2011). According to the stage of AKI, mortality was 55%, 64%, and 73%, respectively. Older age, poor performance status, severity of organ involvement, and sepsis as the underlying cause (compared with TLS or nephrotoxic ATN) were associated with higher mortality. In the presence of MODS and ventilator dependence, mortality increased to 85%–95% among patients with hematologic malignancies (Darmon et al., 2007).

CRRT refers to a group of clearance techniques tailored for hemodynamically unstable patients with renal failure. Although the indications for starting this type of therapy are similar to those used to start patients on IHD, the prescription is different, including the duration and the intensity of clearance and fluid removal (see Figure 8-2). The machines used for each therapy also differ. Patients with unstable hemodynamics cannot tolerate large amounts of fluid removal in a limited amount of time, nor can they tolerate the high electrolyte and solute fluxes that accompany the higher blood flow and dialysate flow rates in IHD. Considering this, the advent of CRRT was an exciting opportunity for intensivists and nephrologists caring for critically ill patients with acute renal failure (Golestaneh, Richter, & Amato-Hayes, 2012). Although vascular access is problematic because of thrombocytopenia and neutropenia, CRRT offers advantages, including smaller intracranial pressure increases and the allowance of large-volume infusions while maintaining the neutral or negative overall fluid balance frequently needed in patients with hematologic cancers (Berghmans et al., 2004; Rosolem et al., 2012).

Summary

AKI is a common complication in patients with malignancy, is associated with a poor prognosis, and presents challenges for timing and dosing of cancer ther-

---

Figure 8-2. Types of Renal Replacement Therapy

→

Slowest and least efficient:	Hybrid (between slow and fast):	Fastest and most efficient:
• CVVHD	• SLED, SLEDD, slow HD	• Intermittent HD
• BFR: 200–250 cc/min	• BFR: 100–300 cc/min	• BFR: 300–500 cc/min
• DFR: 1–3 L/hr	• DFR:100–300 cc/min	• DFR: 600–800 cc/min
• UFR: 50–250 cc/hr	(6–18 L/hr)	(36–48 L/hr)
• Done over 24 hours	• UFR: 50–250 cc/hr	• UFR: 0.5–2 L/hr
	• Done over 3–12 hours	• Done over 3–4 hours

BFR—blood flow rate; CVVHD—continuous venovenous hemodialysis; DFR—dialysate flow rate; HD—hemodialysis; SLED—sustained low-efficiency dialysis; SLEDD—sustained low-efficiency daily dialysis; UFR—ultrafiltration rate

Note. Based on information from Bellomo et al., 2002; Dirkes & Hodge, 2007; Golestaneh et al., 2012; Zobel et al., 1998.

---

apeutics. Various etiologies of cancer-related AKI include hemodynamic, vascular, glomerular, tubular, and interstitial processes. Obstructive renal disease is seen more commonly in patients with cancer than in the general population. TLS and multiple myeloma are cases of malignancy-related AKI that deserve special mention. Hyponatremia, hypercalcemia, and hyperkalemia are frequently seen as complications of malignancy and are considered medical emergencies in severe cases. Therapeutic plasma exchange is used for stabilization of TMA and myeloma cast nephropathy, though its use is controversial in the latter. Leukapheresis is used for severe leukocytosis and hyperviscosity. Decision making regarding initiation of RRT should involve consideration of the risks and benefits, including prognostic considerations as well as the type and intensity of the therapy. Frequent reappraisal of the risk versus benefit of CRRT is necessary once the decision has been made to initiate RRT. CRRT, IHD, and SLED have been used successfully in malignancy-related AKI (Darmon et al., 2007; Soares et al., 2006). Ultimately, the key to managing AKI is to ensure an interprofessional approach to preventive care, disease management, and early intervention (Rosolem et al., 2012).

References

Al-Nouri, Z.L., Reese, J.A., Terrell, D.R., Vesely, S.K., & George, J.N. (2015). Drug-induced thrombotic microangiopathy: A systematic review of published reports. *Blood, 125,* 616–618. doi:10.1182/blood-2014-11-611335

Arrambide, K., & Toto, R.D. (1993). Tumor lysis syndrome. *Seminars in Nephrology, 13,* 273–280.

Bagshaw, S.M., George, C., & Bellomo, R. (2008). A comparison of the RIFLE and AKIN criteria for acute kidney injury in critically ill patients. *Nephrology Dialysis Transplantation, 23,* 1569–1574. doi:10.1093/ndt/gfn009

Bellomo, R., Baldwin, I., Ronco, C., & Golper, T. (2002). *Atlas of hemofiltration.* London, England: W.B. Saunders.

Benoit, D.D., & Hoste, E.A. (2010). Acute kidney injury in critically ill patients with cancer. *Critical Care Clinics, 26,* 151–179. doi:10.1016/j.ccc.2009.09.002

Berghmans, T., Meert, A.P., Markiewicz, E., & Sculier, J.P. (2004). Continuous venovenous haemofiltration in cancer patients with renal failure: A single-centre experience. *Supportive Care in Cancer, 12,* 306–311. doi:10.1007/s00520-003-0588-8

Berghmans, T., & Sculier, J.P. (2004). Is there any usefulness for a specific scoring system in assessing the prognosis of cancer patients admitted to the intensive care unit? *Intensive Care Medicine, 30,* 1849. doi:10.1007/s00134-004-2364-8

Berns, J.S., & Ford, P.A. (1997). Renal toxicities of antineoplastic drugs and bone marrow transplantation. *Seminars in Nephrology, 17,* 54–66.

Bower, M., Robinson, L., & Cox, S. (2015). Endocrine and metabolic complications of advanced cancer. In N. Cherny, M. Fallon, S. Kassa, R. Portenoy, & D.C. Currow (Eds.), *Oxford textbook of palliative medicine* (5th ed., pp. 906–919). England, UK: Oxford University Press.

Buemi, M., Fazio, M.R., Bolignano, D., Coppolino, G., Donato, V., Lacquaniti, A., ... Allegra, A. (2009). Renal complications in oncohematologic patients. *Journal of Investigative Medicine, 57,* 892–901. doi:10.2310/JIM.0b013e3181c5e762

Cairo, M.S., & Bishop, M. (2004). Tumour lysis syndrome: New therapeutic strategies and classification. *British Journal of Haematology, 127,* 3–11. doi:10.1111/j.1365-2141.2004.05094.x

Campbell, G.A., Hu, D., & Okusa, M.D. (2014). Acute kidney injury in the cancer patient. *Advances in Chronic Kidney Disease, 21,* 64–71. doi:10.1053/j.ackd.2013.08.002

Carroll, M.F., & Schade, D.S. (2003). A practical approach to hypercalcemia. *American Family Physician, 67,* 1959–1966.

Coiffier, B., Altman, A., Pui, C.-H., Younes, A., & Cairo, M.S. (2008). Guidelines for the management of pediatric and adult tumor lysis syndrome: An evidence-based review. *Journal of Clinical Oncology, 26,* 2767–2778. doi:10.1200/JCO.2007.15.0177

Darmon, M., & Azoulay, E. (2009). Critical care management of cancer patients: Cause for optimism and need for objectivity. *Current Opinion in Oncology, 21,* 318–326. doi:10.1097/CCO.0b013e32832b68b6

Darmon, M., Guichard, I., Vincent, F., Schlemmer, B., & Azoulay, E. (2010). Prognostic significance of acute renal injury in acute tumor lysis syndrome. *Leukemia and Lymphoma, 51,* 221–227. doi:10.3109/10428190903456959

Darmon, M., Malak, S., Guichard, I., & Schlemmer, B. (2008). Acute tumor lysis syndrome: A comprehensive review. *Revista Brasileira de Terapia Intensiva, 2003,* 278–285. doi:10.1590/S0103-507X2008000300011

Darmon, M., Thiery, G., Ciroldi, M., Porcher, R., Schlemmer, B., & Azoulay, E. (2007). Should dialysis be offered to cancer patients with acute kidney injury? *Intensive Care Medicine, 33,* 765–772. doi:10.1007/s00134-007-0579-1

Dirkes, S., & Hodge, K. (2007). Continuous renal replacement therapy in the adult intensive care unit: History and current trends. *Critical Care Nurse, 27,* 61–81.

Epstein, M. (1992). The hepatorenal syndrome—Newer perspectives. *New England Journal of Medicine, 327,* 1810–1811. doi:10.1056/NEJM199212173272509

Eremina, V., Jefferson, J.A., Kowalewska, J., Hochster, H., Haas, M., Weisstuch, J., ... Quaggin, S.E. (2008). VEGF inhibition and renal thrombotic microangiopathy. *New England Journal of Medicine, 358,* 1129–1136. doi:10.1056/NEJMoa0707330

Finkel, K.W., & Foringer, J.R. (2007). Renal disease in patients with cancer. *Nature Clinical Practice Nephrology, 3,* 669–678.

Gafter-Gvili, A., Ram, R., Gafter, U., Shpilberg, O., & Raanani, P. (2009). Renal failure associated with tyrosine kinase inhibitors—Case report and review of the literature. *Leukemia Research, 34,* 123–127. doi:10.1016/j.leukres.2009.07.009

Ganguli, A., Sawinski, D., & Berns, J.S. (2015). Kidney diseases associated with haematological cancers. *Nature Reviews Nephrology, 11,* 478–490. doi:10.1038/nrneph.2015.81

George, J.N., & Nester, C.M. (2014). Syndromes of thrombotic microangiopathy. *New England Journal of Medicine, 371,* 654–666. doi:10.1056/NEJMra1312353

Ginès, P., & Schrier, R.W. (2009). Renal failure in cirrhosis. *New England Journal of Medicine, 361,* 1279–1290.

Golestaneh, L., Richter, B., & Amato-Hayes, M. (2012). Logistics of renal replacement therapy: Relevant issues for critical care nurses. *American Journal of Critical Care, 21,* 126–130. doi:10.4037 /ajcc2012280

Halfdanarson, T.R., Hogan, W.J., & Moynihan, T.J. (2006). Oncologic emergencies: Diagnosis and treatment. *Mayo Clinic Proceedings, 81,* 835–848. doi:10.4065/81.6.835

Howard, S.C., Jones, D.P., & Pui, C.-H. (2011). The tumor lysis syndrome. *New England Journal of Medicine, 364,* 1844–1854. doi:10.1056/NEJMra0904569

Hsu, C.N., Lee, C.T., Su, C.H., Wang, Y.C., Chen, H.L., Chuang, J.H., & Tain, Y.L. (2016). Incidence, outcomes, and risk factors of community-acquired and hospital-acquired acute kidney injury: A retrospective cohort study. *Medicine, 95,* e3674. doi:10.1097/MD.0000000000003674

Humphreys, B.D., Soiffer, R.J., & Magee, C.C. (2005). Renal failure associated with cancer and its treatment: An update. *Journal of the American Society of Nephrology, 16,* 151–161. doi:10.1681 /ASN.2004100843

Izzedine, H., & Perazella, M.A. (2015). Thrombotic microangiopathy, cancer, and cancer drugs. *American Journal of Kidney Diseases, 66,* 857–868. doi:10.1053/j.ajkd.2015.02.340

Kapoor, M., & Chan, G.Z. (2001). Malignancy and renal disease. *Critical Care Clinics, 17,* 571–598. doi:10.1016/S0749-0704(05)70199-8

Kleeberg, L., Morgera, S., Jakob, C., Hocher, B., Schneider, M., Peters, H., … Sezer, O. (2009). Novel renal replacement strategies for the elimination of serum free light chains in patients with kappa light chain nephropathy. *European Journal of Medical Research, 14,* 47–54. doi:10.1186 /2047-783X-14-2-47

Lam, A.Q., & Humphreys, B.D. (2012). Onco-nephrology: AKI in the cancer patient. *Clinical Journal of the American Society of Nephrology, 7,* 1692–1700. doi:10.2215/CJN.03140312

Lameire, N.H. (2007). The kidney in oncology. *Acta Clinica Belgica, 62,* 141–154. doi:10.1179/acb .2007.025

Lameire, N.H., Flombaum, C.D., Moreau, D., & Ronco, C. (2005). Acute renal failure in cancer patients. *Annals of Medicine, 37,* 13–25. doi:10.1080/07853890510007205

Lameire, N.H., Van Biesen, W., & Vanholder, R. (2008). Acute renal problems in the critically ill cancer patient. *Current Opinion in Critical Care, 14,* 635–646. doi:10.1097/MCC .0b013e32830ef70b

Lameire, N.H., Van Biesen, W., & Vanholder, R. (2010). Electrolyte disturbances and acute kidney injury in patients with cancer. *Seminars in Nephrology, 30,* 534–547. doi:10.1016/j.semnephrol .2010.09.002

Laskin, B.L., Goebel, J., Davies, S.M., & Jodele, S. (2011). Small vessels, big trouble in the kidneys and beyond: Hematopoietic stem cell transplantation-associated thrombotic microangiopathy. *Blood, 118,* 1452–1462. doi:10.1182/blood-2011-02-321315

Launay-Vacher, V., Oudard, S., Janus, N., Gligorov, J., Pourrat, X., Rixe, O., … Deray, G. (2007). Prevalence of renal insufficiency in cancer patients and implications for anticancer drug management: The Renal Insufficiency and Anticancer Medications (IRMA) study. *Cancer, 110,* 1376–1384. doi:10.1182/blood-2011-02-321315

LeGrand, S.B., Leskuski, D., & Zama, I. (2008). Narrative review: Furosemide for hypercalcemia: An unproven yet common practice. *Annals of Internal Medicine, 149,* 259–263. doi:10.7326 /0003-4819-149-4-200808190-00007

Li Cavoli, G., Passantino, D., Tortorici, C., Bono, L., Ferrantelli, A., & Rotolo, U. (2015). Acute interstitial nephritis overlapping chronic renal damage. *Saudi Journal of Kidney Diseases and Transplantation, 26,* 1020–1022. doi:10.4103/1319-2442.164597

Lin, C.Y., & Chen, Y.-C. (2012). Acute kidney injury classification: AKIN and RIFLE criteria in critical patients. *World Journal of Critical Care Medicine, 1,* 40–45. doi:10.5492/wjccm.v1.i2.40

Lumachi, F., Brunello, A., Roma, A., & Basso, U. (2009). Cancer-induced hypercalcemia. *Anticancer Research, 29,* 1551–1555.

Maccariello, E., Valente, C., Nogueira, L., Bonomo, H., Jr., Ismael, M., Machado, J.E., … Soares, M. (2011). Outcomes of cancer and non-cancer patients with acute kidney injury and need of renal replacement therapy admitted to general intensive care units. *Nephrology Dialysis Transplantation, 26,* 537–543. doi:10.1093/ndt/gfq441

Maesaka, J.K., Mittal, S.K., & Fishbane, S. (1997). Paraneoplastic syndromes of the kidney. *Seminars in Oncology, 24,* 373–381.

Mato, A.R., Riccio, B.E., Qin, L., Heitjan, D.F., Carroll, M., Loren, A., … Luger, S.M. (2006). A predictive model for the detection of tumor lysis syndrome during AML induction therapy. *Leukemia and Lymphoma, 47,* 877–883. doi:10.1080/10428190500404662

Maxwell, A.P., Linden, K., O'Donnell, S., Hamilton, P.K., & McVeigh, G.E. (2013). Management of hyperkalemia. *Journal of the Royal College of Physicians of Edinburgh, 43,* 246–251. doi:10.4997/JRCPE.2013.312

Mirrakhimov, A.E., Voore, P., Khan, M., & Ali, A.M. (2015). Tumor lysis syndrome: A clinical review. *World Journal of Critical Care Medicine, 4,* 130–138. doi:10.5492/wjccm.v4.i2.130

Pamuk, G.E., Uyanik, M.S., Demir, M., Tekgündüz, E., Turgut, B., & Soy, M. (2007). Systemic antineutrophil cytoplasmic antibody vasculitis in a patient with chronic lymphocytic leukemia: Quite a rare diagnosis. *Leukemia Research, 31,* 1149–1151. doi:10.1016/j.leukres.2006.08.017

Parikh, C.R., & Coca, S.G. (2006). Acute renal failure in hematopoietic cell transplantation. *Kidney International, 69,* 430–435. doi:10.1038/sj.ki.5000055

Perazella, M.A. (2012). Onco-nephrology: Renal toxicities of chemotherapeutic agents. *Clinical Journal of the American Society of Nephrology, 7,* 1713–1721. doi:10.2215/CJN.02780312

Perazella, M.A., & Markowitz, G.S. (2008). Bisphosphonate nephrotoxicity. *Kidney International, 74,* 1385–1393. doi:10.1038/ki.2008.356

Praga, M., & González, E. (2010). Acute interstitial nephritis. *Kidney International, 77,* 956–961. doi:10.1038/ki.2010.89

Rampello, R., Fricia, T., & Malaguarnera, M. (2006). The management of pediatric and adult tumor lysis syndrome. *Nature Clinical Practice, 3,* 438–447. doi:10.1038/ncponc0581

Riedl, M., Fakhouri, F., Le Quintrec, M., Noone, D.G., Jungraithmayr, T.C., Fremeaux-Bacchi, V., & Licht, C. (2014). Spectrum of complement-mediated thrombotic microangiopathies: Pathogenetic insights identifying novel treatment approaches. *Seminars in Thrombosis and Hemostasis, 40,* 444–464. doi:10.1055/s-0034-1376153

Rogers, M.J. (2003). New insights into the molecular mechanisms of action of bisphosphonates. *Current Pharmaceutical Design, 9,* 2643–2658. doi:10.2174/1381612033453640

Ronco, C., Haapio, M., House, A.A., Anavekar, N., & Bellomo, R. (2008). Cardiorenal syndrome. *Journal of the American College of Cardiology, 52,* 1527–1539. doi:10.1016/j.jacc.2008.07.051

Rosner, M.H., & Dalkin, A.C. (2012). Onco-nephrology: The pathophysiology and treatment of malignancy-associated hypercalcemia. *Clinical Journal of the American Society of Nephrology, 7,* 1722–1729. doi:10.2215/CJN.02470312

Rosolem, M.M., Rabello, L.S.C.F., Lisboa, T., Caruso, P., Costa, R.T., Leal, J.V., … Soares, M. (2012). Critically ill patients with cancer and sepsis: Clinical course and prognostic factors. *Journal of Critical Care, 27,* 301–307. doi:10.1016/j.jcrc.2011.06.014

Salahudeen, A.K., & Bonventre, J.V. (2013). Onconephrology: The latest frontier in the war against kidney disease. *Journal of the American Society of Nephrology, 24,* 26–30. doi:10.1681/ASN.2012070690

Schlondorff, J.S., Mendez, G.P., Rennke, H.G., & Magee, C.C. (2007). Electrolyte abnormalities and progressive renal failure in a cancer patient. *Kidney International, 71,* 1181–1184. doi:10.1038/sj.ki.5002182

Seccareccia, D. (2010). Cancer-related hypercalcemia. *Canadian Family Physician, 56,* 244–246.

Soares, M., Salluh, J.I.F., Carvalho, M.S., Darmon, M., Rocco, J.R., & Spector, N. (2006). Prognosis of critically ill patients with cancer and acute renal dysfunction. *Journal of Clinical Oncology, 24,* 4003–4010. doi:10.1200/JCO.2006.05.7869

Solimando, D.A. (2001). Overview of hypercalcemia of malignancy. *American Journal of Health-System Pharmacy, 58*(Suppl. 3), S4–S7.

Stewart, A.F. (2005). Hypercalcemia associated with cancer. *New England Journal of Medicine, 352,* 373–379. doi:10.1056/NEJMcp042806

Wilson, F.P., & Berns, J.S. (2012). Onco-nephrology: Tumor lysis syndrome. *Clinical Journal of the American Society of Nephrology, 7,* 1730–1739. doi:10.2215/CJN.03150312

Zakarija, A., & Bennett, C. (2005). Drug-induced thrombotic microangiopathy. *Seminars in Thrombosis and Hemostasis, 31,* 681–690. doi:10.1055/s-2005-925474

Zobel, G., Rödl, S., Urlesberger, B., Kuttnig-Haim, M., & Ring, E. (1998). Continuous renal replacement therapy in critically ill patients. *Kidney International, 66*(Suppl. 5), S169–S173.

CHAPTER 9

Cardiovascular Complications

Catherine Sargent, MS, RN, BC, AOCNS®, and
Brenda K. Shelton, DNP, APRN-CNS, RN, CCRN, AOCN®

Introduction

As cancer survival rates rise, the population ages, and targeted/oral therapy use increases, so too does the prevalence of cardiovascular complications that require critical or step-down care (Bonita & Pradhan, 2013; Curigliano, Mayer, Burstein, Winer, & Goldhirsch, 2010; Viale & Yamamoto, 2008; Villarraga, Herrmann, & Nkomo, 2014). These complications range from asymptomatic subclinical abnormalities to life-threatening events and may be acute or progressive in onset, have the potential to be short-lived or long term, and can be reversible or lead to permanent defects (Curigliano et al., 2010; Khawaja, Cafferkey, Rajani, Redwood, & Cunningham, 2014). Lenihan and Cardinale (2012) reported asymptomatic systolic and diastolic left ventricular dysfunction as the most common signs of chronic cardiotoxicity that can lead to heart failure and possible death in patients with cancer. Because of this risk, an interprofessional approach for surveillance and early detection is crucial and should involve both oncology and cardiology healthcare providers.

The incidence of cardiovascular disease associated with cancer and its treatment is greatly underestimated and frequently attributed to other causes (Fadol & Lech, 2011; Polovich, Olsen, & LeFebvre, 2014). Little is known about the extent or the exact mechanisms of injury that cancer treatments inflict on the heart and vessels (Hampton, 2010). Survivors of childhood cancer can experience chronic illnesses and may take medication for hypertension, hyperlipidemia, and diabetes mellitus (Walsh, 2010). In addition, a suspected link exists between specific cancers and the development of cardiovascular disease, but this may be more related to the risk similarities of the two diseases (Rahman, 2009). Squamous cell and pancreatic cancers have most often been associated with coronary artery disease (Rahman, 2009). Although cardiovascular complications in patients with cancer have historically been associated with chemotherapy agents (e.g., anthracyclines, tyrosine kinase inhibitors [TKIs]), these problems can occur with almost any cancer treatment (Force & Kerkelä, 2008). Other risks include a past medical history of diabetes mellitus, HIV, or gastrointestinal malignancies (Leja, 2013). Patients with chest masses or those who have received prior treatments with hormone therapies, corticosteroids, or chest irradiation are also at risk (Leja, 2013; Yusuf, Sami, & Daher, 2011). Patient- and therapy-related risks for cardiovascular complications are summarized in Figure 9-1.

Early identification of cardiovascular complications can be difficult because symptoms, such as shortness of breath, peripheral edema, and fatigue, can be attributed to other malignancies or noncardiac-related causes (Force & Kerkelä, 2008). Many new antineoplastic agents have only been associated with cardiovascular toxicity during the postmarketing period, making the true incidence of complications difficult to quantify. Additionally, cardiotoxicity or overt heart failure may not occur until later in life, typically 20–30 years after therapeutic treatment, and clinicians may not recognize a correlation to previous cancer treatments (Anderson & Sawyer, 2008; Villarraga et al., 2014).

Figure 9-1. Patients at Risk for Cardiotoxicity

Intrinsic Risks
- African American race
- Alcohol consumption, excessive and prolonged
- Drug hypersensitivity reaction
- Electrolyte abnormalities (e.g., hypercalcemia, hypocalcemia, hyperkalemia, hypomagnesemia, hypokalemia)
- Female sex
- Heart disease or hypertension (preexisting)
- Infection or sepsis
- Obesity
- Pregnancy
- Renal dysfunction
- Smoking
- Trisomy 21

Disease-Mediated Risks
- Cardiac involvement of heart
- Malignant infiltration of pericardium
- Damage to the vagus nerve with loss of sympathetic mediation
- Thrombotic risk due to cancer procoagulants
- Malignancy infiltration/erosion into vessels

Therapy Risks
- Type of drug category
- Specific antineoplastic agent
- Toxicity ameliorating strategy (liposomal or pegylated formulation)
- Rate of medication administration
- Delivery schedule
- Combination therapy
- Radiation to chest involving heart or great vessels

Note. Based on information from Hampton, 2010.

This chapter will describe the best practices in management of cardiovascular complications requiring a higher level of medical or nursing care, including the transfer to intensive or step-down care units. It will also detail cardiac complications in cancer care and include a global perspective of how these complications influence oncologic treatment. Cancer invasion of cardiac structures, indirect cardiac complications from the presence of primary tumors or their metastases, and common antineoplastic medications or radiation-induced toxicities also will be reviewed.

Cardiac Injury Related to Cancer

One approach to understanding and classifying a cardiovascular complication is to consider the cardiac subsystem it affects. Normal cardiovascular function involves blood filling the coronary arteries to provide energy and oxygenation for heart function. Coronary artery ischemia or occlusion occurs because of vasospasm or thromboses and has been associated with cancer therapies such as fluoropyrimidines and interleukin-2 (Escalante & Yeung, 2013). Cardiac myocytes initiate electrical automaticity through a coordinated conduction pathway, which results in dysrhythmias when disrupted. Conduction disturbances (dysrhythmias) may occur acutely during treatment or result from long-term damage to conduction pathways (Anderson & Sawyer, 2008). Structural changes in valves or myocytes may occur from direct injury to mitochondrial function in the myocytes, as seen with the development of cardiomyopathy after exposure to specific antineoplastic medications (Bonita & Pradhan, 2013). Excess pericardial fluid also impairs venous return and blood flow through the heart, resulting in inadequate cardiac output. Vascular tone contributes to cardiovascular function by regulating blood flow through the vessels. Abnormalities in vascular tone include hypotension, hypertension, Raynaud disease, and vascular thrombosis (Anderson & Sawyer, 2008; Polovich et al., 2014; Viale & Yamamoto, 2008).

Cardiac Diagnostic Tests

Accurate interpretation of diagnostic tests is essential in understanding cardiovascular complications of cancer and its treatment. Initial diagnostic tests are routinely used to establish baseline function prior to known cardiotoxic antineoplastic therapy. It is normal for patients to have a baseline echocardiogram or multigated acquisition (MUGA) scan prior to administration of anthracyclines or high-dose cyclophosphamide. It also is common for a patient to have a 12-lead electrocardiogram (ECG) with corrected QT (QTc) interval prior to receiving arsenic trioxide or TKIs. Nurses routinely examine baseline or ongoing screening diagnostic test results prior to administering specific antineoplastic therapies and should recognize patient and test variables that influence changes in these results or warrant additional testing. Tests may be affected by patient weight, body position, metabolic disturbances, comorbidities, or operator skill. When using diagnostic tests to evaluate symptoms, the first test is chosen based on the major cardiac subsystem affected. For example, a chest x-ray may be used as a basic screening tool for abnormal structural defects. If an enlarged cardiac silhouette is noted, this can be followed by a heart function test, such as an echocardiogram. More specialized or targeted studies, such as a cardiac magnetic resonance imaging (MRI) scan, serum cardiac troponins, or an exercise stress test, may assist in differential diagnosis of unique disorders. The most common diagnostic tests used for assessment of cardiovascular disease and their indications, common findings, and nursing implications are included in Table 9-1.

Cardiovascular Disorders and Antineoplastic Therapy

The clinical implications of cardiovascular injury in cancer care relate to the type or degree of cardiac dysfunction and the cancer treatment plan. The goal of care is to implement preventive or supportive care therapies against cardiovascular insult while optimizing cancer treatment. Cardiovascular complications can affect cancer treatment plans in a variety of ways. For example, a baseline cardiovascular disease may influence the ability to adequately treat a malignancy, or a cancer treatment may require modification if overlapping risks for a specific complication are present. Treatment-related considerations should be discussed in the context of providing acute and critical care in patients with cancer. Nurses who understand these concepts can better advocate and prioritize care for their patients. In the case of comorbid or concomitant cardiac disease, considerations must be made to evaluate whether specific cardiotoxic antineoplastic therapies can be employed, doses need to be modified, or closer toxicity monitoring is indicated.

Cancer Involvement of Cardiac Structures

Cancer involvement of cardiac structures is rare, with occurrence rates under 1%. It is most commonly associated with atrial myxomas, cardiac sarcomas, and infiltrative lymphoma (Escalante & Yeung, 2013; Leja, 2013). Metastases to the heart have been reported with melanoma and cancers of the breast and lung (Leja, 2013). The most prevalent manifestation is involvement of the pericardium with subsequent pericardial effusion (Story, 2013). The dual pericardial layer impedes metastasis of most cancers into the myocardium. In unusual cases, a tumor manifests in the myocardial wall and compromises wall motion and cardiac output. Intrachamber or intramural thromboses may also be present, complicating treatment. Signs and symptoms may include chest discomfort, dyspnea, edema, effusions, dysrhythmias, and heart failure. Displaced precordial pulses and heart sounds may also be present. These disorders are usually

Table 9-1. Cardiac Diagnostic Tests			
Test	**Description**	**Indications**	**Cancer Care Implications**
Brain natriuretic peptide serum level	Substance produced by a ventricle in heart failure Normal serum < 100 mg/dl, clinically significant if > 300 mg/dl	Evaluates presence and severity of heart failure Monitors effects of medications	Early screening for heart failure or monitoring response to heart failure treatment May be elevated due to other disorders common in patients with cancer (e.g., atrial fibrillation/flutter, chronic obstructive lung disease, sepsis)
Cardiac catheterization and angiogram	Dye injection with fluoroscopic evaluation of primary and collateral blood flow to the heart	Coronary artery syndromes for diagnosis, access to perform reperfusion interventions (e.g., angioplasty, stent placement)	Particularly useful for assessment of intracardiac blood supply and potential resectability Vasospastic coronary artery changes may result in lack of abnormalities during angiogram. Anticoagulation required for the procedure or after management may be contraindicated due to bleeding risks of patients with cancer.
Cardiac enzymes (e.g., creatine phosphokinase, troponin)	Levels of enzymes leaking from myocytes at time of injury	Detects of current acute coronary syndrome	Small elevations in troponin levels may be indicative of increased metabolic stress common in cancer due to anemia, sepsis, chemotherapy, or transfusion reactions. Use of troponin levels to monitor for early risk of cardiotoxicity if collected during administration of cardiotoxic agents

(Continued on next page)

Table 9-1. Cardiac Diagnostic Tests *(Continued)*			
Test	**Description**	**Indications**	**Cancer Care Implications**
Cardiac computed tomography (CT) with or without angiography	Scan of the heart and related structures in the chest	Evaluates heart and surrounding structures including fluid in the pericardial space Detects metastases to the heart or pericardium	Especially useful to describe the blood supply to intracardiac tumors May show fluid accumulation in the posterior plane where other tests do not Able to detect differences between fluid and blood in the pericardial space
Cardiac magnetic resonance imaging	Provides a three-dimensional view of the size, shape, and relationship between the heart and nearby structures	Evaluates all heart structures and specific size, shape, and relationships to each other	High contrast and resolution make it the ideal test to assess cardiac tumors. May be problematic due to cost, availability, contraindications, or patient intolerance
Echocardiogram (echo) (e.g., transthoracic, transesophageal, two-dimensional, three-dimensional, with or without Doppler, stress echo)	Ultrasound of wall thickness, internal diameter, wall motion, and fluid in pericardial space Able to estimate ejection fraction	Detects valve, global wall motion, and pericardial fluid abnormalities; can calculate approximate ejection fraction With additional features, such as color Doppler or post-stress echo, provides more details about ischemia and cardiac function under stress	Not sensitive for the presence of cardiac tumors, missing structures in the posterior atria, and ventricles because the density may be similar to the myocardium Use of transthoracic echo for baseline evaluation for cardiotoxic drugs is effective in the absence of coronary artery disease. Transesophageal echo is useful for evaluation of valve vegetations and intracavitary thrombi. Results may be more reproducible than with multigated acquisition (MUGA) scans. Less accurate in obese patients or those with barrel chest

(Continued on next page)

Test	Description	Indications	Cancer Care Implications
Table 9-1. Cardiac Diagnostic Tests (Continued)			
Electrocardio-gram (e.g., 12-lead, stress)	Pictorial view of conduction pathways	Detects isch-emia, injury, old infarction, electrolyte dis-orders, and pericardial effusion	Nonspecific changes are common in patients with cancer because of increased metabolic demands.
MUGA scan	Accurate reflec-tion of circula-tion of nuclear substance that detects coro-nary blood flow with or without exercise Wall motion abnormalities without uptake indicate old infarction.	Detects signifi-cant compro-mise of cor-onary blood flow Helpful to mon-itor progres-sion of cor-onary artery disease or recovery from myocardial infarction	Segmental ischemia may be better detected by MUGA than echo, and this test may be more useful prior to cardio-toxic medication admin-istration when underly-ing coronary disease is suspected. This is a better test for wall motion than ejec-tion fraction and likely to underestimate ejec-tion fraction, which may lead to earlier dose adjustment or discontin-uation of antineoplastic agents. Small amount of radiation exposure with this test makes it difficult to use as a long-term monitor-ing tool.

Note. Based on information from Anderson & White, 2013; Fee, 2013; Leja, 2013; Shelton, 2014a, 2014b, 2014c; Story, 2013; Truong et al., 2014; Woods, 2013.

suspected based on routine screening tests, such as a chest x-ray, chest computed tomography (CT) scan, or echocardiogram. A contrast-enhanced CT scan, car-diac MRI, or cardiac positron-emission tomography scan can provide greater details. The degree of myocyte injury can be determined by elevations in serum cardiac troponin levels or by ischemic ST changes on a 12-lead ECG. These often do not match typical findings with acute coronary syndrome or pericar-ditis/effusion (Hamo & Bloom, 2015). The presence of thrombi may also pro-duce pulmonary hypertension. Common intracardiac tumors are often sensitive to chemotherapy; thus, initial treatment may include inpatient IV chemotherapy with or without inclusion of thrombolytic infusions. Thrombectomies may be performed when patients are extremis, although all invasive procedures are considered high risk in this population.

Coronary and pulmonary artery occlusions are infrequent but significant cardiac complications of cancer that may occur with large chest masses. Signs and symptoms include ischemic chest pain or ST changes on ECG and may be position dependent. They may also occur transiently and resolve when the chest mass is no longer compressing the cardiac structures. This symptomatology is unique to the presence of chest masses and does not occur with typical coronary artery disease. Patients with chest masses may have fewer symptoms when sitting and leaning forward or while in a prone position. These patients are often admitted to intensive care and intermediate care settings for close observation and continuous cardiac monitoring before and during treatment. They may experience sudden and intractable vascular collapse when general anesthetics are administered, warranting special anesthetic procedures (Andréjak et al., 2011; Azoulay et al., 2011). Nurses can be essential leaders in patient care by initiating and maintaining patient positioning to optimize coronary perfusion or radiation therapy.

Vigilant monitoring for new cardiac symptoms can detect untoward effects of treatment, such as vascular injury, worsening effusions, conduction system dysfunction, or coronary ischemia. Because cardiac involvement in heart structures is uncommon, little is known to help predict typical responses (Leja, 2013). Awareness of possible cardiac complications, risk factors, and implications for care is instrumental in enhancing patient outcomes.

Nonspecific Demands on the Cardiovascular System

The metabolic demands of malignancy encompass issues involving oxygen-carrying capacity, high metabolic and energy demands, and perfusion deficits. Pulmonary complications with impaired oxygenation are common problems for many patients with cancer and can lead to organ ischemia and injury. Nonspecific 12-lead electrocardiographic changes indicating global ischemia, such as flattened or inverted T waves and ST depression, may be present in patients; however, their significance is unclear without other insults. Cancer is associated with a high metabolic rate, causing cachexia, chronic nutrient deficiency, and organ ischemia. Anemia related to disease or treatment may impair oxygen-carrying capacity and tissue perfusion. The cardiac ischemic effect of anemia is inconsistent and may depend on the severity of anemia or other risks; however, it should be considered a potentially treatable etiology in this population. The high incidence of thromboses in patients with cancer has been attributed to cancer procoagulants, inflammation, hyperviscosity, and impaired mobility. Patients with the highest risk for thrombotic complications include those with adenocarcinomas (mucin-producing tumors), acute leukemia (high inflammation), and multiple myeloma (high viscosity) (Story, 2014). The most common cancer types for venous thromboses are brain tumors, acute leukemia, and pancreatic cancer (Story, 2014). These risks predispose patients to myocardial ischemia, vasculitis, and pulmonary embolism with pulmonary hypertension. Inflammatory processes involved in malignancy, chronic or severe infection, and immune treatments for cancer (e.g., interleukin-2) have rarely been associated with cardiac complications such as endocarditis, myocarditis, and pericarditis (Woods, 2013). Although patients may require admission to intensive and intermediate care units for these complications, their infrequency warrants review of general critical care resources for the most current and best management suggestions.

Preexisting Cardiovascular Disease

Preexisting cardiac disease at cancer diagnosis may preclude patients from certain treatment options where cardiotoxic agents are traditionally used or the presence of cardiac comorbidity may prevent use of specific anesthetic agents or surgical procedures. These patients are also at risk for malignancy, making these two disorders common comorbidities. The existence of premorbid cardiovascular disease does not pose added risk for all antineoplastic therapies but may require contemplation in some situations. Uncontrolled cardiac disease conditions (e.g., coronary artery disease, dysrhythmias, heart failure, hypertension, Raynaud disease) will be enhanced by overlapping toxicities from therapy. The presence of cardiac disease may also alter antineoplastic drug selection. For example, a woman with breast cancer may not receive an anthracycline if she also has diabetes or heart disease. Alternatively, medication doses may be changed to decrease cardiovascular risk or enhance patient tolerance while still receiving recommended treatment (Fadol & Lech, 2011; Polovich et al., 2014). An outpatient regimen may be administered in the hospital to monitor for complications, such as dysrhythmias. The demands of other toxicities (e.g., gastrointestinal distress) may indirectly worsen these conditions. For example, patients with chemotherapy-induced diarrhea may also experience fluid and electrolyte imbalances that may exacerbate their chronic dysrhythmias or angina. Poorly controlled hypertension may become more severe, leading to premature discontinuation of antineoplastic medications (e.g., bevacizumab, sunitinib) (Guglin, Aljayeh, Saiyad, Ali, & Curtis, 2009).

Antineoplastic Medications

Cardiovascular toxicity related to antineoplastic medications has been a long-established concern but is felt to be well controlled by dose management strategies. Toxicities range from minor and asymptomatic conduction delays to severe and sudden pump dysfunction with heart failure. The diverse toxicities and mechanisms of injury necessitate a thorough cancer treatment history when patients present with cardiovascular symptoms. Current resources are limited in provision of complete lists of medications with potential cardiotoxic effects; however, specific medication classifications may exhibit class effect toxicities, meaning all agents may cause the clinical effect with varying degrees of severity or at different doses. Table 9-2 provides an overview of currently available agents and their known cardiotoxicities.

Anthracyclines have long been associated with development of left ventricular dysfunction with established maximum recommended doses; however, scientists have recently recognized potential for dose adjustments, albeit with a higher risk of toxicity. Formulations of these agents with liposomal coating or pegylation have been created to reduce the risk of toxicity. The concomitant risks associated with host-related factors, such as preexisting diabetes mellitus or hypertension, have not been clearly quantified. Additionally, other chemotherapeutic agents produce effects that may be more idiosyncratic and less dose related, such as dysrhythmias, QT prolongation, or coronary vasospasm. Many occur acutely, without known cofactors or precipitators. These features have made prevention more challenging.

In addition to the type I cardiotoxicity identified with anthracyclines, type II cardiotoxicity causes reversible injury without microtubule destruction of the myocytes. Symptoms and myocardial dysfunction occur, but cellular damage is not evident. The exact mechanisms differentiating type I and II injury remain elusive but are loosely associated with class effects. On some occasions, the typical clinical trajectory based on known effects of a specific agent is not as anticipated. Type I injury has been associated with anthracyclines, alkylating agents (e.g., cyclophosphamide, cisplatin), and microtubule inhibitors (e.g., taxanes). Type II cardiotoxicity has been associated with ErbB2 receptor inhibitors that target the MAPK/ERK or AKT/P13K signaling pathways. Their action is time limited based on the half-life of the drug, making toxicities reversible. Of note, no known dose-related thresholds exist that cause a type II injury to become a type I injury; however, mixed injury has been noted in some high-risk individuals, particularly if they receive more than one cardiotoxic agent.

Alkylating Agents

Cardiotoxicity with cisplatin is caused by the release of oxygen radicals, which can result in acidosis, ischemia, and arterial vasospasm with cumulative dosing (Polovich et al., 2014). Additionally, hypomagnesemia from cisplatin damage to the renal tubules can produce prolongation of the QT interval, resulting in bradycardia, atrial dysrhythmias, or life-threatening ventricular dysrhythmias (Slovacek, Ansorgova, Macingova, Haman, & Petera, 2008). Cyclophosphamide is another commonly used alkylating agent that has demonstrated cardiovascular toxicity. Although toxicity risk is rare in standard or cumulative doses, it is increased with higher doses (more than 1.5 mg/m^2/day), such as in hematopoietic stem cell transplantation (HSCT). Cardiotoxicity is thought to occur secondary to endothelial damage or from the release of free radicals. Rare cases of acute lethal pericarditis, pericardial effusions, cardiac tamponade, hemorrhagic myocardial necrosis, and

Table 9-2. Drugs Causing Cardiotoxicity

Agent	Dysrhythmias	Hypotension	Hypertension	Raynaud Disease	Coronary Artery Disease	Heart Failure	Cardiomyopathy	Pericardial Effusion/ Tamponade	VTE
Chemotherapy									
Amsacrine	X					X			
Belinostat	X								
Bleomycin				X			X		
Busulfan	X		X					X	
Capecitabine	X			X	X				
Carmustine	X	X							
Cisplatin	X		X	X	X	X			
Cladribine	X								
Cyclophospha- mide						X	X	X	
Cytarabine	X					X		X	
Dacarbazine		X							
Daunorubicin	X					X	X	X	
Docetaxel	X	X				X			
Doxorubicin	X					X	X	X	
Epirubicin hydrochloride	X					X	X		
Eribulin	X								

(Continued on next page)

Table 9-2. Drugs Causing Cardiotoxicity (Continued)

Agent	Dysrhythmias	Hypotension	Hypertension	Raynaud Disease	Coronary Artery Disease	Heart Failure	Cardiomyopathy	Pericardial Effusion/ Tamponade	VTE
Chemotherapy (cont.)									
Estramustine			X			X			
Etoposide	X	X							
5-Azacitidine	X	X						X	
5-Fluorouracil	X				X				
Gemcitabine hydrochloride	X	X			X			X	
Idarubicin						X			
Ifosfamide	X	X	X			X			
Methotrexate	X	X				X		X	X
Mitomycin C	X					X			
Mitoxantrone						X			
Paclitaxel	X	X			X			X	
Teniposide		X							
Trabectedin						X	X		
Vinblastine				X					
Vincristine				X	X				
Vinorelbine tartrate	X		X		X				

(Continued on next page)

Table 9-2. Drugs Causing Cardiotoxicity (Continued)

Agent	Dysrhythmias	Hypotension	Hypertension	Raynaud Disease	Coronary Artery Disease	Heart Failure	Cardiomyopathy	Pericardial Effusion/Tamponade	VTE
Hormonal Agents									
Abiraterone acetate	X		X						
Anastrozole						X			
Enzalutamide			X						
Letrozole						X			
Palbociclib									X
Tamoxifen	X				X				X
Monoclonal Antibodies/Biologics									
Ado-trastuzumab emtansine						X	X		
Alemtuzumab	X								
Bevacizumab			X		X	X			X
Blinatumomab		X	X						
Bortezomib		X				X			
Brentuximab		X							
Cetuximab	X	X							
Denileukin diftitox	X	X							

(Continued on next page)

Table 9-2. Drugs Causing Cardiotoxicity (Continued)

Agent	Dysrhythmias	Hypotension	Hypertension	Raynaud Disease	Coronary Artery Disease	Heart Failure	Cardiomyopathy	Pericardial Effusion/ Tamponade	VTE
Monoclonal Antibodies/Biologics (cont.)									
Dinutuximab		X							
Eltrombopag									X
Interferon-alfa				X					
Interleukin-2	X	X				X			
Interleukin-11	X								
Ipilimumab		X				X		X	X
Lenalidomide	X		X		X	X			
Ofatumumab	X	X			X				
Pertuzumab	X					X			
Pomalidomide					X				
Ramucirumab			X						
Retinoic acid						X		X	
Rituximab	X	X			X				
Siltuximab		X							
Sipuleucel-T	X		X						
Thalidomide	X								X
Tositumomab		X							
Trastuzumab	X	X				X			

(Continued on next page)

Table 9-2. Drugs Causing Cardiotoxicity (Continued)

Agent	Dysrhythmias	Hypotension	Hypertension	Raynaud Disease	Coronary Artery Disease	Heart Failure	Cardiomyopathy	Pericardial Effusion/ Tamponade	VTE
Targeted Therapies									
Afatinib									
Alectinib	X					X	X		
Axitinib			X						
Belinostat	X	X							
Bosutinib								X	
Cabozantinib		X	X						
Carfilzomib		X	X		X	X			X
Ceritinib	X							X	
Cobimetinib						X			
Crizotinib	X								
Dabrafenib	X					X	X		X
Dasatinib	X					X		X	
Erlotinib					X				
Ibrutinib	X		X						
Imatinib						X			
Lapatinib	X					X			
Lenvatinib	X		X		X	X			
Motesanib	X								
Nilotinib	X								

(Continued on next page)

Table 9-2. Drugs Causing Cardiotoxicity (Continued)

Agent	Dysrhythmias	Hypotension	Hypertension	Raynaud Disease	Coronary Artery Disease	Heart Failure	Cardiomyopathy	Pericardial Effusion/ Tamponade	VTE
Targeted Therapies (cont.)									
Osimertinib	X								
Panobinostat	X				X				
Pazopanib	X		X						X
Ponatinib	X		X		X	X			X
Ramucirumab		X	X			X	X		X
Regorafenib			X		X	X			
Ruxolitinib			X						
Sorafenib	X		X		X	X			
Sunitinib	X		X		X	X			X
Telatinib	X								
Trametinib	X		X			X	X		X
Vandetanib	X				X	X			
Vatalanib	X								
Vemurafenib	X								
Miscellaneous									
Arsenic trioxide	X								
Asparaginase									X
Darbepoetin			X						X
Epoetin alfa			X						X

(Continued on next page)

Table 9-2. Drugs Causing Cardiotoxicity (Continued)

Agent	Dysrhythmias	Hypotension	Hypertension	Raynaud Disease	Coronary Artery Disease	Heart Failure	Cardiomyopathy	Pericardial Effusion/ Tamponade	VTE
Miscellaneous (cont.)									
Eribulin	X								
Lanreotide	X								
Pegaspargase									X
Romidepsin	X								
Sargramostim								X	
Vorinostat	X								X
Ziv-aflibercept			X						X

VTE—venous thromboembolism

Note. Based on information from Adão et al., 2013; De Jesus-Gonzalez et al., 2012; Polovich et al., 2014; Stephens, 2013; Truven Health Analytics Inc., 2017.

cardiomyopathy have also occurred (Polovich et al., 2014). In addition, cases of congestive heart failure and dysrhythmias in patients receiving ifosfamide have been reported. The causes of the ifosfamide-induced cardiotoxicity are thought to be similar to the class effects of cyclophosphamide. Its mechanism of action is thought to be caused by a delay in elimination of cardiotoxic metabolites secondary to nephrotoxicity (Yeh & Bickford, 2009). Cardiotoxicity from ifosfamide is considered transient and reversible (Khakoo & Yeh, 2008).

Anthracyclines

A class effect of almost all anthracycline agents is type I myocyte damage, leading to myocyte atrophy with heart failure. The estimated risk of all types of anthracycline-induced cardiotoxicity is 30%–40% (Hampton, 2010; Herrmann & Lerman, 2014). Three well-defined presentation patterns of anthracycline-induced cardiotoxicity exist and are dependent on length of exposure and possible acute reactivity (Herrmann et al., 2014; Lipshultz, Alvarez, & Scully, 2008). The first pattern is acute cardiotoxicity, which presents within hours to days after administration as a drug-induced rhythm disturbance (i.e., supraventricular tachycardia, ventricular ectopy, myopericarditis, cardiomyopathy, or death). According to Bonita and Pradhan (2013), this acute inflammatory cardiotoxicity is not a predictor of future development of heart failure and is thought to be reversible on agent discontinuation. Type I cardiotoxicity is a typical anthracycline cardiotoxicity from direct injury and myocyte remodeling by free radicals that produces irreversible dilated cardiomyopathy (Lipshultz et al., 2008). It may be early onset, occurring within a year, or late onset (chronic toxicity), occurring after one year. Early-onset cardiotoxicity typically occurs within one year following exposure to an anthracycline and is dependent on the total received cumulative dose. Recommended maximum lifetime doses have been established for most anthracyclines; however, science now shows that it is a continuous process with increasing risk as the dose increases. For example, the recommended maximum dose of doxorubicin is 550 mg/m^2; however, congestive heart failure has also been noted in patients treated with doxorubicin at doses starting at 360 mg/m^2 (Anderson & Sawyer, 2008).

The severity of toxicity ranges from stable, asymptomatic abnormalities in left ventricular function to progressive, overt congestive heart failure. Studies have demonstrated that asymptomatic changes in ejection fraction often precede overt symptoms (Anderson & White, 2013; Polovich et al., 2014). Small studies using troponin measurement during drug administration suggest that early troponin leak may be indicative of myocyte injury (Anderson & White, 2013). Anthracycline-induced cardiomyopathy is irreversible and progressive in nature, and symptoms are often gradual and dose dependent, with increased incidence with cumulative doses.

Antimetabolites

The antimetabolite agent 5-fluorouracil (5-FU) has been shown to cause angina-like chest pain with or without myocardial infarctions, dysrhythmias, heart failure, or cardiogenic shock. Although the exact mechanism is unknown, it is believed to be cardiotoxicity related to 5-FU and caused by coronary vasospasm (Polovich et al., 2014), coronary artery thrombosis or vasospasm, or direct effect on the myocardium (Yeh & Bickford, 2009). Incidence of cardiotoxicity is 1.2%–7.6% with bolus administration and up to approximately 20% with continuous infusion (Viale & Yamamoto, 2008). Capecitabine, the fluoropyrimidine prodrug of 5-FU, may also cause cardiotoxicity in patients. By comparison, the incidence of cardiotoxicity with capecitabine is 3%–9%, with onset of angina-like pain within hours to several days following initiation of therapy. With both agents, the risk of cardiotoxicity is dose or infusion-rate dependent.

Taxanes

With the taxane agent paclitaxel, cardiotoxicity is commonly seen as asymptomatic bradycardia in approximately 30% of patients and as cardiac ischemia or myocardial infarction in rarer instances (5%) (Bonita & Pradhan, 2013; Polovich et al., 2014; Yusuf, Razeghi, & Yeh, 2008). Other cardiotoxicities include asymptomatic ventricular tachycardia, hypotension, atypical chest pain, pericardial effusion, and myocardial ischemia (rare). When paclitaxel is combined with an anthracycline, the risk for cardiotoxicity increases (Anderson & Sawyer, 2008; Bonita & Pradhan, 2013). It has also been postulated that Kolliphor® EL (formerly Cremophor® EL), in which paclitaxel is formulated, may account for the development of cardiotoxicity caused by histamine release (Polovich et al., 2014). Docetaxel can cause hypotension, sinus tachycardia, atrial flutter, dysrhythmias, unstable angina, and hypertension.

Immunotherapy Agents

Immunotherapy agents have not been identified as having intrinsic cardiotoxic effects but have been associated with cardiac complications. Interferon alfa can cause hypotension, hypertension, tachycardia, Raynaud phenomenon, and angina and myocardial ischemia in severe cases (Polovich et al., 2014). Toxicity is typically reversible once treatment has been discontinued; however, combination therapy with hydroxyurea may increase cardiovascular risk (Schering Corporation, 2012). Denileukin diftitox, an immune conjugate, can cause vascular leak syndrome, also known as capillary leak syndrome. As a result of vasodilation, hypotension and dysrhythmias may occur within hours following treatment. Interleukin-2 is a cytokine that commonly results in cardiovascular compromise similar to septic shock. It can lead to capillary leak syndrome, vasodilation, hypotension, compensatory tachycardia, dysrhythmias, myocardial ischemia, cardiomyopathy, myocarditis, or death (Polovich et al., 2014; Viale & Yamamoto, 2008). Side effects are dose related, self-limiting, and typically reversible on discontinuation. Hypotension occurs in up to 71% of all patients, with 3% experiencing grade 4 toxicity (Prometheus Laboratories Inc., 2012).

Monoclonal Antibodies

Bevacizumab-induced cardiotoxicity can produce significant hypertension in 5%–8% of patients and may last as long as several weeks after discontinuation (Genentech, Inc., 2012). Other cardiotoxicities include thrombosis, hemorrhage, and a low incidence (1.7%–14%) of grade 3 or 4 congestive heart failure, predominantly in anthracycline-pretreated patients (Curigliano et al., 2010; Polovich et al., 2014). Cetuximab is another monoclonal antibody with known cardiac toxicities. Although incidence is extremely low, cardiotoxicity can be serious, leading to cardiac arrest, especially in patients with head and neck cancer (Bristol-Myers Squibb Co. & ImClone LLC, 2012). The etiology of cardiotoxicity with cetuximab is well defined; however, it may also be caused by hypomagnesemia, which can result in dysrhythmias related to QT prolongation (Polovich et al., 2014). Rituximab-related cardiotoxicity is considered infusion related and is especially common with the first dose. It has occasionally been associated with hypotension, dysrhythmias, myocardial infarction, ventricular fibrillation, and cardiogenic shock. The mechanism of action is postulated to be caused by cytokine release (Biogen-Idec, Inc., & Genentech, Inc., 2013). The incidence of cardiotoxicity with trastuzumab as a single agent is 7%. When combined with paclitaxel, the incidence increases to 11%. It increases further to 28% with concurrent administration of an anthracycline or cyclophosphamide (Bonita & Pradhan, 2013; Polovich et al., 2014). The exact mechanism of action for cardiotoxicity with trastuzumab is unclear, but it has been theorized that the HER2 pathway occurs, impacting normal regulation of cardiac contractility and function (Curigliano et al., 2010). Cardiac dysfunction with trastuzumab includes decreased left ventricular ejection fraction, congestive heart failure, cardiomyopathy, and thrombosis. All agents affecting the ErbB receptors (e.g., HER2, epidermal growth factor receptor [EGFR], vascular endothelial growth factor receptors [VEGFRs]) may cause cardiotoxicity because the same pathways are essential for cardiomyocyte function (Cheng & Force, 2010).

Targeted Therapy

Targeted therapy agents were initially thought to be less toxic than traditional chemotherapy; however, several of these agents, especially the TKIs and multikinase inhibitors (MKIs), have been associated with an increased risk of cardiovascular effects. Toxicity is caused by similar targets found in both tumor cells and cardiomyocytes, such as HER2, EGFR, VEGFR, and platelet-derived growth factor receptor (Cheng & Force, 2010; Force & Kerkelä, 2008; Lenihan & Kowey, 2013). Numerous parallels exist between the signaling pathways that drive tumor genesis and those that regulate hypertrophy and survival of cardiomyocytes, especially in a stressed heart. Cardiotoxicities seen with TKIs and MKIs include conduction abnormalities, prolonged QT interval, left ventricular dysfunction, heart failure, and hypertension (Lenihan & Kowey, 2013; Ryberg, 2013). On-target and off-target toxicity are the two mechanisms of cardiotoxicity related to TKIs and MKIs. In on-target toxicity, the kinase targeted in the cancer cell provides important maintenance function in both the heart and vasculature, leading to left ventricular dysfunction (Cheng & Force, 2010). Target inhibition thus causes adverse effects on the heart. In on-target toxicity, the *HER2* gene plays a critical role in cardiomyocyte proliferation during fetal development and in cell survival during adulthood. It also protects against anthracycline-induced toxicity. In off-target cardiotoxicity, a kinase that is not supposed to be inhibited becomes inhibited. If this specific kinase plays a role in the function of the heart, inhibition leads to toxicity (Cheng & Force, 2010). Sunitinib is a known MKI that can cause off-target cardiotoxicity.

Hormonal Agents

Hormonal agents have long been associated with an increased risk of cardiovascular disease. Tamoxifen, an estrogen agonist/antagonist agent, has been found to cause ventricular dysrhythmias, heart failure, or QT prolongation with bradycardia in rare cases (Polovich et al., 2014). Abiraterone acetate, a steroidal antiandrogen drug, can cause fluid retention that leads to hypertension, chest pain, dysrhythmias, and heart failure. With the aromatase inhibitors, such as fulvestrant and anastrozole, cardiovascular-related toxicities include vasodilation, myocardial ischemia, heart failure, and thromboembolic events (Litsas, 2011). When compared to tamoxifen, aromatase inhibitors pose a higher risk of cardiovascular toxicities; however, tamoxifen tends to have a greater risk of thromboembolic events. For these reasons, caution should be used for any patient with preexisting cardiovascular disease being considered for hormonal therapy.

Radiation Therapy

In 2017, more than 600,000 patients were diagnosed with a cancer involving the chest, with many receiving chest radiation as treatment (American Cancer Society, 2017). The predominant diagnoses were breast and lung cancers, followed by lymphoma, head and neck, and esophageal cancers. Risk factors for radiation-induced cardiotoxicity can be divided into two sections.

The first group of risk factors is patient related and includes younger age at the time of treatment, hypertension, hyperlipidemia, diabetes, obesity/increased body mass index (BMI), history of tobacco use, metabolic syndrome for a longer time after exposure, and primary cardiac tumors (Martinou & Gaya, 2013). Obesity/increased BMI is believed to be a risk factor because of "deep setup errors," resulting in the inclusion of additional heart volume in the radiation field (Martinou & Gaya, 2013, p. 180). Patients at highest risk for developing radiation-induced cardiotoxicity are those treated at a young age for curable malignancies, such as Hodgkin lymphoma and early-stage breast cancer, especially left-sided. A 2006 study by the Early Breast Cancer Trialists' Collaborative Group concluded that the risk of death from heart disease increases by 3% per 1 Gy (Clark, 2006).

The second group of risk factors is related to radiation treatment and includes total dose of radiation (doses higher than 30 Gy or 25 Gy with concurrent anthracyclines), dose per fraction more than 2 Gy, volume of the heart irradiated, and concomitant administration of cardiotoxic chemotherapeutic agents (Bovelli, Plataniotis, & Roila, 2010; Herrmann et al., 2014; Martinou & Gaya, 2013; Yahalom & Portlock, 2008). Newer radiation delivery methods have decreased the incidence of radiation-induced cardiotoxicity in recent years (Yusuf et al., 2011).

Ionizing radiation to any vascular location not only places the patient at increased risk for early atherosclerosis but also can cause damage to blood vessels, leading to inflammatory changes that ultimately can cause fibrosis (Herrmann et al., 2014). When this fibrosis occurs to heart tissue, it can lead to coronary artery disease, conduction defects, dysrhythmias, valvular dysfunction (e.g., mitral insufficiency), acute or delayed pericarditis, pericardial effusions, cardiomyopathy, or myocardial ischemia (Anderson & Sawyer, 2008; Yahalom & Portlock, 2008). Most cardiotoxicities are late effects, except for pericarditis, pericardial effusions, and dysrhythmias, which can occur during or immediately following treatment.

Most studies on long-term cardiac complications of radiation were reported more than 20 years ago and come from research conducted on young children with Hodgkin lymphoma. Nurses need to be aware that radiation treatment, especially to the mediastinal area, places the patient at increased risk for the development of radiation-induced cardiotoxicity. The use of cardiac blocks to shield the heart from radiation remains controversial. Although blocks may reduce cardiotoxicity risk, they have been associated with an increased risk of local recurrence (Martinou & Gaya, 2013). The advent of intensity-modulated radiation has demonstrated successful treatment of internal mammary nodes for patients with breast cancer while minimizing radiation exposure to the heart.

Because of the increased risk for the development of radiation-induced cardiotoxicity, guidelines suggest lifelong monitoring for patients at cardiac risk. The European Association of Cardiovascular Imaging and the American Society of Echocardiography (Lancellotti et al., 2013) have recommended evaluation and surveillance starting at five years following treatment for high-risk patients and at 10 years for all other patients. Tests may include serial stress echocardiography, radionucleotide angiography, and serial blood tests, such as fasting lipid profile, which has been shown to be reliable for screening high-risk patients for coronary artery disease.

Selected Cardiovascular Disorders

Pericardial Disease (Pericarditis/Pericardial Effusion)

Direct involvement of the pericardium or infiltration into pericardial fluid occurs rarely with malignancy but often warrants a higher level of care, including interventions to drain fluid or monitor for decompensation during treatment. Pericarditis from radiation scarring or pericardial effusion from disease, medication, or mass effect is most common, with a reported incidence of 5%–50% in patients with malignancies (Borlaug & DeCamp, 2015). Borlaug and DeCamp (2015) reported overall pericardial disease incidence at 1%–20%; however, the authors believed this to be an underestimation.

Pathogenesis

Pericardial disease may include acute or constrictive pericarditis, pericardial effusion, or pericardial tamponade. Pericarditis is an inflammatory disorder produced by an irritating factor, such as inflammatory mediators or immune therapies. Inflammation may cause swelling and global dysfunction of the myocytes, producing dysrhythmias, coronary vasospasm, or impaired inotropy. Pericardial effusion is accumulation of increased pericardial fluid within the space between the visceral and parietal pericardial layers. Increased fluid changes the space from negative to more positive. This positive pressure provides resistance for returning venous blood from the vena cava, causing venous backup and congestion. The reduced flow of blood into the atrium results in lower cardiac output and hypoperfusion throughout the body.

When the positive pressure is extreme enough to prevent almost all blood from entering the right atrium from the body, right atrial and ventricular collapse occurs and blood flow through the heart is minimized or nonexistent, leading to no cardiac output and subsequent cardiac arrest. This excessive pressure and the physiology of cardiac chamber collapse are correlated to cardiac tamponade. Pulseless electrical activity is a common arrest rhythm for these patients, as the actual muscle is not impaired, nor is the conduction system damaged.

Risk Factors

Patients with cancer who are most likely to develop pericardial disease are those with large chest and mediastinal malignancies or specific subtypes of leukemia and those receiving chemobiotherapeutic agents that cause capillary permeability (e.g., cytosine arabinoside) or are associated with effusions (e.g., docetaxel) (Story, 2013; Woods, 2013). Inflammatory diseases, such as rheumatoid conditions (e.g., systemic lupus erythematosus), and administration of interferon, interleukin-2, and interleukin-11 have been associated with pericarditis or effusion (Story, 2013). Pericardial effusions may be related to increased production of fluid (malignant infiltration), impaired or obstructed pericardial fluid drainage (large chest masses), or a combination of these etiologies (Story, 2013). Nonmalignant etiologies of pericardial effusion include anemia, anticoagulants, congestive heart failure, hydrochlorothiazide diuretics, hypothyroidism, infections, and uremia (Shelton, 2014c). Antineoplastic medications associated with pericardial effusion include anthracyclines (e.g., bleomycin, daunorubicin, doxorubicin), cyclophosphamide, cytarabine, dasatinib, imatinib, or methotrexate (Story, 2013; Woods, 2013).

Assessment

Patients with pericardial disease frequently present with unique signs and symptoms dependent on the severity of impaired venous return and cardiac output. Pericarditis produces more distinct chest pain than other disorders, a higher risk of dysrhythmias, and less pronounced changes in cardiac output. Pericardial effusions increase the volume in the space between the visceral and parietal pericardium, changing the pressure within this cavity. Symptoms may be subtler, despite the higher acuity of the disorder. Chest pain is more dull and diffuse, and symptoms may include impediment of venous return with edema, weight gain, or hepatic congestion with concurrent reduced cardiac output and poor peripheral pulses, slowed capillary refill, and decreased urine output. The Beck triad describes the three most consistent symptoms of pericardial effusion and impending tamponade, which are muffled heart sounds, arterial hypotension, and bilateral jugular venous distension. Symptoms of pericardial effusion depend on the rapidity of fluid accumulation onset. Many patients with malignant effusions have slow fluid collection and may present with right heart failure symptoms and large-volume effusions (Shelton, 2014c). More rapid fluid trapping in the pericardial space occurs with drug-induced effusions and may present as acute low ejection fraction and cardiogenic shock. As the pericardial effusion increases, the pulse pressure narrows and pulsus paradoxus or hypotension becomes more predominant. Pericardial tamponade is a culmination of limited or no fluid entering or leaving the heart. Hypoperfusion, the primary symptom, is first noted in the distal lower extremities and progressively involves the upper extremities. Extremities are cool to the touch and potentially cyanotic, pulses are diminished, and capillary refill is prolonged. Although poor perfusion in many circumstances causes altered mental status, the small amount of blood being ejected from the heart goes into the carotid, and many patients have surprising maintenance of cognitive function in the face of perfusion deficits, such as a nondetectable blood pressure.

The echocardiogram is the diagnostic test with the greatest sensitivity and specificity. It can detect the amount of fluid in the pericardial space, the degree of atrial or ventricular collapse from impaired venous return, and the functional ejection fraction or cardiac output. Other diagnostic tests used to assist in the differential diagnosis or confirmation include a wide mediastinum and enlarged cardiac silhouette on chest x-ray, diffuse precordial lead ST elevation of ECG, pericardial fluid detectable on CT scan, and cardiac MRI (Shelton, 2014c; Story 2013; Woods, 2013). A summary of common clinical findings and diagnostic test results with pericardial disorders is described in Table 9-3.

Management

Monitoring for disease progression toward tamponade is essential whether observing early effusions or caring for patients after definitive interventions, such as pericardial drainage. Pericarditis is always treated conservatively with anti-inflammatory medications and ECG monitoring for dysrhythmias.

Pericardial effusions may be observed, actively drained, or managed with anti-neoplastic therapy. Pericardial fluid drainage may be accomplished with needle pericardiocentesis, percutaneous pericardial catheter, operative pericardial win-

Table 9-3. Differentiation of Pericardial Disease			
Assessment Type	Pericarditis	Pericardial Effusion	Pericardial Tamponade
Symptoms			
Chest discomfort	Sharp, localized Exacerbated by deep breath Relieved by sitting up and leaning forward	Dull, diffuse Nonpositional	Absent, or a sensation of "heaviness"
Cough	Absent	Present with pulmonary congestion	Persistent but variable severity
Dyspnea	Mild to moderate	Moderate to severe	Severe air hunger
Signs			
Blood pressure	Narrow pulse pressure	Reduced systolic blood pressure, reduced pulse pressure, pulsus paradoxus > 10 mm Hg	Nondetectable, or barely discernable by Doppler Only discernable systolic, no diastolic pressure
Cardiac rhythm	Tachycardia	Tachycardia but bradycardia or heart block with deep inspiration	Same as pericardial effusion but potentially periods of asystole, sinus pause Electrical alternans Pulseless electrical activity
Central venous pressure	Normal	Moderate elevation	High
Heart sounds	Pericardial rub	Muffled heart sounds or pericardial rub that is position dependent	Absent
			(Continued on next page)

Assessment Type	Pericarditis	Pericardial Effusion	Pericardial Tamponade
Table 9-3. Differentiation of Pericardial Disease *(Continued)*			
Signs *(cont.)*			
Hepatojugular reflex	Negative	Positive	Jugular venous distension (JVD) persistent and not influenced by hepatic compression
JVD and jugular venous pulsations (JVP)	Nonflat neck veins and slight increase in JVP	Bulging neck veins with JVP near mandible	Bulging neck veins with JVP producing continuous wave up the neck to the chin
Mental status	Normal	Anxious, restless but usually oriented	Altered sensorium and level of consciousness relates to diminished cardiac output
Peripheral edema	Trace dependent edema	Moderate edema of extremities	Dependent upon the rapidity of symptom onset
Point of maximal impulse	Normal	Shifted to the left (toward the axilla) or downward (toward sixth intercostal space)	Difficult to palpate, but may be shifted as with pericardial effusion
Pulse equality and strength	Pulses decreased in periphery, particularly lower extremities	Carotid and other central pulses may be diminished. Pulses more pronounced decrease in periphery, particularly lower extremities	Minimal carotid pulse, absent lower extremity pulses
Urine output	Normal	Oliguria	Anuria

(Continued on next page)

Assessment Type	Pericarditis	Pericardial Effusion	Pericardial Tamponade
Table 9-3. Differentiation of Pericardial Disease *(Continued)*			
Diagnostic Test Findings			
Chest x-ray	Normal	Widened mediastinum	Same as pericardial effusion
Echocardiogram	Global wall motion abnormality with minimal impairment to ejection fraction	Excess fluid in pericardial space Wall motion impairment with possible collapse of right atrium or ventricle Reduced ejection fraction	Wall motion impairment with collapsed right ventricle Reduced or absent ejection fraction
Electrocardiogram (ECG)	Low-voltage QRS Precordial chest lead ST elevation or ST depression	Low-voltage QRS Precordial chest lead ST elevation	Low-voltage QRS ECG ST changes may be nonspecific, depressed, or elevated
Troponin levels	Mild to moderate elevations	Low to mild elevations	Same as pericardial effusions

Note. Based on information from Shelton, 2014c; Story, 2013.

dow, or pericardiectomy. Needle pericardiocentesis is used only in emergencies, when adequate time or expertise is unavailable to safely drain the pericardium under ultrasound and controlled catheter insertion (Woods, 2013). Some individuals advocate catheter drainage and removal, while others leave the catheter in place for longer-term drainage. Some individuals report using the catheter to insert antineoplastic therapy into the pericardial space. Agents given intrapericardially include bleomycin, cisplatin, corticosteroids, cytarabine, daunorubicin, doxorubicin, doxycycline, minocycline, mitomycin, mitoxantrone, thiotepa, and teniposide (Shelton, 2014c; Story, 2013). Insufficient evidence exists to guide nursing management of an indwelling pericardial catheter, although its reported use is highest among patients undergoing cardiac surgery or with cancer. Straight drainage with a sealed and attached closed drainage system is ideal but may not be practical for patients with malignant effusions more likely to involve large volumes or continuous drainage for extended periods of time (Shelton, 2014c). The bag should be maintained below the level of the heart to enable constant drainage and reduce the risk for occlusion. Institutional protocols should provide direction for staff regarding whether nurses are permitted to flush pericardial drains as well as for catheter maintenance procedures (Woods, 2013). The catheter is anchored by sutures or adhesive securing devices, and accidental removal is common because of the weight of the drainage bag and tendency for the straight and rigid catheter to dislodge. A pericardial window removes a section of pericardium and inserts a screen-like window, allowing fluid to drain into the mediastinum. This procedure is preferred with longer life expectancy and when pleuropericardial effusions are treated (Shelton, 2014c). Pericardial fluid in the mediastinum necessitates more comprehensive follow-up with systemic antineoplastic therapy when malignant cells are in the pericardial fluid. This may include systemic chemotherapy with or without chest irradiation. If the pericardial disorder clearly involves malignant infiltration, systemic chemotherapy or radiation therapy may be used to reduce the tumor size and effects. The therapy is determined based on the cancer's sensitivity and responsiveness to treatment.

Dysrhythmias

Dysrhythmia is an abnormal heart rate or rhythm and is further defined by origin and lethality. Because monitoring is often intermittent and few studies are available that describe characteristics of this phenomenon, the exact prevalence of rhythm disturbances related to cancer or its treatment is unknown (Guglin et al., 2009). Common rhythm disturbances may include sinus bradycardia, sinus tachycardia, atrial flutter, atrial fibrillation, supraventricular tachycardia, and junctional rhythm. Infrequently, ventricular tachycardia, or heart block, can occur (Polovich et al., 2014).

Pathogenesis

Common rhythm disturbances may occur because of the presence of cancer or the result of hormonal or sympathetic triggers, concomitant medical problems (e.g., acid–base disturbance), or the adverse effects or toxicity of medications and treatment. The pathogenesis of conduction disturbances ranges from direct injury to conduction pathways to indirect toxic effects from multiple etiologies. Patients with cancer and without intrinsic cardiac comorbidities or common cardiac toxicities may still experience dysrhythmias from indirect effects, such as catecholamine surges or medication- and electrolyte-induced QT prolongation.

Risk Factors

Direct cardiac involvement with tumors is rare; however, with greater and longer survival rates, patients are more likely to develop long-term radiation injury to the conduction system or treatment-related cardiomyopathy. Both result in dysrhythmias years after initial cancer diagnosis and treatment. Increased tumor response rates for children with cancer have led to higher numbers of survivors requiring conduction system support with pacemakers and implantable defibrillators (Coviello & Knobf, 2013). Cancers involving the adrenal gland, such as pheo-chromocytoma, are naturally linked to dysrhythmias and hypertension because of excess catecholamines excreted by the tumor. Tumors located in the stomach and lower esophagus may affect the vagus nerve, which normally counteracts the effects of sympathetic hormones on the heart. Damage to the vagus nerve can lead to refractory tachycardia and hypertension. Indirect effects of tumors in the lungs or infectious lung complications produce atrial irritability and a propensity for atrial tachycardia, flutter, and fibrillation. This risk can be enhanced by elec-trolyte disturbances, such as the hypomagnesemia and hypokalemia that occurs with chemotherapy injury to the kidneys or with chemotherapy-induced diar-rhea (Shelton, 2014a). The most common rhythm disturbance is sinus tachycardia because it occurs with prevalent complications, such as deconditioning, anemia, and sepsis (Shelton, 2014a). Many antineoplastic and oncologic support drugs have been identified as QT prolongation precipitators. QT prolongation is asso-ciated with high risk of torsade de pointes, a lethal ventricular tachycardia. Table 9-4 lists medications commonly used in oncologic practice as well as disorders known to cause or exacerbate QT prolongation.

Assessment

When assessing a patient with possible dysrhythmia, a key history, physical symptoms, and examination findings may be noted. These are categorized as either involved in the cardiovascular system or as the indirect effects of altered car-diac output. Assessment of any rhythm considered abnormal should first involve assessment of tolerance or stability. Because the body will normally shunt avail-able blood to essential organs when cardiac output is impaired, the initial assess-ment for patients with dysrhythmias should include evaluation for compromised lungs, heart, or brain. Unstable dysrhythmias may present with cool extremities, faint or near-absent peripheral pulses, hypotension, chest discomfort with isch-emic ECG changes, dyspnea, hypoxemia, presyncope, or altered mental status and sensorium. These signs warrant immediate intervention rather than contin-ued assessment of the rhythm type or etiology. More stable rhythms originating in the sinus node, atria, junction, and ventricle have different treatment implica-tions.

In addition to visual review of the ECG, other diagnostic tests may be helpful in assessing dysrhythmias and identifying site of origin or clinical significance. A 12-lead ECG may help to define the specific rhythm disturbance. Electrophysi-ologic testing may be used to locate the origin of persistent dysrhythmias, such as atrial flutter or paroxysmal atrial tachycardia, and provide an opportunity for direct ablation; however, patients with cancer more commonly have dysrhyth-mias with multifactorial etiologies. Laboratory tests that may provide information about the degree of cardiac injury associated with the rhythm may include car-diac troponin or brain natriuretic peptide (BNP) levels. Wall motion and ejection fraction during dysrhythmias can be determined with echocardiogram or MUGA scans, although irregular or rapid rhythms impair the quality of these tests.

Table 9-4. Etiologies of QT Prolongation

Etiology	Examples
Anesthetics	Fluranes Propofol
Antiarrhythmics	Amiodarone Dofetilide Procainamide Sotalol
Anticonvulsants	Valproic acid
Antidepressants	Selective serotonin reuptake inhibitors (e.g., citalopram, escitalopram) Tricyclic antidepressants (e.g., amitriptyline)
Antifungals	Fluconazole Itraconazole Posaconazole Voriconazole
Antihistamines (H_1 and H_2)	Diphenhydramine Ranitidine
Antimicrobials (fluoroquinolones)	Ciprofloxacin Levofloxacin
Antimicrobials (macrolides)	Erythromycin
Antineoplastic agents (general)	Arsenic trioxide
Antineoplastic agents (BCR-ABL inhibitors)	Dasatinib Imatinib Nilotinib
Antineoplastic agents (multikinase inhibitors)	Sorafenib Sunitinib
Antineoplastic agents (tyrosine kinase inhibitors)	ErbB2 receptor inhibitors (e.g., erlotinib, lapatinib)
Butyrophenones	Droperidol Haloperidol
Decongestants	Ephedrine Pseudoephedrine
Electrolyte abnormalities	Hypocalcemia Hypokalemia Hypomagnesemia

(Continued on next page)

Table 9-4. Etiologies of QT Prolongation *(Continued)*	
Etiology	**Examples**
Host characteristics	Bradycardia Female
Lifestyle factors	Caffeine
Miscellaneous	Barium Disopyramide Pentamidine
Motility stimulants	Metoclopramide
Opiates	Methadone Morphine
Phenothiazine	Compazine Thorazine
Proton pump inhibitors	Omeprazole
Selective estrogen receptor antagonists	Astemizole
Serotonin inhibitor antiemetics	Ondansetron Palonosetron
Stimulants	Amphetamines

Note. Based on information from Attin & Davidson, 2010; Briasoulis et al., 2011; Cahoon, 2009; Chen, 2009; Drew et al., 2010.

Management

Treatment of dysrhythmias depends on the seriousness of the rhythm disturbance, the specific conduction problem, and the potential etiology. The priority is to assess the patient's tolerance and hemodynamic stability during the abnormal rhythm. Life-threatening rhythms defined by symptoms of instability should be treated immediately through electrical therapy. Bedside defibrillation, synchronous cardioversion, and transcutaneous pacing may be employed until access to the electrophysiology laboratory is available. At times, the level of immune compromise and bleeding risk of patients with cancer may warrant continued temporary interventions, such as transvenous pacing or externalized automatic cardioverter devices. Patients with more stable dysrhythmias may be treated medically. Table 9-5 includes a summary of common antidysrhythmic medications used for management of nonventricular tachycardias and their oncologic implications.

After emergent issues have been resolved or the dysrhythmia is temporarily suppressed, the etiology should be sought and controlled. For patients having antineoplastic drug–induced dysrhythmias, this may result in permanent drug discontinuation. At times, if the rhythm problem is a class effect, such as with fluorouracil agents, all medications in the class may be avoided. Rhythm disturbances related to tumor compression or involvement of the heart and lungs may resolve when the cancer is quiescent. Other long-term therapies that may be implemented for chronic dysrhythmias in stable patients with reasonable life expectancies include electro-

Table 9-5. Antidysrhythmic Medications and Oncologic Implications

Drug	Dose	Category	Implications
Adenosine	6 mg IV rapid push followed by a fluid bolus, wait 1–2 minutes, and if no response, may administer 12 mg by rapid IV push followed by a fluid bolus. Central line administration may be given at half the recommended dose.	Purine analog	Can cause several seconds of asystole; patient may experience crushing chest pain; supraventricular tachycardia will recur 50%–60% of the time; half-life less than five seconds; patients on theophylline may require larger doses, whereas dipyridamole potentiates its effects.
Amiodarone	In cases of stable ventricular or supraventricular tachycardia, the loading dose is 150 mg IV over 10 minutes, followed by 1 mg/min infusion of 6 hours (completing the load), and then 0.5 mg/min for 18 additional hours. Discontinuation or conversion to oral is recommended by this time.	Miscellaneous	Most common immediate adverse effect is hypotension, counteracted partly by infusion rather than IV push; bolus dose acceptable to administer in normal saline and via polyethylene bag, but infusion should be mixed with dextrose in a glass bottle; long-term adverse effects that may be potentiated by other oncologic therapies include pulmonary fibrosis, hepatic transaminase elevations, and peripheral neuropathies. Long half-life of drug limits use in patients with high risk for heart block.

(Continued on next page)

Table 9-5. Antidysrhythmic Medications and Oncologic Implications *(Continued)*			
Drug	**Dose**	**Category**	**Implications**
Digoxin	10–15 mcg/kg lean body weight administered as a loading dose over 2–4 hours, followed by a daily dose of 0.125–0.5 mg/day	Digitalis glycoside	Rate and conduction effect seen within 5–30 minutes; peak effect within 90 minutes and 3 hours; correct hypokalemia, hypocalcemia, and hypomagnesemia to reduce risk of toxicity.
Diltiazem	Bolus dose of 0.25 mg/ kg (average 20–25 mg) over 2 minutes; if not controlled after 15 minutes, may give an additional 0.35 mg/kg over 2–5 minutes. Follow with 5–20 mg/hr continuous infusion. *(Most patients with cancer and many older adults are extremely sensitive to this agent, and doses usually are half the recommended dose.)*	Calcium channel blocker	Less incidence of myocardial depression than verapamil
Esmolol	Load with 250–500 mcg/ kg for 1 minute, followed by continuous infusion of 25–50 mcg/ kg/min, titrated upward in these increments every 5–10 minutes until a maximum of 300 mcg/kg/min.	Selective beta-blocker	Very rapid onset and short duration; should be diluted to 10 mg/ml before administration; do not use in patients with significant atrioventricular block or bradycardia.
Labetalol	20 mg IV over 2 minutes, followed by 40–80 mg IV at 10-minute intervals until the blood pressure drops; maximum dose is 2 mg/min or 300 mg total daily dose.	Alpha beta-blocker	Alpha and beta effects lead to blocking receptors in both heart and vasculature with decreased work on the heart as well as direct cardiac effects.

(Continued on next page)

Table 9-5. Antidysrhythmic Medications and Oncologic Implications (Continued)

Drug	Dose	Category	Implications
Metoprolol	5 mg IV push over 1–2 minutes. This dose may be repeated two additional times 5–15 minutes apart.	Selective beta-blocker	Onset of action is approximately 5 minutes, and duration varies among individuals; no clear reversal agent exists, but some clinicians prescribe IV glucagon as an antidote in potential overdose. Effective beta-blockade is determined by a heart rate ≤ 70 beats/min without stress-related increases (e.g., exercise, fever).
Verapamil	5 mg IV push over 2 minutes, 5–10 mg after 15–30 minutes; maximum dose is 30 mg. *(Most patients with cancer and many older adults are extremely sensitive to this agent, and doses usually are half the recommended dose.)*	Calcium channel blocker	Observe blood pressure closely; reverse effects with calcium chloride 0.5–1 g slowly for best absorption; consider not using this agent in patients with Wolff-Parkinson-White syndrome.

physiologic ablation, a permanent pacemaker, or an automatic implanted cardioverter defibrillator. When patients with cancer have a deterioration of their condition, discussion regarding inactivation of these devices should be included in the goals of care. Many patients are not continuously dependent on device activity and may wish to have it deactivated while undergoing a natural death.

Cardiomyopathy and Heart Failure

Pathogenesis

Although cardiomyopathy and heart failure are commonly used interchangeably, they are not synonymous (Yancy et al., 2013). The Comprehensive Heart Failure Practice Guidelines, developed by the Heart Failure Society of America, defined heart failure as "a syndrome caused by cardiac dysfunction, generally resulting from myocardial muscle dysfunction or loss and characterized by either

LV [left ventricular] dilation or hypertrophy or both" (Lindenfeld et al., 2010, p. 480). Cardiomyopathy describes a group of heterogeneous myocardial disorders that comprise ventricular dilation and decreased myocardial contractility in the absence of abnormal loading conditions, such as hypertension and valvular disease (Yancy et al., 2013). Cardiomyopathy can be classified as primary or secondary or as ischemic or nonischemic. Cardiomyopathy related to ischemic heart failure is caused by coronary artery disease or myocardial infarctions, where a lack of blood flow to the myocardium damages the heart muscle, resulting in myocyte atrophy and cardiomyopathy.

Although patients with cancer may experience ischemic heart failure, nonischemic heart failure is more common. Nonischemic cardiomyopathy associated with cancer therapies has also been described as toxic cardiomyopathy (Yancy et al., 2013). The etiology of nonischemic cardiomyopathy related to cancer treatment is typically considered to be the result of direct toxicity to the myocytes. The exception to this pathogenesis is when secondary heart failure occurs because of anatomic changes, such as pulmonary hypertension from chest masses or pulmonary emboli or from stress-induced heart failure with severe or chronic anemia (Viale & Yamamoto, 2008).

Nonischemic cardiomyopathy may be classified as being dilated or restrictive. Restrictive heart failure is also known as hypertrophic cardiomyopathy, which is almost exclusively a hereditary condition that leads to sudden dysrhythmic death. Dilated cardiomyopathy may present as congestive or noncongestive, which is an essential differentiating symptomatology because it dictates treatment. Cardiomyopathy and congestive heart failure are similar; however, one has congestion, while the other disorder does not. Both cases may exhibit enlarged heart, hypokinetic wall motion, and inadequate ejection.

Risk Factors

Anthracycline-induced cardiotoxicity has been appreciated since the 1960s, when heart failure was first reported with childhood leukemia (Khawaja et al., 2014; Walsh, 2010). It is the most thoroughly documented cause of chemotherapy-induced cardiomyopathy (Polovich et al., 2014). This class of chemotherapeutic agents is widely used and includes daunorubicin, doxorubicin, epirubicin, idarubicin, and mitoxantrone. Although the mechanisms of anthracycline-induced cardiotoxicity are not fully understood, several have been proposed, with the most recognized as a generation of free radicals that can cause oxidative stress and cardiomyocyte cell death (Bonita & Pradhan, 2013).

Risk factors for anthracycline-induced cardiotoxicity include a history of hypertension, increasing age (older than 65 years) or young age (younger than 15 years), being female, and having preexisting cardiovascular disease, such as coronary artery disease (Anderson & Sawyer, 2008). Other risk factors are length of exposure to agent, history of diabetes, adjuvant taxane therapy, African American ancestry, and combination chemotherapy with large or repeated doses of known cardiotoxic agents.

The best predictor of type I cardiotoxicity is total cumulative doses. The suggested lifetime cumulative dose for doxorubicin is 550 mg/mm² (Polovich et al., 2014; Yeh & Bickford, 2009). Less than 1% of patients experience acute cardiotoxicity immediately following infusion of an anthracycline (Yeh & Bickford, 2009). Doxorubicin-induced heart failure occurs in 3%–5% of patients who have received 400 mg/m² and increases to 7%–26% incidence at a cumulative dose of 550 mg/m² (Yeh & Bickford, 2009). If the dose exceeds 700 mg/m², the risk for developing cardiotoxicity ranges from 18%–48%, with exponential increases with each dose increment (Yeh & Bickford, 2009). For daunorubicin, the incidence of toxicity ranges from 0%–41% at doses less than 600 mg/m². Epirubicin, idarubicin, and mitoxantrone can cause cardiotoxicity, but when compared to doxorubicin, these agents have shown reduced risk (Bonita & Pradhan, 2013; Viale & Yamamoto, 2008). The total cumulative dose of epirubicin has been established at 400 mg/m², and monitoring for cardiotoxicity with mitoxantrone is recommended at doses greater than 100 mg/m² (Polovich et al., 2014). Marked cardiac dysfunction can occur in relatively low doses of anthracyclines. For example, cardiotoxicity has been reported at doses as low as 240 mg/m² of doxorubicin, especially in patients with preexisting comorbidities (Anderson & Sawyer, 2008). Liposomal formulations provide a lipid layer around the free drug, with the intention to reduce toxicity. Doxorubicin, daunorubicin, and pegylated doxorubicin formulations have been found to have a better safety profile but can still cause cardiotoxicity. Other commonly used chemotherapeutic agents known to cause type I, irreversible damage to the heart include cisplatin, cyclophosphamide, 5-FU, and paclitaxel (Khawaja et al., 2014; Polovich et al., 2014). Cyclophosphamide at high doses (greater than 1.5 mg/m²), as seen with blood marrow transplant rather than cumulative dosing, can lead to interstitial hemorrhage with myocytes (Polovich et al., 2014). Hemorrhagic myocarditis cases have been reported but rarely occur.

Assessment

Dyspnea and fatigue are common but subtle symptoms of heart failure (Yancy et al., 2013). Both symptoms are frequently attributed to cancer or its treatment and may delay thorough evaluation for heart failure. The New York Heart Association (1964) Functional Classification of Heart Failure is a widely used method to evaluate significance of disease. The classification system range is 1–4, with class 1 being no limitations in physical activity and no heart failure symptoms, and class 4 being discomfort with any physical activity and heart failure symptoms while at rest. Other symptoms that may indicate diagnosis of heart failure include dyspnea at rest or with exertion, exercise intolerance, orthopnea, paroxysmal nocturnal dyspnea, nocturnal cough, edema (especially in the lower extremities), and ascites or scrotal edema (King, Kingery, & Casey, 2012; Lindenfeld et al., 2010). Other symptoms less specific for heart failure are pulmonary edema, wheezing, cough, fatigue, early satiety, nausea and vomiting, abdominal swelling or bloating, confusion, fluid retention, and decreased urinary output (King et al., 2012; Lindenfeld et al., 2010). Specific cardiac symptoms of heart failure include a full, bounding pulse, brady/tachycardia, elevated jugular venous pressure, arrhythmias, and S_3 gallop or murmur. Many of these compensatory symptoms are the body's attempt to enhance perfusion to the tissue despite the inability of the heart to adequately pump. See Figure 9-2 for the clinical manifestations of heart failure and cardiomyopathy.

Clinical evaluation of patients suspected of or having heart failure or cardiomyopathy can be broken into three groups (Lindenfeld et al., 2010). The first group comprises patients at risk for developing heart failure, such as a patient receiving a cardiotoxic agent for the first time. The second group comprises patients suspected of having heart failure based on symptoms. Patients with already known symptomatology of heart failure make up the third group. Besides a careful and detailed history and physical examination, patients should also have an echocardiogram to determine cardiac structure and function (Lindenfeld et al., 2010), especially those who may be asymptomatic. MUGA scans may be used to evaluate cardiac damage but may not determine early reversible cardiac changes (Yusuf et al., 2008). BNP or N-terminal pro-BNP laboratory studies may be used to assess patients, particularly in patients with left ventricular heart failure (Polovich et al., 2014). However, BNP levels frequently increase with age and are higher in women, African Americans, and patients with renal failure (King et al., 2012). Another laboratory study used to detect myocardiocyte injury is serum troponin level. This study may be used to evaluate damage caused by anthracycline-induced cardiotoxicity. Both cardiac troponin levels and BNP have been suggested as effective monitoring approaches for immediate and ongoing cardiotoxicity (Polovich et al., 2014).

Figure 9-2. Clinical Manifestations for Cardiomyopathy/Heart Failure

Signs	Symptoms
• Tachycardia	• Fatigue
• Tachypnea	• Weakness
• Hypotension	• Dyspnea (orthopnea or paroxysmal nocturnal)
• Abnormal heart sounds (i.e., S_3 gallop)	
• Decreased oxygenation (PaO_2 less than 92%)	• Increased abdominal girth
• Abnormal lung sounds	• Cough
• Edema of lower extremities	• Sudden weight gain
• Jugular vein distension	• Poor appetite
• Hepatomegaly	• Mental status changes
• Changes in skin appearance	• Activity intolerance

PaO_2—partial pressure of oxygen

Note. Based on information from King et al., 2012; Lindenfeld et al., 2010; Polovich et al., 2014; Viale & Yamamoto, 2008.

An ECG can be used to determine cardiac status and detect abnormalities in cardiac electrophysiology. Daily weights, especially in high-risk patients, should be performed, as weight is a highly sensitive and specific predictor of decompensating heart failure (Yancy et al., 2013). Other recommended laboratory tests for evaluating patients for heart failure may include a basic or comprehensive metabolic profile, magnesium, fasting lipid profile, complete blood count, uric acid, liver function tests, urinalysis, and thyroid function (King et al., 2012; Lindenfeld et al., 2010).

Management

Three main aims exist in the management of cardiomyopathy and heart failure. The first aim is to reduce the workload on the heart and may include monitoring oxygenation and administering supplemental oxygen as needed or maintaining a slightly higher hemoglobin than with other patients to enhance the oxygen-carrying capacity. Recommendations by the American Heart Association and the American College of Cardiology for a patient who develops cardiotoxicity during or following therapy include placing the patient on an angiotensin-converting enzyme inhibitor (ACE) or angiotensin receptor blocker (ARB) plus a statin (Weber et al., 2013; Yancy et al., 2013). Diuretics, beta-blockers, and nitrates may also be used; however, these drugs may worsen the risk of hypotension, especially if the patient becomes infected, febrile, or septic. Actual pharmacologic management of heart failure is dependent on the patient's symptoms. The next aim is to enhance pump function by administering medications that reduce the workload of the heart. Digoxin or an ACE inhibitor may be used for this purpose. Continuous positive airway pressure therapy has also been used for acute management of heart failure because it will immediately reduce venous return and workload on the heart. The third aim is to minimize the risk or progression of injury with cardioprotectants. Dexrazoxane is an iron chelator that binds with free radical or anthracycline-bound ferric ions, thus decreasing cardiomyocyte damage; however, it has only been studied with doxorubicin and is thought to decrease antitumor efficacy. Potential risk may outweigh benefits (Polovich et al., 2014). Statin use has been shown to reduce the risk of cardiac injury (Herrmann et al., 2014). Coenzyme Q10 has demonstrated cardioprotectant properties by reduction in oxidative stress and free radical formation (Brown & Giampa, 2010).

Nonpharmacologic interventions for the care of a patient with heart failure include assessment of daily weights (Bui & Fonarow, 2012), breath and heart sounds, and presence of edema, especially in the lower extremities. Electrolytes should be evaluated to determine potassium and calcium levels, as abnormal levels may interfere with cardiac function (Polovich et al., 2014). Patient and family education is essential in minimizing complications and includes strategies to manage at home, reportable signs and symptoms, tobacco cessation, and regular exercise.

Prior to the initiation of treatment, a comprehensive history and physical should be performed to determine and establish baseline cardiovascular risk and the need for more intensive monitoring protocols. Reassessment of cardiotoxicity risk is recommended at 6- and 12-month intervals following completion of treatment and as early as 3 months for patients at high-risk for cardiotoxicity (Herrmann et al., 2014). Figure 9-3 presents an algorithm for when to seek a cardio-oncology consultation.

Hypotension

Pathogenesis

In a scientific statement from the American College of Cardiology, the American Society of Hypertension, and the International Society of Hypertension,

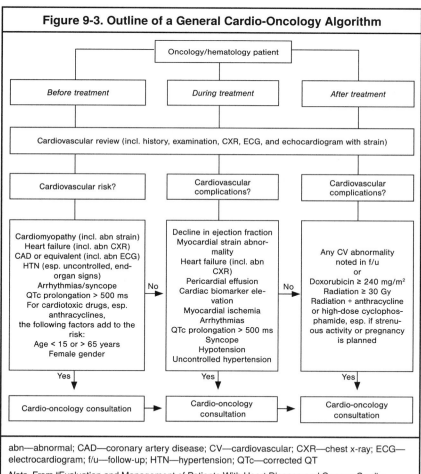

Figure 9-3. Outline of a General Cardio-Oncology Algorithm

abn—abnormal; CAD—coronary artery disease; CV—cardiovascular; CXR—chest x-ray; ECG—electrocardiogram; f/u—follow-up; HTN—hypertension; QTc—corrected QT

Note. From "Evaluation and Management of Patients With Heart Disease and Cancer: Cardio-Oncology," by J. Herrmann, A. Lerman, N.P. Sandhu, H.R. Villarraga, S.L. Mulvagh, and M. Kohli, 2014, *Mayo Clinic Proceedings, 89,* p. 1294. Copyright 2014 by Mayo Foundation for Medical Education and Research. Reprinted with permission.

hypotension was defined as a systolic blood pressure (SBP) less than 90 mm Hg, a drop in systolic blood pressure greater than 40 mm from baseline, or a mean arterial pressure (MAP) less than 60–70 mm Hg (Rosendorff et al., 2015). In patients with baseline low blood pressure, other indicators of perfusion may be needed to identify clinically significant hypotension. Orthostatic hypotension can be classified as primary or secondary or as acute or chronic and is defined as a decrease in SBP of greater than or equal to 20 mm Hg and/or a decrease in diastolic blood pressure (DBP) of greater than or equal to 10 mm Hg within 30 seconds to 3 minutes of active standing, during a head tilt test of 60°, or in a patient with symptoms (Gauer, 2011; Ricci, De Caterina, & Fedorowski, 2015). In patients with a history of hypertension, hypotension may occur with blood pressure changes greater than or equal to 30 mm Hg from gradual impairment of adaptive mechanisms. Additionally, two broad pathologic categories for hypotension are structural (neurogenic), such as with Parkinson disease or because of complications with diabetes or end-stage renal disease, and functional (non-neurogenic) causes of the autonomic nervous system (Ricci et al., 2015). Examples of functional impairment causing orthostatic hypotension include underlying cardiovascular disease, renal failure, history of multiple myeloma, spinal cord injuries, paraneoplastic syndromes, treatment with vasodilators, tricyclic antidepressants, use of diuretics, several chemotherapeutic agents, decreased circulating blood volume, venous pooling, and heart failure (Ricci et al., 2015).

Risk Factors

In patients with cancer, hypotension occurs infrequently and is typically associated with vasodilation, volume depletion, or poor perfusion (Sharp, 2014). Several causes of hypotension exist related to cancer and its treatment, including blood or fluid loss from bleeding, infection or sepsis, severe hypersensitivity, hepatic failure, increased intracranial pressure or spinal injury leading to heart block or bradycardia, hormonal abnormalities (e.g., adrenal insufficiency, hypothyroidism), heart failure (e.g., myocardial infarction, congestive heart failure, cardiac tamponade), or drug-induced causes (Gauer, 2011; Ricci et al., 2015). Specific chemotherapeutic agents associated with hypotension include alemtuzumab, cetuximab, denileukin diftitox, docetaxel, etoposide, 5-azacitidine, gemcitabine, ifosfamide, interferon alfa, interleukin-2, ipilimumab, paclitaxel, rituximab, and thalidomide (Polovich et al., 2014; Yusuf et al., 2008).

Assessment

Many patients may be asymptomatic or experience few nonspecific symptoms, making assessment for clinically significant hypotension beyond the systolic blood pressure essential. MAP may provide the most accurate reflection of perfused pressure and is calculated by multiplying the DBP by 2, adding this value to the SBP, then dividing this sum by 3 (2D + S/3). In a patient with a normal blood pressure of 90/60, the mean pressure is 70 mm Hg, but when the diastolic drops and the blood pressure measures 90/45, the mean pressure is 60 mm

Hg. It is estimated that the brain requires 65–70 mm Hg of perfused pressure and the kidneys need 60–65 mm Hg, making the usual goal blood pressure when providing interventions about 65 mm Hg. Mental status or urine output is used to evaluate if the goal is adequate for the patient. Setting an ideal pressure and using MAP to establish goal blood pressure is common critical care practice and is especially important in patients with low normal SBP, low DBP, or at risk for hypovolemia (e.g., bleeding or dehydration) and vasodilation (e.g., sepsis or liver failure).

Patients with orthostatic hypotension frequently experience wide swings in blood pressure, especially in the morning or with postural changes. Symptoms in patients with cancer can be exacerbated by dehydration, venous pooling, fever, urination, and immobilization. In addition to the presence of low blood pressure, signs of poor perfusion are considered necessary for diagnosis and include lightheadedness, blurred vision, dizziness, nausea, fatigue, and "coat hanger" pain that can ultimately lead to syncope (Ricci et al., 2015).

Management

The goal of hypotension treatment is to stop or decrease the dose or rate of any offending medication; assess the patient's baseline blood pressure and the change from baseline; assess for orthostatic changes, mentation, and urinary output; administer fluids; and evaluate the need for fluids, vasopressors, or inotropic agents. It is usually considered standard to expect a urine output of at least 0.5 ml/kg reference or dry weight, although patients with altered renal function may have reduced urine output at baseline and are at high risk for compromise after minimal insult.

Fluid administration for treatment of hypotension is standard practice, even while providing more definitive therapy that targets the etiology of the hypotension. Recent research with large-volume fluid resuscitation in sepsis suggests that administration of lactated Ringer's solution is preferred because it reduces the risk of hyperchloremia seen with 0.9% normal saline infusion (Madhusudan, Vijayaraghavan, & Cove, 2014). Fluid boluses for management of presumed volume depletion or vasodilation-induced hypotension are recommended as 30 ml/kg reference or dry weight, unless specific contraindications such as heart failure exist (Madhusudan et al., 2014). When fluid unresponsiveness has been established, vasopressor or inotropic agents are considered. The selection of vasoactive agents is dependent on the cause of hypotension and the presence of cardiac dysfunction (Zhou et al., 2015). The current preferred agent in distributive shock is norepinephrine, although the addition of vasopressin at a fixed dose of 0.4 units/hour is advocated (Zhou et al., 2015).

Hypertension

Hypertension is one of the most common chronic diseases and is estimated to affect approximately one-fourth of adults in the Unites States (James et al., 2014; Rosendorff et al., 2015). The prevalence of hypertension in patients with cancer has steadily increased because of a number of new targeted therapy agents

(Force & Kerkelä, 2008; Lenihan & Kowey, 2013). Emerging data propose that the occurrence of hypertension, especially with the tyrosine kinase inhibitors, is a pharmacodynamic marker of response to anti-VEGF therapy. Stage 1 hypertension has been defined as an SBP of 140 mm Hg or greater or a DBP of 90 mm Hg or greater. Stage 2 is defined as 160/100 mm Hg or greater (James et al., 2014; Weber et al., 2013). The mechanisms of action are multifactorial and have been associated with functional and structural cardiac and vascular abnormalities, which may promote hypertrophy, myocardial fibrosis, and loss of contractility of the heart muscle, as well as potentiate pathophysiologic changes of the left ventricle, leading to heart failure (Curigliano et al., 2010; Nazer, Humphreys, & Moslehi, 2011; Weber et al., 2013).

Pathogenesis

Rosendorff et al. (2015) described several pathophysiologic mechanisms of hypertension and the development of coronary artery disease, including increased sympathetic nervous system and renin–angiotensin–aldosterone system activity, deficiencies in the release or activity of vasodilators, and increased expression of growth factors and inflammatory cytokines in the arterial tree. Hemodynamic effects and structural and functional abnormalities in conductive and resistance arteries lead to increased vascular stiffness and endothelial dysfunction. In patients with comorbidities, hypertension can lead to production of vasoactive cytokines that promote vasoconstriction, endothelial dysfunction, inflammation, and increased oxidative stress in the vasculature, increasing both blood pressure and coronary artery disease risk (Rosendorff et al., 2015).

Risk Factors

Risk factors for hypertension include preexisting hypertension or cardiovascular disease, renal insufficiency, African American descent, hyperthyroidism, Cushing syndrome, tobacco use, obesity, increased intracranial pressure, and hypomagnesemia (James et al., 2014; Polovich et al., 2014; Rosendorff et al., 2015). Smokers with hypertension have a five times higher risk of developing severe hypertension and have a higher mortality rate than nonsmokers (Rosendorff et al., 2015). Obesity, defined as a BMI of 30 kg/m^2 or higher, increases the risk of developing hypertension about three times over nonobese individuals. Magnesium has been found to act as a natural antihypertensive agent, making it important to maintain magnesium levels as close to normal as possible.

Assessment

The gold standard for diagnosis of hypertension is manual auscultation, when it is verified that blood pressure is greater than 130/90 mm Hg on two separate occasions at least two weeks apart (James et al., 2014). In patients with cancer, situations exist that cause unequal blood pressure in the upper extremities. Superior vena cava syndrome can cause marked increased blood pressure in the right arm (Shelton, 2013). Other tests used to diagnosis and monitor hypertension include electrocardiography and laboratory studies, such as electrolytes, fasting glucose concentration, serum creatinine and blood urea nitrogen, lipid panel, complete blood counts, and liver function tests.

Management

The primary goal of antihypertensive therapy is the prevention of cardiovascular complications and death through the identification of risk factors. Early and aggressive initiation of antihypertensives can help maintain treatment schedules and decrease risk of significant cardiovascular complications (see Table 9-6). Additionally, it has been proposed that some antihypertensives may have cardioprotective effects, especially with ACE inhibitors and beta-blockers. ACE inhibitors are considered the antihypertensive drug of choice in obesity-related hypertension because of their ability to increase insulin sensitivity, which helps to decrease the risk of developing diabetes (Rosendorff et al., 2015). A second recommendation for treatment of hypertension includes lifestyle modifications, such as smoking cessation, limiting alcohol intake, maintaining ideal body weight, and reducing sodium intake, which is considered a first-line modification. Pharmacologic management of hypertension is recommended when blood pressure is greater than 140/90 mm Hg or when lifestyle modifications have been ineffective. In adults aged 80 years or older, pharmacologic treatment should be started when blood pressure is 150/90 mm Hg or higher, and sooner if the individual has chronic kidney disease or diabetes.

Resistant hypertension, also known as malignant hypertension, is defined as an extremely high blood pressure that develops suddenly and can lead to organ damage. This condition is considered a medical emergency and requires immediate treatment. A patient with malignant hypertension has a blood pressure frequently greater than 180/120 mm Hg or a diastolic blood pressure greater than 130 mm Hg accompanied by symptoms of papilledema, central nervous system (CNS) manifestations, cardiac decompensation, and progressive deterioration of renal function (George & Neilson, 2008). Malignant hypertension has been associated with African American males and patients with renal cell carcinoma, kidney failure, and renal hypertension. Causes of malignant hypertension include kidney disease; collagen vascular disease, such as scleroderma; spinal cord injuries; tumors of the adrenal gland; illicit drugs, such as cocaine; and certain medications, such as birth control pills and monoamine oxidase inhibitors. Patients should be assessed for CNS symptoms, such as blurred vision, dizziness, severe headache, change in mental status, and headache, as these typically occur first. Cardiovascular decompensation and renal failure typically follow the CNS symptom (George & Neilson, 2008). A patient may complain of chest pain, nausea or vomiting, cough, shortness of breath, decreased urinary output, or seizure. A chest x-ray may reveal congested lungs and an enlarged heart, which increases the risk for pericardial effusions, cardiac tamponade, and myocardial infarction. Nursing implications include the monitoring of patients at risk, early identification, and treatment of this disorder.

Table 9-6. Drug Selection in Hypertensive Patients With or Without Other Major Conditions

Patient Type	First Drug	Add Second Drug if Needed to Achieve a BP < 140/90 mm Hg	If Third Drug Is Needed to Achieve a BP < 140/90 mm Hg
When Hypertension Is the Only or Main Condition			
Black patients (African ancestry): All ages	CCB[a] or thiazide diuretic	ARB[b] or ACE inhibitor (If unavailable can add alternative first drug choice)	Combination of CCB + ACE inhibitor or ARB + thiazide diuretic
White or other non-black patients: Younger than 60	ARB[b] or ACE inhibitor	CCB[a] or thiazide diuretic	Combination of CCB + ACE inhibitor or ARB + thiazide diuretic
White or other non-black patients: 60 years and older	CCB[a] or thiazide diuretic (Although ACE inhibitors or ARBs are also usually effective)	ARB[b] or ACE inhibitor (or CCB or thiazide if ACE inhibitor or ARB used first)	Combination of CCB + ACE inhibitor or ARB + thiazide diuretic
When Hypertension Is Associated With Other Conditions			
Hypertension *and* diabetes	ARB or ACE inhibitor (Note: In black patients, it is acceptable to start with a CCB or thiazide)	CCB or thiazide diuretic (Note: In black patients, if starting with a CCB or thiazide, add an ARB or ACE inhibitor)	The alternative second drug (thiazide or CCB)
Hypertension *and* chronic kidney disease	ARB or ACE inhibitor (Note: In black patients, good evidence for renal protective effects of ACE inhibitors)	CCB or thiazide diuretic[c]	The alternative second drug (thiazide or CCB)

(Continued on next page)

Table 9-6. Drug Selection in Hypertensive Patients With or Without Other Major Conditions (Continued)

Patient Type	First Drug	Add Second Drug if Needed to Achieve a BP < 140/90 mm Hg	If Third Drug Is Needed to Achieve a BP < 140/90 mm Hg
Hypertension and clinical coronary artery disease[d]	β-blocker plus ARB or ACE inhibitor	CCB or thiazide diuretic	The alternative second drug (thiazide or CCB)
Hypertension and stroke history[e]	ACE inhibitor or ARB	Thiazide diuretic or CCB	The alternative second drug (thiazide or CCB)
Hypertension and heart failure	Patients with symptomatic heart failure should usually receive an ARB or ACE inhibitor + β-blocker + diuretic + spironolactone regardless of blood pressure. A dihydropyridine CCB can be added if needed for BP control.		

[a] CCBs are generally preferred, but thiazides may cost less.

[b] ARBs can be considered because ACE inhibitors can cause cough and angioedema, although ACE inhibitors may cost less.

[c] If eGFR < 40 ml/min, a loop diuretic (e.g., furosemide or torsemide) may be needed.

[d] Note: If history of myocardial infarction, a β-blocker and ARB/or ACE inhibitor are indicated regardless of blood pressure.

[e] Note: If using a diuretic, there is good evidence for indapamide (if available).

ACE—angiotensin-converting enzyme; ARB—angiotensin receptor blocker; BP—blood pressure; CCB—calcium channel blocker; eGFR—estimated glomerular filtration rate

Note. From "Clinical Practice Guidelines for the Management of Hypertension in the Community: A Statement by the American Society of Hypertension and the International Society of Hypertension," M.A. Weber, E.L. Schiffrin, W.B. White, S. Mann, L.H. Lindholm, J.G. Kenerson, ... S.B. Harrap, 2014, *Journal of Clinical Hypertension, 16,* p. 21. Copyright 2014 by John Wiley and Sons. Reprinted with permission.

Summary

While cancer survivorship has increased, so too has awareness of the potential for cardiovascular complications from the cancer and its treatment. Oncology nurses need to be knowledgeable about the risk for cardiac complications to help identify patients at risk for the development of cardiovascular toxicities, especially because cardiovascular toxicity is a dose-limiting toxicity of cancer treatment.

References

Adão, R., de Keulenaer, G., Leite-Moreira, A., & Brás-Silva, C. (2013). Cardiotoxicity associated with cancer therapy: Pathophysiology and prevention. *Revista Portuguesa de Cardiologia, 32,* 395–409. doi:10.1016/j.repce.2012.11.019

American Cancer Society. (2017). *Cancer facts and figures 2017.* Retrieved from https://www.cancer.org/content/dam/cancer-org/research/cancer-facts-and-statistics/annual-cancer-facts-and-figures/2017/cancer-facts-and-figures-2017.pdf

Anderson, B., & Sawyer, D.B. (2008). Predicting and preventing the cardiotoxicity of cancer therapy. *Expert Review of Cardiovascular Therapies, 6,* 1023–1033. doi:10.1586/14779072.6.7.1023

Anderson, S., & White, B.W. (2013). Anthracyclines, trastuzumab, and cardiomyopathy. In A.P. Fadol (Ed.), *Cardiac complications of cancer therapy* (pp. 13–30). Pittsburgh, PA: Oncology Nursing Society.

Andréjak, C., Terzi, N., Thielen, S., Bergot, E., Zalcman, G., Charbonneau, P., & Jounieaux, V. (2011). Admission of advanced lung cancer patients to intensive care unit: A retrospective study of 76 patients. *BMC Cancer, 11,* 159. doi:10.1186/1471-2407-11-159

Attin, M., & Davidson, J.E. (2010). Using QRS morphology and QTc interval to prevent complications and cardiac death. *Critical Care Nursing Quarterly, 34,* 246–253. doi:10.1097/CNQ.0b013e318221477c

Azoulay, E., Soares, M., Darmon, M., Benoit, D., Pastores, S., & Afessa, B. (2011). Intensive care of the cancer patient: Recent achievements and remaining challenges. *Annals of Intensive Care, 1,* 1–13. doi:10.1186/2110-5820-1-5

Biogen-Idec, Inc., & Genentech, Inc. (2013). *Rituxan® (rituximab)* [Package insert]. South San Francisco, CA: Genentech, Inc.

Bonita, R., & Pradhan, R. (2013). Cardiovascular toxicities of cancer chemotherapy. *Seminars in Oncology, 40,* 156–167. doi:10.1053/j.seminoncol.2013.01.004

Borlaug, B.A., & DeCamp, M.M. (2015). Pericardial disease associated with malignancy [Literature review current through May 2017]. Retrieved from http://www.uptodate.com/contents/pericardial-disease-associated-with-malignancy

Bovelli, D., Plataniotis, G., & Roila, F. (2010). Cardiotoxicity of chemotherapeutic agents and radiotherapy-related heart disease: ESMO clinical practice guidelines. *Annals of Oncology, 21*(Suppl. 5), v277–v282. doi:10.1093/annonc/mdq200

Briasoulis, A., Agarwal, V., & Pierce, W.J. (2011). QT prolongation and torsade de pointes induced by fluoroquinolones: Infrequent side effects from commonly used medications. *Cardiology, 120,* 103–110. doi:10.1159/000334441

Bristol-Myers Squibb Co. & ImClone LLC. (2012). *Erbitux® (cetuximab)* [Package insert]. Princeton, NJ: Author.

Brown, L.S., & Giampa, S. (2010). Alternative avenues: Supplements and nutraceuticals for treating cardiovascular disease. *Today's Dietitian.* Retrieved from http://www.todaysdietitian.com/heart_health_index.shtml

Bui, A.L., & Fonarow, G.C. (2012). Home monitoring for heart failure management. *Journal of the American College of Cardiology, 59*, 97–104. doi:10.1016/j.jacc.2011.09.044

Cahoon, W.D., Jr. (2009). Acquired QT prolongation. *Progress in Cardiovascular Nursing, 24*, 30–33. doi:10.1111/j.1751-7117.2009.00021.x

Chen, M.H. (2009). Cardiac dysfunction induced by novel targeted anticancer therapy: An emerging issue. *Current Cardiology Reports, 11*, 167–174. doi:10.1007/s11886-009-0025-9

Cheng, H., & Force, T. (2010). Why do kinase inhibitors cause cardiotoxicity and what can be done about it? *Progress in Cardiovascular Diseases, 53*, 114–120. doi:10.1016/j.pcad.2010.06.006

Clarke, M. (2006). Meta-analyses of adjuvant therapies for women with early breast cancer: The Early Breast Cancer Trialists' Collaborative Group overview. *Annals of Oncology, 17*(Suppl. 10), 54–62. doi:10.1093/annonc/mdl238

Coviello, J.S., & Knobf, M.T. (2013). Screening and management of cardiovascular risk factors in cancer survivors. In A.P. Fadol (Ed.), *Cardiac complications of cancer therapy* (pp. 267–296). Pittsburgh, PA: Oncology Nursing Society.

Curigliano, G., Mayer, E.L., Burstein, H.J., Winer, E.P., & Goldhirsch, A. (2010). Cardiac toxicity from systemic cancer therapy: A comprehensive review. *Progress in Cardiovascular Diseases, 53*, 94–104. doi:10.1016/j.pcad.2010.05.006

De Jesus-Gonzalez, N., Robinson, E., Moslehi, J., & Humphreys, B.D. (2012). Management of antiangiogenic therapy-induced hypertension. *Hypertension, 60*, 607–615. doi:10.1161/HYPERTENSIONAHA.112.196774

Drew, B.J., Ackerman, M.J., Funk, M., Gibler, W.B., Kligfield, P., Menon, V., … Zareba, W. (2010). Prevention of torsade de pointes in hospital settings: A scientific statement from the American Heart Association and the American College of Cardiology Foundation. *Circulation, 121*, 1047–1060. doi:10.1161/CIRCULATIONAHA.109.192704

Escalante, C.P., & Yeung, S.-C.J. (2013). Cardiac emergencies in cancer patients. In M.S. Ewer & E.T. Yeh (Eds.), *Cancer and the heart* (2nd ed., pp. 243–262). Shelton, CT: People's Medical Publishing House.

Fadol, A.P., & Lech, T. (2011). Cardiovascular adverse events associated with cancer therapy. *Journal of the Advanced Practitioner in Oncology, 2*, 229–242. doi:10.6004/jadpro.2011.2.4.2

Fee, A.E. (2013). Acute coronary syndromes in patients with cancer. In A.P. Fadol (Ed.), *Cardiac complications of cancer therapy* (pp. 55–75). Pittsburgh, PA: Oncology Nursing Society.

Force, T., & Kerkelä, R. (2008). Cardiotoxicity of the new cancer therapeutics—Mechanisms of, and approaches to, the problem. *Drug Discovery Today, 13*, 778–784. doi:10.1016/j.drudis.2008.05.011

Gauer, R. (2011). Evaluation of syncope. *American Family Physician, 84*, 640–650.

Genentech, Inc. (2012). *Avastin® (bevacizumab)* [Package insert]. South San Francisco, CA: Author.

George, A., & Neilson, E. (2008). Cellular and molecular biology of the kidney. In A.S. Fauci, E. Braunwald, D.L. Kasper, S.L. Hauser, D.L. Longo, J.L. Jameson, & J. Loscalzo (Eds.), *Harrison's principles of internal medicine* (17th ed., pp. 1741–1747). New York, NY: McGraw-Hill Medical.

Guglin, M., Aljayeh, M., Saiyad, S., Ali, R., & Curtis, A.B. (2009). Introducing a new entity: Chemotherapy-induced arrhythmia. *Europace, 11*, 1579–1586. doi:10.1093/europace/eup300

Hamo, C.E., & Bloom, M.W. (2015). Getting to the heart of the matter: An overview of cardiac toxicity related to cancer therapy. *Clinical Medicine Insights: Cardiology, 9*(Suppl. 2), 47–51. doi:10.4137/CMC.S19704

Hampton, T. (2010). Cancer therapy can be hard on the heart. *JAMA, 303*, 1019–1020. doi:10.1001/jama.2010.269

Herrmann, J., & Lerman, A. (2014). An update on cardio-oncology. *Trends in Cardiovascular Medicine, 24*, 285–295. doi:10.1016/j.tcm.2014.07.003

Herrmann, J., Lerman, A., Sandhu, N.P., Villarraga, H.R., Mulvagh, S.L., & Kohli, M. (2014). Evaluation and management of patients with heart disease and cancer: Cardio-oncology. *Mayo Clinic Proceedings, 89*, 1287–1306. doi:10.1016/j.mayocp.2014.05.013

James, P.A., Oparil, S., Carter, B.L., Cushman, W.C., Dennison-Himmelfarb, C., Handler, J., … Ortiz, E. (2014). 2014 evidence-based guidelines for the management of high blood pressure in adults: Report from the panel members appointed to the Eighth Joint National Committee (JNC 8). *JAMA, 311,* 507–520. doi:10.1001/jama.2013.284427

Khakoo, A.Y., & Yeh, E.T. (2008). Therapy insight: Management of cardiovascular disease in patients with cancer and cardiac complications of cancer therapy. *Nature Clinical Practice Oncology, 5,* 655–667. doi:10.1038/ncponcl225

Khawaja, M.Z., Cafferkey, C., Rajani, R., Redwood, S., & Cunningham, D. (2014). Cardiac complications and manifestations of chemotherapy for cancer. *BMJ Heart, 100,* 1133–1140. doi:10.1136/heartjnl-2014-305859

King, M., Kingery, J., & Casey, B. (2012). Diagnosis and evaluation of heart failure. *American Family Physician, 84,* 1161–1168.

Lancellotti, P., Nkomo, V.T., Badano, L.P., Bergler-Klein, J., Bogaert, J., Davin, L., … Yang, P.C. (2013). Expert consensus for multi-modality imaging evaluation of cardiovascular complications of radiotherapy in adults: A report from the European Association of Cardiovascular Imaging and the American Society of Echocardiography. *European Heart Journal—Cardiac Imaging, 14,* 721–740. doi:10.1093/ehjci/jet123

Leja, M.J. (2013). Cardiovascular anatomy and cardiac malignancy. In A.P. Fadol (Ed.), *Cardiac complications of cancer therapy* (pp. 1–11). Pittsburgh, PA: Oncology Nursing Society.

Lenihan, D.J., & Cardinale, D.M. (2012). Late cardiac effects of cancer treatment. *Journal of Clinical Oncology, 30,* 3657–3664. doi:10.1200/JCO.2012.45.2938

Lenihan, D.J., & Kowey, P.R. (2013). Overview and management of cardiac adverse events associated with tyrosine kinase inhibitors. *Oncologist, 18,* 900–908. doi:10.1634/theoncologist.2012-0466

Lindenfeld, J., Albert, N.M., Boehmer, J.P., Collins, S.P., Ezekowitz, J.A., Givertz, M.M., … Walsh, M.N. (2010). Executive summary: HFSA 2010 comprehensive heart failure practice guideline. *Journal of Cardiac Failure, 16,* 475–539. doi:10.1016/j.cardfail.2010.04.005

Lipshultz, S.E., Alvarez, J.A., & Scully, R.E. (2008). Anthracycline associated cardiotoxicity in survivors of childhood cancer. *Heart, 94,* 525–533. doi:10.1136/hrt.2007.136093

Litsas, G. (2011). Nursing perspectives on fulvestrant for the treatment of postmenopausal women with metastatic breast cancer. *Clinical Journal of Oncology Nursing, 15,* 674–681. doi:10.1188/11.CJON.674-681

Madhusudan, P., Vijayaraghavan, B.K.T., & Cove, M.E. (2014). Fluid resuscitation in sepsis: Reexamining the paradigm. *BioMed Research International, 2014,* Article ID 984082. doi:10.1155/2014/984082

Martinou, M., & Gaya, A. (2013). Cardiac complications after radial radiotherapy. *Seminars in Oncology, 40,* 178–185. doi:10.1053/j.seminoncol.2013.01.007

Nazer, B., Humphreys, B.D., & Moslehi, J. (2011). Effects of novel angiogenesis inhibitors for the treatment of cancer on the cardiovascular system: Focus on hypertension. *Circulation, 124,* 1687–1691. doi:10.1161/CIRCULATIONAHA.110.992230

New York Heart Association Criteria Committee. (1964). *Diseases of the heart and blood vessels: Nomenclature and criteria for diagnosis* (6th ed.). Boston, MA: Little, Brown.

Polovich, M., Olsen, M., & LeFebvre, K.B. (Eds.). (2014). *Chemotherapy and biotherapy guidelines and recommendations for practice* (4th ed.). Pittsburgh, PA: Oncology Nursing Society.

Prometheus Laboratories Inc. (2012). *Proleukin® (aldesleukin)* [Package insert]. San Diego, CA: Author.

Rahman, A.M. (2009). Ischemic heart disease in cancer patients. In S.-J. Yeung, C.P. Escalante, & R.F. Gagel (Eds.), *Medical care of the cancer patient* (pp. 471–483). Shelton, CT: People's Medical Publishing House.

Ricci, F., De Caterina, R., & Fedorowski, A. (2015). Orthostatic hypotension: Epidemiology, prognosis, and treatment. *Journal of the American College of Cardiology, 66,* 848–860. doi:10.1016/j.jacc.2015.06.1084

Rosendorff, C., Lackland, D.T., Allison, M., Aronow, W.S., Black, H.R., Blumenthal, R.S., … White, W.B. (2015). Treatment of hypertension in patients with coronary artery disease: A scientific statement from the American Heart Association, American College of Cardiology, and American Society of Hypertension. *Journal of the American College of Cardiology, 65,* 1998–2038. doi:10.1016/j.jacc.2015.02.038

Ryberg, M. (2013). Cardiovascular toxicities of biological therapies. *Seminars in Oncology, 40,* 168–177. doi:10.1053/j.seminoncol.2013.01.002

Schering Corporation. (2012). *Intron° A (interferon-alfa 2b, recombinant)* [Package insert]. Kenilworth, NJ: Author.

Sharp, K. (2014). Hypotension. In D. Camp-Sorrell & R.A. Hawkins (Eds.), *Clinical manual for the oncology advanced practice nurse* (3rd ed., pp. 419–425). Pittsburgh, PA: Oncology Nursing Society.

Shelton, B.K. (2013). Superior vena cava syndrome. In M. Kaplan (Ed.), *Understanding and managing oncologic emergencies: A resource for nurses* (2nd ed., pp. 385–410). Pittsburgh, PA: Oncology Nursing Society.

Shelton, B.K. (2014a). Dysrhythmias. In D. Camp-Sorrell & R.A. Hawkins (Eds.), *Clinical manual for the oncology advanced practice nurse* (3rd ed., pp. 371–390). Pittsburgh, PA: Oncology Nursing Society.

Shelton, B.K. (2014b). Myocardial infarction/acute coronary syndromes. In D. Camp-Sorrell & R.A. Hawkins (Eds.), *Clinical manual for the oncology advanced practice nurse* (3rd ed., pp. 427–444). Pittsburgh, PA: Oncology Nursing Society.

Shelton, B.K. (2014c). Pericarditis, pericardial effusion, and pericardial tamponade. In D. Camp-Sorrell & R.A. Hawkins (Eds.), *Clinical manual for the oncology advanced practice nurse* (3rd ed., pp. 445–460). Pittsburgh, PA: Oncology Nursing Society.

Slovacek, L., Ansorgova, V., Macingova, Z., Haman, L., & Petera, J. (2008). Tamoxifen-induced QT interval prolongation. *Journal of Clinical Pharmacy and Therapeutics, 33,* 453–455. doi:10.1111/j.1365-2710.2008.00928.x

Stephens, J.M.L. (2013). Cardiopulmonary complications. In S.A. Ezzone (Ed.), *Hematopoietic stem cell transplantation: A manual for nursing practice* (2nd ed., pp. 201–236). Pittsburgh, PA: Oncology Nursing Society.

Story, K.T. (2013). Cardiac tamponade. In M. Kaplan (Ed.), *Understanding and managing oncologic emergencies: A resource for nurses* (2nd ed., pp. 43–68). Pittsburgh, PA: Oncology Nursing Society.

Story, K.T. (2014). Deep venous thrombosis. In D. Camp-Sorrell & R.A. Hawkins (Eds.), *Clinical manual for the oncology advanced practice nurse* (3rd ed., pp. 349–361). Pittsburgh, PA: Oncology Nursing Society.

Truong, J., Yan, A.T., Cramarossa, G., & Chan, K.K.W. (2014). Chemotherapy-induced cardiotoxicity: Detection, prevention, and management. *Canadian Journal of Cardiology, 30,* 869–878. doi:10.1016/j.cjca.2014.04.029

Truven Health Analytics, Inc. (2017). Micromedex. Retrieved from http://truvenhealth.com/products/micromedex

Viale, P.H., & Yamamoto, D.S. (2008). Cardiovascular toxicity associated with cancer treatment. *Clinical Journal of Oncology Nursing, 12,* 627–638. doi:10.1188/08.CJON.627-638.

Villarraga, H.R., Herrmann, J., & Nkomo, V.T. (2014). Cardio-oncology: Role of echocardiography. *Progress in Cardiovascular Diseases, 57,* 10–18. doi:10.1016/j.pcad.2014.05.002

Walsh, M.C. (2010). Impact of treatment-related cardiac toxicity on lymphoma survivors: An institutional approach for risk reduction and management. *Clinical Journal of Oncology Nursing, 14,* 505–507. doi:10.1188/10.CJON.505-507

Weber, M.A., Schiffrin, E.L., White, W.B., Mann, S., Lindholm, L.H., Kenerson, J.G., ... Harrap, S.B. (2013). Clinical practice guidelines for the management of hypertension in the community: A statement by the American Society of Hypertension and the International Society of Hypertension. *Journal of Clinical Hypertension, 16,* 14–26. doi:10.1111/jch.12237

Woods, M.L. (2013). Cardiac inflammatory conditions and cardiac tamponade in patients with cancer. In A.P. Fadol (Ed.), *Cardiac complications of cancer therapy* (pp. 77–93). Pittsburgh, PA: Oncology Nursing Society.

Yahalom, J., & Portlock, C.S. (2008). Long-term cardiac and pulmonary complications of cancer therapy. *Hematology/Oncology Clinics of North America, 22,* 305–318. doi:10.1016/j.hoc.2008.01.010

Yancy, C.W., Jessup, M., Bozkurt, B., Butler, J., Casey, D.E., Drazner, M.H., ... Wilkoff, B.L. (2013). 2013 ACCF/AHA guideline for the management of heart failure: Executive summary:

A report of the American College of Cardiology Foundation/American Heart Association task force on practice guidelines. *Circulation, 128,* 1810–1852. doi:10.1161/CIR.0b013e31829e8807

Yeh, E.T.H., & Bickford, C.L. (2009). Cardiovascular complications of cancer therapy: Incidence, pathogenesis, diagnosis, and management. *Journal of the American College of Cardiology, 53,* 2231–2247. doi:10.1016/j.jacc.2009.02.050

Yusuf, S.W., Razeghi, P., & Yeh, E. (2008). The diagnosis and management of cardiovascular disease in cancer patients. *Current Problems in Cardiology, 33,* 163–193. doi:10.1016/j.cpcardiol.2008.01.002

Yusuf, S.W., Sami, S., & Daher, I.N. (2011). Radiation-induced heart disease: A clinical update. *Cardiology Research and Practice, 2011,* Article ID 317659. doi:10.4061/2011/317659

Zhou, F.H., Mao, Z., Zeng, X.T., Kang, H.J., Liu, H., Pan, L., & Hou, P.C. (2015). Vasopressors in septic shock: A systematic review and network meta-analysis. *Therapeutics and Clinical Risk Management, 11,* 1047–1059. doi:10.2147/TCRM.S80060

CHAPTER 10

Oncologic Emergencies

Lisa Parks, MS, ANP-BC

Introduction

Oncologic emergencies are life-threatening conditions that require immediate recognition and intervention to prolong survival and improve quality of life. These emergencies can occur any time after a cancer diagnosis. In the setting of recurrent malignancy, oncologic emergencies can occur years after cancer surveillance has been transferred from a medical oncologist to a primary care provider. As a nurse, it is important to assess for oncologic emergencies by determining a patient's cancer history or current treatments. This chapter will discuss the most common oncologic emergencies and their associated treatments.

Metabolic Emergencies

Hypercalcemia

Pathophysiology

Hypercalcemia is a metabolic emergency that occurs in 20%–30% of patients with advanced cancer during the disease course (Pi et al., 2015). Breast and lung cancer and multiple myeloma are the most common cancers associated with hypercalcemia of malignancy (Lewis, Hendrickson, & Moynihan, 2011). Many physiologic mechanisms can lead to hypercalcemia, including a systemic release of parathyroid hormone–related peptide (PTHrP) from the tumor and also parathyroid hormone (PTH) that leads to the overproduction of calcium from increased bone and calcium reabsorption. Bony metastases may also cause a local paracrine effect by stimulating osteoclasts, leading to bone resorption and destruction. Tumor production of vitamin D analogs in Hodgkin and non-

Hodgkin lymphoma can produce elevated calcitriol and increase production of serum calcium.

Signs and Symptoms

See Table 10-1 for signs and symptoms of hypercalcemia of malignancy.

Table 10-1. Signs and Symptoms of Hypercalcemia of Malignancy	
System	**Signs and Symptoms**
Cardiovascular	Shortened ST segments and QT intervals, widened T waves, bundle branch patterns, depressed ST segments, second-degree heart block, brady arrhythmias, complete heart block, cardiac arrest
Dermatologic	Pruritus
Gastrointestinal	Nausea, anorexia, vomiting, constipation, ileus, peptic ulcer disease, pancreatitis
Neurologic	Muscle weakness, fatigue, hyporeflexia, apathy, disturbances of perception and behavior, lethargy, stupor, and coma
Renal	Polyuria, polydipsia, volume depletion, progressive renal insufficiency, nephrocalcinosis, nephrolithiasis
Note. Based on information from Wagner & Arora, 2014.	

Diagnosis

Hypercalcemia is defined as a total serum calcium concentration greater than 10 mg/dl or an ionized calcium concentration greater than 5.6 mg/dl (Wagner & Arora, 2014). Ionized calcium is the most reliable test to detect hypercalcemia and is considered elevated at greater than 1.29 mmol/L (Lewis et al., 2011). High levels may be tolerated if calcium increase is gradual.

Treatment

The 30-day mortality rate of hospitalized patients with cancer and hypercalcemia can be as high as 50% (Lewis et al., 2011). Because patients with hypercalcemia have intravascular volume depletion, hydration is the initial management. Thiazide diuretics should be avoided, as they increase calcium reabsorption from the urine. Bisphosphonates block bone resorption by osteoclasts but do not lower calcium rapidly enough to replace aggressive hydration. With bisphosphonates, calcium declines within 48–96 hours of infusion and nadirs at one week (Lewis et al., 2011). Calcitonin lowers the calcium within 12–24 hours but should not be used as a single agent because of rebound hypercalcemia. Glucocorticoids mediate the release of cytokines and prostaglandins that stimulate osteoclasts. Steroids also inhibit calcitriol production by macrophages and lower calcium within three to five days (Lewis et al., 2011). Table 10-2 details treatment.

Nursing Implications

Patients with cancer and hypercalcemia should be admitted to a bed with a cardiac monitor. IV fluids should be initiated with fluid resuscitation of 500–1,000 ml in the first hour and continuing at 150–250 ml/hour until urine output is achieved. Neurologic checks should be conducted every two hours. A basic malignancy workup should include chest x-ray, complete blood count, and comprehensive metabolic panel. PTH level should be drawn. Nurses also should consider a renal consult (Lewis et al., 2011).

Hyponatremia

Pathophysiology

Hyponatremia is the most common electrolyte disorder in patients with cancer and is defined as a sodium level less than 135 mmol/L (Pi et al., 2015; Rosner &

Table 10-2. Treatment of Hypercalcemia		
Medication	**Usual Dose**	**Nursing Implications**
Normal saline	Rapid infusion of 300–500 ml/hr until euvolemic	Caution in patients with heart failure
Furosemide	20–40 mg IV every 12–24 hours	Only after adequate hydration
Pamidronate	60–90 mg IV	Renal dosing adjustment for creatinine clearance
Zoledronic acid	4 mg IV	Consider alternative treatment in patients with renal failure.
Calcitonin	4–8 IU/kg subcutaneous or IV every 12 hours	Tachyphylaxis occurs quickly.
Steroids	Hydrocortisone 100 mg IV every 6 hours or prednisone 60 mg orally daily	Role usually limited to lymphomas. Anticipate hyperglycemia.
Mithramycin and gallium	–	Historical interest only
Denosumab	Under investigation	Currently approved only for the prevention of skeletal-related events from bone metastases
Note. Based on information from Pi et al., 2015.		

Dalkin, 2014). Patients on chemotherapy may be staged with the Common Terminology Criteria for Adverse Events from the National Cancer Institute Cancer Therapy Evaluation Program. Grades 1 and 2 on this scale are considered mild to moderate with sodium values of 131–134 mmol/L. Grade 3 is severe with sodium values of 121–130 mmol/L. Grade 4 is considered life threatening with a sodium value less than 120 mmol/L (Pi et al., 2015). Cancers commonly associated with hyponatremia are lung, breast, head, neck, gastrointestinal, genitourinary, endocrine, sarcoma, and lymphoma.

The most common etiology of hyponatremia is syndrome of inappropriate antidiuretic hormone secretion (SIADH). Antineoplastic drugs can cause hyponatremia, and the mechanism of action for these drugs (cyclophosphamide, vinblastine, and vincristine) may involve SIADH (De las Peñas et al., 2016).

Patients with cancer, hyponatremia, and SIADH have several criteria for diagnosis, which are categorized as essential or supplemental.

Essential criteria include a decreased serum osmolality and a urine osmolality greater than 100 mOsm/kg. Patients are euvolemic with normal thyroid and adrenal function. Urine sodium is greater than 30 mEq/L on a normal daily sodium intake and with no recent use of diuretics.

Supplemental criteria used to diagnose SIADH are a plasma uric acid less than 4 mg/dl and a blood urea nitrogen of less than 10 mg/dl, the inability to correct hyponatremia, a worsening hyponatremia after receiving 1–2 L of 0.9% normal saline IV, or a correction of hyponatremia with fluid restriction. Other criteria include a plasma arginine vasopressin level elevated relative to plasma osmolality and an abnormal result on test of water loss (less than 80% excretion of 20 ml water/kg over four hours or an inadequate urinary dilution of less than 100 mOsm/kg water) (De las Peñas et al., 2016).

Any disturbance of sodium can affect hemodynamic stability. Diet is the sole provider of sodium, which is excreted by the kidneys (Keane, 2014). Hyponatremia is a disruption of water and sodium balance, which is regulated by thirst and antidiuretic hormone. Most patients with hyponatremia are asymptomatic, suggesting that it develops slowly (Keane, 2014).

Signs and Symptoms

In cancer, hyponatremia can be caused by diarrhea and vomiting, either because of the disease itself or because of chemotherapy or radiation therapy. Sodium is an essential electrolyte for controlling fluid balance and exists as a positively charged ion. Sodium ions control the movement of fluid into the extracellular space (Abu Zeinah, Al-Kindi, Hassan, & Allam, 2015). The mechanism in which fluid is lost or reabsorbed by the body is controlled by antidiuretic hormone (Keane, 2014). Hyponatremia can manifest in several body systems. In the gastrointestinal tract, it can appear as nausea. In the neurologic system, cerebral edema, lethargy, disorientation, seizures, coma, and gait disturbances can all be symptoms of hyponatremia and lead to falls, dizziness, and headaches (De las Peñas et al., 2016).

Diagnosis

Hyponatremia is described as either hypovolemic, euvolemic, or hypervolemic based on extracellular fluid status. To determine the type of hyponatremia, plasma osmolality and urine sodium excretion should be obtained (Rosner & Dalkin, 2014). Table 10-3 details hyponatremia classification and diagnosis.

Treatment

Treatment is based on symptoms and symptom severity. Medications that may cause hyponatremia should be discontinued. Treating underlying malignancy and medical conditions may improve hyponatremia (see Table 10-4).

Nursing Implications

Nurses should maintain strict oral and parenteral intake and output. Daily weights should be obtained to monitor fluid volume status. Skin turgor should be

Table 10-3. Classification and Diagnosis of Hyponatremia			
Laboratory Value	**Hypovolemic**	**Euvolemic**	**Hypervolemic**
Serum sodium	–	< 135 mmol/L	–
Serum osmolality	–	< 280 mOsm/kg	–
Urine osmolality	–	> 100 mOsm/kg	–
Total body water	Decreased; total body sodium very low	Increased; total body sodium normal	Greatly increased; total body sodium increased
Urine sodium	Renal sodium loss > 20 mmol/L; extrarenal sodium loss < 20 mmol/L	–	Renal failure > 20 mmol/L; cirrhosis < 20 mmol/L
Supportive labs	Uric acid normal or elevated; blood urea nitrogen (BUN) elevated	Uric acid normal or low; BUN normal or low	Brain natriuretic peptide elevated
Signs	Dehydration; weight loss; dry mucous membranes	No dehydration or edema	Edema; ascites; weight gain

Note. Based on information from Pi et al., 2015.

Table 10-4. Treatment of Hyponatremia			
Management	Dose	Duration	Additional Comments
Hypovolemic (Mild to Moderate Hyponatremia)			
0.9% normal saline (154 mmol Na/L)	Rate is based on severity and volume repletion needed.	Resolution of hyponatremia	First-line treatment
Sodium chloride tablets (1 g = 17 mmol Na/L)	Dose is based on mEq needed; 1–3 g orally every 6–12 hours	Resolution of hyponatremia	Calculation: mEq NaCl needed = 0.6 × weight (kg) × (desired Na – actual Na)
Fludrocortisone	0.1 mg orally three times daily	Days	May be beneficial for cerebral salt wasting and subarachnoid hemorrhage at risk for vasospasms Side effects: Hypokalemia, fluid overload, hypertension
Euvolemic and Hypervolemic (Mild to Moderate Hyponatremia)			
Fluid restriction	Restrict fluids to < 500–1,000 ml/day or target 500 ml/day less than the average urine output.	Days until hyponatremia resolves	First line
Demeclocycline	600–1,200 mg/day orally in divided doses	Effects may not be seen for 3–4 days.	Second line Does not require concomitant fluid restriction Side effects: Gastrointestinal intolerance, nephrotoxicity (higher doses), liver dysfunction
Urea	15–30 g/day orally in divided doses	Days until hyponatremia resolves	Second line Dissolve in orange juice for taste. Side effects: azotemia, liver dysfunction

(Continued on next page)

			Additional
Management	**Dose**	**Duration**	**Comments**

Table 10-4. Treatment of Hyponatremia *(Continued)*

Euvolemic and Hypervolemic (Mild to Moderate Hyponatremia) *(cont.)*

Management	Dose	Duration	Additional Comments
Conivaptan	Infuse 20 mg bolus over 30 minutes followed by 20 mg continuously over 24 hours for up to 4 days.	Days until hyponatremia resolves; max is 4 days after the loading dose.	Third line Dose adjustment is required for mild hepatic dysfunction. Drug interactions with CYP3A4 inhibitors and inducers Side effects: Infusion site reaction, head-ache, hypotension, nausea, constipation
Tolvaptan	15 mg/day orally; may be increased up to 60 mg daily	Days until hyponatremia resolves; max is 30 days due to increased risk for liver injury.	Third line Drug interactions with CYP3A4 inhibitors and inducers No dose adjustments for renal (not studied in creatinine clear-ance < 10ml/min) or hepatic dysfunction Side effects: Dry mouth, polyuria, constipation, hyper-glycemia
Severe Hyponatremia			
3% sodium (513 mmol Na/L)	Infuse 1–2 ml/kg/hour until resolu-tion of symptoms, then 0.5 ml/kg/hour.	Hours until reso-lution of clinical symptoms	Total correction should be < 10 mmol/L within 24 hours. Monitor sodium every 2–4 hours in the first 24 hours.

Note. Based on information from Pi et al., 2015.

assessed to accurately record hydration status. Signs of edema, hypertension, and hyponatremia should be monitored, and neuromuscular changes, such as changes in levels of consciousness, fatigue, and muscular weakness, should be assessed. For those with mental status changes, safety precautions should be instituted, such as bed alarms, bed in low locked position, and side rails up. Mouth care needs to be provided because decreased saliva production creates dry mouth.

Hypoglycemia

Pathophysiology

Patients with cancer can develop hypoglycemia through several pathways. Rapidly proliferating neoplasms can rapidly consume glucose. Mesenchymal tumors, such as sarcoma, gastrointestinal stromal tumor, and solitary fibrous tumor, can produce insulin-like growth factors (IGFs). IGF-2 increases glucose use by the tissues. Levels of IGF-1 have been reported in lung cancer (Lewis et al., 2011). Tumors can also infiltrate organs that function in glucose metabolism.

Signs and Symptoms

Neurologic symptoms of hypoglycemia include confusion, delirium, blurred vision, seizures, and coma. Catecholamine response to hypoglycemia can result in diaphoresis, palpitations, and dilation of the pupils.

Diagnosis

Hypoglycemia is defined as a blood glucose less than 70 mg/dl (Hammer & Voss, 2012). High insulin and C-peptide levels implicate islet cell tumors. Elevated IGF-2 to IGF-1 ratio indicates a mesenchymal tumor.

Treatment

Treatment of cancer-related hypoglycemia can include surgical removal of the tumor or chemotherapy and radiation for unresectable tumors. Glucagon administration of 1 mg IV or intramuscularly, dextrose infusion, and discontinuing nonselective beta-blockers, which blunt adrenergic response to low blood sugar, is the treatment for hypoglycemia (Storey & Von Ah, 2012).

Nursing Implications

If the patient's blood glucose is less than 70 mg/dl, give the patient 15 g of fast-acting carbohydrates, such as the following (Ballin, 2016):
- Glucose tablets
- Glucose gel tube
- ½ cup (4 oz) of juice or regular soft drink
- 1 tablespoon sugar, honey, or corn syrup
- 2 tablespoons raisins
- 8 oz of nonfat or 1% milk
- 5–6 pieces of hard candy

Once initial carbohydrate dose has been administered to the patient, proceed with the following:
1. Recheck blood sugar after 15 minutes.
2. If hypoglycemia persists, give the patient another 15 g of carbohydrates.
3. When blood glucose returns to normal, give the patient a small snack.
4. If the patient is unable to take anything by mouth, administer an amp of D50 or start a D50 IV drip.

Hyperkalemia

Pathophysiology

Hyperkalemia in the patient with cancer may be caused by acute kidney injury, rhabdomyolysis, or tumor lysis syndrome (TLS). A less common cause is adrenal insufficiency associated with metastatic disease or drugs, such as ketoconazole, metyrapone, calcineurin inhibitors in stem cell transplant patients, nonsteroidal anti-inflammatory agents, trimethoprim, and heparin (Rosner & Dalkin, 2014). Pseudohyperkalemia should be considered in any patient with marked leukocytosis and thrombocytosis, such as chronic lymphocytic leukemia, acute myelocytic leukemia, or essential thrombocytosis (Wagner & Arora, 2014). Elevated potassium levels can occur in the absence of clinical symptoms or electrocardiogram (ECG) changes. A shift of potassium out of platelets or leukocytes after a blood draw and when a blood clot has formed causes this elevation. A serum to plasma potassium gradient above 0.4 mEq/L is diagnostic of pseudohyperkalemia (Wagner & Arora, 2014).

Signs and Symptoms

Hyperkalemia in the cardiovascular system may cause bradyarrhythmias, ventricular fibrillation, and asystole. ECG changes include peaked T waves, PR interval prolongation, and QRS widening. Neurologic symptoms related to hyperkalemia include altered mental status, confusion, and paresthesia. Muscle cramps and weakness may be signs of hyperkalemia in the musculoskeletal system (Ballin, 2016).

Diagnosis

Hyperkalemia is defined as a potassium level greater than 5.5 mEq/L (Henneman, Guirguis, Grace, Patel, & Shah, 2016).

Treatment

Table 10-5 outlines the administration, dosage, onset of action, duration of effect, mechanism of action, and other variables associated with hyperkalemia treatment.

Nursing Implications

A thorough head-to-toe nursing assessment is critical to determine any physiologic changes. The nurse should assess cardiac status, frequently listening to the heart and reviewing the cardiac monitor for any dysrhythmias. Vascular perfusion should be monitored with assessment of peripheral pulses and capillary refill. A neurologic assessment should be performed for fatigue, sleepiness, altered mental status, headache, muscle weakness or cramping, and paresthesia. The respiratory system should also be assessed with breath sounds, respiratory rate and depth, and oxygen saturation levels. Vital signs and intake and output should be frequently monitored (Crawford, 2014).

Patient education should focus on limiting oral intake of potassium and protein and increasing fluid intake to promote adequate urinary output. Patients should be cautioned about salt substitutes, which are high in potassium, and taught how to read food package labels and avoid foods high in potassium (Kovesdy, 2015).

Table 10-5. Treatment of Hyperkalemia

Treatment	Dose	Route of Administration	Onset of Action	Duration of Effect	Mechanism of Action	Additional Comments
Calcium chloride or calcium gluconate	6.8 mmol of calcium = 10 ml of calcium chloride or 30 ml calcium gluconate	IV (Calcium chloride is caustic and may damage peripheral veins.)	1–3 minutes	30–60 minutes	Membrane potential stabilization	It does not affect serum potassium level. Effect is measured by normalization of electrocardiogram changes. Dose can be repeated if no effects noted. Caution is advised in patients on digoxin.
Hypertonic saline (3%–5%)	50–250 ml	IV	5–10 minutes	2 hours	Membrane potential stabilization	Efficacy is shown only in hyponatremic patients.
Sodium bicarbonate	50–100 mEq	IV or PO	5–10 minutes	2 hours	Redistribution	Efficacy in dialysis patients is questioned.
Insulin	10 units regular	IV	30 minutes	4–6 hours	Redistribution	Administer with 50 g of glucose IV to prevent hyperglycemia.
Beta-2 agonists	10–20 mg aerosol (nebulized) or 0.5 mg in 100 ml D5W IV	IV or nebulized	30 minutes	2–4 hours	Redistribution	Effect is independent of insulin and aldosterone. Practice caution in patients with coronary artery disease.

(Continued on next page)

Table 10-5. Treatment of Hyperkalemia *(Continued)*

Treatment	Dose	Route of Administration	Onset of Action	Duration of Effect	Mechanism of Action	Additional Comments
Diuretics	40 mg furosemide or equivalent dose of loop diuretic; potentially higher dose with advanced kidney disease	IV or PO	Varies with start of diuresis	Until diuresis	Excretion	Loop diuretics are given for acute intervention. Loop or thiazide diuretics are given for chronic management.
Fludrocortisone acetate	0.4–1 mg/day	PO	—	—	Excretion	In patients with aldosterone deficiency Larger doses may be needed to effectively lower potassium. Sodium retention, edema, and hypertension may occur.
Cation-exchange resins	25–50 g	PO or per rectum with or without sorbitol	1–2 hours	4–6 hours	Excretion	Sodium polystyrene sulfonate Calcium polystyrene sulfonate
Dialysis	—	Hemodialysis or peritoneal dialysis	Within minutes after starting treatment	Until end of dialysis or longer	Removal	Additional effects of serum sodium, bicarbonate, calcium, magnesium

Note. Based on information from Viera & Wouk, 2015.

Hypokalemia
Pathophysiology

The etiology of hypokalemia includes medications that can cause tubular damage, such as cisplatin, ifosfamide, amphotericin B, and aminoglycoside antibiotics. Diuretic use may contribute to hypokalemia, hyponatremia, and hypomagnesemia (Rosner & Dalkin, 2014). Patients with hypercalcemia may develop hypokalemia from the kaliuretic effect of an elevated calcium level or from diuretics. Many medications promote potassium loss, such as antibiotics with high anion content, antifungal agents, insulin, corticosteroids, diuretics, beta-agonists, and epinephrine. Hypokalemia is often associated with hypomagnesemia and difficulty weaning from mechanical ventilation (Scotto, Fridline, Menhart, & Klions, 2014). Table 10-6 details hypokalemia causes and mechanisms of action.

Signs and Symptoms

Hypokalemia affects almost every system of the body. Some symptoms may be minor, while others can be life threatening. Hypokalemia can affect the cardiovascular system by causing ECG changes. For example, U waves become prominent and T waves can be flattened or inverted. ST segment depression and T and U wave fusion can occur with the appearance of QT prolongation. Arrhythmias can also develop, including atrial tachycardia with or without block, premature ventricular contraction, ventricular tachycardia and/or fibrillation, and torsade de

Table 10-6. Hypokalemia Causes and Mechanisms of Action	
Cause	**Mechanism of Action**
Inadequate potassium intake	Poor nutrition, anorexia
Excessive gastrointestinal losses	Chemotherapy-induced vomiting Chemotherapy-induced or tumor-associated diarrhea Post-ureterosigmoid diversion
Kidney losses	Diuretics Hypercalcemia Hypomagnesemia Postobstructive diuresis Medications Lysozymuria with acute leukemia Mineralocorticoid excess Primary hyperaldosteronism due to tumor Renin-producing tumors Ectopic adrenocorticotropin syndrome Intracellular shifts Pseudohypokalemia Use of growth factors and vitamin B_{12} therapy

Note. Based on information from Viera & Wouk, 2015.

pointes, as well as severe hypertension and sudden cardiac death (Asmar, Mohandas, & Wingo, 2012).

Diagnosis

Hypokalemia is defined as a potassium level less than 3.5 mmol/L (Scotto et al., 2014).

Treatment

For mild to moderate hypokalemia (serum potassium 3–3.5 mEq/L), assess and treat any underlying disorder. Potassium chloride in divided doses of 60–80 mEq/day may be administered. Recheck the serum potassium level after replacement therapy and adjust further treatment. For severe hypokalemia (serum less potassium than 3 mEq/L), administer potassium chloride 10 mEq increments every three to four hours or IV potassium chloride 10–20 mEq every hour. Recheck serum potassium every two to four hours (Viera & Wouk, 2015).

Nursing Implications

It is important for patients with a cardiac history to maintain potassium of at least 4 mEq (Viera & Wouk, 2015). Serum glucose, magnesium, and creatinine levels should be monitored and an creatinine ECG obtained for a baseline and with any change in symptoms. Patients should be instructed on dietary supplementation.

Tumor Lysis Syndrome

Pathophysiology

TLS occurs when cancer cells release their contents into the bloodstream, causing an influx of electrolytes and nucleic acids into the body circulation. The sudden development of hyperkalemia, hyperuricemia, and hyperphosphatemia can have critical effects on the myocardium, kidneys, and central nervous system. Hypocalcemia from hyperphosphatemia is included in this metabolic disturbance (Maloney & Denno, 2011).

Signs and Symptoms

TLS is diagnosed when one or more of the following occur: acute renal failure, which is defined as a rise in creatinine to at least 1.5 times the upper limit of normal not attributed to other factors; arrhythmias, including sudden cardiac death; and seizures (Lewis et al., 2011). TLS is more common in rapidly proliferative hematologic malignancies, such as acute lymphoblastic leukemia, acute myeloid leukemia, and Burkitt lymphoma. It has also been demonstrated in solid tumors, such as small cell lung cancer, germ cell tumors, inflammatory breast cancer, and melanoma (Wagner & Arora, 2014). Liver metastases increase the risk of TLS, and it also can occur after chemotherapy, radiation, surgery, or ablation procedures. The onset of TLS can be delayed by days to weeks in a patient with a solid tumor (Lewis et al., 2011).

Diagnosis

A laboratory definition of TLS using the Cairo-Bishop Classification includes the following (Lewis et al., 2011):

- Uric acid greater than 8 mg/dl or 25% increase from baseline
- Potassium greater than 6 mEq/L or 25% increase from baseline
- Phosphorus greater than 6.5 mg/dl or 25% increase from baseline
- Calcium less than 7 mg/dl or 25% decrease from baseline

Treatment

Major metabolic issues resulting in TLS include renal insufficiency and hypovolemia, hyperuricemia, hyperphosphatemia, hyperkalemia, and hypocalcemia.

Renal insufficiency and hypovolemia can be treated with 3 L of daily normal saline. This should be used cautiously in those with congestive heart failure. Dialysis may be required for oliguric renal failure.

Hyperuricemia can be treated with allopurinol 100 mg/m^2 every eight hours to a maximum dose of 800 mg. Rasburicase 0.15–0.2 mg/kg per day IV may be used but is very costly.

Hyperphosphatemia may be treated by limiting dairy and bread products. Phosphate binders may be used, such as aluminum hydroxide or aluminum carbonate 30 ml every six hours. If no response to oral therapy occurs, dialysis may be required.

Hyperkalemia may be treated with 10 units of regular insulin by IV, dextrose 50 ml of 50% dextrose by IV, and an infusion of 50–75 ml of 10% dextrose over one hour. Nebulized albuterol 20 mg and calcium gluconate 1,000 mg IV may be given.

Hypocalcemia may be treated with 1,000 mg calcium gluconate (Lewis et al., 2011).

Nursing Implications

Hydration and administration of allopurinol and rasburicase are important preventive measures. Knowledge of normal ranges of laboratory values helps the oncology nurse assess for TLS. Renal function during treatment must be monitored. Oncology nurses need to educate patients and their caregivers on TLS prevention and treatment (Maloney & Denno, 2011).

Infectious Emergencies

Neutropenic Fever

Pathophysiology

Neutropenia is most commonly seen as an effect of cytotoxic therapy. For most outpatient chemotherapy regimens, the nadir (lowest point) in the absolute neutrophil count (ANC) occurs 5–10 days after the last dose (White & Ybarra, 2014).

Inpatient regimens, especially those used to treat hematologic malignancies, produce a more intense presentation and duration. Chemotherapy classes with the highest risk of inducing neutropenia are anthracyclines, taxanes, topoisomerase inhibitors, platinums, gemcitabine, vinorelbine, and alkylators (e.g., cyclophosphamide, ifosfamide) (Lewis et al., 2011). Gram-positive cocci are responsible for most of the culture-positive cases of neutropenic fever, including *Staphylococcus aureus, Staphylococcus epidermis, Streptococcus pneumoniae, Streptococcus pyogenes, Streptococcus viridans, Enterococcus faecalis,* and *Enterococcus faecium. Corynebacterium* is the most likely gram-positive bacillus. Gram-negative bacilli include *Escherichia coli, Klebsiella* species, and *Pseudomonas aeruginosa. Candida* is the most common fungal infection (Lewis et al., 2011).

Signs and Symptoms
Infection is responsible for half of all neutropenic fever cases. Fever is defined as a single oral temperature of 38.3°C (101°F) or temperatures of 38°C (100.4°F) or higher measured an hour apart (White & Ybarra, 2014). Skin and soft tissue infections may not be associated with erythema or induration. Abscesses will not accumulate in the absence of pus-generating neutrophils. Pulmonary infections may not result in audible or radiographically visible infiltrates.

Diagnosis
The risk of infection dramatically rises when ANC is less than 1,000/mm^3. At least 20% of patients with an ANC less than 100/mm^3 are bacteremic (Lewis et al., 2011).

Treatment
The Infectious Diseases Society of America created febrile neutropenia guidelines to define high-risk patients (White & Ybarra, 2014). High-risk patients are those with hypotension, acute abdominal pain, neurologic changes, or suspicion of pneumonia who have neutropenia anticipated to last longer than a week with an ANC of 100/mm^3 or less. These patients require hospitalization for close monitoring and IV antibiotics. Monotherapy should only be used with broad-spectrum agents, such as a fourth-generation cephalosporin, carbapenem, or piperacillin-tazobactam. Vancomycin can be added for skin infections, pneumonia, or the suspicion of an infected vascular device but should never be used as monotherapy. Antibiotic therapy should be continued until ANC is above 500/mm^3 (Wagner & Arora, 2014). The addition of antifungal coverage should be considered in high-risk patients who remain febrile after four to seven days of broad-spectrum antibiotics (Wagner & Arora, 2014).

Nursing Implications
Nurses should perform a thorough physical examination, especially with the gums, pharynx, perineum, and anus. Palpation of the maxillary and frontal sinuses and inspection of vascular access sites should also be performed.

Two sets of blood cultures should be drawn. If an intravascular device is present, one set of cultures should be obtained through it, while the others should be through each lumen of a multiport catheter.

Urinalysis and urine culture should be obtained. The lack of neutrophils may prevent the development of pyuria. A chest x-ray also should be obtained to evaluate respiratory symptoms.

Cardiovascular Emergencies

Pericardial Effusion and Cardiac Tamponade

Pathophysiology

Malignant pericardial effusions develop through direct or metastatic involvement of the pericardial sac. Tumors with sites of origin adjacent to the heart (e.g., lung and breast cancer, mediastinal lymphoma) contribute because of direct extension of the tumor. Thoracic irradiation causes effusions as well. Immunosuppression can also allow infections to develop in the pericardial space (Lewis et al., 2011).

Signs and Symptoms

Pericardial effusions can be asymptomatic. An effusion of 350 ml or larger is a poor prognostic indicator (Lewis et al., 2011). Tamponade classically presents with the Beck triad: hypotension, elevated jugular venous pressure, and a muffled precordium (West & Cannon, 2013). Most patients complain of dyspnea and chest discomfort.

Diagnosis

Tachycardia and pulsus paradoxus are present. Chest x-rays may show cardiomegaly. An ECG may show low voltage from the shifting axis of the heart as it moves like a pendulum within the fluid-filled sac. Right ventricular collapse during early diastole is indicated on the ECG (Lewis et al., 2011).

Treatment

Pericardiocentesis can be used to drain the pericardial sac. Cancer-induced pericardial effusions are more likely to recur. A pericardial window or pericardiectomy may be indicated for these patients. Decompression can produce hemodynamic instability requiring pressor support. The risk of decompensation increases with hematologic malignancies and is in direct proportion to pericardial fluid volume (West & Cannon, 2013).

Nursing Implications

Nursing care is aimed at addressing symptoms. The head of the bed should be elevated to 90°. Oxygen, IV fluids, and medications should be administered to maintain cardiac output. Pain management and energy conservation for patients are critical and should include hemodynamic and cardiac monitoring (West & Cannon, 2013).

Superior Vena Cava Syndrome

Pathophysiology

Primary or metastatic tumors can cause compression of the superior vena cava (SVC), which returns all blood from the head, neck, and upper extremities to the right atrium of the heart (Lewis et al., 2011).

Signs and Symptoms

The extent and acuity of the SVC obstruction define a patient's symptoms. Obstruction is better tolerated when collateral veins develop in the azygos and internal mammary vessels. Varicose veins may be present on the patient's chest, as well as edema in the face, arms, and periorbital area. Stridor may develop as edema narrows the luminal diameter of the pharynx and larynx. Cancers associated with SVC syndrome include lung, primary mediastinal lymphoma, breast, lymphoblastic lymphoma, thymoma, and germ cell tumors (Lewis et al., 2011).

Diagnosis

The standard for localizing obstruction is selective venography. Computed tomography (CT) and magnetic resonance imaging (MRI) are preferable because of their noninvasiveness (Lewis et al., 2011).

Treatment

Patients who have neurologic symptoms or a compromised airway need immediate treatment. Previously, all cases of SVC syndrome were considered medical emergencies. No association exists between symptom duration and long-term treatment outcomes for SVC syndrome cases using chemotherapy, radiation therapy, or stenting. Endovascular stenting can provide palliation, while chemotherapy may be the only necessary treatment in patients presenting with nonemergent symptoms (Straka et al., 2016).

Nursing Implications

Frequent assessment of the patient's airway and respiratory effort is necessary. Nasal and laryngeal edema may develop and require intubation. Neurologic function should be assessed for cerebral edema and may require medication, such as mannitol. Cerebral edema may present as headache, confusion, dizziness, obtundation, and mental status changes. Hemodynamic monitoring, including vital signs, central venous pressure, and arterial line monitoring, is used to assess for emergent versus nonemergent symptoms (Straka et al., 2016).

Neurologic Emergencies

Malignant Spinal Cord Compression

Pathophysiology

All tumor types have the potential to cause malignant spinal cord compression (MSCC). MSCC can occur as the initial cancer presentation in 5%–25% of cases and requires prompt treatment to relieve pain and preserve neurologic function (Lewis et al., 2011).

MSCC is defined as the compressive indentation, displacement, or encasement of the thecal sac that surrounds the spinal cord or cauda equina because of cancer. Metastases to vertebral bone can lead to bone weakening and vertebral collapse with displacement of the bone fragments into the epidural space. Rarely, metastases can occur directly to the spinal cord and meninges. The most common locations of MSCC are the thoracic spine and the lumbosacral area (Lewis et al., 2011).

Signs and Symptoms

Clinical presentation of MSCC can vary depending on severity, location, and duration of compression. The most common initial symptom is back pain. MSCC is often the first sign of cancer and is most common with lung cancer, multiple myeloma, and non-Hodgkin lymphoma. Once symptoms other than pain are present, progression is rapid. Motor weakness, sensory impairment, and autonomic dysfunction may develop. Cauda equina syndrome may present as urinary retention and overflow incontinence (Pi et al., 2016).

Diagnosis

The standard for MSCC diagnosis is an MRI and should include the entire thecal sac (Lewis et al., 2011).

Treatment

Glucocorticoids, surgery, and external beam radiation therapy are used to manage MSCC. Systemic therapy can be used in patients with chemotherapy-sensitive tumors. Corticosteroids are integral in initial therapy. If spinal instability is present, surgical decompression is indicated. Radiation therapy has a critical role in MSCC treatment, including in patients who have undergone surgical decompression. Radiation extends one to two vertebral bodies above and below the compression site. Therapy is usually given with 30 Gy in 10 fractions. For patients with a poor prognosis and significant pain, external beam radiation therapy with 1–2 fractions of 8 Gy can palliate without extended treatment (Lewis et al., 2011).

Nursing Implications

A thorough pain assessment should be completed, including severity, location, duration, and radiation. Neurologic assessment for motor weakness and sensory impairment should be documented. Changes in urination should be reported, such as incontinence and retention. Corticosteroids may be administered to alleviate symptoms (Scott, 2015).

Increased Intracranial Pressure

Pathophysiology

Elevated intracranial pressure (ICP) secondary to cancer can cause neurologic injury. Most intracranial tumors are metastatic. Untreated patients have a median survival of four weeks (Lewis et al., 2011).

Metastases frequently travel to the brain through the bloodstream. Tumor microemboli lodge into the distal arteries and small capillaries of the gray-white matter. Metastatic distribution follows brain blood flow, with most occurring in the cerebrum, then the cerebellum, and finally the brain stem. ICP is increased by the tumor mass effect and cerebral edema from neoplastic disruption of the blood–brain barrier caused by local production of vascular endothelial growth factor (Lewis et al., 2011).

Signs and Symptoms

Clinical presentation depends on tumor location, size, and growth. The most common symptom is a headache. The classic tumor-related headache is worse in the morning and improves throughout the day. Seizures are caused by supratentorial lesions. Strokes occur if the tumor embolizes, bleeds, or compresses an artery. Cushing response is a triad of hypertension with widened pulse pressure, bradycardia, and an irregular respiratory rate. This is a late effect and indicates impending herniation.

Diagnosis

Diagnostic tests include chemistry, complete blood count, antiepileptic drug level (if appropriate), oxygen saturation, and an MRI or CT scan. An MRI of the brain provides assessment of circulation, anatomy, and brain tumor characteristics (Lee & Armstrong, 2008).

Treatment

The goals of treatment are to determine the cause of increased ICP and to reduce it so that cranial blood flow adequately oxygenates the brain and herniation is prevented. Corticosteroids are used to reduce cerebral edema in patients with subtle signs of increased ICP. If the tumor is large with associated mass effect, surgical debulking may be required (Lewis et al., 2011).

Nursing Implications

Nursing implications include the following (Shah & Christensen, 2012):
• Use the Glasgow Coma Scale every 30 minutes to monitor, detect, and report changes in condition.

- Assess papillary response and vision.
- Elevate the head of the bed to 30° to decrease ICP by improving venous flow and reducing the risk of aspiration.
- Administer stool softeners to decrease the possibility of using the Valsalva maneuver, which may increase ICP.
- Assess for neurogenic pulmonary edema (oxygen saturation less than 95%), tachypnea, crepitus on auscultation, use of respiratory accessory muscles, cyanosis, and pink frothy sputum.
- Monitor for bradycardia, widening pulse pressure, and irregular breathing indicative of the Cushing triad.
- Monitor mean arterial pressure instead of systolic blood pressure. Adequate cerebral perfusion should be greater than 70 mm Hg.
- Monitor for signs of vasospasm, such as agitation and worsening level of consciousness.

Hematologic Emergency: Hyperviscosity Syndrome

Pathophysiology

Increased blood viscosity can result from elevated cellular components seen in hyperproliferative states, such as leukemia and multiple myeloma. These cancers are characterized by clonal proliferation of plasma cells and the production of monoclonal proteins, known as paraproteins. Hyperviscosity syndrome (HVS) is the result of impaired blood flow in the microvasculature (Kwaan, 2013).

Signs and Symptoms

Symptoms for HVS are detailed in Figure 10-1.

Diagnosis

HVS is present when viscosity levels reach 4–5 centipose (cP) when the normal level is 1.4–1.8 cP (Mullen & Mendez, 2008). The presence of M protein and immunoglobulins A, D, and G should be assessed.

Treatment

Symptomatic HVS requires aggressive IV hydration and plasmapheresis to reduce the blood protein concentration. Plasmapheresis reduces the viscosity of the blood by reducing the immunoglobulin concentration. The long-term management of HVS is achieved by control of the underlying disease (Mullen & Mendez, 2008).

Figure 10-1. The Clinical Spectrum for Symptomatology in Hyperviscosity Syndrome

Mild Impaired Microcirculation
• Neurologic: Headache, dizziness, impaired mentation up to coma
• Visual: Blurring up to blindness
• Pulmonary: Shortness of breath

Severe Thromboembolic Events
• Central nervous system: Transient ischemic attacks up to stroke
• Heart: Myocardial ischemia up to acute myocardial infarction

Peripheral Arterial Occlusion
• Venous thromboembolism: Often unusual sites
• Budd-Chiari syndrome

Pulmonary Embolism
• Bleeding complications: Impaired hemostatic function

Note. Based on information from Kwaan, 2013.

Nursing Implications

After stabilization of the patient, the role of the nurse is support and education. Nurses should facilitate patient discussions regarding treatment options with the hematologist. Patients should be educated on how to manage symptoms during treatment. Patients with multiple myeloma need close monitoring of paraprotein, immunoglobulin, chemistry, and complete blood count levels (Mullen & Mendez, 2008).

Summary

Oncologic emergencies are a series of critical conditions that can affect a patient with cancer at any point after diagnosis, including years after treatment. A complete oncologic history of the patient may key the critical care oncology nurse into identifying and treating the conditions discussed in this chapter. The goal of treatment is to improve quality of life and overall survival.

References

Abu Zeinah, G.F., Al-Kindi, S.G., Hassan, A.A., & Allam, A. (2015). Hyponatremia in cancer: Association with type of cancer and mortality. *European Journal of Cancer Care, 24,* 224–231. doi:10.1111/ecc.12187

Asmar, A., Mohandas, R., & Wingo, C.S. (2012). A physiologic-based approach to the treatment of a patient with hypokalemia. *American Journal of Kidney Diseases, 60,* 492–497. doi:10.1053/j.ajkd .2012.01.031

Ballin, M.C. (2016). Hypoglycemia: A serious complication for the older adult with diabetes. *American Journal of Nursing, 116*(2), 34–39. doi:10.1097/01.NAJ.0000480493.33351.97

Crawford, A.H. (2014). Hyperkalemia: Recognition and management of a critical electrolyte disturbance. *Journal of Infusion Nursing, 37,* 167–175. doi:10.1097/NAN.0000000000000036

De las Peñas, R., Ponce, S., Henao, F., Herrero, C.C., Carcereny, E., Álvarez, Y., ... López, R.L. (2016). SIADH-related hyponatremia in hospital day care units: Clinical experience and management with tolvaptan. *Supportive Care in Cancer, 24,* 499–507. doi:10.1007/s00520-015-2948 -6

Hammer, M.J., & Voss, J.G. (2012). Malglycemia and cancer: Introduction to a conceptual model [Online exclusive]. *Oncology Nursing Forum, 39,* E275–E287. doi:10.1188/12.ONF.E275-E287

Henneman, A., Guirguis, E., Grace, Y., Patel, D., & Shah, B. (2016). Emerging therapies for the management of chronic hyperkalemia in the ambulatory care setting. *American Journal of Health-System Pharmacy, 73,* 33–44. doi:10.2146/ajhp150457

Keane, M. (2014). Recognising and managing acute hyponatraemia. *Emergency Nurse, 21*(9), 32–36. doi:10.7748/en2014.02.21.9.32.e1128

Kovesdy, C.P. (2015). Management of hyperkalemia: An update for the internist. *American Journal of Medicine, 128,* 1281–1287. doi:10.1016/j.amjmed.2015.05.040

Kwaan, H.C. (2013). Hyperviscosity in plasma cell dyscrasias. *Clinical Hemorheology and Microcirculation, 55,* 75–83. doi:10.3233/CH-131691

Lee, E.L.T., & Armstrong, T.S. (2008). Increased intracranial pressure. *Clinical Journal of Oncology Nursing, 12,* 37–41. doi:10.1188/08.CJON.37-41

Lewis, M.A., Hendrickson, A.W., & Moynihan, T.J. (2011). Oncologic emergencies: Pathophysiology, presentation, diagnosis, and treatment. *Cancer, 64,* 287–314. doi:10.3322/caac.20124

Maloney, K., & Denno, M. (2011). Tumor lysis syndrome: Prevention and detection to enhance patient safety. *Clinical Journal of Oncology Nursing, 15,* 601–603. doi:10.1188/11.CJON.601-603

Mullen, E., & Mendez, N. (2008). Hyperviscosity syndrome in patients with multiple myeloma. *Oncology Nursing Forum, 35,* 350–352. doi:10.1188/08.ONF.350-352

Pi, J., Kang, Y., Smith, M., Earl, M., Norigian, Z., & McBride, A. (2015). A review in the treatment of oncologic emergencies. *Journal of Oncology Pharmacy Practice, 22,* 1–14. doi:10.1177 /1078155215605661

Rosner, M.H., & Dalkin, A.C. (2014). Electrolyte disorders associated with cancer. *Advances in Chronic Kidney Disease, 21,* 7–17. doi:10.1053/j.ackd.2013.05.005

Scott, B.J. (2015). Neuro-oncologic emergencies. *Seminars in Neurology, 35,* 675–682. doi:10.1055 /s-0035-1564684

Scotto, C.J., Fridline, M., Menhart, C.J., & Klions, H.A. (2014). Prevention hypokalemia in critically ill patients. *American Journal of Critical Care, 23,* 145–149. doi:10.4037/ajcc2014946

Shah, L., & Christensen, M. (2012). Ineffective cerebral perfusion related to increased intracranial pressure secondary to subarachnoid haemorrhage: An examination of nursing interventions. *Singapore Nursing Journal, 39,* 15–24.

Storey, S., & Von Ah, D. (2012). Impact of malglycemia on clinical outcomes in hospitalized patients with cancer: A review of the literature. *Oncology Nursing Forum, 39,* 458–465. doi:10.1188/12 .ONF.458-465

Straka, C., Ying, J., Kong, F.-M., Willey, C.D., Kaminski, J., & Nathan Kim, D.W. (2016). Review of evolving etiologies, implications and treatment strategies for the superior vena cava syndrome. *Springer Plus, 5,* 1–13. doi:10.1186/s40064-016-1900-7

Viera, A.J., & Wouk, N. (2015). Potassium disorders: Hypokalemia and hyperkalemia. *American Family Physician, 92,* 487–495.

Wagner, J., & Arora, S. (2014). Oncologic metabolic emergencies. *Emergency Medicine Clinics of North America, 32,* 509–525. doi:10.1016/j.emc.2014.04.003

West, P.J., & Cannon, M. (2013). Heartaches: Malignant pericardial effusions. *Oncology Nursing Forum, 40*, 315–317. doi:10.1188/13.ONF.315-317

White, L., & Ybarra, M. (2014). Neutropenic fever. *Emergency Medicine Clinics of North America, 32*, 549–561. doi:10.1016/j.emc.2014.04.002

CHAPTER 11

Respiratory Failure

Cindy Byrd, DNP, RN, ACNP-BC,
and Lisa Koser, DNP, RN, ACNP-BC, CPNP-AC

Introduction

Respiratory failure is one of the leading causes of admission to the intensive care unit (ICU) and occurs when the body is unable to maintain oxygenation and/or ventilation (Barjaktarevic & Wang, 2017). Failure occurs in one or both main functions of the respiratory system, either oxygenation (hypoxic respiratory failure) or elimination of carbon dioxide (hypercarbic respiratory failure). The lungs' primary function is gas exchange, including the transport of oxygen from inspired air to the circulating blood for oxygenation and elimination of carbon dioxide (Barjaktarevic & Wang, 2017).

The respiratory system can be divided into two equally important parts: the lungs, which act as a balloon by expanding and contracting with each breath, and the airways, or pipes, which act as the tunnels for transportation of inspired air. Respiratory failure results from alterations or other forces that impede the function of this system. For example, a patient with hepatic failure with a large amount of ascites may develop respiratory failure from increased intra-abdominal pressure, which affects intrathoracic pressure and results in decreased ventilation and/or perfusion.

Causes of Respiratory Failure

Type 1—Hypoxic Respiratory Failure

Patients with type 1 respiratory failure present with a low arterial partial pressure of oxygen (PaO_2). Hypoxic respiratory failure is categorized as PaO_2 less than

60 mm Hg on an arterial blood gas (ABG) test and will frequently have a normal or low partial pressure of carbon dioxide ($PaCO_2$). Multiple causes of hypoxic respiratory failure exist and are often classified by the origin of inciting factors. The most common causes are ventilation/perfusion mismatch and intrapulmonary shunting (Krüger & Ludman, 2014).

Ventilation/perfusion mismatch describes the perfusion of oxygen and carbon dioxide across the alveolar–capillary border. The differences in these two gases must be maintained by the ventilation of the alveoli and the perfusion of the pulmonary capillaries (Levitzky, 2013). An alteration in this regulation causes a mismatch, impairing exchange of oxygen and causing hypoxia. An example of ventilation/perfusion mismatch is when a patient has pneumonia. Fluid is in the alveoli from infection, prohibiting the diffusion of oxygen across the alveolar membrane.

Intrapulmonary shunting describes an extreme form of ventilation/perfusion mismatch. Usually, adequate perfusion exists, but areas of lung tissue are not ventilated. Shunting occurs because of alveolar hypoventilation, alveolar collapse, or flooding caused by infection, blood, or fluid (Krüger & Ludman, 2014). Patients often have hypoxia with elevated $PaCO_2$. Examples of ventilation/perfusion mismatch include the following:

- Acute asthma
- Acute respiratory distress syndrome (ARDS)
- Chronic obstructive pulmonary disease (COPD)
- Pneumonia
- Pulmonary edema
- Pulmonary embolism
- Pulmonary fibrosis

Type 2—Hypercarbic Respiratory Failure

Patients with type 2 respiratory failure present with hypoxia (PaO_2 less than 60 mm Hg) and hypercapnia, which is a $PaCO_2$ greater than 50 mm Hg that occurs because of the body's inability to excrete carbon dioxide (CO_2), leading to systemic disturbances (Gurka & Balk, 2014). The most common causes of type 2 respiratory failure are often classified by the underlying disease process (e.g., acute asthma, COPD).

Hypercarbic respiratory failure is caused by decreased alveolar ventilation and minute ventilation, as related to demand and increased dead space ventilation. Minute ventilation is the amount of gas inhaled or exhaled from a person's lungs in one minute (V [minute ventilation] = Vt [tidal volume] × f [respiratory rate]) (Gurka & Balk, 2014). Dead space ventilation describes the ventilated portions of the respiratory tract not perfused by pulmonary circulation (Levitzky, 2013).

Hypoventilation is described as slow, shallow breathing that cannot adequately meet the body's metabolic demands (Wagner, Powell, & West, 2010). It is common in the following (Fayyaz & Lessnau, 2016):

- Chest wall deformities (e.g., kyphoscoliosis, fibrothorax, post-thoracoplasty procedures)
- Decreased neurologic states (e.g., traumatic brain injury, stroke, metabolic encephalopathy, coma)
- Neuromuscular disorders (e.g., Guillain-Barré syndrome, myasthenia gravis, amyotrophic lateral sclerosis)
- Obesity (e.g., hypoventilation syndrome)
- Opioid overdose (decreased respiratory drive)

Type 3 and Type 4 Respiratory Failure

Two additional classifications of respiratory failure include type 3 perioperative respiratory failure and type 4 respiratory failure in the setting of shock (Krüger & Ludman, 2014). Perioperative respiratory failure is seen after surgery, and the principal alteration in this type is caused by decreased functional residual capacity (FRC) from anesthesia. FRC is the volume of air present in the lungs after passive expiration (Johnson & Abraham, 2015). A low FRC leads to increased atelectasis, often resulting in type 1 or 2 respiratory failure. Type 3 respiratory failure is attributed to upper abdominal incisions, airway secretions, supine positioning, obesity, and ascites (Krüger & Ludman, 2014).

Type 4 respiratory failure is caused by decreased perfusion to organs seen in states of shock. Shock is a state of increased oxygen demand and/or a compromised ability to deliver oxygen to tissues, potentially leading to acute respiratory failure (ARF) (Krüger & Ludman, 2014). Patients with type 4 respiratory failure are electively intubated and ventilated as part of treatment for shock. The goal of ventilation is to stabilize gas exchange and lower oxygen consumption.

Clinical Manifestations

Clinical manifestations of respiratory failure vary based on type, underlying medical conditions, and etiology. Respiratory failure can be avoided with early recognition and treatment of the underlying cause. The bedside clinician may note subtle changes in a patient's condition that can prompt further investigation into potentially reversible causes.

Dyspnea is often the presenting symptom associated with respiratory failure and may be manifested as an increased respiratory rate, increased use of accessory muscles, inability to carry on a conversation, or as a late sign of altered mental status.

Diagnostic Studies

An initial diagnostic evaluation for ARF should begin with a detailed history and physical examination. Understanding the events leading up to the evaluation allows the clinician to begin a focused workup, which most often begins with a chest x-ray. An interpreter can comment on any bony abnormalities (e.g., rib fractures, chest wall deformities), lobar collapse, pneumothorax, pneumonia, pulmonary edema, ARDS, and COPD. A chest x-ray can reveal gross abnormalities; however, this method frequently falls behind a patient's clinical presentation and thus should not be used as a sole diagnostic tool.

A pulse oximeter provides continuous, noninvasive measurements of respiratory status. It uses the principles of Beer's Law and Lambert's Law by differing the absorption of light by the hemoglobin to measure concentration (Lee, 2016). The pulse oximeter can calculate blood oxygen saturation levels (SpO_2) at a rate of 25–30 times per second (Lee, 2016).

Pulse oximetry can have decreased reliability in patients with poor perfusion, such as patients on multiple vasopressors for shock caused by hypotension. Other factors that can affect accuracy include nail polish, abnormal hemoglobin, dyes (methylene blue and indocyanine green absorb), and pulsatile veins, as seen in tricuspid regurgitation and venous congestion (Lee, 2016).

Capnography and end-tidal CO_2 ($ETCO_2$) monitoring measure expired CO_2 levels. This technology allows for continuous CO_2 tracing, can help detect periods of apnea as demonstrated by an elevated CO_2, and may help decipher subtle respiratory changes. The use of waveform capnography in nonintubated patients and $ETCO_2$ in intubated patients can help decrease the number of ABG draws and provide alternative ways to monitor respiratory status. A change in $ETCO_2$ can indicate a change in CO_2 production, minute ventilation, or dead space ventilation. Some metabolic examples of increased CO_2 production are hyperthermia, total parenteral nutrition, malignant hyperthermia, thyrotoxicosis, and bicarbonate infusion (Lee, 2016). Examples of decreased CO_2 production include hypothermia and sedation.

An ABG test can give the clinician a good understanding of the patient's overall clinical status, including information on pH, PaO_2, and bicarbonate levels. These numbers play an integral role in the clinician's determination of the best action for patients with ARF. For example, a severe respiratory acidosis revealed on an ABG test is the result of profound hypercarbia and may facilitate earlier interventions. This situation may have gone unrecognized without an ABG.

Radiologic testing should be dictated based on a thorough history and physical examination of the patient. A computed tomography (CT) scan of the chest with IV dye may be indicated in a patient with a suspected pulmonary issue. A CT of the chest without contrast may be indicated if pneumonia is suspected. A bedside echocardiogram may be indicated if the origin of respiratory distress is thought to be cardiac in nature. This can determine cardiac output as well as global function of the heart. Patients with declining respiratory status should not be sent off the floor to radiology for diagnostic testing until definitive treatment of their respiratory status is completed.

Noninvasive Ventilation in Acute Respiratory Failure

Noninvasive ventilation describes the delivery of positive-pressure ventilation without the use of an endotracheal tube (ETT) or invasive airway. Positive-pressure ventilation can be further divided into continuous positive airway pressure (CPAP) and noninvasive positive-pressure ventilation (NIPPV). CPAP does not provide active assistance but a constant positive airway pressure throughout inspiration and expiration. NIPPV, also known as biphasic positive airway pressure, provides inspiratory positive airway pressure, positive end-expiratory pressure (PEEP), or exploratory positive airway pressure (Nava & Hill, 2009).

Noninvasive ventilation can be used in patients with ARF to prevent muscle fatigue by reducing inspiratory respiratory workload and thus possibly avoiding intubation. The use of inspiratory positive pressure assists with lung inflation by increasing alveolar inflation and ventilation, resulting in an increase in tidal volume with each breath. Increasing tidal volume improves oxygenation, decreases the work of breathing, and reverses acidosis by improving carbon dioxide elimination (Hill, Brennan, Garpestad, & Nava, 2007). Noninvasive ventilation can also help decrease cardiac workload by reducing preload and afterload secondary to increased intrathoracic pressure caused by positive-pressure ventilation (Hill et al., 2007).

Indications and Contraindications

Indications for NIPPV use in ARF include hypoxia and hypercapnic respiratory failure. The most common causes of these failures are pneumonia, COPD exacerbation, acute asthma exacerbation, congestive heart failure exacerbation, and neuromuscular disorders. Patients who often benefit from NIPPV use include those who have been weaned from invasive ventilation but still require some support prior to standard oxygen therapy (Agarwal, Aggarwal, Gupta, & Jindal, 2007).

Absolute contraindications include the inability of the patient to initiate breaths, including patients in cardiopulmonary and respiratory arrest or those too physically weak. Other relative contraindications include medical instability, uncooperative or agitated mood, unresponsive behavior, inability to protect airway or clear own secretions, and recent upper gastrointestinal surgery with an anastomosis (Nava & Hill, 2009).

Equipment

NIPPV requires that the patient have a mask (e.g., helmet device, full face, partial, nasal) with a good seal to deliver positive pressure. The mask is connected with tubing to a device that can deliver positive pressure and oxygen.

Monitoring

All patients with ARF should be placed on cardiopulmonary monitoring prior to initiation of therapy, including pulse oximetry and possibly $ETCO_2$ monitoring. Patients who experience claustrophobia often do not tolerate positive-pressure ventilation and require support and encouragement. Intolerance can lead to agitation and uncoordinated breathing between the patient and device. Increased intrathoracic pressures caused by positive pressure can cause complications such as hemodynamic instability and pneumothoraces. Vomiting or inability to control secretions put patients at risk for aspiration and possible development of pneumonia or pneumonitis.

Patient tolerance of noninvasive ventilation should be closely monitored. Successful initiation often requires explanation of the procedure as well as strategies to enhance tolerance. Patients often already have anxiety from shortness of breath with an increased work of breathing. Securing a mask on an already anxious patient only increases this anxiety. To improve patient tolerance, the mask should be slowly secured to the patient's face over several minutes. It can initially be held close to the patient's face, allowing the patient to experience the force of air. The mask can be moved closer to the face with each breath until the patient is able to tolerate it with a good seal.

ABG is often obtained at baseline prior to initiation of positive-pressure ventilation and within the first few hours to assess treatment effectiveness. Frequent cardiopulmonary and neurologic assessment is necessary to detect intolerance or worsening respiratory failure. Failure of noninvasive ventilation is often detected within the first few hours of treatment initiation. Manifestations of therapy failure include unchanged or worsening cardiopulmonary or neurologic assessment or ABG results.

Endotracheal Intubation

Indications

Endotracheal intubation, often referred to as intubation, is indicated in patients with inadequate oxygenation or ventilation who have failed conservative management. An ETT is placed into the trachea, allowing for improved oxygenation and ventilation. Indications include the need for general anesthesia, airway obstruction, multisystem organ dysfunction in critically ill patients, failure to protect own airway, and inadequate oxygenation or ventilation (Joynt & Choi, 2014).

Contraindications

Few contraindications for endotracheal intubation exist and are often limited to very high upper airway injuries or obstructions that make the passage of the ETT impossible or worsen the injury. These patients would require the use of a surgical airway, including tracheostomy or cricothyrotomy, based on condition and provider.

Equipment and Preparation

Prior to the intubation procedure, the patient, equipment, and provider must be prepared. Providers must have extensive knowledge of the procedure, including any possible complications and their treatment options. About half of the patients undergoing intubation will experience a complication (Jaber et al., 2006).

A critical step prior to performing orotracheal intubation is to gather appropriate equipment, including gloves, a face mask with eye shield, suction with suction catheter and supplies, a bag-valve mask attached to oxygen, a laryngoscope with functioning light and blades, the anticipated size of the ETT (e.g., half-size smaller, stylet, holder or tape), a 10 ml syringe, an $ETCO_2$ monitor or detector, a stethoscope, a ventilator with circuit, and medications for intubation, emergencies, and sedation after the procedure.

Two primary types of laryngoscope blades are used for direct laryngoscopy: the Macintosh and Miller blades. The Macintosh blade is curved and fits in the vallecula, indirectly lifting the epiglottis. The Miller blade is straight and directly lifts the epiglottis. Both blades come in variable sizes, ranging from 00 to 4. The choice and size of the blade depend on patient anatomy, provider expertise, and personal preference.

ETTs come in a variety of sizes and are chosen based on patient size and condition. Tube size is based on internal diameter and ranges from 2 to 10 mm with a length of up to 30 cm. The most common adult sizes include 7, 7.5, or 8 mm. Each ETT has visual markings every centimeter on the outside of the tube that measure from that point to the distal end. These markings assist in depth of ETT placement. Adult patient tube depth most commonly ranges from 20 cm to 25 cm.

ETTs can have a cuff at the distal end of the tube or be uncuffed. Cuffed tubes are most appropriate for adult patients and are either high or low volume. These cuffs create a seal between the ETT and the tissue in the trachea. After insertion, this cuff will need to be inflated to prevent leakage of air or aspiration of gastric contents during ventilation (Sole et al., 2009). ETT cuffs are commonly inflated to and maintained at 20–30 cm H_2O. Cuffs inflated to less than 20 cm H_2O can create an increased risk of aspiration secondary to leakage of gastric content into the lungs, causing ventilator-associated pneumonia (Sole et al., 2009). Conversely, if cuff pressures are high, tracheal wall damage and surrounding tissue damage can occur and cause further complications (Sole et al., 2009). The cuff does not secure the tube in place. Below the cuff at the distal end of the tube is a small oval, or Murphy eye, which provides an opening if the distal end of the ETT is occluded (Davies, 2001).

Equipment must be checked prior to the procedure to ensure that all items are functioning correctly and prepared for use. Suction must be connected and provide adequate power. The laryngoscope blade light must be bright and secured. Each ETT balloon should be tested by inflating the cuff to check for leaks and deflating. The stylet should be placed in the ETT to ensure that it is the correct length. The ETT should then be shaped like a hockey puck to facilitate placement into the airway.

The patient should also be prepared for the procedure. Functioning vascular access should be obtained for medication administration and potential complications. The patient should be placed on a cardiopulmonary monitor, including pulse oximetry. If not contraindicated, the patient should be positioned so their ears are level with the sternum. This is typically accomplished by raising the head of the bed to the correct position. The patient should then be placed in the "sniffing position" by placing a small pillow or towel roll under the occiput. These maneuvers align the axes of the oral cavity, pharynx, and larynx to provide optimal visualization of the airway.

The patient should be preoxygenated with 100% oxygen for at least three minutes prior to the procedure via nonrebreather or bag-valve-mask ventilation. This increases the time from apnea to desaturations and decreases the need for positive-pressure ventilation, reducing the risk of gastric content aspiration. All oral devices should be removed just prior to medication administration, including dentures or bridges; however, if positive-pressure ventilation is needed, reinserting dentures may facilitate a good seal during bag-valve-mask ventilation.

Endotracheal Intubation Medications

Patients will often require medications for intubation procedures, including analgesia, sedation, and neuromuscular blockade. Medication-assisted intubation allows for improved patient comfort, amnesia to the event, and improved visualization of the vocal cords. Medications should also be available for postprocedure sedation and analgesia.

Prior to medication administration, the provider should assess for predictors of difficult intubation, including a history of difficult intubation, inability to freely move the neck secondary to suspected or known trauma or medical conditions, micrognathia, limited opening of the mouth, and anything causing anatomic distortion. If the patient is suspected or known to be a difficult intubation, the provider should have a backup plan.

Endotracheal Intubation Procedure

As previously mentioned, the patient should be in the optimal position prior to medication administration. The person intubating will be positioned at the head of the bed. Intubation can begin after ensuring that equipment is ready and the patient has been given the prescribed medication regimen with effect.

A laryngoscope is designed to fit in the left hand, as the mouth is opened with the right hand with a scissor-type motion. The laryngoscope is then gently placed into the middle to right side of the mouth, displacing the tongue to the left. The blade is gently advanced to locate the epiglottis. Optimal placement of the laryngoscope is determined based on blade selection. The laryngo-scope is then lifted upward and forward at about a 45° angle, being careful to not hit the teeth and cause dental injury. This angle should allow for vocal cord visualization.

Once visualization is obtained, the ETT should then be placed in the right hand and inserted into the right side of the mouth without losing visualization. The ETT should be gently advanced between the vocal cords until the appropriate cord marker is at the level of the vocal cords, ensuring the balloon is a few centi-meters past the vocal cords. Once the ETT is in the proper place, the stylet should be removed and the balloon inflated with enough air to create a seal with the sur-rounding tissue. This is usually approximately 10 ml in adults. Proper ETT place-ment should be confirmed by a primary and secondary evaluation.

Complications during this procedure include hypoxia, hypercapnia, laryngo-spasm, and bronchospasms. Patients can also have vomiting with possible aspira-tions of the gastric contents, causing pneumonia or pneumonitis. Manipulations of the mouth and airway with the laryngoscope can cause traumatic injury to the teeth and surrounding structures.

Endotracheal Tube Confirmation

After placement of the ETT, a manual resuscitation bag can be used to provide manual ventilations. Initial primary ETT placement should be with an $ETCO_2$ detector or monitor, placing the connector between the ETT and resuscitation bag (Nolan et al., 2015). CO_2 can be adequately detected after six breaths. Patients in cardiopulmonary arrest do not produce CO_2 without optimal chest compres-sions, making this method unreliable in some instances; a secondary method should be used.

Secondary methods for ETT confirmation include physical examination and chest x-ray. A stethoscope should be used to first listen over the gastric area. If no sounds are noted with ventilations, listen over both lung fields for equal and bilat-eral breath sounds (Sitzwohl et al., 2010). If breath sounds are diminished on one side, typically the left, the ETT may be positioned in the right mainstem bron-chus. If this is suspected, the ETT can be slowly withdrawn until equal bilateral breath sounds are noted. The ETT is then secured.

Once the patient can be ventilated and bilateral breath sounds are noted, a chest x-ray should be obtained to confirm proper placement. The ETTs contain a radiopaque line that will be visible on chest x-ray. ETT in adults patient most commonly ranges between 20–25 cm. A chest x-ray can be obtained to confirm proper placement. On the chest x-ray, the ETT tip should be approximately 3–5 cm above the carina.

After initial and secondary ETT placement confirmation, the tube should be secured to prevent displacement. Many commercial devices are available and spe-cifically created for adult ETTs. Tape also can be used (Gardner et al., 2005). Lung sounds must be assessed anytime the ETT is manipulated or moved to ensure proper placement. ETT displacement is one of the most serious complications of the procedure and must be rapidly recognized to prevent further complications.

Mechanical Ventilation

Once the patient has been intubated, the next decision concern is determining the type of ventilation. New technology in ventilators has led to complex modes of ventilation. A ventilator is designed to assist respirations or to fully augment respirations (Chatburn & Mireles-Cabodevila, 2016). Different variables must be decided once a patient is placed on a ventilator, including mode of ventilation, respiratory rate, tidal volume, PEEP, and percentage of delivered fraction of inspired oxygen (FiO$_2$).

Modes of Ventilation

Mode refers to the method in which breaths are triggered, cycled, and limited (Celli, 2017). *Trigger* is either the inspiratory effort or a time-based signal, which determines what the ventilator senses to begin a breath. *Cycle* refers to the factors that determine the end of inspiration. For example, in volume-cycled ventilation, inspiration ends when a target volume is delivered (Celli, 2017).

Assist-Control Mode Ventilation

This mode of ventilation is initiated by the patient's inspiratory effort or, if no effort exists, delivers a breath within a specified time. The provider designates the respiratory rate and the tidal volume in this mode, and these parameters are guaranteed to be delivered. The tidal volume of each breath is the same regardless of whether it is a patient-triggered breath or a ventilator-delivered breath (Celli, 2017). Difficulties can occur when patients are tachypneic or awake and are dyssynchronous with the ventilator.

Synchronized Intermittent Mechanical Ventilation

The primary difference between synchronized intermittent mechanical ventilation (SIMV) and assist-control mode ventilation is that the former allows the patient to breathe spontaneously between delivered breaths. A rate and tidal volume are set in this mode as well. Mandatory breaths are delivered in synchrony with the patient's respiratory effort. SIMV allows patients with intact respiratory drive to exercise their respiratory muscles while on mechanical ventilation (Celli, 2017).

Spontaneous Ventilation

Spontaneous modes of ventilation include pressure support ventilation (PSV) and pressure control ventilation (PCV). PSV is a patient-triggered mode in which the patient initiates a breath and the ventilator determines how much support is needed based on effort (Celli, 2017). This mode requires careful attention by staff to ensure that adequate ventilation is being maintained, as rate and tidal volume are variable (i.e., ensuring that minute ventilation is adequate). This mode is often used when weaning patients from mechanical ventilation.

PCV is a time-triggered mode with multiple variables. During the inspiration phase, a specific pressure is imposed at the opening of inspiration (Celli, 2017). Providers and staff must ensure minute ventilation and tidal volume are adequate. This mode is also used to wean patients from mechanical ventilation. See Table 11-1 for terms associated with mechanical ventilation.

Weaning From Mechanical Ventilation

The decision to liberate patients from mechanical ventilation should be assessed daily by the critical care team. Mechanical ventilation places a patient at increased risk for complications such as ventilator-associated pneumonia; therefore, the patient should be extubated as soon as possible.

The weaning process comprises three diagnostic tests performed in sequence: measurement of parameters, a weaning trial, and a trial of extubation (Tobin, 2016). Each critical care group will perform these functions differently, but the premise is always the same. Objective measures of a patient's ability to be liberated from mechanical ventilation and clinical judgment are useful tools to determine successful extubation.

Prior to extubation, a respiratory therapist can ascertain the rapid shallow breathing index and negative inspiratory force and combine these with the clinical examination. Once these parameters have been obtained, patients are often placed on a spontaneous breathing trial (SBT). SBTs should be conducted with

Term	Definition	Normal Value
Table 11-1. Terms Associated With Mechanical Ventilation		
Peak airway pressure	The highest level of pressure applied to the lungs during inhalation; increases with airway resistance	< 40 cm H_2O
Plateau pressure	The pressure applied to small airways and alveoli measured during inspiration	< 30 cm H_2O
Positive end-expiratory pressure	Helps to prevent alveolar derecruitment and with oxygenation	5–10 cm H_2O
Tidal volume	The amount of air that enters the lung during inhalation	6–8 ml/kg ideal body weight

Note. Based on information from Krüger & Ludman, 2014.

inspiratory pressure augmentation (5–8 cm H_2O) (Schmidt et al., 2017). SBT comprises placing the patient on spontaneous ventilation with inspiratory pressure augmentation. The period varies from institution to institution but is approximately one hour in duration. A determination for extubation should be based on the patient's respiratory rate, oxygen saturation, and overall status as well as on input from each team member. Although an optimal rate of reintubation has not been clearly outlined, studies have documented rates at approximately 5%–15% (Johnson & Abraham, 2015). Higher reintubation rates may be reflective of weaning that is too aggressive, and rates lower than 5% may not be aggressive enough.

Extubation and critical care are best completed by an interprofessional team because of the knowledge and quality of care such a team possesses. For example, the respiratory therapist can provide important information surrounding current ventilator support and potential barriers, and the nurse can advocate for the patient and disclose concerns to the team. See Table 11-2 for considerations for extubation/liberation from mechanical ventilation.

Table 11-2. Considerations for Extubation/Liberation From Mechanical Ventilation		
Considerations for Extubation	Definition	Reference Range
Respiratory rate (RR)	Number of breaths per minute	< 30 respirations per minute
Negative inspiratory force	Measurement of respiratory muscle strength and respiratory reserve	−20 to −30 cm H_2O
Rapid shallow breathing index	RR/tidal volume (liters)	< 105 respirations per minute
Vital capacity	The amount of gas expelled by a patient after maximal inhalation	4–6 ml/kg
Secretions	Amount of secretions suctioned from patient	Minimal
Resolution of cause of initial respiratory failure	Treatment of cause (i.e., pneumonia treated, pulmonary embolism treated)	–
Hemodynamic status	Stability of blood pressure and vasopressor usage	Vasopressor requirements stable and not escalating

Note. Based on information from Johnson & Abraham, 2015.

Summary

Respiratory failure requiring mechanical ventilation is one of the leading causes of admission to the ICU. Understanding invasive and noninvasive methods of respiratory support is important in treating these patients. The critical care oncology nurse should be versed on the different modes of mechanical ventilation and how to wean patients off ventilation. Aggressive pulmonary toileting is very important in the management of these patients.

References

Agarwal, R., Aggarwal, A.N., Gupta, D., & Jindal, S.K. (2007). Role of noninvasive positive-pressure ventilation in postextubation respiratory failure: A meta-analysis. *Respiratory Care, 52,* 1472–1479.

Barjaktarevic, I., & Wang, T. (2017). Acute respiratory failure. In J.-L. Vincent, E. Abraham, P. Kochanek, F.A. Moore, & M.P. Fink (Eds.), *Textbook of critical care* (7th ed., pp. 33–37). Philadelphia, PA: Elsevier Saunders.

Celli, B.R. (2017). Mechanical ventilatory support. In J. Loscalzo (Ed.), *Harrison's pulmonary and critical care medicine* (3rd ed., pp. 294–300). New York, NY: McGraw-Hill Education.

Chatburn, R.L., & Mireles-Cabodevila, E. (2016). Design and function of mechanical ventilators. In A. Webb, D. Angus, S. Finfer, L. Gattinoni, & M. Singer (Eds.), *Oxford textbook of critical care* (2nd ed., pp. 419–429). doi:10.1093/med/9780199600830.003.0092

Davies, R.G. (2001). The importance of a Murphy Eye. *Anesthesia, 56,* 906–924. doi:10.1046/j.1365-2044.2001.02230-16.x

Fayyaz, J., & Lessnau, K.-D. (2016, September 26). Hypoventilation syndromes. Retrieved from http://emedicine.medscape.com/article/304381-overview

Gardner, A., Hughes, D., Cook, R., Henson, R., Osborne, S., & Gardner, G. (2005). Best practice in stabilisation of oral endotracheal tubes: A systematic review. *Australian Critical Care, 18,* 158–165. doi:10.1016/S1036-7314(05)80029-3

Gurka, D.P., & Balk, R.A. (2014). Acute respiratory failure. In J.E. Parrillo & R.P. Dellinger (Eds.), *Critical care medicine: Principles of diagnosis and management in the adult* (4th ed., pp. 629–644). St. Louis, MO: Elsevier Saunders.

Hill, N., Brennan, J., Garpestad, E., & Nava, S. (2007). Noninvasive ventilation in acute respiratory failure. *Critical Care Medicine, 35,* 2404–2407. doi:10.1097/01.CCM.0000284587.36541.7F

Jaber, S., Amraoui, J., Lefrant, J.-Y., Arich, C., Cohendy, R., Landreau, L., … Eledjam, J.-J. (2006). Clinical practice and risk factors for immediate complications of endotracheal intubation in the intensive care unit: A prospective, multiple-center study. *Critical Care Medicine, 34,* 2355–2361. doi:10.1097/01.CCM.0000233879.58720.87

Johnson, A., & Abraham, J. (2015). Monitoring for respiratory dysfunction. In K.J. Booker (Ed.), *Critical care nursing: Monitoring and treatment for advanced nursing practice* (pp. 35–56). doi:10.1002/9781118992845.ch3

Joynt, G.M., & Choi, G.Y.S. (2014). Airway management and acute airway obstruction. In A.D. Bersten & N. Soni (Eds.), *Oh's intensive care manual* (7th ed., pp. 341–353). Philadelphia, PA: Elsevier.

Krüger, W., & Ludman, A.J. (2014). *Core knowledge in critical care medicine.* London, England: Springer-Verlag.

Lee, R. (2016). Pulse oximetry and capnography. In A. Webb, D. Angus, S. Finfer, L. Gattinoni, & M. Singer (Eds.), *Oxford textbook of critical care* (2nd ed., pp. 331–334). New York, NY: Oxford University Press.

Levitzky, M.G. (2013). *Pulmonary physiology* (8th ed.). New York, NY: McGraw-Hill Education.

Nava, S., & Hill, N. (2009). Non-invasive ventilation in acute respiratory failure. *Lancet, 374,* 250–259. doi:10.1016/S0140-6736(09)60496-7

Nolan, J.P., Hazinski, M.F., Aickin, R., Bhanji, F., Billi, J.E., Callaway, C.W., ... Zideman, D.A. (2015). Part 1: Executive summary: 2015 International Consensus on Cardiopulmonary Resuscitation and Emergency Cardiovascular Care Science With Treatment Recommendations. *Resuscitation, 95,* e1–e31. doi:10.1016/j.resuscitation.2015.07.039

Schmidt, G.A., Girard, T.D., Kress, J.P., Morris, P.E., Ouellette, D.R., Alhazzani, W., ... Truwit, J.D. (2017). Liberation from mechanical ventilation in critically ill adults: Executive summary of an official American College of Chest Physicians/American Thoracic Society clinical practice guideline. *Chest, 151,* 160–165. doi:10.1016/j.chest.2016.10.037

Sitzwohl, C., Langheinrich, A., Schober, A., Krafft, P., Sessler, D.I., Herkner, H., ... Kettner, S.C. (2010). Endobronchial intubation detected by insertion depth of endotracheal tube, bilateral auscultation, or observation of chest movements: Randomised trial. *BMJ, 341,* c5943. doi:10.1136/bmj.c5943

Sole, M.L., Penoyer, D.A., Su, X.G., Jimenez, E., Kalita, S.J., Poalillo, E., ... Ludy, J.E. (2009). Assessment of endotracheal cuff pressure by continuous monitoring: A pilot study. *American Journal of Critical Care, 18,* 133–143. doi:10.4037/ajcc2009441

Tobin, M.J. (2016). Assessment and technique of weaning. In A. Webb, D. Angus, S. Finfer, L. Gattinoni, & M. Singer (Eds.), *Oxford textbook of critical care* (2nd ed., pp. 470–473). New York, NY: Oxford University Press.

Wagner, P.D., Powell, F.L., & West, J.B. (2010). Ventilation, blood flow, and gas exchange. In R.J. Mason, V.C. Broaddus, & T.R. Martin (Eds.), *Murray and Nadel's textbook of respiratory medicine* (5th ed., pp. 53–88). Philadelphia, PA: Elsevier Saunders.

CHAPTER 12

Sepsis

Anna Vioral, PhD, MEd, RN, OCN®, BMTCN®

Introduction

Shock occurs as a response to poor tissue oxygenation when the cardiovascular system fails to adequately perfuse tissues. The impaired oxygen delivery to tissues and organs results in widespread impairment of cellular metabolism, leading to a life-threatening emergency. The cause, pathophysiologic process, or clinical manifestation classifies shock. For example, shock caused by heart failure is known as cardiogenic (O'Leary, 2015). Alterations in the vascular smooth muscle result in neurogenic or vasogenic shock. Insufficient intravascular fluid volume occurs with hypovolemic shock. A widespread hypersensitivity reaction leads to anaphylactic shock. Septic shock occurs when large amounts of toxins produced by bacteria are released into the body. The overwhelming infection leads to low blood pressure and blood flow, altered coagulation, cellular ischemia, hypoxia, and multiorgan system failure. Early recognition and treatment is vital to survival. Without prompt interventions, mortality rates significantly increase.

Patients with cancer develop systemic neutropenic sepsis as a complication of their disease or anticancer treatments. These immunocompromised patients often require emergency admissions and care in the intensive care unit (ICU); therefore, critical care nurses must understand the underlying concepts related to neutropenic sepsis in this patient population. Prompt and early recognition and treatment of neutropenic sepsis may impact outcomes. Nurses are essential in detecting these early signs. This chapter reviews the epidemiology and incidence of sepsis, describes the pathophysiology of neutropenia and sepsis, discusses assessment criteria of sepsis, explains the treatment and management of sepsis, and summarizes implications for critical care nurses caring for patients with cancer.

Definitions

Although the terms *septicemia*, *sepsis*, *sepsis syndrome*, and *septic shock* are often used interchangeably, the classic definitions of sepsis were published in 1992 by the American College of Chest Physicians (ACCP) and the Society of Critical Care Medicine (SCCM), who convened to clarify terminology and definitions of sepsis syndromes (Bone et al., 1992). In 2001, ACCP, SCCM, the European Society of Intensive Care Medicine (ESICM), the American Thoracic Society, and the Surgical Infection Society attempted to update these definitions at the International Sepsis Definitions Conference. A consensus document was developed concluding that not enough evidence existed to support new definitions (Levy et al., 2003); however, to better define the pathophysiology of sepsis, the document did expand the list of signs and symptoms reflective of the bedside experience. Table 12-1 provides definitions consistently used until 2016 for bacteremia, systemic inflammatory response

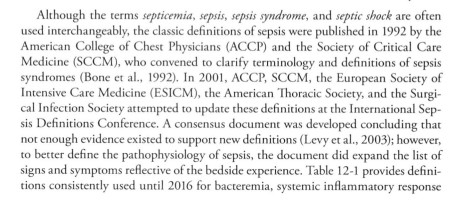

Table 12-1. Definitions of Sepsis	
Term	**Definition**
Bacteremia	The presence of viable bacteria in the blood
Systemic inflammatory response syndrome (SIRS)	The systemic inflammatory response to a variety of clinical insults, manifested by two or more of the following: • Temperature greater than 100.4°F (38°C) or less than 96.4°F (36°C) • Heart rate greater than 90 beats per minute • Respiratory rate greater than 20 breaths per minute or $PaCO_2$ less than 32 mm Hg • White blood cell count greater than 12,000/mm³, less than 4,000/mm³, or greater than 10% bands
Sepsis	SIRS because of infection
Severe sepsis	Sepsis associated with organ dysfunction, hypoperfusion, or hypotension. Hypoperfusion and perfusion abnormalities may include lactic acidosis, oliguria, or acute alteration in mental status.
Septic shock	Acute circulatory failure with hypotension, despite adequate fluid resuscitation, along with presence of perfusion abnormalities and persistent hemodynamic instability
Multiple organ dysfunction syndrome	A continuation of the sepsis syndrome characterized by the presence of altered function of more than one organ such that homeostasis cannot be measured without immediate intervention

Note. Based on information from Bone et al., 1992; Levy et al., 2003.

syndrome (SIRS), sepsis, severe sepsis, septic shock, and multiple organ dysfunction syndrome (MODS) (Bone et al., 1992; Levy et al., 2003).

After nearly two decades, ESICM and SCCM convened in 2014 with a task force of 19 critical care, infectious disease, surgical, and pulmonary specialists to reexamine the current definitions of sepsis (Singer et al., 2016). Through an expert consensus process, new definitions were generated and a deeper understanding of sepsis biology and organ dysfunction was provided. Sepsis terminology was also more clearly defined with a focus on early detection to decrease morbidity and mortality. Now, sepsis is defined as "a life-threatening organ dysfunction caused by dysregulated host response to infection" (Singer et al., 2016, p. 801). Septic shock is now referred to as "a subset of sepsis that results in profound circulatory, cellular, and metabolic abnormalities" (Singer et al., 2016, p. 801). SIRS remains in the definition but is no longer used to diagnose sepsis. The quick sepsis-related organ failure assessment (SOFA or qSOFA) provides a prompt way to identify patients with suspected infections who are at a greater risk of poor outcomes outside the ICU. The three criteria used in qSOFA are blood pressure, respiratory rate, and mental status. MODS is now referred to as organ dysfunction that occurs with an active change in a qSOFA score of greater than or equal to two points. Nurses must gain familiarity with sepsis terms prior to clinically caring for patients.

Epidemiology

Sepsis has become increasingly common, and the clinical consensus definitions have allowed for epidemiology studies. Severe sepsis afflicts as many as 3 million U.S. adults annually and results in an estimated 750,000 deaths (Whittaker et al., 2015). Approximately 4.2% of patients in the hospital develop septicemia (Elixhauser, Friedman, & Stranges, 2011).

The National Center for Healthcare Statistics found from its National Hospital Discharge Survey that the number of hospital stays because of sepsis had more than doubled between 2000 and 2008 (Hall, Williams, DeFrances, & Golosinskiy, 2011). In 2009, septicemia was the sixth most common principal reason for hospitalization in the United States, accounting for 836,000 hospital stays (Elixhauser et al., 2011). An additional 829,500 stays had a secondary diagnosis of septicemia (Elixhauser et al., 2011). Septicemia hospital stays accounted for 4% of all inpatient costs, totaling nearly $15.4 billion in aggregate hospital costs (Elixhauser et al., 2011). The hospital mortality rate for septicemia was about 16%, which is more than eight times higher than other stays (Hall et al., 2011). ICUs receive many patients with sepsis because of its wide spectrum of disease severity at presentation and high morbidity and mortality.

Mayr, Yende, and Angus (2014) associated sepsis with the highest mortality rate of 50%. Approximately 50% of sepsis survivors suffer long-term sequelae and complications. The adverse long-term outcomes significantly influence quality of life and overall survival. Survivors report moderate to severe limitations with at least one dimension of activities of daily living, including mobility and self-care (Iwashyna, Ely, Smith, & Langa, 2010). Acute respiratory distress syndrome (ARDS), myocardial dysfunction, acute kidney injury, and liver failure are also significant sequelae of sepsis (Iwashyna et al., 2010). Older adult survivors experience three times as many complications with persistent cognitive and functional impairments (Iwashyna et al., 2010). Despite medical advances leading to improved outcomes, many new developments have also led to septic complications.

Etiology and Risk Factors

The etiology of sepsis originates from infectious pathogens in the bloodstream. Gram-negative organisms represent the most common microorganisms; however, gram-positive organisms have increased over time because of the greater use of invasive procedures and indwelling devices and the increasing proportion of hospital-acquired infections (Guidet, Aegerter, Gauzit, Meshaka, & Dreyfuss, 2005; Mayr et al., 2014). Anaerobes, fungi, parasites, and other bacteria and organisms also contribute to sepsis. Other etiologic factors include more frequent use of broad-spectrum antibiotics, resulting in increased bacterial resistance over time; duration of mechanical ventilation; and prolonged hospitalization (Mayr et al., 2014).

A determinant to the outcome of sepsis correlates to the type of organism causing the sepsis. Table 12-2 shows the most predominant organisms reported from the most recent study on international prevalence of infection (Vincent et al., 2009).

Although the most prevalent organisms are *Staphylococcus aureus* (20.5%), *Pseudomonas* species (19.9%), *Escherichia coli* (16.0%), and fungi (19%), about

Table 12-2. Common Infection Sources	
Site	**Frequency (%)**
Respiratory	77.6
Bacteremia (unspecified site)	41.0
Genitourinary	28.3
Abdominal	16.7
Wounds	16.5
Device related	2.2
Central nervous system	1.2
Endocarditis	1.4
Other	15.3
Note. Based on information from Mayr et al., 2010; Vincent et al., 2009.	

one-third of patients with sepsis did not have positive blood cultures (Guidet et al., 2005; Mayr et al., 2014; Vincent et al., 2009). Cohen, Cristofaro, Carlet, and Opal (2004) completed a large meta-analysis of 510 studies examining mortality rates related to gram-negative and gram-positive bacteremia. The most common bloodstream infections were from coagulase-negative staphylococci and *Escherichia coli*, but these also had relatively low mortality rates (20% and 19%, respectively). The *Candida* and *Acinetobacter* species had relatively higher mortality rates (43% and 40%, respectively). Gram-positive pneumonia from *Staphylococcus aureus* also had a higher mortality rate (41%) compared to *Streptococcus pneumoniae* (13%). The highest mortality rate was associated with gram-negative bacillus *Pseudomonas aeruginosa* (77%) (Cohen et al., 2004). The origin site of infection also influences mortality rates. Common sources of infection with associated mortality rates are summarized in Table 12-3, with the respiratory system cited as the most common site (Mayr et al., 2010; Vincent et al., 2009).

Additional risk factors contributing to the etiology of sepsis include age, gender, race, environment, and chronic health conditions. Although patients younger than one year old have an increased risk of developing sepsis (Angus et al., 2001), more than half of sepsis cases occur in adults older than age 65 (Mayr et al., 2010). This may be attributed to a decline in immune function, leading to B- and T-cell impairment (Mayr et al., 2010). More than half of older adult patients who develop sepsis also have at least one chronic health condition, reside in long-term care facilities, suffer from malnourishment, or take immunosuppressant medications (Mayr et al., 2010).

Gender also contributes to sepsis, with men more likely to develop sepsis than women (Martin, Mannino, Eaton, & Moss, 2003). Community-acquired respiratory bacteremia occurs more frequently in younger patients and men (Hartman, Linde-Zwirble, Angus, & Watson, 2013), while patients older than age 65 and women develop more urinary tract infections (Mayr et al., 2010). Studies have reported higher rates of sepsis among African Americans and those with genetic polymorphisms in the host response to infection (Berkowitz & Martin, 2007; Henckaerts et al., 2009). Environmental risk factors for sepsis include higher rates of respiratory infections in colder months and more frequent genitourinary infections in hotter months (Danai, Sinha, Moss, Haber, & Martin, 2007).

Patients with underlying comorbidities experience a higher risk of developing sepsis. For example, studies have reported the most prevalent coexisting conditions for developing sepsis include immunodeficiency (22%), hypertension (7%–18%), diabetes mellitus (12%–18%), cancer (8%–18%), congestive heart failure (8%–15%), and chronic obstructive pulmonary disease (9%–12%) (Angus et al., 2001; Annane, Aegerter, Jars-Guincestre, & Guidet, 2003; Martin et al., 2003). Patients with malignancies have a nearly 10-fold increase in relative risk of developing sepsis compared to those without cancer (Danai, Moss, Mannino, & Martin, 2006). Cancer diagnoses with the highest risk for developing sepsis include hematologic malignancies, such as leukemia, lymphoma, and multiple myeloma, and solid tumors, such as lung and pancreatic cancer. Patients with these malig-

Table 12-3. Organisms Associated With Mortality	
Organism	**Frequency (%)**
Gram-Positive	
Staphylococcus (S.) aureus	20.5
Enterococcus	10.9
S. epidermidis	10.8
Methicillin-resistant *S. aureus*	10.2
S. pneumoniae	4.1
Other	6.4
Gram-Negative	
Pseudomonas species	19.9
Escherichia coli	16.0
Klebsiella species	12.7
Acinetobacter species	8.8
Enterobacter	7.0
Other	17.0
Anaerobes	4.5
Other Bacteria	1.5
Fungi	
Candida	17.0
Aspergillus	1.4
Other fungi	1.0
Parasites	0.7
Other Organisms	3.9
Note. Based on information from Vincent et al., 2009.	

nancies often have disease in their bone marrow and receive intensive cytotoxic medications, which further compromise the ability to fight infection. Complications from cancer and its treatment also place this patient population at a greater risk for developing neutropenic sepsis.

Pathophysiology

The sepsis triad refers to inflammation, coagulation, and fibrinolysis. Infection occurs when an organism or microbe enters the bloodstream. In the normal pathophysiology of an infection, when a microorganism such as bacteria, fungus, or a virus invades the body, an intact immune system recognizes the organism and mounts an immune response. Neutrophils, macrophages, monocytes, lymphocytes, and antibodies phagocytize the organism, preventing colonization. When the organism colonizes and reproduces within a host, however, the localized inflammatory response cannot manage the infection, resulting in sepsis as a systemic response (Gobel, Peterson, & Hoffner, 2013).

Sepsis occurs either directly from the site of infection or from toxic substances released by the bacteria directly into the bloodstream. The toxic substances act as triggering molecules in sepsis. Gram-negative microorganisms release endothelial toxins, and gram-positive microorganisms release exotoxins from the cell walls of dead bacteria after phagocytosis occurs by the neutrophils (Gobel et al., 2013). These toxins alter the endothelium that activates the complement system and the coagulation cascade. The activation of the complement system releases vasoactive mediators, such as kinins, histamines, interleukins (ILs), and tumor necrosis factor-alpha (TNF-α), leading to vasodilation (Gobel et al., 2013; Jones & Puskarich, 2009).

Vasoactive mediators further activate the coagulation cascade, leading to aggregation of platelets and fibrin formation (Gobel et al., 2013; Jones & Puskarich, 2009). Intravascular and extravascular fibrin formations are characteristic in sepsis. The systemic inflammatory response leads to significant coagulopathy and disseminated intravascular coagulation (DIC). A downregulation of the anticoagulation pathways and impaired fibrinolysis occur, resulting in microvascular fibrin thrombosis.

Initially, both proinflammatory and anti-inflammatory cytokines function to fight off infection and modulate the immune response; however, as sepsis progresses without adequate treatment, more fibrin formation, platelet aggregation, and decreased tissue perfusion cause septic shock. This involves profound circulatory, cellular, and metabolic abnormalities with a greater risk of mortality.

In a proinflammatory response, the polymorphonuclear leukocytes, macrophages, monocytes, and platelets release proinflammatory mediators in the form of cytokines, including IL-1, IL-2, IL-6, IL-8, IL-15, TNF-α, granulocyte–colony-stimulating factor, complement, kinins, prostaglandins, leukotrienes, endorphins, histamine, serotonin, and the clotting cascade (Meyers, 2008). These cytokines are potent vasodilators, are pyrogens, and mediate inflammation. As these increase in the bloodstream in response to septic shock, they also stimulate the release of additional inflammatory mediators.

As a compensatory response, the anti-inflammatory mediators release cytokines, including IL-4, IL-10, IL-11, IL-13, transforming growth factor-beta, and soluble TNF receptors, to suppress gene function and synthesis of IL-1 and TNF (Chuang et al., 2007). Continuous increased cytokine release promotes further cell-leukocyte adhesion, release of proteases and arachidonate antimetabolites, and activation of the clotting cascade (Gobel et al., 2013). This combination effect eventually causes hypovolemia, hypotension, hypoxia, lactic acidosis, tissue ischemia, DIC, oliguria, and organ failure. Figure 12-1 illustrates the schema of sepsis.

Figure 12-1. Schema of Sepsis

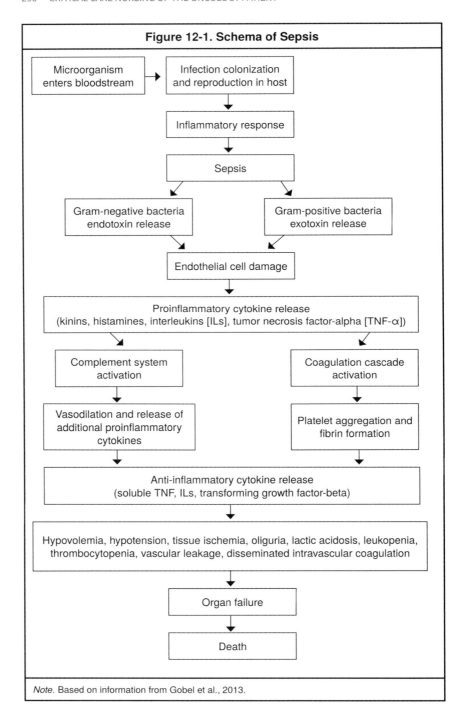

Note. Based on information from Gobel et al., 2013.

Neutropenic Sepsis

In patients who develop sepsis, cancer is one of the most common comorbidities and has some of the worst outcomes. Sepsis incidence in patients with cancer is estimated to be 25% and has an associated mortality rate of approximately 28% (Shelton, 2018).

This increased incidence of sepsis in patients with cancer can be attributed to many causes. For example, patients with cancer often experience malignancy-related immunosuppression. Hematologic malignancies, such as leukemia, lymphoma, and multiple myeloma, develop cancer in the bone marrow cells, which weakens the immune system. Solid tumors, such as breast, lung, and colon cancer, may metastasize to the bone marrow and cause disease-related immunosuppression. Both humoral and cellular immunity can be modified or compromised from the malignancy.

Patients with hematologic and solid tumor malignancies receive intensive cytotoxic medications, radiation therapy, and other immune-modulating therapies that cause immunosuppression. The effect from these therapies begins anywhere between 7 and 14 days from treatment initiation and lasts 21–28 days. Patients receiving intense treatment schedules or repetitive therapies often experience effects beyond these parameters. Patients with cancer often have additional chronic comorbidities, which compromise their ability to combat infection. Immunosuppression from malignancy and treatment leads to neutropenia or granulocytopenia, the most important risk factor in sepsis development. This is referred to as neutropenic sepsis and prevails as a potentially fatal complication for patients with cancer. Sepsis occurs in approximately 10%–20% of patients who experience neutropenia (Courtney et al., 2007). Approximately one in five patients are admitted to the ICU for septic syndromes (Vincent et al., 2006). ICU nurses must develop an understanding of neutropenia, assessment criteria, and management of patients experiencing febrile neutropenia and neutropenic sepsis.

Hematopoiesis

The production of all blood cells derives from the hematopoietic stem cells in the adult bone marrow and is called hematopoiesis. This process begins with the multipluripotent stem cell, which gives rise to the proliferation and differentiation of a cellular lineage. Stem cell proliferation and differentiation occur in response to the body's needs when encountering exogenous and endogenous demands (Polovich, Olsen, & LeFebvre, 2014). Figure 12-2 illustrates how the pluripotent stem cell gives rise to either the myeloid or lymphoid progenitor lineage (Polovich et al., 2014).

Figure 12-2. Hematopoiesis

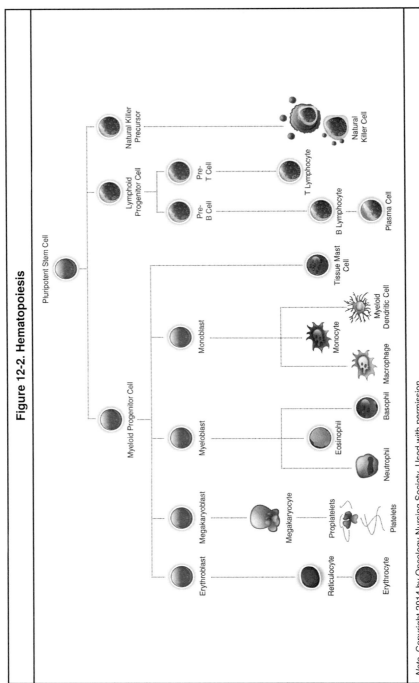

Lymphoid Progenitor Lineage

The lymphoid progenitor lineage produces B lymphocytes (B cells), T lymphocytes (T cells), and natural killer cells (NK cells). B cells originate and mature in the bone marrow, whereas T cells mature in the thymus after leaving the bone marrow. B cells have a major role in humoral adaptive immunity through the production of antibodies (immunoglobulins or plasma cells). T cells have a major role in cell-mediated immunity by directly killing infected cells. NK cells kill selected tumor cells and viruses without requiring activation.

Myeloid Progenitor Lineage

The myeloid progenitor gives rise to the megakaryocyte-erythrocyte progenitor and the granulocyte-monocyte progenitor. The megakaryocyte-erythrocyte progenitor produces the erythroid-lineage cells necessary for oxygenation and red blood cell formation and the megakaryocytes that form platelets and assist with coagulation. The granulocyte-monocyte progenitor produces the granulocyte lineages to generate neutrophils, basophils, eosinophils, monocyte-macrophage lineages, and dendritic cell lineages. Monocytes migrate into tissues and develop into macrophages, which then remove antigens and present antigens to lymphocytes to destroy pathogens. Polymorphonuclear granulocytes, or leukocytes, have granules with enzymes that are released during infections and allergic reactions. They comprise 60%–70% of the body's leukocytes and encompass neutrophils, basophils, and eosinophils (Polovich et al., 2014). Eosinophils comprise 2%–5% of the leukocytes that phagocytize microorganisms, such as parasites, and also are a major source of inflammatory mediators, such as prostaglandins, cytokines, and leukotrienes. Basophils constitute less than 0.2% of leukocytes and play a key role in allergic reactions in the degranulation process through the release of histamine.

Neutrophils only live about 4–12 hours but respond quickly to bacterial invasion, providing the body's first line of defense. As the most common leukocyte, they contain 35%–76% of circulating white blood cells (WBCs). Without a sufficient supply, the body cannot mount an inflammatory response. Neutrophils leave the bone marrow through pores between the marrow and venous blood vessels (Polovich et al., 2014). Once released into the bloodstream, they adhere to the endothelial cells lining the blood vessels and then move to the infection sites (Polovich et al., 2014). Because of the short life span of neutrophils, the bone marrow must continually produce them. Patients with cancer receiving cytotoxic medications experience bone marrow suppression, which prevents the neutrophil maturation process and induces neutropenia.

Neutropenia

Neutropenia is a term used to define an abnormally low number of neutrophils in the bloodstream. Patients with cancer experience a decrease in neutrophils related to their disease, treatments, or infection. Neutropenia has significant negative clinical outcomes for patients with cancer and is one of the greatest predictors of life-threatening infections (O'Leary, 2015). Neutropenia generally occurs 7–14 days after a patient receives cytotoxic medications but may last more than six weeks. The term *nadir* refers to the lowest level of blood cell counts for patients undergoing chemotherapy. Patients with a greater degree or longer duration of neutropenia have a greater risk for complications and neutropenic sepsis. To determine the risk for neutropenia, nurses must calculate an absolute neutrophil count (ANC), or the number of mature WBCs in circulation. Obtaining a complete blood count (CBC) with differential and platelet count provides the necessary data to calculate ANC. Table 12-4 provides an example of reference ranges for CBC with differential and platelet count.

WBC count represents the total number of WBCs in the peripheral blood, but this is not the ANC. To calculate the ANC, add the number of neutrophils and bands, multiply by the total WBC count, and then divide by 100. The total WBC count may be reported as 4.5 k/uL or 4,500/mm³. Figure 12-3 provides an example of how to calculate the ANC.

The National Cancer Institute Cancer Therapy Evaluation Program (2010) outlines the grading criteria for neutropenia in the Common Terminology Criteria for Adverse Events. This tool grades the depth of neutropenia but does not always directly correlate with sepsis incidence.

Table 12-4. Common Terminology Criteria for Adverse Events Grading for Absolute Neutrophil Count

Grade	Absolute Neutrophil Count (/mm³)
1	≥ 1,500
2	< 1,500
3	< 1,000
4	< 500

Note. Based on information from National Cancer Institute Cancer Therapy Evaluation Program, 2010.

Figure 12-3. Absolute Neutrophil Count Calculation

$$\frac{(\text{Segmented neutrophils} + \text{bands}) \times \text{total white blood cell count}}{100} = \text{absolute neutrophil count}$$

Example:
Segmented neutrophils = 18
Bands = 2
White blood cells = 2.1 k/uL × 1,000 = 2,100/mm³

(18 + 2) × 2,100 = 42,000 divided by 100 = 420

Note. Based on information from Zitella, 2014.

Assessment Criteria

Sepsis results when the body fails to mount an adequate immune response to an overwhelming infection (e.g., bacterial, viral, fungal) (Gobel et al., 2013). Patients with cancer have a baseline compromised immune system, thus patients with febrile neutropenia often spiral into septic shock as a potentially life-threatening emergency.

A patient history provides useful information and may identify a septic cause or contributing factors. Assessing a patient for neutropenia involves a thorough history of potential factors that may increase the risk of neutropenia, including any previous chemotherapy, immunotherapy, radiation, medications, and comorbidities; however, a thorough head-to-toe physical assessment provides crucial data to identify neutropenia signs and symptoms.

Common signs and symptoms of infection include redness, swelling, pus formation, productive cough, and urinary frequency, hesitancy, or burning. These occur because of the arrival of neutrophils to infection sites. Patients with neutropenia do not produce sufficient amounts of mature neutrophils to mount an immune response; therefore, they lack the classic signs and symptoms of infection. The respiratory, gastrointestinal, genitourinary, and integumentary systems present as the most common infection sites.

Many patients with neutropenia do not develop cough or sputum, even with pneumonia. Respiratory alkalosis may manifest with dyspnea, rales, hypoxemia, pulmonary edema, and ARDS (Gobel et al., 2013). The abdomen is a common site for peritonitis, typhlitis, and *Clostridium difficile* in patients with neutropenia. Abdominal pain may indicate bowel obstruction, perforation, or organ abnormalities with the spleen, liver, pancreas, gallbladder, or appendix. Patients may develop oliguria or mental status changes with urinary tract infections rather than urinary frequency, hesitancy, or burning. The integumentary system requires thorough assessment of indwelling catheters, exit sites, and mucosal membranes for edema, drainage, erythema, tenderness, and ulceration. Cold, clammy, and cyanotic skin changes are caused by a lack of tissue oxygenation (Gobel et al., 2013). Patients may develop jaundice from hyperbilirubinemia and elevated serum liver transaminases (Gobel et al., 2013).

Vital signs often provide the most invaluable information regarding sepsis in a patient with neutropenia. An elevated temperature is the earliest and most common sign of infection. The National Comprehensive Cancer Network® (NCCN®, 2017b) defines a fever in a patient with neutropenia as a onetime oral temperature greater than 101°F (38.3°C) or an oral temperature of 100.4°F (38°C) lasting one hour. A temperature less than 96°F (36°C) results from endotoxin release from gram-negative organisms and indicates sepsis (NCCN, 2017b). Rectal temperatures may cause injury to the rectal mucosa and should be avoided.

Other vital signs indicating sepsis include tachycardia, tachypnea, hypotension, and decreased oxygen saturations. Patients often experience high cardiac output with vasodilation and slightly elevated blood pressure during early sepsis (Gobel et al., 2013). Inadequate assessment and treatment results in capillary leak with edema, a decrease in blood pressure, and decreased blood flow and tissue perfusion, resulting in organ dysfunction (Gobel et al., 2013). A thorough patient assessment helps to identify sepsis and adequately complete diagnostic evaluation and implementation of treatment management strategies.

The Third International Consensus Task Force sought to identify sepsis from uncomplicated infection (Singer et al., 2016). They developed qSOFA to identify the best clinical criteria in infected patients who were most likely to be experiencing sepsis. This qSOFA method requires a prompt bedside assessment to identify patients with suspected infection who are at greater risk for a poorer outcome in the ICU (Singer et al., 2016). Three criteria are used, including low blood pressure (systolic blood pressure less than or equal to 100 mm Hg), increased respiratory rate (greater than or equal to 22 breaths per minute), and altered mentation (Glasgow Coma Scale less than 15) (Dellinger et al., 2008; Singer et al., 2016).

Diagnostic Evaluation

Positive cultures from blood or an involved organ remain the gold standard of diagnosing sepsis. Cultures include blood, urine, sputum, wound, spinal fluids, stool, and other body fluids and should be obtained prior to initiating antimicrobial therapy, as they determine the pathogenic organisms responsible for sepsis. According to NCCN (2017b), two sets of cultures should initially be obtained and repeated every 24 hours for ongoing fevers or based on clinical findings. WBCs and neutrophils are necessary to grow bacteria in the culture medium. Patients with neutropenia have minimal WBCs and neutrophils; therefore, administering antibiotics before obtaining cultures may suppress the cultures from growing microorganisms. Unfortunately, patients with neutropenic sepsis may not develop positive blood cultures, further increasing morbidity and mortality.

A variety of laboratory and diagnostic tests also assist in the diagnosis of sepsis. A CBC with differential may indicate potential for sepsis. A WBC count greater than 12,000/mm³ or less than 4,000/mm³ or a differential with greater than 10% bands indicates an increased potential for sepsis (Gobel et al., 2013). An ANC less than 1,000/mm³ poses a significant risk for infection. Longer durations of neutropenia (more than seven days) significantly increase the risk of septic shock. A complete metabolic panel (CMP) with liver function tests (LFTs) may reveal elevated blood urea nitrogen (BUN) and creatinine, reflecting dehydration or decreased renal function. Blood glucose levels tend to rise in early sepsis and septic shock, but hypoglycemia develops with prolonged sepsis because of hepatic failure and loss of compensatory mechanisms (Gobel et al., 2013).

Lactic acid has become a valuable biochemical biomarker in the diagnosis and treatment of sepsis. In normal conditions, cellular energy is extracted aerobically by the citric acid cycle (Mikkelsen et al., 2009). Conversely, when the body experiences inadequate tissue perfusion, anaerobic metabolism increases lactate productions. When cellular metabolism is strained, lactic acid accumulates in the muscles, skeleton, brain, red blood cells, and kidneys (Mikkelsen et al., 2009); thus, using lactate as an indicator of impaired metabolism may help further diagnose, risk stratify, and treat patients with sepsis.

Because of the increased coagulopathies and disseminated intravascular coagulation associated with sepsis, partial thromboplastin time, prothrombin time, fibrinogen, platelets, and D-dimer levels must be monitored. Elevated serum lactate indicates tissue hypoperfusion and metabolic acidosis associated with increased morbidity and mortality. Arterial blood gases reflect oxygenation and evaluate for respiratory alkalosis and metabolic acidosis.

Additional tests may further diagnose sources of infection and potential organ dysfunction. For example, chest radiographs (x-rays) may rule out lung infections and pneumonia. However, patients with neutropenic sepsis may not have enough neutrophils to radiographically visualize infiltrates. Often, additional chest computed tomography (CT) scans or venograms isolate the infections or pulmonary embolus. Electrocardiograms and echocardiograms may determine a cardiac source of infection. Abdominal x-rays or ultrasounds may identify intra-abdominal and biliary sources of infection. A CT scan of the head or lumbar puncture may detect neurologic infections. Accurate and detailed head-to-toe assessments integrated with diagnostic evaluation enable the clinician to determine the proper treatment plan.

Treatment Management Strategies

Several treatment management strategies have been established for patients with neutropenic sepsis, including prevention and early detection, early goal-directed therapy, cardiovascular and pulmonary support, and antibiotic therapy.

Prevention and Early Detection

Infection prevention is the primary focus of caring for a patient with neutropenia. Current interventions to promote optimal outcomes include infection control, colony-stimulating factors, vaccinations, antimicrobial therapies, respiratory care, and oral care (NCCN, 2017a; O'Leary, 2015; Rosselet, 2013; Zitella, Gobel, O'Leary, & Belansky, 2009). Handwashing remains the most effective way to reduce the risk of infection (Allegranzi & Pittet, 2009; Centers for Disease Control and Prevention, 2016; Irwin, Erb, Williams, Wilson, & Zitella, 2013).

NCCN (2017a) guidelines also recommend colony-stimulating factors includ-ing filgrastim (granulocyte–colony stimulating factor, Neupogen®), pegfilgras-tim (Neulasta®), tbo-filgrastim (Granix®), and sargramostim (granulocyte mac-rophage–colony stimulating factor, Leukine®). Colony-stimulating factors do not stimulate the immune system to produce increased neutrophils but do acceler-ate the maturation of immature neutrophils in the bone marrow (Polovich et al., 2014). They also do not reduce infection-related mortality or overall survival (Bohlius, Herbst, Reiser, Schwarzer, & Engert, 2008), but they can reduce the risk, severity, and duration of severe and febrile neutropenia (Polovich et al., 2014).

Other recommended preventive measures for neutropenic sepsis comprise annual influenza and pneumococcal vaccinations and protection of integumen-tary and mucosal membranes, including providing meticulous central venous access device care, limiting invasive procedures, using electric razors, perform-ing frequent oral care at least three to four times daily, and cleansing the peri-anal area after toileting (Brown, 2015; NCCN, 2017b; O'Leary, 2015; Shelton, 2018).

Neutropenic precautions and diets have minimal evidence and lack effec-tiveness. Recent studies demonstrated no significant differences in infection rates between patients on a regular diet and those consuming low microbial diets (Foster, 2014; Gardner et al., 2008; van Tiel et al., 2007). National guide-lines now recommend the following prudent basic food safety practices, such as avoiding uncooked meats, fresh salad bars, seafood, and eggs (Foster, 2014; Gardner et al., 2008; van Tiel et al., 2007). Strict reverse-flow hospital rooms and isolation have not shown a decreased incidence of infections; however, patients should avoid those with colds or respiratory infections and large crowds (Zitella et al., 2009).

Early Goal-Directed Therapy

Despite prevention and early detection efforts, patients with cancer may develop sepsis. The key to managing sepsis in this population is prompt interven-tion. Initial resuscitation efforts should occur within the first six hours of diag-nosis (Chamberlain, Willis, & Bersten, 2011; Dellinger et al., 2008). A patient requires blood cultures and antibiotics within one hour of fever onset (Gaieski et al., 2010; van Vliet, Potting, Sturm, Donnelly, & Blijlevens, 2011). Cultures should also be taken from other sources, such as urine and sputum. Initiating IV fluids, vasopressors, blood transfusions, and inotropic agents has been shown to improve survival (Puskarich, Marchick, Kline, Steuerwald, & Jones, 2009). Many institutions have implemented the use of sepsis care bundles that specify to mea-sure lactate levels, obtain blood cultures, administer broad-spectrum antibiotics, and give crystalloids within three hours from the time of presentation (Dellinger et al., 2013). On transfer to the ICU, patients require a central venous access device, an arterial line for vasopressors, and supportive monitoring. According to Dellinger et al. (2008), initial resuscitation goals should include the following:

- Sustain a mean arterial pressure (MAP) greater than or equal to 65 mm Hg.
- Keep urine output greater than or equal to 0.5 ml/kg/hr.
- Retain a central venous or mixed venous oxygen saturation greater than 70% or 65%, respectively.
- Initiate mechanical ventilation if partial pressure of arterial oxygen falls below 60 mm Hg.

Cardiovascular and Pulmonary Support

Septic shock alters tissue perfusion, causing decreased oxygen and nutrients to the tissues, and resulting in cellular and organ dysfunction. The cardiovascular system responds by decreasing vascular tone, triggering myocardial depression, and shifting plasma volume into the interstitial space, resulting in decreased intravascular volume, hypotension, and organ dysfunction (Dellinger et al., 2008; Gobel et al., 2013). Hemodynamic therapy aims to restore effective tissue perfusion to normalize cellular and organ dysfunction.

Initial cardiovascular goals include replacing intravascular volume with isotonic crystalloids. Once fluid volume is restored, vasopressors, such as dopamine, norepinephrine, vasopressin, and phenylephrine, are added to maintain a mean arterial presure greater than 65 mm Hg to preserve tissue perfusion (Gobel et al., 2013). These medications increase cardiac contractibility and vasoconstriction, resulting in increased perfusion and blood pressure. Patients with severe refractory sepsis may also require inotropic medications, such as dobutamine, to cause a greater contractility and heart rate. The inflammatory cytokines involved in sepsis may cause insult to the alveolar capillary wall, leading to alveolar fluid retention, pulmonary edema, ARDS, and acute lung injury. Severe inflammation causes increased hypoxia and respiratory failure, requiring mechanical ventilation.

Antibiotic Therapy

Neutropenia increases the risk for more frequent and severe infections that require aggressive treatment. The microorganisms commonly associated with invasive bloodstream infections in patients with neutropenia derive from damaged normal microflora that has colonized. Common infection sites include the skin, central venous access devices, central nervous system, sinuses, oropharynx, nasopharynx, lungs, esophagus, abdomen, and urinary tract. ANC determines the magnitude of physical signs and symptoms of inflammation and infection. For example, patients with severe neutropenia (ANC less than 500/mm^3) typically do not present with localizing erythema, swelling, exudate, ulcerations, or tenderness. Bacterial infections account for 90% of cases in patients with neutropenia (Anderson-Reitz, 2018); therefore, an increased body temperature is often the earliest and only sign of infection. The most common bacterial pathogens are included in Figure 12-4.

Figure 12-4. Common Bacterial Pathogens

Gram-Positive Pathogens
- Coagulase-negative staphylococci
- *Staphylococcus aureus* (methicillin-resistant strain)
- *Enterococcus* (vancomycin-resistant strain)
- Viridans streptococci
- *Streptococcus pneumoniae*
- *Streptococcus pyogenes*

Gram-Negative Pathogens
- *Escherichia coli*
- *Klebsiella* species
- *Enterobacter* species
- *Pseudomonas aeruginosa*
- *Citrobacter* species
- *Acinetobacter* species

Note. Based on information from Freifeld et al., 2011.

Other common infections include yeast (*Candida albicans*) and fungus (*Aspergillus*). The reactivation of viruses, such as herpes simplex and cytomegalovirus, may also occur, requiring a rapid workup and administration of empiric systemic antimicrobial therapy. Early detection of the source and organisms with immediate initiation of appropriate antibiotic therapy improves overall outcomes.

Neutropenic patients with cancer who develop septic shock require immediate management interventions with cultures and IV antibiotic therapy. To effectively affect outcomes, antibiotics should be administered within three hours from the time of presentation in the emergency department and within one hour from the time of presentation for nonemergency department admissions (Mokart et al., 2014). Making a microbial diagnosis in sepsis ensures administration of effective antimicrobial therapy; however, positive blood cultures only occur in approximately one-third of septic cases (Bow, 2013; Freifeld et al., 2011; Rosselet, 2013). Selection of empiric therapy depends on patient history, allergies, drug intolerances, underlying comorbidities, and clinical presentation.

NCCN (2017b) recommends initial antimicrobial therapy with a single, broad-spectrum agent focusing primarily on gram-negative pathogens. Although no specific drug or period of treatment can be unequivocally recommended for all patients, the correct initial empirical antimicrobial therapy is critical to survival outcomes. Inappropriate therapy reduces survival outcomes from 52% to 10.3% (Kumar et al., 2009; Ram et al., 2012). A summary of the common antimicrobial therapies administered for neutropenic sepsis is shown in Table 12-5.

Initial antimicrobial therapy should include antipseudomonal beta-lactam, such as a third- or fourth-generation cephalosporin. Additional agents may include coverage for gram-positive pathogens for skin, central venous access devices, and coagulase-negative staphylococci bloodstream infections. For continued febrile episodes, a broader approach with an aminoglycoside or fluoroquinolone may be required. Figure 12-5 illustrates a schema for antimicrobial therapy recommendations.

Table 12-5. Neutropenic Sepsis Antimicrobial Therapy

Antibiotic Class	Antimicrobial Coverage	Antimicrobial Agent(s)
Penicillins	*Actinomyces* *Clostridium* *Meningococcemia* *Proteus* *Salmonella* *Streptococcus* *Staphylococcus* Broad-spectrum *Pseudomonas*	Tazobactam Clavulanate
Carbapenems	Respiratory Skin/structure Gynecologic	Imipenem Meropenem Ertapenem Doripenem
Cephalosporins	Enterobacter (e.g., *Escherichia* *[E.] coli*, *Klebsiella*, *Proteus*, *Serratia*) *Staphylococcus aureus* *Haemophilus influenzae*	Ceftazidime Cefepime Ceftriaxone
Monobactams	–	Aztreonam
Glycopeptides	*Staphylococcus aureus*	Vancomycin
Lipopeptides	–	Daptomycin
Oxazolidinones	–	Linezolid
Fluoroquinolones	Resistant enterobacteria	Ciprofloxacin Levofloxacin
Aminoglycosides	Gram-negative enterobacteria (e.g., *Serratia*, *Proteus*, *Kleb-* *siella*, *E. coli*) *Pseudomonas* *Erwinia*	Gentamicin Tobramycin Amikacin
Other antibacte- rials	Gastrointestinal bacilli	Clindamycin
	Campylobacter *Chlamydia* conjunctivitis *Corynebacterium diphtheria* *Legionella* *Mycoplasma pneumoniae*	Erythromycin
	Bacteroides *Clostridium difficile*	Metronidazole

(Continued on next page)

Table 12-5. Neutropenic Sepsis Antimicrobial Therapy *(Continued)*		
Antibiotic Class	**Antimicrobial Coverage**	**Antimicrobial Agent(s)**
Antifungals	*Candida* *Aspergillus* *Cryptococcus* *Fusarium*	Azoles • Itraconazole • Voriconazole • Posaconazole Echinocandins • Caspofungin • Micafungin
Antivirals	Herpes simplex Varicella zoster Cytomegalovirus Cytomegalovirus retinitis	Acyclovir Valacyclovir Ganciclovir Cidofovir Foscarnet

Note. Based on information from National Comprehensive Cancer Network, 2017b; Zitella, 2014.

Modification of the initial antimicrobial therapy occurs when the patient fails to defervesce in an expected timeframe, a microorganism is resistant to initial therapy, the infection progresses, and/or toxicity or end-organ damage occurs (Bow, 2013). Persistent fevers may require the addition of a systemic antifungal agent, anaerobic coverage, and/or antiviral therapy. Patients that develop invasive fungal infections in the ICU, such as invasive candidiasis and aspergillosis, experience 40% and 80% mortality, respectively. Nursing intervention in the prevention, early detection, and the management of neutropenic sepsis significantly affects the morbidity and mortality of these patients.

Nursing Implications

Neutropenic sepsis remains the most common reason for admission to the ICU with associated respiratory failure. Studies over the past two decades have reported ICU mortality rates for neutropenic sepsis ranging from 43%–98% (Hampshire, Welch, McCrossan, Francis, & Harrison, 2009; McGrath, Chatterjee, Whiteley, & Ostermann, 2010; Soares et al., 2010).

Prompt early recognition and treatment of neutropenic sepsis may impact outcomes. Nurses have a pivotal role in detecting early signs of sepsis and minimizing the delay of fever onset to initiation of antimicrobial therapy. This requires timely initiation of empirical broad-spectrum antimicrobial therapy at the onset of fever, ideally within one hour (de Naurois et al., 2010; Freifeld et al., 2011). Adminis-

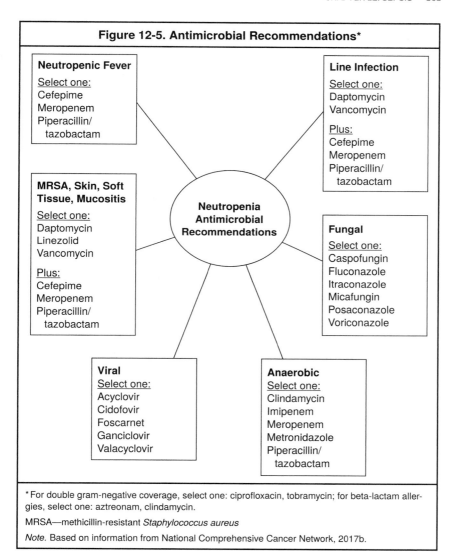

Figure 12-5. Antimicrobial Recommendations*

Neutropenic Fever
Select one:
Cefepime
Meropenem
Piperacillin/
 tazobactam

MRSA, Skin, Soft Tissue, Mucositis
Select one:
Daptomycin
Linezolid
Vancomycin

Plus:
Cefepime
Meropenem
Piperacillin/
 tazobactam

Neutropenia Antimicrobial Recommendations

Line Infection
Select one:
Daptomycin
Vancomycin

Plus:
Cefepime
Meropenem
Piperacillin/
 tazobactam

Fungal
Select one:
Caspofungin
Fluconazole
Itraconazole
Micafungin
Posaconazole
Voriconazole

Viral
Select one:
Acyclovir
Cidofovir
Foscarnet
Ganciclovir
Valacyclovir

Anaerobic
Select one:
Clindamycin
Imipenem
Meropenem
Metronidazole
Piperacillin/
 tazobactam

* For double gram-negative coverage, select one: ciprofloxacin, tobramycin; for beta-lactam allergies, select one: aztreonam, clindamycin.

MRSA—methicillin-resistant *Staphylococcus aureus*

Note. Based on information from National Comprehensive Cancer Network, 2017b.

tration of effective antimicrobial therapy in severe sepsis and septic shock within one hour of documented hypotension was associated with an 80% survival rate (Kumar et al., 2006). Conversely, for each hour of delay with effective antibacterial therapy in the first six hours, a 7.6% reduction in survival occurred (Kumar et al., 2006); however, timely administration remains problematic. The mean time for implementation of initial antimicrobial therapy in a febrile patient with neutropenia ranges from 4–14 hours (Kumar et al., 2006; Szwajcer, Czaykowski, & Turner, 2011).

Summary

Sepsis and septic shock in patients with neutropenia occur rapidly as life-threatening emergencies. A better understanding of the factors influencing the risk combined with prompt early detection and intervention improves outcomes. Nurses remain pivotal in early detection, monitoring, and treatment of neutropenic sepsis with evidence-based interventions. Developing protocols for neutropenic fever remains the cornerstone for preventing and treating neutropenic sepsis and significantly reducing morbidity and mortality.

References

Allegranzi, B., & Pittet, D. (2009). Role of hand hygiene in healthcare-associated infection prevention. *Journal of Hospital Infection, 73*, 305–315. doi:10.1016/j.jhin.2009.04.019

Anderson-Reitz, I. (2018). Complications of hematopoietic cell transplantation. In C.H. Yarbro, D. Wujcik, & B.H. Gobel (Eds.), *Cancer nursing: Principles and practice* (8th ed., pp. 591–610). Burlington, MA: Jones & Bartlett Learning.

Angus, D.C., Linde-Zwirble, W.T., Lidicker, J., Clermont, G., Carcillo, J., & Pinsky, M.R. (2001). Epidemiology of severe sepsis in the United States: Analysis of incidence, outcome, and associated costs of care. *Critical Care Medicine, 29*, 1303–1310. doi:10.1097/00003246-200107000 -00002

Annane, D., Aegerter, P., Jars-Guincestre, M.C., & Guidet, B. (2003). Current epidemiology of septic shock: The CUB-Réa network. *American Journal of Respiratory and Critical Care Medicine, 168*, 165–172. doi:10.1164/rccm.2201087

Berkowitz, D.M., & Martin, G.S. (2007). Disparities in sepsis: What do we understand? *Critical Care Medicine, 35*, 958–960. doi:10.1097/01.CCM.0000257226.48893.02

Bohlius, J., Herbst, C., Reiser, M., Schwarzer, G., & Engert, A. (2008). Granulopoiesis-stimulating factors to prevent adverse effects in the treatment of malignant lymphoma. *Cochrane Database of Systematic Reviews, 2008*(4). doi:10.1002/14651858.CD003189.pub4

Bone, R.C., Balk, R.A., Cerra, F.B., Dellinger, R.P., Fein, A.M., Knaus, W.A., ... Sibbald, W.J. (1992). Definitions for sepsis and organ failure and guidelines for the use of innovative therapies in sepsis. *Chest, 101*, 1644–1655. doi:10.1378/chest.101.6.1644

Bow, E.J. (2013). Infection in neutropenic patients with cancer. *Critical Care Clinics, 29*, 411–441. doi:10.1016/j.ccc.2013.03.002

Brown, C.G. (2015). Mucositis. In C.G. Brown (Ed.), *A guide to oncology symptom management* (2nd ed., pp. 469–483). Pittsburgh, PA: Oncology Nursing Society.

Centers for Disease Control and Prevention. (2016). Preventing infections in cancer patients. Retrieved from http://www.cdc.gov/cancer/preventinfections

Chamberlain, D.J., Willis, E.M., & Bersten, A.B. (2011). The severe sepsis bundles as processes of care: A meta-analysis. *Australian Critical Care, 24*, 229–243. doi:10.1016/j.aucc.2011.01.003

Chuang, C.C., Wang, S.T., Chen, W.C., Chen, C.C., Hor, L.I., & Chuang, A.Y. (2007). Increases in serum macrophage migration inhibitory factor in patients with severe sepsis predict early mortality. *Shock, 27*, 503–506. doi:10.1097/SHK.0b013e31802c024b

Cohen, J., Cristofaro, P., Carlet, J., & Opal, S. (2004). New method of classifying infections in critically ill patients. *Critical Care Medicine, 32*, 1510–1526. doi:10.1097/01.CCM.0000129973 .13104.2D

Courtney, D.M., Aldeen, A.Z., Gorman, S.M., Handler, J.A., Trifilio, S.M., Parada, J.P., ... Bennett, C.L. (2007). Cancer-associated neutropenic-fever: Clinical outcome and economic costs of emergency department care. *Oncologist, 12,* 1019–1026. doi:10.1634/theoncologist.12-8-1019

Danai, P.A., Moss, M., Mannino, D.M., & Martin, G.S. (2006). The epidemiology of sepsis in patients with malignancy. *Chest, 129,* 1432–1440. doi:10.1378/chest.129.6.1432

Danai, P.A., Sinha, S., Moss, M., Haber, M.J., & Martin, G.S. (2007). Seasonal variation in the epidemiology of sepsis. *Critical Care Medicine, 35,* 410–415. doi:10.1097/01.CCM.0000253405.17038.43

Dellinger, R.P., Levy, M.M., Carlet, J.M., Bion, J., Parker, M.M., Jaeschke, R., ... Vincent, J.-L. (2008). Surviving Sepsis Campaign: International guidelines for management of severe sepsis and septic shock. *Intensive Care Medicine, 34,* 17–60. doi:10.1007/s00134-007-0934-2

Dellinger, R.P., Levy, M.M., Rhodes, A., Annane, D., Gerlach, H., Opal, S.M., ... Moreno, R. (2013). Surviving Sepsis Campaign: International guidelines for management of severe sepsis and septic shock: 2012. *Critical Care Medicine, 41,* 580–637. doi:10.1097/CCM.0b013e31827e83af

de Naurois, J., Novitzky-Basso, I., Gill, M.J., Marti, F.M., Cullen, M.H., & Roila, F. (2010). Management of febrile neutropenia: ESMO clinical practice guidelines. *Annals of Oncology, 21*(Suppl. 5), v252–v256. doi:10.1093/annonc/mdq196

Elixhauser, A., Friedman, B., & Stranges, E. (2011). *Agency for healthcare research and quality: Septicemia in U.S. hospitals, 2009.* Retrieved from https://www.hcup-us.ahrq.gov/reports/statbriefs/sb122.jsp

Foster, M. (2014). Reevaluating the neutropenic diet: Time to change. *Clinical Journal of Oncology Nursing, 18,* 239–241. doi:10.1188/14.CJON.239-241

Freifeld, A.G., Bow, E.J., Sepkowitz, K.A., Boeckh, M.J., Ito, J.I., Mullen, C.A., ... Wingard, J.R. (2011). Clinical practice guideline for the use of antimicrobial agents in neutropenic patients with cancer: 2010 update by the Infectious Diseases Society of America. *Clinical Infectious Diseases, 52,* e56–e93. doi:10.1093/cid/cir073

Gaieski, D.F., Mikkelsen, M.E., Band, R.A., Pines, J.M., Massone, R., Furia, F.F., ... Goyal, M. (2010). Impact of time to antibiotic on survival in patients with severe sepsis or septic shock in whom early goal-directed therapy was initiated in the emergency department. *Critical Care Medicine, 38,* 1045–1053. doi:10.1097/CCM.0b013e3181cc4824

Gardner, A., Mattiuzzi, G., Faderl, S., Borthakur, G., Garcia-Manero, G., Pierce, S., ... Estey, E. (2008). Randomized comparison of cooked and noncooked diets in patients undergoing remission induction therapy for acute myeloid leukemia. *Journal of Clinical Oncology, 26,* 5684–5688. doi:10.1200/JCO.2008.16.4681

Gobel, B.H., Peterson, G.J., & Hoffner, B. (2013). Sepsis and septic shock. In M. Kaplan (Ed.), *Understanding and managing oncologic emergencies: A resource for nurses* (2nd ed., pp. 287–335). Pittsburgh, PA: Oncology Nursing Society.

Guidet, B., Aegerter, P., Gauzit, R., Meshaka, P., & Dreyfuss, D. (2005). Incidence and impact of organ dysfunctions associated with sepsis. *Chest, 127,* 942–951. doi:10.1378/chest.127.3.942

Hall, M.J., Williams, S.N., DeFrances, C.J., & Golosinskiy, A. (2011, June). *Inpatient care for septicemia or sepsis: A challenge for patients and hospitals* (Issue Brief No. 62). Retrieved from http://www.cdc.gov/nchs/data/databriefs/db62.htm

Hampshire, P.A., Welch, C.A., McCrossan, L.A., Francis, K., & Harrison, D.A. (2009). Admission factors associated with hospital mortality in patients with haematological malignancy admitted to UK adult, general critical care units: A secondary analysis of the ICNARC Case Mix Programme database. *Critical Care, 13,* R137. doi:10.1186/cc801613-R137

Hartman, M.E., Linde-Zwirble, W.T., Angus, D.C., & Watson, R.S. (2013). Trends in the epidemiology of pediatric severe sepsis. *Pediatric Critical Care Medicine, 14,* 686–693. doi:10.1097/PCC.0b013e3182917fad

Henckaerts, L., Nielsen, K.R., Steffensen, R., Van Steen, K., Mathieu, C., Giulietti, A., ... Van den Berghe, G. (2009). Polymorphisms in innate immunity genes predispose to bacteremia and death in the medical intensive care unit. *Critical Care Medicine, 37,* 192–201. doi:10.1097/CCM.0b013e31819263d8

Irwin, M., Erb, C., Williams, C., Wilson, B.J., & Zitella, L.J. (2013). *Putting evidence into practice: Improving oncology patient outcomes: Prevention of infection.* Pittsburgh, PA: Oncology Nursing Society.

Iwashyna, T.J., Ely, E.W., Smith, D.W., & Langa, K.M. (2010). Long-term cognitive impairment and functional disability among survivors of severe sepsis. *JAMA, 304,* 1787–1794. doi:10.1001/jama.2010.1553

Jones, A.E., & Puskarich, M.A. (2009). Sepsis-induced tissue hypoperfusion. *Critical Care Clinics, 25,* 769–779. doi:10.1016/j.ccc.2009.06.003

Kumar, A., Ellis, P., Arabi, Y., Roberts, D., Light, B., Parrillo, J.E., … Chateau, D. (2009). Initiation of inappropriate antimicrobial therapy results in a fivefold reduction of survival in human septic shock. *Chest, 136,* 1237–1248. doi:10.1378/chest.09-0087

Kumar, A., Roberts, D., Wood, K.E., Light, B., Parrillo, J.E., Sharma, S., … Cheang, M. (2006). Duration of hypotension before initiation of effective antimicrobial therapy is the critical determinant of survival in human septic shock. *Critical Care Medicine, 34,* 1589–1596. doi:10.1097/01.CCM.0000217961.75225.E9

Levy, M.M., Fink, M.P., Marshall, J.C., Abraham, E., Angus, D.C., Cook, D., … Ramsay, G. (2003). 2001 SCCM/ESICM/ACCP/ATS/SIS International Sepsis Definitions Conference. *Critical Care Medicine, 31,* 1250–1256. doi:10.1097/01.CCM.0000050454.01978.3B

Martin, G.S., Mannino, D.M., Eaton, S., & Moss, M. (2003). The epidemiology of sepsis in the United States from 1979 through 2000. *New England Journal of Medicine, 348,* 1546–1554. doi:10.1056/NEJMoa022139

Mayr, F.B., Yende, S., & Angus, D.C. (2014). Epidemiology of severe sepsis. *Virulence, 5,* 4–11. doi:10.4161/viru.27372

Mayr, F.B., Yende, S., Linde-Zwirble, W.T., Peck-Palmer, O.M., Barnato, A.E., Weissfeld, L.A., & Angus, D.C. (2010). Infection rate and acute organ dysfunction risk as explanations for racial differences in severe sepsis. *JAMA, 303,* 2495–2503. doi:10.1001/jama.2010.851

McGrath, S., Chatterjee, F., Whiteley, C., & Ostermann, M. (2010). ICU and 6-month outcome of oncology patients in the intensive care unit. *Quarterly Journal of Medicine, 103,* 397–403. doi:10.1093/qjmed/hcq032

Meyers, J.S. (2008). Proinflammatory cytokines and sickness behavior: Implications for depression and cancer-related symptoms. *Oncology Nursing Forum, 35,* 802–807. doi:10.1188/08.ONF.802-807

Mikkelsen, M.E., Miltiades, A.N., Gaieski, D.F., Goyal, M., Fuchs, B.D., Shah, C.V., … Christie, J.D. (2009). Serum lactate is associated with mortality in severe sepsis independent of organ failure and shock. *Critical Care Medicine, 37,* 1670–1677. doi:10.1097/CCM.0b013e31819fcf68

Mokart, D., Saillard, C., Sannini, A., Chow-Chine, L., Brum, J.-P., Faucher, M., … Leone, M. (2014). Neutropenic cancer patients with severe sepsis: Need for antibiotics in the first hour. *Intensive Care Medicine, 40,* 1173–1174. doi:10.1007/s00134-014-3374-9

National Cancer Institute Cancer Therapy Evaluation Program. (2010). *Common terminology criteria for adverse events* [v.4.03]. Retrieved from http://evs.nci.nih.gov/ftp1/CTCAE/About.html

National Comprehensive Cancer Network. (2017a). *NCCN Clinical Practice Guidelines in Oncology (NCCN Guidelines®): Myeloid growth factors* [v.1.2017]. Retrieved from https://www.nccn.org/professionals/physician_gls/PDF/myeloid_growth.pdf

National Comprehensive Cancer Network. (2017b). *NCCN Clinical Practice Guidelines in Oncology (NCCN Guidelines®): Prevention and treatment of cancer-related infections* [v.2.2017]. Retrieved from http://www.nccn.org/professionals/physician_gls/PDF/infections.pdf

O'Leary, C. (2015). Neutropenia and infection. In C.G. Brown (Ed.), *A guide to oncology symptom management* (2nd ed., pp. 483–504). Pittsburgh, PA: Oncology Nursing Society.

Polovich, M., Olsen, M., & LeFebvre, K.B. (Eds.). (2014). *Chemotherapy and biotherapy guidelines and recommendations for practice* (4th ed.). Pittsburgh, PA: Oncology Nursing Society.

Puskarich, M.A., Marchick, M.R., Kline, J.A., Steuerwald, M.T., & Jones, A.E. (2009). One year mortality of patients treated with an emergency department based early goal directed therapy protocol for severe sepsis and septic shock: A before and after study. *Critical Care, 13,* R167. doi:10.1186/cc8138

Ram, R., Farbman, L., Leibovici, L., Raanani, P., Yeshurun, M., Vidal, L., … Paul, M. (2012). Characteristics of initial compared with subsequent bacterial infections among hospitalised haematooncological patients. *International Journal of Antimicrobial Agents, 40,* 123–126. doi:10.1016 /j.ijantimicag.2012.05.001

Rosselet, R.M. (2013). Hematologic effects. In S.A. Ezzone (Ed.), *Hematopoietic stem cell transplantation: A manual for nursing practice* (2nd ed., pp. 155–172). Pittsburgh, PA: Oncology Nursing Society.

Shelton, B.K. (2018). Infection. In C.H. Yarbro, D. Wujcik, & B.H. Gobel (Eds.), *Cancer nursing: Principles and practice* (8th ed., pp. 817–850). Burlington, MA: Jones & Bartlett Learning.

Singer, M., Deutschman, C.S., Seymour, C.W., Shankar-Hari, M., Annane, D., Bauer, M., … Angus, D.C. (2016). The Third International Consensus Definitions for Sepsis and Septic Shock (Sepsis-3). *JAMA, 315,* 801–810. doi:10.1001/jama.2016.0287

Soares, M., Caruso, P., Silva, E., Teles, J.M.M., Lobo, S.M.A., Friedman, G., … Salluh, J.I.F. (2010). Characteristics and outcomes of patients with cancer requiring admission to intensive care units: A prospective multicenter study. *Critical Care Medicine, 38,* 9–15. doi:10.1097/CCM .0b013e3181c0349e

Szwajcer, D., Czaykowski, P., & Turner, D. (2011). Assessment and management of febrile neutropenia in emergency departments within a regional health authority—A benchmark analysis. *Current Oncology, 18,* 280–284. doi:10.3747/co.v18i6.841

van Tiel, F.H., Harbers, M.M., Terporten, P.H.W., van Boxtel, R.T.C., Kessels, A.G., Voss, G.B.W.E., & Schouten, H.C. (2007). Normal hospital and low-bacterial diet in patients with cytopenia after intensive chemotherapy for hematologic malignancy: A study of safety. *Annals of Oncology, 18,* 1080–1084. doi:10.1093/annonc/mdm082

van Vliet, K., Potting, C.M., Sturm, P.D., Donnelly, J.P., & Blijlevens, N.M. (2011). How prompt is prompt in daily practice: Early initiation of empirical antibacterial therapy for febrile neutropenic patient. *European Journal of Cancer Care, 20,* 679–685. doi:10.1111/j.1365-2354.2011 .01264.x

Vincent, J.-L., Rello, J., Marshall, J., Silva, E., Anzueto, A., Martin, C.D., … Reinhart, K. (2009). International study of the prevalence and outcomes of infection in intensive care units. *JAMA, 302,* 2323–2329. doi:10.1001/jama.2009.1754

Vincent, J.-L., Sakr, Y., Sprung, C.L., Ranieri, V.M., Reinhart, K., Gerlach, H., … Payen, D. (2006). Sepsis in European intensive care units: Results of the SOAP study. *Critical Care Medicine, 34,* 344–353. doi:10.1097/01.CCM.0000194725.48928.3A

Whittaker, S.-A., Fuchs, B.D., Gaieski, D.F., Christie, J.D., Goyal, M., Meyer, N.J., … Mikkelsen, M.E. (2015). Epidemiology and outcomes in patients with severe sepsis admitted to the hospital wards. *Journal of Critical Care, 30,* 78–84. doi:10.1016/j.jcrc.2014.07.012

Zitella, L.J. (2014). Infection. In C.H. Yarbro, D. Wujcik, & B.H. Gobel (Eds.), *Cancer symptom management* (4th ed., pp. 131–157). Burlington, MA: Jones & Bartlett Learning.

Zitella, L., Gobel, B.H., O'Leary, C., & Belansky, H. (2009). Prevention of infection. In L.H. Eaton & J.M. Tipton (Eds.), *Putting evidence into practice: Improving oncology patient outcomes* (pp. 273–283). Pittsburgh, PA: Oncology Nursing Society.

CHAPTER **13**

Delirium

Leanne M. Boehm, PhD, RN, ACNS-BC, and
Aimee S. Hoskins, BSN, RN

Introduction

Delirium is a common and dangerous complication seen in patients with cancer. Once thought of as a normal course of confusion (e.g., intensive care unit [ICU] psychosis), ICU delirium is associated with detrimental short- and long-term adverse outcomes for critically ill patients. This chapter will define delirium and its associated outcomes, review the latest research for monitoring and management, and detail evidence-based tools crucial to identifying and responding to the needs of the delirious patient with cancer.

Etiology, Prevalence, and Subtypes

Delirium includes disturbances in attention and awareness in conjunction with a change in cognition not better accounted for by a preexisting, established, or evolving dementia. The disturbance is characterized by fluctuations during the day and develops over a short period (American Psychiatric Association, 2013). Delirium is a sign of acute brain dysfunction and should be taken as seriously as other organ dysfunctions, such as liver, heart, or kidney failure. The exact etiology of this acute and fluctuating disturbance of consciousness and cognition is still under investigation. Several hypotheses exist for ICU delirium etiology but require further study. A leading theory is that delirium is related to neurotransmitter imbalances. Various neurotransmitters may play a role in the development of delirium, but primary suppositions include the influence of excess dopamine, norepinephrine, and glutamate release; deficient acetylcholine and melatonin availability; and effects of alterations in histamine, gamma-aminobutyric acid, and 5-hydroxytryptamine on neuronal excitability (Maldonado, 2013). Imbalance in any of these neurotransmitters may cause neuronal instability and unpredictable neurotransmission. Routine actions performed within the hospital can influence neurotransmission, most commonly medications administered to the patient (e.g., benzodiazepines, anticholinergics, glucocorticoids) (Maldonado, 2013).

Although the exact etiology of delirium is still under investigation, it is a common problem. As much as 80% of mechanically ventilated (MV) patients, the sickest population within the ICU, develop delirium (Girard, Pandharipande, & Ely, 2008). Multiple ICU delirium risk factors have been reported (see Figure 13-1), with patients averaging 11 such factors (Ely, Gautam, et al., 2001). Risk factors with the strongest link to ICU delirium include preexisting dementia, hypertension, alcoholism, coma, benzodiazepine use, and a high severity of illness (Barr et al., 2013).

The three subtypes of delirium include hyperactive, hypoactive, and mixed. Hyperactive delirium (i.e., positive delirium screen with a hyperactive level of consciousness [LOC]) presents as a restlessness or agitation that may involve pulling at IV lines or the removal of artificial airways. It can escalate to a combativeness in which patients may become a danger to themselves or others (Morandi & Jackson, 2011). Conversely, patients with hypoactive delirium (i.e., positive delirium screen with a somnolent LOC) are more difficult to arouse or have difficulty maintaining arousal (e.g., appear to be sleeping or resting) (Morandi & Jackson, 2011). If patients are not drawing attention to themselves, as is the case with

---

Figure 13-1. Risk Factors for Delirium

Predisposing Factors	Precipitating Factors	Iatrogenic Factors
Patient factors	Factors of critical illness	Environment
• Demographics: Age	• Acute physiology/diagnosis	• Isolation
• Genetic: Apolipoprotein E4 polymorphism	• Anemia	• Daylight family visits
• Chronic comorbidities	• Anxiety	• Sleep disturbances
– Alcoholism	• Arterial pH/acidosis	Medications
– Cognitive impairment	• Coma	• Antipsychotics
– Depression	• Fever/infections/sepsis	• Benzodiazepines
– Hypertension	• High severity of illness	• Dopamine
– Vision or hearing impairment	• Hypotension	• Epidural use
• Lifestyle: Smoking	• Medical admission	• Opioids
	• Metabolic disturbances	• Propofol
	• Respiratory disease	Immobilization
		• Number of IV infusions
		• Number of tubes/catheters
		• Restraints

Note. Based on information from Girard et al., 2008; Vasilevskis et al., 2010.

hyperactive delirium, the clinical team may suppose no problem exists; however, a delirium assessment may reveal inattention, fluctuations in LOC, or disorganized thinking that may indicate an abnormality. Hypoactive delirium, the most prevalent delirium subtype, is frequently missed in clinical practice (Ely, Siegel, & Inouye, 2001). Mixed delirium represents patients that fluctuate and experience both hyperactive and hypoactive states of delirium (Pandharipande, Cotton, et al., 2007; Peterson et al., 2006).

Outcomes Associated With Intensive Care Unit Delirium

Outcomes associated with ICU delirium have a profound effect on the quality of life of individuals with critical illness, including increased time on mechanical ventilation, prolonged length of stay, a higher likelihood of death, and long-term cognitive impairment (Ely, Gautam, et al., 2001; Pandharipande et al., 2013). Each day of ICU delirium is correlated with a 10% reduction in survival at 6 and 12 months following hospital discharge (Ely et al., 2004; Pisani et al., 2009). Similarly, the presence of delirium is associated with fewer days alive and free of mechanical ventilation. This is a strong predictor of hospital length of stay (Ely, Gautam, et al., 2001). Delirium duration is associated with more than 50% of ICU survivors having long-term cognitive impairment, with a third of those having severe cognitive impairment akin to that of traumatic brain injury or Alzheimer disease (Pandharipande et al., 2013). Duration and severity of delirium are also correlated with higher ICU and hospital costs (Milbrandt et al., 2004).

Monitoring for Intensive Care Unit Delirium

If not routinely monitored for, ICU delirium often goes undetected. The Clinical Practice Guidelines for the Management of Pain, Agitation, and Delirium (PAD) in Adult Patients in the Intensive Care Unit, an integrated how-to manual for developing patient-centered protocols to guide practice and improve outcomes in critical care, recommend that all adult ICU patients be monitored for delirium every shift and as needed using either the Confusion Assessment Method for the Intensive Care Unit (CAM-ICU) or the Intensive Care Delirium Screening Checklist (ICDSC) (Barr et al., 2013; Bergeron, Dubois, Dumont, Dial, & Skrobik, 2001). These tools have been validated in both MV and non-MV ICU patients. If delirium is identified, it should be acted on quickly to reduce the burden of long-term adverse outcomes. An essential component of any delirium assessment is the evaluation of LOC, as fluctuations and alterations in LOC are delirium symptoms. Researchers recommend either the Richmond Agitation and

Sedation Scale (RASS) or the Riker Sedation-Agitation Scale (SAS) for the assessment of LOC in all ICU patients, regardless of the use of psychoactive medications (Ely et al., 2003; Riker, Picard, & Fraser, 1999). RASS and SAS provide clear descriptors of LOC states and a common language for communication.

Confusion Assessment Method for the Intensive Care Unit

CAM-ICU is a spot-check assessment for delirium that takes less than two minutes. If a patient can respond to vocal stimulation without need for physical stimulation (i.e., RASS −3 to +4 or SAS 3 to 7), CAM-ICU can be performed to assess for content of consciousness (i.e., delirium) (Ely, Inouye, et al., 2001; Ely, Margolin, et al., 2001). CAM-ICU assesses the following:
- Fluctuation in mental status or change from baseline
- Inattention
- Altered LOC
- Disorganized thinking

For a patient to be considered delirious, features 1, 2, and *either* 3 or 4 must be present (see Figure 13-2). Fluctuations in mental status (i.e., feature 1) do not exclude those related to sleep or administration of psychoactive medications (e.g., sedatives, analgesics, antipsychotics). Inattention (i.e., feature 2) is the cardinal feature of delirium and can be assessed using either a "Letter A" or "Picture" screening test. For more infomation on CAM-ICU, as well as answers to common questions and case scenarios for application, visit www.icudelirium.org.

Intensive Care Delirium Screening Checklist

ICDSC is an eight-item checklist that evaluates for the presence or absence inattention, disorientation, hallucination, delusion or psychosis, psychomotor agitation or retardation, inappropriate speech or mood, sleep–wake disturbances, and fluctuation of these symptoms (Bergeron et al., 2001). The presence of four or more symptoms during a specified evaluation period (i.e., 8- or 12-hour shift) indicates the presence of delirium.

Management Recommendations

Agitation may result from inadequately treated pain, anxiety, delirium, or ventilator dyssynchrony (Barr et al., 2013). Symptoms of extreme pain (e.g., restlessness, ventilator dyssynchrony, crying out) are similar to agitated LOC and hyperactive delirium. Conversely, oversedation is similar to somnolent LOC and hypoactive delirium. Management for delirium differs depending on the results of pain, LOC, and delirium assessments. For example, pain management may be most appropriate for hyperactive delirium accompanied by symptoms of extreme

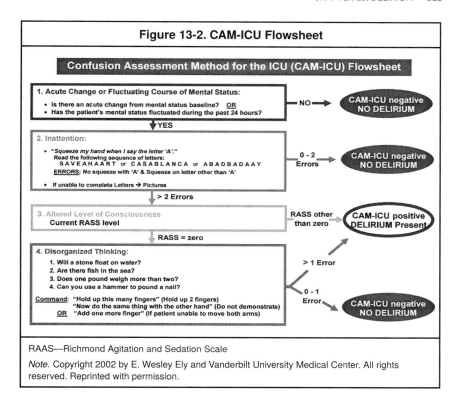

Figure 13-2. CAM-ICU Flowsheet

RAAS—Richmond Agitation and Sedation Scale

Note. Copyright 2002 by E. Wesley Ely and Vanderbilt University Medical Center. All rights reserved. Reprinted with permission.

pain, and reduction or cessation of sedative medications may be most appropriate for hypoactive delirium.

In general, delirium is an early warning sign of distress in the body. Prevention and management are largely focused on reducing risk and treating etiologic conditions. No one-size-fits-all approach exists, but the methods in this chapter can help clinicians address delirium and reduce adverse outcomes associated with delirium duration in patients with cancer.

Avoiding benzodiazepines and maintaining a more awake LOC, especially in patients at high risk for delirium (i.e., preexisting dementia, alcoholism, hypertension), may reduce prevalence and delirium duration (Barr et al., 2013). As an alternative to benzodiazepines, dexmedetomidine infusion administered for sedation may also be associated with a lower prevalence of delirium and is recommended for sedation in ICU patients with delirium unrelated to alcohol or benzodiazepine withdrawal (Pandharipande, Pun, et al., 2007; Riker et al., 2009). Clinicians should consider comfort strategies that involve analgesics as a primary treatment for sedation in MV patients (Barr et al., 2013). PAD guidelines suggest that patients participate in their own care (i.e., be awake and able to follow commands), unless contraindicated by a clinical condition (Barr et al., 2013).

Antipsychotic medications (e.g., haloperidol, quetiapine, olanzapine) are therapeutic agents commonly used for the treatment of agitation in the ICU; however, no current published evidence exists that treatment with haloperidol reduces delirium duration. Treatment with atypical antipsychotics (e.g., quetiapine) may reduce delirium duration in adult ICU patients (Barr et al., 2013). QTc interval should be monitored for any patients receiving antipsychotic medication. Antipsychotics should not be administered to patients at significant risk of torsade de pointes (e.g., baseline prolonged QTc, history of torsade de pointes, concomitant medications known to prolong QTc) (Barr et al., 2013).

When delirium is present, the THINK or Dr. DRE mnemonic can guide team discussion of delirium etiology and management approaches (Brummel et al., 2013):

- **T**oxic situation (e.g., organ failure [new], shock, dehydration, deliriogenic medications)
- **H**ypoxemia, hypercarbia
- **I**nfection (e.g., consider new nosocomial infection), inflammation, immobility
- **N**onpharmacologic interventions (e.g., treat pain, mobilize, reorient, lower noise, promote sleep)
- **K**$^+$ (potassium) or other electrolyte abnormalities
  Or
- **D**iseases (e.g., sepsis, organ failure)
- **D**rug **R**emoval (e.g., stop deliriogenic medications such as benzodiazepines, daily sedation interruption)
- **E**nvironment (e.g., remove restraints, orient, mobilize, reduce isolation, restore day/night pattern)

For an algorithm to guide interprofessional discussion of delirium management approaches based on pain, agitation, and delirium assessment results, see Figure 13-3 or visit www.icudelirium.org. Suggested actions are also included based on whether the patient is delirious, not delirious, or comatose.

Script for Interprofessional Communication: The Brain Roadmap

Assessment scales provide a common language for the communication of PAD findings (Pun, Balas, & Davidson, 2013). These scales are necessary to assess for the presence and intensity of PAD, to evaluate the response to treatment, and to help the interprofessional team determine therapeutic approaches. The Brain Roadmap is a script that can be used during interprofessional rounds, 1:1 rounds, or in emergency situations to clearly and concisely (approximately 10 seconds) communicate patient mental status with other clinicians (Brummel et al., 2013). Essential components of this map include pain assessment, LOC (target and actual), delirium assessment, and related medications (e.g., sedatives, analgesics,

Figure 13-3. Delirium Management Algorithm

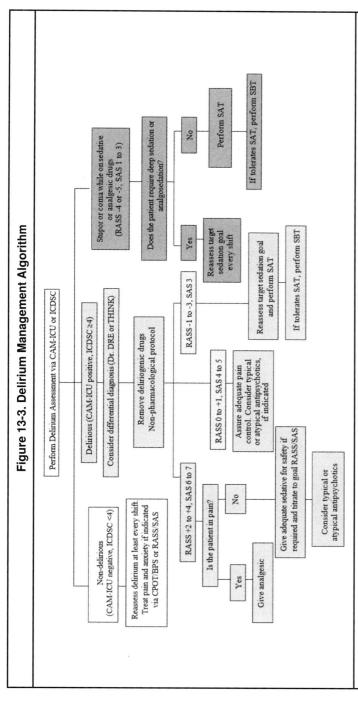

BPS—Behavioral Pain Scale; CAM-ICU—Confusion Assessment Method for the Intensive Care Unit; CPOT—Critical-Care Pain Observation Tool; ICDSC—Intensive Care Delirium Screening Checklist; RASS—Richmond Agitation and Sedation Scale; SAS—Sedation-Agitation Scale; SAT—spontaneous awakening trial; SBT—spontaneous breathing trial

Note. From "Management of Delirium in the ICU," by Delirium and Cognitive Impairment Study Group. Retrieved from http://www.icudelirium.org/delirium/management .html. Copyright 2013 by Vanderbilt University Medical Center. Reprinted with permission.

antipsychotics) (Brummel et al., 2013). The Brain Roadmap involves investigating and reporting the following:
- **Where is the patient going?** Report target LOC (RASS or SAS).
- **Where is the patient now?**
  - Report pain score (one of the following):
    * Numeric Rating Scale (NRS)
    * Behavioral Pain Scale (BPS)
    * Critical-Care Pain Observation Tool (CPOT)
  - Report actual LOC (RASS or SAS).
  - Report delirium assessment (CAM-ICU or ICDSC).
- **How did the patient get there?** Report sedatives, analgesics, or antipsychotics the patient is currently receiving or has received over the past 24 hours.

Following presentation of this information, it is possible for an interprofessional discussion of LOC target adjustments, changes in patient clinical status, potential etiology of changes, sedative medication changes or cessation, or opportunities for nonpharmacologic interventions for delirium (e.g., early mobility) (Brummel et al., 2013).

Interprofessional Care Approach: The ABCDEF Bundle

Barr et al. (2013) recommended the use of an interdisciplinary ICU team approach to care that included provider education, standing protocols and order sets, and quality rounding checklists to facilitate guidelines for management of PAD. The authors designed the multicomponent ABCDEF Bundle (see Figure 13-4) to bring cohesion to the recommended evidence-based practices in the PAD guidelines.

The bundle serves as a template for PAD guideline implementation that provides order to and alignment for currently existing people, processes, and technology to improve collaboration among disciplines and standardize processes of care in the ICU. Overall, the bundle reduces cognitive and physical dysfunction and dramatically improves the care of and outcomes for critically ill patients (Balas et al., 2014). High-value patient outcomes related to bundle components include improved likelihood of survival, reduced length of hospital stay, and improved physical function (Morandi, Brummel, & Ely, 2011).

Pain: Assess, Prevent, and Manage

Critically ill patients, including those with cancer, routinely experience pain, often related to procedures such as endotracheal suctioning, wound care, and turning. Leaving pain untreated can result in delirium and other complications (Barr et al., 2013). PAD guidelines recommend routine monitoring of pain using NRS for patients able to self-report or either BPS or CPOT for patients unable to

---

Figure 13-4. ABCDEF Bundle

A	• Assess, prevent and manage pain
B	• Both SATs and SBTs - coordinate Wake up and Breathe approach
C	• Choice of analgesia and sedation - thoughtful sedative/analgesic administration & meds to avoid
D	• Delirium: Assess, prevent and manage
E	• Early mobility - optimize mobility and advance as clinically able
F	• Family engagement and empowerment

SAT—spontaneous awakening trial; SBT—spontaneous breathing trial

Note. From "For Medical Professionals," by Delirium and Cognitive Impairment Study Group. Retrieved from http://www.icudelirium.org/medicalprofessionals.html. Copyright 2013 by Vanderbilt University Medical Center. Reprinted with permission.

---

communicate pain. These are considered the most valid and reliable pain scales for adult ICU patients based on rigorous psychometric testing (Barr et al., 2013).

Spontaneous Awakening and Breathing Trials

Awakening and breathing coordination is the daily performance of a spontaneous awakening trial (SAT; cessation of sedative medications) recommended by PAD guidelines followed by a spontaneous breathing trial (SBT; trial of independent breathing with minimal ventilator support) (Barr et al., 2013). This "wake-up and breathe" approach capitalizes on a more alert, cooperative patient during an SBT. In one study, use of this coordinated intervention resulted in reduced hospital length of stay, reduced prevalence of coma, a 14% absolute risk reduction in death at one year, and reduced incidence of cognitive impairment at three months (Girard et al., 2008). The Wake Up and Breathe flowchart for the coordination process and screening/failure criteria can be found at www.icudelirium.org.

Analgesia and Sedation

Maintaining patient comfort is an essential component of oncologic and critical care therapy. Ensuring patient comfort involves appropriate assessment and management of pain, anxiolysis, and prevention and treatment of delirium. Achieving appropriate balance of analgesia and sedation while reducing the risk of delirium can be challenging. PAD guidelines emphasize the treatment of pain and goal-directed delivery of sedatives (i.e., RASS or SAS targets) to avoid oversedation and promotion of earlier liberation from mechanical ventilation (Barr et al., 2013).

If additional sedatives are required for anxiolytics despite adequate analgesia, nonbenzodiazepine strategies (e.g., propofol, dexmedetomidine) are recommended to improve clinical outcomes in MV patients. Recommendations for goal-directed delivery of sedatives include RASS targets of 0 to −2 or SAS targets of 3 to 4 if clinically indicated.

Delirium: Assess, Prevent, and Manage

Routine screening for delirium using the most valid and reliable assessment tools (i.e., CAM-ICU or ICDSC) is recommended. Delirium screening improves the recognition of delirium, provides a method of concise communication of cognitive function, and signals the need for clinicians to evaluate and change aspects of critical care therapy to improve cognitive function (Devlin et al., 2007, 2008; Pun et al., 2005).

Early Mobility

Physical weakness and functional impairment during and following critical illness is a highly prevalent problem and a fundamental reason for early mobility as a component of the ABCDEF Bundle (Kress & Hall, 2014). Early mobility has been found to be both feasible and safe to perform with critically ill patients in the earliest days of ICU care and is the only nonpharmacologic intervention known to reduce delirium duration (Bailey et al., 2007; Pohlman et al., 2010; Schweickert et al., 2009). Successful application of early mobilization relies on a patient to be awake enough to participate. A "wake-up, breathe, and move" approach comprising sedative cessation or more awake LOC goals is recommended to ensure patient capability to participate in and advance through early mobility activities (e.g., active range of motion, dangle at edge of bed, active transfers, ambulation). Early mobility may require coordination with other disciplines depending on the patient's respiratory and functional status (e.g., respiratory therapy, physical/occupational therapy), but this can be performed by any trained member of the interprofessional team. A simple screening method for determining safe initiation is the MOVE screen (Schweickert et al., 2009):

- **M**yocardial stability
  - No evidence of active myocardial ischemia in the last 24 hours
  - No dysrhythmia requiring new antidysrhythmic agent in the last 24 hours
- **O**xygenation adequate on FiO_2 less than or equal to 0.60 and positive end-expiratory pressure less than 10 cm H_2O
- **V**asopressor(s) minimal: no increase in vasopressor(s) in the last 2 hours
- **E**ngages to voice: patient responds to verbal stimulation

Family Engagement and Empowerment

Critical illness and cancer influence the patient and his or her support system. It is important to meet the needs of the patient's social support network. Needs will vary, but emotional and social support, education, and resources are common. Communication with the support system early in a hospitalization should focus on building rapport and setting realistic expectations for ICU and oncology care and outcomes. Providing information on supportive services (e.g., support groups, websites, clergy, social work) can empower the patient's support system to seek out resources based on unique needs. Family members and friends serve an important role at the bedside by encouraging and assisting with completion of components of the ABCDEF Bundle, such as reorientation, cognitive stimulation, provision of glasses or other sensory needs, promotion of sleep hygiene, and encouragement of early mobilization when appropriate. Reminding family members and friends to take care of their own needs is important (e.g., proper nutrition and adequate sleep). Some members of the patient's social network may require counseling on the prevention of caregiver burnout and on personal health and emotional needs.

Summary

Delirium is a common and significant problem in the ICU with many etiologies and risk factors in patients with cancer. With early identification, PAD guidelines provide an integrated and evidence-based approach to addressing the pain, agitation, and delirium that frequently coexist in critical illness and cancer. Assessment of each of these syndromes allows for the targeting of therapeutic interventions to minimize morbidity and improve quality of life with patients with cancer who survive critical illness. Based on current evidence, a multicomponent approach to management is most appropriate. The ABCDEF Bundle is an interprofessional set of practices that can serve as a template for PAD guideline implementation.

References

American Psychiatric Association. (2013). *Diagnostic and statistical manual of mental disorders* (5th ed.). Washington, DC: Author.

Bailey, P., Thomsen, G.E., Spuhler, V.J., Blair, R., Jewkes, J., Bezdjian, L., ... Ramona, O. (2007). Early activity is feasible and safe in respiratory failure patients. *Critical Care Medicine, 35,* 139–145. doi:10.1097/01.CCM.0000251130.69568.87

Balas, M.C., Vasilevskis, E.E., Olsen, K.M., Schmid, K.K., Shostrom, V., Cohen, M.Z., ... Burke, W.J. (2014). Effectiveness and safety of the awakening and breathing coordination, delirium monitoring/management, and early exercise/mobility bundle. *Critical Care Medicine, 42,* 1024–1036. doi:10.1097/CCM.0000000000000129

Barr, J., Fraser, G.L., Puntillo, K., Ely, E.W., Gélinas, C., Dasta, J.F., … Jaeschke, R. (2013). Clinical practice guidelines for the management of pain, agitation, and delirium in adult patients in the intensive care unit. *Critical Care Medicine, 41,* 263–306. doi:10.1097/CCM .0b013e3182783b72

Bergeron, N., Dubois, M.J., Dumont, M., Dial, S., & Skrobik, Y. (2001). Intensive care delirium screening checklist: Evaluation of a new screening tool. *Intensive Care Medicine, 27,* 859–864.

Brummel, N.E., Vasilevskis, E.E., Han, J.H., Boehm, L., Pun, B.T., & Ely, E.W. (2013). Implementing delirium screening in the ICU: Secrets to success. *Critical Care Medicine, 41,* 2196–2208. doi:10.1097/CCM.0b013e31829a6f1e

Devlin, J.W., Fong, J.J., Schumaker, G., O'Connor, H., Ruthazer, R., & Garpestad, E. (2007). Use of a validated delirium assessment tool improves the ability of physicians to identify delirium in medical intensive care unit patients. *Critical Care Medicine, 35,* 2721–2724.

Ely, E.W., Gautam, S., Margolin, R., Francis, J., May, L., Speroff, T., … Inouye, S.K. (2001). The impact of delirium in the intensive care unit on hospital length of stay. *Intensive Care Medicine, 27,* 1892–1900. doi:10.1007/s00134-001-1132-2

Ely, E.W., Inouye, S.K., Bernard, G.R., Gordon, S., Francis, J., May, L., … Dittus, R. (2001). Delirium in mechanically ventilated patients: Validity and reliability of the confusion assessment method for the intensive care unit (CAM-ICU). *JAMA, 286,* 2703–2710.

Ely, E.W., Margolin, R., Francis, J., May, L., Truman, B., Dittus, R., … Inouye, S.K. (2001). Evaluation of delirium in critically ill patients: Validation of the Confusion Assessment Method for the Intensive Care Unit (CAM-ICU). *Critical Care Medicine, 29,* 1370–1379.

Ely, E.W., Shintani, A., Truman, B., Speroff, T., Gordon, S.M., Harrell, F.E., Jr., … Dittus, R.S. (2004). Delirium as a predictor of mortality in mechanically ventilated patients in the intensive care unit. *JAMA, 291,* 1753–1762. doi:10.1001/jama.291.14.1753

Ely, E.W., Siegel, M.D., & Inouye, S.K. (2001). Delirium in the intensive care unit: An underrecognized syndrome of organ dysfunction. *Seminars in Respiratory and Critical Care Medicine, 22,* 115–126. doi:10.1055/s-2001-13826

Ely, E.W., Truman, B., Shintani, A., Thomason, J.W.W., Wheeler, A.P., Gordon, S., … Bernard, G.R. (2003). Monitoring sedation status over time in ICU patients: Reliability and validity of the Richmond Agitation-Sedation Scale (RASS). *JAMA, 289,* 2983–2991. doi:10.1001/jama.289 .22.2983

Girard, T.D., Kress, J.P., Fuchs, B.D., Thomason, J.W.W., Schweickert, W.D., Pun, B.T., … Ely, E.W. (2008). Efficacy and safety of a paired sedation and ventilator weaning protocol for mechanically ventilated patients in intensive care (Awakening and Breathing Controlled trial): A randomised controlled trial. *Lancet, 371,* 126–134. doi:10.1016/S0140-6736(08)60105-1

Girard, T.D., Pandharipande, P.P., & Ely, E.W. (2008). Delirium in the intensive care unit. *Critical Care, 12*(Suppl. 3), S3. doi:10.1186/cc6149

Kress, J.P., & Hall, J.B. (2014). ICU-acquired weakness and recovery from critical illness. *New England Journal of Medicine, 371,* 1626–1635. doi:10.1056/NEJMc1406274

Maldonado, J.R. (2013). Neuropathogenesis of delirium: Review of current etiologic theories and common pathways. *American Journal of Geriatric Psychiatry, 21,* 1190–1222. doi:10.1016/j.jagp.2013.09.005

Milbrandt, E.B., Deppen, S., Harrison, P.L., Shintani, A.K., Speroff, T., Stiles, R.A., … Ely, E.W. (2004). Costs associated with delirium in mechanically ventilated patients. *Critical Care Medicine, 32,* 955–962.

Morandi, A., Brummel, N.E., & Ely, E.W. (2011). Sedation, delirium and mechanical ventilation: The ABCDE approach. *Current Opinion in Critical Care, 17,* 43–49. doi:10.1097/MCC .0b013e3283427243

Morandi, A., & Jackson, J.C. (2011). Delirium in the intensive care unit: A review. *Neurologic Clinics, 29,* 749–763. doi:10.1016/j.ncl.2011.08.004

Pandharipande, P.P., Cotton, B.A., Shintani, A.K., Thompson, J., Costabile, S., Pun, B.T., … Ely, E.W. (2007). Motoric subtypes of delirium in mechanically ventilated surgical and trauma intensive care unit patients. *Intensive Care Medicine, 33,* 1726–1731. doi:10.1007/s00134-007-0687-y

Pandharipande, P.P., Girard, T.D., Jackson, J.C., Morandi, A., Thompson, J.L., Pun, B.T., ... Ely, E.W. (2013). Long-term cognitive impairment after critical illness. *New England Journal of Medicine, 369,* 1306–1316. doi:10.1056/NEJMoa1301372

Pandharipande, P.P., Pun, B.T., Herr, D.L., Maze, M., Girard, T.D., Miller, R.R., ... Ely, E.W. (2007). Effect of sedation with dexmedetomidine vs lorazepam on acute brain dysfunction in mechanically ventilated patients: The MENDS randomized controlled trial. *JAMA, 298,* 2644–2653. doi:10.1001/jama.298.22.2644

Peterson, J.F., Pun, B.T., Dittus, R.S., Thomason, J.W.W., Jackson, J.C., Shintani, A.K., & Ely, E.W. (2006). Delirium and its motoric subtypes: A study of 614 critically ill patients. *Journal of the American Geriatrics Society, 54,* 479–484. doi:10.1111/j.1532-5415.2005.00621.x

Pisani, M.A., Kong, S.Y.J., Kasl, S.V., Murphy, T.E., Araujo, K.L.B., & Van Ness, P.H. (2009). Days of delirium are associated with 1-year mortality in an older intensive care unit population. *American Journal of Respiratory and Critical Care Medicine, 180,* 1092–1097. doi:10.1164/rccm.200904-0537OC

Pohlman, M.C., Schweickert, W.D., Pohlman, A.S., Nigos, C., Pawlik, A.J., Esbrook, C.L., ... Kress, J.P. (2010). Feasibility of physical and occupational therapy beginning from initiation of mechanical ventilation. *Critical Care Medicine, 38,* 2089–2094. doi:10.1097/CCM.0b013e3181f270c3

Pun, B.T., Balas, M.C., & Davidson, J. (2013). Implementing the 2013 PAD guidelines: Top ten points to consider. *Seminars in Respiratory and Critical Care Medicine, 34,* 223–235. doi:10.1055/s-0033-1342985

Pun, B.T., Gordon, S.M., Peterson, J.F., Shintani, A.K., Jackson, J.C., Foss, J., ... Ely, E.W. (2005). Large-scale implementation of sedation and delirium monitoring in the intensive care unit: A report from two medical centers. *Critical Care Medicine, 33,* 1199–1205.

Riker, R.R., Picard, J.T., & Fraser, G.L. (1999). Prospective evaluation of the Sedation-Agitation Scale for adult critically ill patients. *Critical Care Medicine, 27,* 1325–1329.

Riker, R.R., Shehabi, Y., Bokesch, P.M., Ceraso, D., Wisemandle, W., Koura, F., ... Rocha, W.G. (2009). Dexmedetomidine vs midazolam for sedation of critically ill patients: A randomized trial. *JAMA, 301,* 489–499. doi:10.1001/jama.2009.56

Schweickert, W.D., Pohlman, M.C., Pohlman, A.S., Nigos, C., Pawlik, A.J., Esbrook, C.L., ... Kress, J.P. (2009). Early physical and occupational therapy in mechanically ventilated, critically ill patients: A randomised controlled trial. *Lancet, 373,* 1874–1882. doi:10.1016/S0140-6736(09)60658-9

Vasilevskis, E.E., Pandharipande, P.P., Girard, T.D., & Ely, E.W. (2010). A screening, prevention, and restoration model for saving the injured brain in intensive care unit survivors. *Critical Care Medicine, 38*(Suppl. 10), S683–S691. doi:10.1097/CCM.0b013e3181f245d3

CHAPTER 14

Nutritional Support

Ainsley Malone, MS, RD, LD, CNSC, FAND, FASPEN

Introduction

Regardless of the oncologic condition, critical illness and injury result in profound metabolic alterations, beginning at the time of insult and persisting until wound healing and recovery. Whether the event involves sepsis, respiratory distress, or surgery, the systemic response is activated and has severe nutritional consequences. If not addressed, these consequences will result in significantly negative clinical outcomes.

This makes nutritional support of the critically ill patient with cancer essential. It is well known that malnourished patients will likely have worse outcomes compared to their well-nourished counterparts (Aapro et al., 2014). Malnourishment combined with insidious catabolism increases morbidity and mortality. This chapter will provide insight into the metabolic response to illness, describe nutrition status assessment, outline nutritional support modalities and their complications, and provide current evidence-based recommendations for nutrition care of the critically ill patient.

Metabolic Response to Stress

The metabolic response to critical illness, injury, sepsis, or major surgery is complex and involves many metabolic pathways. During this response, accelerated catabolism of lean body or skeletal mass occurs, which clinically results in net negative nitrogen balance and muscle wasting. Metabolic response includes both ebb and flow phases. The ebb phase, occurring immediately following injury, is associated with hypovolemia, shock, and tissue hypoxia. Insulin levels fall in response to an increase in glucagon, most likely as a signal to increase hepatic glucose production. Increased cardiac output, oxygen consumption, body temperature, energy expenditure, and total body protein catabolism characterize the flow phase, which follows fluid resuscitation and restoration of oxygen transport. Physiologically, a marked increase occurs in glucose production, free fatty acid release, circulating levels of insulin, catecholamines (epinephrine and norepinephrine released by the adrenal medulla), glucagon, and cortisol. The magnitude of the hormonal response appears to be associated with the severity of injury (Cuthbertson, 1930).

Metabolic stress is associated with an altered hormonal state that results in an increased flow of substrate and poor use of carbohydrate, protein, fat, and oxygen (Kinney, Duke, Long, & Gump, 1970). Counterregulatory hormones, elevated after injury and sepsis, play a key role in the accelerated proteolysis. Glucagon promotes gluconeogenesis, amino acid uptake by the liver, ureagenesis, and protein catabolism (Kinney et al., 1970). Cortisol enhances skeletal muscle catabolism and promotes hepatic use of amino acids for gluconeogenesis.

The cumulative effect of this metabolic response is a profound reliance on protein for fuel and significant loss of lean body mass. Patients with cancer experience some of the same metabolic abnormalities, which magnify the overall response. Cytokines, including tumor necrosis factor-alpha, interleukin-1, and interleukin-6, mediate these metabolic alterations.

Nutrition Status and Assessment

Malnutrition is common in patients with cancer (Kern & Norton, 1988). In a recent observational study of patients with cancer undergoing treatment, 41.6% were identified as moderately malnourished, and 26.4% were severely malnourished (Shpata et al., 2015). Malnourished patients with cancer are much more likely to experience negative outcomes, including reduced quality of life, reduced treatment effectiveness, increased postoperative complications, and death (Datema, Ferrier, & Baatenburg de Jong, 2011; Hill, Kiss, Hodgson, Crowe, & Walsh, 2011; Norman et al., 2010; Van Cutsem & Arends, 2005). For patients with cancer in the intensive care unit (ICU), the risk of malnutrition-related negative outcomes is exacerbated. Management of critical illness, coupled with the challenges in nutrient delivery, can lead to nutritional deterioration. This highlights the need for early nutrition assessment, identification, and intervention, especially in a population already at a high nutritional risk.

Nutrition Care Pathway

In 2015, the American Society for Parenteral and Enteral Nutrition (ASPEN) published *Improve Patient Outcomes*, a clinician's guide to identifying and treating the malnourished patient. The first step in identifying a malnourished patient with cancer in the ICU is to perform a nutrition screening. This screening must be completed within 24 hours of admission to the hospital, as required by the Joint Commission. In many settings, screening is completed by the admitting nurse (Patel et al., 2014). If a patient is hospitalized and then transferred to the ICU, a nutrition rescreening will be performed, usually by a dietitian (ASPEN, 2015). In either process, if a patient is determined to be at significant nutritional risk, the dietitian will perform a complete nutrition assessment. A nutrition assessment is defined as "a comprehensive approach to defining the nutrition state that uses a combination of the following: medical, nutrition, and medication histories; physical examination; anthropometric measurements; and laboratory data" (ASPEN, 2015, p. 4). Key parameters include, among others, weight status, nutrient intake, evidence of muscle and subcutaneous fat loss, edema, and functional status (Jensen, Hsiao, & Wheeler, 2012).

Malnutrition Diagnosis

The historical definition of malnutrition has recently been reevaluated. In 2009, an international group of nutrition leaders developed an etiologic basis for the definition of malnutrition for hospitalized adult patients. This approach recognized the key role of inflammation and focused on three etiologies: starvation-related malnutrition, chronic disease–related malnutrition, and acute disease–related malnutrition (Jensen, Bistrian, Roubenoff, & Heimburger, 2009).

Using the revised definition, ASPEN and the Academy of Nutrition and Dietetics published a consensus document outlining specific criteria for diagnosing severe and nonsevere malnutrition (White, Guenter, Jensen, Malone, & Schofield, 2012) (see Figure 14-1).

Each etiology is defined by specific criteria and severity thresholds. For example, critically ill patients with cancer could present with chronic disease–related malnutrition because of their underlying cancer and its treatment, or if malnutrition develops while in the ICU, acute illness and injury would be the etiology.

Figure 14-1. Consensus Characteristics to Identify Adult Malnutrition

- Insufficient energy intake
- Weight loss
- Loss of muscle mass
- Loss of subcutaneous fat
- Localized or generalized fluid accumulation
- Diminished handgrip strength

Note. Based on information from White et al., 2012.

Nutritional Support Interventions

The preferred route for nutrient delivery is an orally consumed diet of whole foods; however, critically ill patients often are unable to eat because of endotracheal intubation, ventilator dependence, or the absence of gastrointestinal (GI) function in those undergoing complex surgical procedures. Furthermore, oral feeding may be delayed by chewing or swallowing impairment or by anorexia caused by pain-relieving medications. Patients who can eat may not be able to meet the increased energy and nutrient requirements associated with metabolic stress and recovery. Peterson et al. (2010) reported that patients frequently consumed, at best, only 50% of their estimated requirements postextubation. Critically ill patients with cancer often will require a combination of oral nutritional supplements, enteral nutrition (EN), and parenteral nutrition (PN). When EN fails to meet nutritional requirements or when GI feeding is contraindicated, PN support should be initiated.

Timing and Route of Feeding

EN is the preferred route of feeding for the critically ill patient with good GI function who cannot eat food. Feedings should be initiated within 24–48 hours of ICU admission (McClave et al., 2016). Overt signs of GI motility, including passing of flatus and the presence of bowel sounds, are not required for EN initiation (McClave et al., 2016). This practice is intended for hemodynamically stable patients with mean arterial pressures greater than 50 mm Hg. In the setting of hemodynamic instability (i.e., large volume requirements or use of high-dose catecholamine agents), EN should be withheld until the patient is fully resuscitated or stable to minimize risk of ischemic or reperfusion injury (McClave et al., 2016). EN is safe in patients receiving vasopressors when hemodynamic stability is achieved and may offer a benefit. One study reported improved outcomes in those who were fed less than 48 hours after ICU admission and on vasopressor agents compared to those who were fed more than 48 hours after admission (Khalid, Doshi, & DiGiovine, 2010). In malnourished patients, advanced feedings are recommended within 48–72 hours of initiation to achieve more than 80% of goal energy and protein intakes (McClave et al., 2016). This approach may prevent increases in GI permeability (Jabbar, Chang, Dryden, & McClave, 2003) and improve clinical outcomes (Jie et al., 2012). Either gastric or small-bowel feedings can be used in patients requiring EN. In most patients, it is acceptable to initiate EN in the stomach (McClave et al., 2016). Small-bowel feedings are indicated for individuals considered at high aspiration risk (e.g., history of aspiration, reduced level of consciousness, supine positioning, neurologic deficits, gastroesophageal reflux) (McClave et al., 2016). Nasojejunal or surgically placed feeding tubes can be placed intraoperatively for patients undergoing complicated oncologic surgery procedures, such as those involving the pancreaticobiliary system, the esophagus, or GI tract.

PN is indicated for patients when EN is unsuccessful or contraindicated. Supplemental PN is appropriate after seven days of enteral feeding when goal requirements cannot be met or early EN is not feasible (McClave et al., 2016). This recommendation applies to patients not at nutritional risk. For the malnourished patient with cancer, PN should be initiated as soon as possible following ICU admission to supplement EN or provide full nutrition when EN is not feasible (August & Huhmann, 2009; McClave et al., 2016).

Enteral Formulas

EN formulas can be classified as standard, elemental, or specialized. Standard formulas often meet a patient's nutritional requirements and frequently cost less than elemental or specialized formulas.

Standard Formulas

Standard formulas are used in most patients who require tube feedings. The nutrient sources provided are essentially equal to those consumed by healthy individuals. Additional product types include those with higher protein content, supplemental fiber, and those with a greater nutrient concentration.

Dietary fiber comprises the edible parts of plants resistant to digestion and absorption in the human small intestine (American Association of Cereal Chemistry, n.d.). Fiber formulas can be considered in enterally fed patients who develop diarrhea; however, fiber is not recommended as an initial formula in critically ill patients because of reduced peristalsis (McClave et al., 2016).

Elemental Formulas

Elemental formulas are those with predigested or hydrolyzed macronutrients. The primary indication for these formulas is the presence of GI dysfunction, including persistent diarrhea (McClave et al., 2016). Elemental formulas are indicated in patients with malabsorption, pancreatic dysfunction, short bowel syndrome, or other evidence of GI disease; however, in those with normal GI function, standard enteral formulas should be routinely used.

Specialized Formulas

Specialized formulas encompass a wide range of products and are designed for a variety of clinical conditions or disease states. Evidence supporting routine use is limited (Malone & Farnejad, 2016).

Renal formulas are best used when dialysis is delayed or not planned. In this setting, a calorically dense, reduced-protein and reduced-electrolyte formula is appropriate. However, patients undergoing renal replacement therapy often have significantly increased protein requirements that are unachievable with a renal formula (Scheinkestel et al., 2003). Standard calorically dense formulas are frequently appropriate for these patients.

EN formulas for diabetes mellitus have been designed to assist in the control of blood glucose levels. The routine use of a diabetic formula does not appear to be warranted; however, in specific instances when blood glucose control becomes problematic despite adequate insulin usage, diabetic formulas may offer an advantage in facilitating improved glucose control (Malone & Farnejad, 2016).

An EN formula specifically designed for acute respiratory distress syndrome (ARDS) offers a modified lipid component designed to potentially modulate the inflammatory cascade that occurs in this setting. Limited evidence exists supporting improved clinical outcomes with this formula type; therefore, it is not recommended for routine use in patients with ARDS (McClave et al., 2016).

Immune-enhancing formulas (IEFs) are designed to enhance the immune system by offering specific nutrients, such as arginine, nucleotides, and n-3 fatty acids, known to promote beneficial effects, such as reduced infectious and wound complications and decreased hospital length of stay (Marik & Zaloga, 2010). Evidence exists of IEFs benefiting patients undergoing complex surgical procedures, including oncologic procedures. Perioperative use of IEFs is recommended for those undergoing complex surgical procedures and those with traumatic brain injury (McClave et al., 2016).

Complications of Enteral Nutrition

The most frequently encountered complications with EN involve GI issues, such as nausea and vomiting, diarrhea, and elevated gastric residual volumes (GRVs) (Malone, Seres, & Lord, 2012).

Nausea and Vomiting

Nausea and/or vomiting occurs in approximately 12%–20% of patients who receive EN (Malone et al., 2012). Multiple etiologies exist for nausea and vomiting with EN (Malone & Farnejad, 2016). In the critically ill patient, delayed gastric emptying is common, with a reported incidence between 50% and 80% (Fruhwald & Kainz, 2010). If delayed gastric emptying is suspected, consider reducing or discontinuing all narcotic medications or administering a prokinetic agent (e.g., metoclopramide, erythromycin). Multiple studies have demonstrated improved gastric emptying with prokinetic therapy (Hersch et al., 2015; Ridley & Davies, 2011). If adequate feeding volumes cannot be achieved because of persistent delayed gastric emptying, the placement of a small-bowel feeding tube is highly recommended and will result in improved EN delivery (Metheny, Davis-Jackson, & Stewart, 2010).

Gastric Residual Volumes

The GRV measurement in the patient receiving enteral tube feeding has long been recommended as a determinant of EN tolerance. The rationale for this is the belief that GRV indirectly assesses gastric emptying and can ultimately be used to assess risk of regurgitation and subsequent aspiration (McClave et al., 2016); however, inherent flaws exist. The argument for using GRV does not account for the 1,500–3,000 ml of daily combined salivary and gastric secretions. In addition, studies have shown that GRVs do not correlate with altered gastric emptying (McClave et al., 2016). Current nutrition care guidelines suggest that GRVs should not be used as a part of routine care to monitor EN in ICU patients. The authors instead recommended routine daily physical examination, review of abdominal radiology, and evaluation of risk factors for aspiration (McClave et al., 2016). Recognizing that GRV assessment may still be used in many facilities, the guideline authors recommended avoiding holding EN for GRVs less than 500 ml in the absence of other signs of intolerance (McClave et al., 2016).

Abdominal Distension

Abdominal distension and increased GRVs are two common reasons for EN interruption (De Jonghe et al., 2001; Montejo et al., 2002). Distension and its associated symptoms of bloating and cramping commonly occur because of GI ileus, obstruction, obstipation, ascites, and diarrheal illness. Initial use of a fiber-supplemented formula may also occasionally contribute to abdominal distension. Distension because of ileus or mechanical bowel obstruction may often be diagnosed from a flat and upright abdominal x-ray; however, this method may miss fluid-filled loops of bowel and ascites. If intestinal appearance and function are normal, EN may be continued despite the distension. However, the discontinuation of feedings may be necessary if motility is poor or if the bowel is markedly dilated.

Diarrhea

Diarrhea is the most commonly reported GI side effect in patients receiving EN and occurs frequently in critically ill patients (Lebak, Bliss, Savik, & Patten-Marsh, 2003). In a recent observational study of 150 mechanically ventilated ICU patients, a 73% diarrhea incidence was identified (Dionne et al., 2015). Stool volume can be directly measured by using a fecal management system. Stool volume of greater than 500 ml or more than three liquid stools per day is the standard definition of diarrhea (Lebak et al., 2003). Common causes in patients receiving EN include medications (e.g., liquid medications in a sorbitol base, antibiotics), infection (e.g., *Clostridium difficile*, nonclostridial bacteria), and intolerance (Malone et al., 2012).

If clinically significant diarrhea develops during EN, the following management options should be considered (Malone et al., 2012): medical assessment of the patient for infectious or inflammatory causes, fecal impaction, or use of medications that induce diarrhea; the addition of fiber to the EN regimen; use of an antidiarrheal agent once *Clostridium difficile* has been ruled out or is being treated; or continuation of EN as tolerated and initiation of PN. A systematic approach can be very effective in managing diarrhea (Greenwood, 2010).

Parenteral Nutrition

PN comprises IV dextrose, crystalline amino acids (CAAs), and lipids. CAAs provide the protein source in PN formulations and yield 4 kcal/g. IV fat emulsions (IVFEs) are used as a source of energy, essential fats and linoleic and linolenic acids. PN formulas may be prepared in a two-in-one or three-in-one format. The two-in-one preparation combines dextrose and CAA base solutions with other additives in containers (single or multiple) for infusion. IVFE is infused separately, either daily or intermittently, as a piggyback infusion. In a three-in-one preparation, all three macronutrients are compounded together in the same container. Higher dextrose concentrations (greater than 10%) are reserved for central PN because of their propensity for causing thrombophlebitis in the peripheral vein (Mirtallo & Patel, 2012). Evidence demonstrates a potential negative impact with the use of high omega-6 fatty acids, the primary fatty acid of currently available parenteral fat emulsions (Battistella et al., 1997). High intakes of omega-6 fatty acids are associated with aggravation of inflammatory states, such as ARDS and sepsis. Guidelines recommend withholding IV lipids in the nonmalnourished patient for seven days; however, evidence is lacking (McClave et al., 2016). IVFE should be avoided in patients with triglyceride-induced pancreatitis or with serum triglycerides greater than 400 mg/dl (Kumpf & Gervasio, 2012).

Electrolytes are added to the PN formula to meet individual patient requirements. Electrolyte requirements can vary greatly depending on body weight, organ function, degree of catabolism, presence of malnutrition, electrolyte losses, and administered medications. Trace elements are provided daily in a combination product for most patients to meet individual requirements. Patients with advanced liver disease may have copper and manganese removed, as they are metabolized by the liver and can accumulate.

For those with excessive GI or fistula losses, additional amounts of zinc are added. Glutamine, an amino acid important for immune function, has recently received attention as an additive to PN formulas. Because of its instability, a product that can be added to PN formulas is not currently commercially available. Glutamine supplementation has been studied in the critically ill population with significantly negative results and is not recommended for use in the ICU (Heyland et al., 2013; McClave et al., 2016).

The PN formula can also be used as a medium for the delivery of certain medications; however, this should not be used as a routine practice because of limited compatibility information (Ayers et al., 2014). Specifically, insulin and famotidine can be directly added to the PN formula.

Complications of Parenteral Nutrition

Complications with PN are common, but they can be minimized with judicious management, specifically by those with significant expertise (Naylor, Griffiths, & Fernandez, 2004). Common acute complications include hyperglycemia, electrolyte abnormalities, liver function abnormalities, and central line–associated bloodstream infection (CLABSI) (Kumpf & Gervasio, 2012). Of all potential complications, CLABSI carries the greatest risk of morbidity and mortality. Central line care is of utmost importance, including the use of a bundled care approach, which comprises hand hygiene, maximal barrier protection, chlorhexidine skin antisepsis, optimal site selection, and the daily review of line necessity (O'Grady et al., 2011).

Hyperglycemia

Hyperglycemia is the most common acute metabolic complication with PN. Multiple causes exist for the development of hyperglycemia, including stress metabolism, medications (e.g., steroids), underlying diabetes, obesity, and frequent large doses of IV dextrose (McMahon, 2004). It is important to achieve adequate glycemic control prior to the start of PN to minimize excessive hyperglycemia (Mirtallo & Patel, 2012). A glucose range of 140–180 mg/dl is recommended by multiple organizations (McClave et al., 2016). Efforts to manage glucose during PN administration include providing reduced amounts of PN dextrose until glycemic control is achieved, identifying and removing additional dextrose sources, and providing insulin as needed to achieve desired glucose levels. Insulin can be provided in the PN formula as sliding scale coverage or via a continuous infusion. With many critically ill patients, a continuous insulin infusion is preferable because of the labile nature of metabolic status. Insulin doses can more easily and safely be titrated via a continuous infusion outside of the PN infusion. Close attention to clinical status is imperative with all patients receiving insulin while on PN. As clinical status improves, glucose elevations can resolve quickly. Hypoglycemia risk increases if insulin adjustments are not made in a timely fashion (McMahon, Nystrom, Braunschweig, Miles, & Compher, 2013).

Electrolyte Abnormalities

Electrolyte abnormalities frequently occur in critically ill patients receiving PN. In a European observational study of ICU patients receiving PN, approximately 14% experienced abnormalities in serum electrolytes (Braga et al., 2001). Perhaps one of the greatest contributors to electrolyte abnormalities in PN patients is the presence of refeeding syndrome. This is a constellation of metabolic and physiologic shifts of fluid, electrolytes, and minerals that occurs because of aggressive nutritional repletion of a malnourished patient (Crook, Hally, & Panteli, 2001; Solomon & Kirby, 1990). The incidence of refeeding-induced electrolyte abnormalities varies with the population and degree of malnutrition. Abnormalities of phosphorus, potassium, and magnesium are most frequent in those who experience refeeding, with hypophosphatemia as the most common (Martinez et al., 2006). Interventions to minimize electrolyte abnormalities with PN include recognition of malnutrition-induced refeeding, repletion of low levels prior to the start of PN, and aggressive supplementation of low potassium, phosphorus, and magnesium levels during PN therapy.

Liver Function Abnormalities

Acute changes in liver function tests are common in patients receiving PN. If abnormalities occur, they generally take place within two weeks of PN initiation. This elevation reflects steatosis and generally is benign. Mild elevation of aminotransferases typically resolves with initiation of EN nutrition or discontinuation of PN. If they remain elevated during PN therapy, management strategies include minimizing overfeeding and changing PN from a continuous to a cycled infusion (Kumpf & Gervasio, 2012).

Summary

Critical illness is a profound metabolic and physical stress for any patient, including the patient with cancer. Nutritional support is a key component of treatment during a patient's course in the ICU. Prevention and/or treatment of malnutrition is imperative to minimize malnutrition-related negative outcomes. EN is the preferred modality, reserving PN for when EN is unavailable or contraindicated. Complications for either therapy can be minimized through recognition of the most prevalent adverse effects and management provided by an expert healthcare team.

References

Aapro, M., Arends, J., Bozzetti, F., Fearon, K., Grunberg, S.M., Herrstedt, J., … Strasser, F. (2014). Early recognition of malnutrition and cachexia in the cancer patient: A position paper of a European School of Oncology Task Force. *Annals of Oncology, 25,* 1492–1499. doi:10.1093/annonc/mdu085

American Association of Cereal Chemistry. (n.d.). Dietary fiber. Retrieved from http://www.aaccnet .org/initiatives/definitions/Pages/DietaryFiber.aspx

American Society for Parenteral and Enteral Nutrition. (2015). *Improve patient outcomes: ASPEN's step-by-step guide to addressing malnutrition.* Silver Spring, MD: Author.

August, D.A., & Huhmann, M.B. (2009). ASPEN clinical guidelines: Nutrition support therapy during adult anticancer treatment and in hematopoietic cell transplantation. *Journal of Parenteral and Enteral Nutrition, 33,* 472–500. doi:10.1177/0148607109341804

Ayers, P., Adams, S., Boullata, J., Gervasio, J., Holcombe, B., Kraft, M.D., … Guenter, P. (2014). ASPEN parenteral nutrition safety consensus recommendations: Translation into practice. *Nutrition in Clinical Practice, 29,* 277–282. doi:10.1177/0884533614531294

Battistella, F.D., Widergren, J.T., Anderson, J.T., Siepler, J.K., Weber, J.C., & MacColl, K. (1997). A prospective, randomized trial of intravenous fat emulsion administration in trauma victims requiring parenteral nutrition. *Journal of Trauma and Acute Care Surgery, 43,* 52–58.

Braga, M., Gianotti, L., Gentilini, O., Parisi, V., Salis, C., & Di Carlo, V. (2001). Early postoperative enteral nutrition improves gut oxygenation and reduces costs compared with total parenteral nutrition. *Critical Care Medicine, 29,* 242–248.

Crook, M.A., Hally, V., & Panteli, J.V. (2001). The importance of the refeeding syndrome. *Nutrition, 17,* 632–637.

Cuthbertson, D. (1930). Effect of injury on metabolism. *Biochemical Journal, 2,* 1244.

Datema, F.R., Ferrier, M.B., & Baatenburg de Jong, R.J. (2011). Impact of severe malnutrition on short-term mortality and overall survival in head and neck cancer. *Oral Oncology, 47,* 910–914. doi:10.1016/j.oraloncology.2011.06.510

De Jonghe, B., Appere-De-Vechi, C., Fournier, M., Tran, B., Merrer, J., Melchior, J.C., & Outin, H. (2001). A prospective survey of nutritional support practices in intensive care unit patients: What is prescribed? What is delivered? *Critical Care Medicine, 29,* 8–12.

Dionne, J., Saunders, L., Duan, E., Sullivan, K., Takaoka, A., Heels-Ansdell, D., … Cook, D. (2015). Diarrhea during critical illness. *Critical Care Medicine, 43,* 95. doi:10.1097/01.ccm.0000474202 .28311.e4

Fruhwald, S., & Kainz, J. (2010). Effect of ICU interventions on gastrointestinal motility. *Current Opinion in Critical Care, 16,* 159–164. doi:10.1097/MCC.0b013e3283356679

Greenwood, J. (2010). Management of diarrhea algorithm. Retrieved from http://criticalcarenutrition .com/docs/tools/Diarrhea.pdf

Hersch, M., Krasilnikov, V., Helviz, Y., Zevin, S., Reissman, P., & Einav, S. (2015). Prokinetic drugs for gastric emptying in critically ill ventilated patients: Analysis through breath testing. *Journal of Critical Care, 30,* 655.e7–655.e13. doi:10.1016/j.jcrc.2014.12.019

Heyland, D., Muscedere, J., Wischmeyer, P.E., Cook, D., Jones, G., Albert, M., … Day, A.G. (2013). A randomized trial of glutamine and antioxidants in critically ill patients. *New England Journal of Medicine, 368,* 1489–1497. doi:10.1056/NEJMoa1212722

Hill, A., Kiss, N., Hodgson, B., Crowe, T.C., & Walsh, A.D. (2011). Associations between nutritional status, weight loss, radiotherapy treatment toxicity and treatment outcomes in gastrointestinal cancer patients. *Clinical Nutrition, 30,* 92–98. doi:10.1016/j.clnu.2010.07.015

Jabbar, A., Chang, W.K., Dryden, G.W., & McClave, S.A. (2003). Gut immunology and the differential response to feeding and starvation. *Nutrition in Clinical Practice, 18,* 461–482. doi:10 .1177/0115426503018006461

Jensen, G.L., Bistrian, B., Roubenoff, R., & Heimburger, D.C. (2009). Malnutrition syndromes: A conundrum vs. a continuum. *Journal of Parenteral and Enteral Nutrition, 33,* 710–716.

Jensen, G.L., Hsiao, P.Y., & Wheeler, D. (2012). Nutrition screening and assessment. In C.M. Mueller (Ed.), *The ASPEN adult nutrition support core curriculum* (2nd ed., pp. 155–169). Silver Spring, MD: American Society for Parenteral and Enteral Nutrition.

Jie, B., Jiang, Z.M., Nolan, M.T., Zhu, S.N., Yu, K., & Kondrup, J. (2012). Impact of preoperative nutritional support on clinical outcome in abdominal surgical patients at nutritional risk. *Nutrition, 28,* 1022–1027. doi:10.1016/j.nut.2012.01.017

Kern, K.A., & Norton, J.A. (1988). Cancer cachexia. *Journal of Parenteral and Enteral Nutrition, 12,* 286–298. doi:10.1177/0148607188012003286

Khalid, I., Doshi, P., & DiGiovine, B. (2010). Early enteral nutrition and outcomes of critically ill patients treated with vasopressors and mechanical ventilation. *American Journal of Critical Care, 19,* 261–268. doi:10.4037/ajcc2010197

Kinney, J.M., Duke, J.H., Long, C.L., & Gump, F.E. (1970). Tissue fuel and weight loss after injury. *Journal of Clinical Pathology, 4,* 65–67.

Kumpf, V.J., & Gervasio, J. (2012). Complications of parenteral nutrition. In C.M. Mueller (Ed.), *Adult nutrition support core curriculum* (2nd ed., pp. 284–297). Silver Spring, MD: American Society for Parenteral and Enteral Nutrition.

Lebak, K.J., Bliss, D.Z., Savik, K., & Patten-Marsh, K.M. (2003). What's new on defining diarrhea in tube-feeding studies? *Clinical Nursing Research, 12,* 174–204. doi:10.1177/1054773803012002005

Malone, A.M., & Farnejad, F. (2016). Organ failure and specialized enteral formulas. In D.S. Seres & C.W. Van Way (Eds.), *Nutrition support for the critically ill* (pp. 157–172). Charm, Switzerland: Humana Press.

Malone, A.M., Seres, D.S., & Lord, L. (2012). Challenges and complications with enteral nutrition. In C.M. Mueller (Ed.), *Adult nutrition support core curriculum* (2nd ed., pp. 218–232). Silver Spring, MD: American Society for Parenteral and Enteral Nutrition.

Marik, P.E., Zaloga, G.P. (2010). Immunonutrition in high-risk surgical patients: A systematic review and analysis of the literature. *Journal of Parenteral and Enteral Nutrition, 34,* 378–386. doi:10.1177/0148607110362692

Martinez, M.J., Martinez, M.A., Montero, M., Campelo, E., Castro, I., & Inaraja, M.T. (2006). Hypophosphatemia in postoperative patients with total parenteral nutrition: Influence of nutritional support teams. *Nutricion Hospitalaria, 21,* 657–660.

McClave, S.A., Taylor, B.E., Martindale, R.G., Warren, M.M., Johnson, D.R., Braunschweig, C., … Compher, C. (2016). Guidelines for the provision and assessment of nutrition support therapy in the adult critically ill patient: Society of Critical Care Medicine (SCCM) and American Society for Parenteral and Enteral Nutrition (ASPEN). *Journal of Parenteral and Enteral Nutrition, 40,* 159–211. doi:10.1177/0148607115621863

McMahon, M.M. (2004). Management of parenteral nutrition in acutely ill patients with hyperglycemia. *Nutrition in Clinical Practice, 19,* 120–128. doi:10.1177/0115426504019002120

McMahon, M.M., Nystrom, E., Braunschweig, C., Miles, J., & Compher, C. (2013). ASPEN clinical guidelines: Nutrition support of adult patients with hyperglycemia. *Journal of Parenteral and Enteral Nutrition, 37,* 23–36. doi:10.1177/0148607112452001

Metheny, N.A., Davis-Jackson, J., & Stewart, B.J. (2010). Effectiveness of an aspiration risk-reduction protocol. *Nursing Research, 59,* 18–25. doi:10.1097/NNR.0b013e3181c3ba05

Mirtallo, J.M., & Patel, M. (2012). Overview of parenteral nutrition. In C.M. Mueller (Ed.), *Adult nutrition support core curriculum* (2nd ed., pp. 233–244). Silver Spring, MD: American Society for Parenteral and Enteral Nutrition.

Montejo, J.C., Grau, T., Acosta, J., Ruiz-Santana, S., Planas, M., García-de-Lorenzo, A., … López-Martínez, J. (2002). Multicenter, prospective, randomized, single-blind study comparing the efficacy and gastrointestinal complications of early jejunal feeding with early gastric feeding in critically ill patients. *Critical Care Medicine, 30,* 796–800.

Naylor, C.J., Griffiths, R.D., & Fernandez, R.S. (2004). Does a multidisciplinary total parenteral nutrition team improve patient outcomes? A systematic review. *Journal of Parenteral and Enteral Nutrition, 28,* 251–258.

Norman, K., Stobäus, N., Smoliner, C., Zocher, D., Scheufele, R., Valentini, L., ... Pirlich, M. (2010). Determinants of handgrip strength, knee extension strength and functional status in cancer patients. *Clinical Nutrition, 29,* 586–591. doi:10.1016/j.clnu.2010.02.007

O'Grady, N.P., Alexander, M., Burns, L.A., Dellinger, E.P., Garland, J., Heard, S.O., ... Saint, S. (2011). Guidelines for the prevention of intravascular catheter-related infections. *Clinical Infectious Diseases, 52,* e162–e193. doi:10.1093/cid/cir257

Patel, V., Romano, M., Corkins, M.R., DiMaria-Ghalili, R.A., Earthman, C., Malone, A.M., ... Guenter, P. (2014). Nutrition screening and assessment in hospitalized patients: A survey of current practice in the United States. *Nutrition in Clinical Practice, 29,* 483–490.

Peterson, S.J., Tsai, A.A., Scala, C.M., Sowa, D.C., Sheean, P.M., & Braunschweig, C.L. (2010). Adequacy of oral intake in critically ill patients 1 week after extubation. *Journal of the American Dietetic Association, 110,* 427–433. doi:10.1016/j.jada.2009.11.020

Ridley, D.E., & Davies, A.R. (2011). Practicalities of nutrition support in the intensive care unit: The usefulness of gastric residual volume and prokinetic agents with enteral nutrition. *Nutrition, 27,* 509–512. doi:10.1016/j.nut.2010.10.010

Scheinkestel, C.D., Adams, F., Mahony, L., Bailey, M., Davies, A.R., Nyulasi, I., & Tuxen, D.V. (2003). Impact of increasing parenteral protein loads on amino acid levels and balance in critically ill anuric patients on continuous renal replacement therapy. *Nutrition, 19,* 733–740.

Shpata, V., Kreka, B., Kreka, M., Nurçe, A., Refatllari, B., & Prendushi, X. (2015). MON-PP097: Malnutrition and cancer cachexia during anticancer therapy, call for interdisciplinary approach to cancer patients. *Clinical Nutrition, 34*(Suppl. 1), S164. doi:10.1016/S0261-5614(15)30529-X

Solomon, S.M., & Kirby, D.F. (1990). The refeeding syndrome: A review. *Journal of Parenteral and Enteral Nutrition, 14,* 90–97. doi:10.1177/014860719001400190

Van Cutsem, E., & Arends, J. (2005). The causes and consequences of cancer-associated malnutrition. *European Journal of Oncology Nursing, 9*(Suppl. 2), S51–S63. doi:10.1016/j.ejon.2005.09.007

White, J.V., Guenter, P., Jensen, G.L., Malone, A.M., & Schofield, M. (2012). Consensus statement: Academy of Nutrition and Dietetics and American Society for Parenteral and Enteral Nutrition: Characteristics recommended for the identification and documentation of adult malnutrition (undernutrition). *Journal of Parenteral and Enteral Nutrition, 36,* 275–283.

CHAPTER 15

Early Mobility in the Intensive Care Unit

Yolanda Michelle VanRiel, PhD, RN-BC, OCN®, CNE, ANEF, and
Donald D. Kautz, RN, PhD, CRRN, ACNS-BC

Introduction

Patients may be admitted to the intensive care unit (ICU) because of complications of cancer, including tumor lysis syndrome, superior vena cava syndrome, neutropenia, or chemotherapy-related issues. These patients may also have comorbid syndromes that become life threatening and necessitate an ICU stay, such as diabetes mellitus, cardiac disease, or chronic lung disease, or may experience extreme fatigue, anemia, cachexia, and pain caused by inflammation, infection, or metastasis.

An extended ICU stay can lead to long-term disability from muscle atrophy, also called ICU-acquired weakness (ICU-AW). The incidence of ICU-AW ranges from 30%–100%, depending on diagnosis (Wieske et al., 2015). In critically ill patients with cancer, muscle weakness may also lead to a cascade of complications. On average, every day that a patient spends in a bed in the ICU, they will require an additional 1.5 days in a non-ICU bed (Hunter, Johnson, & Coustasse, 2014). Additionally, long-term use of a ventilator has been associated with cognitive and functional decline (Vollman, 2013). Early mobility is one way to combat these complications.

This chapter will explore the complications of immobility, the ways in which a progressive mobility protocol overcomes these complications, the barriers that exist to early mobility, and the evidence supporting the use of mobility teams in the ICU to ensure that protocols are being correctly implemented.

Complications of Immobility

Physical deconditioning in patients with cancer can become life threatening. An admission to the ICU means that the patient is already compromised, and immobility can lead to other complications, including muscle mass loss, ventilator-associated pneumonia, atelectasis, and plasma volume loss. Immobility causes a 5% loss of muscle mass each day, and this can be worse in older adults, whose functional ability decreases within two days of hospitalization (Freeman & Maley, 2013). Heart muscle wasting can also occur, causing lethal arrhythmias and mortality (Santos-Hiss et al., 2011). Skin breakdown is a complication of immobility, which can lead to infections, sepsis, and a much longer ICU stay. In addition, a less mobile patient with significant functional deficits requires care from more nurses and longer nursing hours. Although these complications are frequent in ICUs, they may be prevented in a patient with cancer through early, progressive mobility. The earlier a patient is mobilized, the sooner his or her body adjusts to fluid shifts, which can cause orthostatic hypotension. A mobile patient with cancer also tends to take bigger breaths, which increases tidal volume and prevents atelectasis and ventilator-associated pneumonia; therefore, progressive mobility can lead to shorter ventilator days. The sooner that these patients become independent, the less care they need.

Progressive Mobility

If patients with cancer are extremely debilitated, nurses should begin mobilization with active and passive range-of-motion exercises, especially in those who may have anemia, cachexia, and fatigue from their chemotherapy or radiation therapy in addition to their presenting problem leading to ICU admission. Continuous lateral rotation can be performed on an unconscious patient, which helps prevent debility. Most ICU beds also can place a patient into the chair or chair egress positions. The chair position places the patient upright at 90° with feet hanging down, similar to the positioning of one sitting in a chair. The chair egress position is used for patients who have trunk control and can move their legs against gravity. The footboard is removed from the bed and the patient can bear weight on the floor. Both the chair and chair egress positions are excellent weight-bearing exercises that a nurse can institute without the help of another staff member. Sitting in either of these positions challenges the patient's body to remain hemodynamically stable with fluid shifts. If available, a ceiling lift can also be used to lift a patient out of bed and into a recliner. It has been shown that a sit-to-stand lift can be used to get the patient from sitting in the chair to standing.

Barriers and Solutions to Progressive Mobility

Many barriers exist to early patient mobility, including lack of staff and equipment. Patients with multiple IV lines, multiple tubes, and on a ventilator require several staff personnel to ensure that they will not inadvertently extubate or that their IVs will not accidently get pulled out. It takes a team of people to get patients on a ventilator out of bed. Ceiling lift tracks may not be present in the room, further complicating mobility. Nurses also may be afraid to mobilize patients because of unstable vital signs, hemodynamic instability, or vasopressor use. Research has shown that progressive activity is safe and should be instituted early (Freeman & Maley, 2013).

A patient with cancer who is critically ill may not be able to respond. Nurses may feel they cannot get a patient out of bed because the patient is delirious or uncooperative. In this scenario, nurses should use proper sedation and agitation assessments, such as the Confusion Assessment Method for the Intensive Care Unit or the Richmond Agitation-Sedation Scale. Mobility protocols should be a mandatory competency for ICU nurses.

A terminally ill patient admitted to the ICU may appear to be at the end of life, and staff may devalue early mobilization and err on the side of patient comfort. Progressive mobility is inappropriate for this patient population. Severe fatigue may lead to spiritual and emotional distress. A patient with cancer and his or her family may see an ICU admission as the end, but the patient may likely recover and live for some time. Helping them understand the cancer trajectory is essential in a progressive mobility program.

Pain is another barrier to early mobility. A critically ill patient with cancer may have chronic pain from metastases or acute pain from cancer-related surgery. Diallo and Kautz (2014) noted that nurses have an obligation to provide state-of-the-art care and to advocate for vulnerable patients in the ICU. Just as immobility can complicate an ICU stay and delay discharge, so too can inadequately treated pain. Nurses can use the Critical-Care Pain Observation Tool to assess pain in unresponsive patients and use the Faces Pain Scale–Revised and the Iowa Pain Thermometer in those who can respond. Involving patients in pain management strategies to encourage progressive mobility increases their independence and may increase the effectiveness of other treatments.

Mobility Teams

ICUs are complicated places full of critically ill patients and life-supportive therapies, which result in emotional peaks and valleys for patients with cancer, their family members, and the ICU staff. Because of the complexity of the patients and the equipment used to treat them, the ICU needs a dedicated mobility team, including a physical therapist and assistant, occupational therapist, respiratory therapist, and an RN. Developing a team is essential to implement progressive mobility protocols with every patient and to ensure that transfers and activity sessions are conducted safely and productively. Atkins and Kautz (2015) described how one hospital implemented mobility teams with the help of managers. At the hospital, respiratory therapists were typically assigned to patients in multiple ICUs and could not be available for ICU mobility; therefore, the respiratory therapy manager became the mobility representative for the respiratory department. Also, physical therapists made rounds each morning with the oncologist, intensivist, nutritionists, pharmacists, social workers, chaplain, and the unit coordinator to ensure everyone knew the patient's condition and to collaborate on the patient's mobility plan each day. Progressive mobility with a critically ill patient with cancer may mean the difference between the patient recovering from or succumbing to cancer complications and treatment. It is essential for patients and families to understand that cancer fatigue and muscle weakness are treatable and that a realistic goal combines progressive mobility in the ICU, an active rehabilitation program after discharge, and medical treatment for fatigue.

Physical and occupational therapists do exercises with each patient with a respiratory therapist present to protect the patient's airway and to ensure that the endotracheal tube and ventilator are stable. An RN is always present during progressive activity sessions to ensure patient stability and monitor heart rate, blood pressure, and any central venous access devices and other tubes and lines. Scheduling a time for activity sessions permits the nurse to premedicate the patient for pain, which is often undertreated in ICU patients, especially older adults (Diallo & Kautz, 2014). Scheduling a time for sessions also ensures that the patient will not be out of the ICU for diagnostic tests or in the middle of another treatment.

Reames, Price, King, and Dickinson (2016) found that a workflow redesign of patient care technicians, interprofessional teamwork, and a culture focused on meeting mobility standards were necessary to implement an evidence-based ICU mobility protocol. With this redesign, data revealed that mobility increased from 1.4 episodes per 24 hours prior to the mobility initiative to 4.7 episodes per 24 hours after 12 months of the initiative. The authors noted that the most meaningful aspect of the initiative was seeing patients walking in the ICU and challenging themselves to take extra steps, all of which promoted a culture change in the unit.

Summary

In the past, a patient with cancer who was off a ventilator and not on medications requiring titration was considered ready for discharge from the ICU. Today, progressive mobility exercises demand that a patient moves as soon as possible in the ICU under close monitoring by a mobility team. Once a mobility team becomes the standard of care in all ICUs, there will be fewer complications, shorter stays, more satisfied nurses, and happier and more satisfied patients and families. The time for change is now.

The authors gratefully acknowledge the vision, inspiration, and editorial assistance of the late Ms. Elizabeth Tornquist, MA, FAAN, and the wonderful assistance of Mrs. Dawn Wyrick, administrative specialist in the School of Nursing at the University of North Carolina at Greensboro, with this chapter.

References

Atkins, J.R., & Kautz, D.D. (2015). ICU progressive mobility. *Nursing Critical Care, 10,* 19–21. doi:10.1097/01.CCN.0000471006.01956.e1

Diallo, B., & Kautz, D.D. (2014). Better pain management for elders in the intensive care unit. *Dimensions of Critical Care Nursing, 33,* 316–319. doi:10.1097/DCC.0000000000000074

Freeman, R., & Maley, K. (2013). Mobilization of intensive care cardiac surgery patients on mechanical circulatory support. *Critical Care Nursing Quarterly, 36,* 73–88. doi:10.1097/CNQ .0b013e31827532c3

Hunter, A., Johnson, L., & Coustasse, A. (2014). Reduction of intensive care unit length of stay: The case of early mobilization. *Health Care Manager, 33,* 128–135. doi:10.1097/HCM .0000000000000006

Reames, C.D., Price, D.M., King, E.A., & Dickinson, S. (2016). Mobilizing patients along the continuum of critical care. *Dimensions of Critical Care Nursing, 35,* 10–15. doi:10.1097/DCC .0000000000000151

Santos-Hiss, M.D.B., Melo, R.C., Neves, V.R., Hiss, F.C., Verzola, R.M.M., Silva, E., … Catai, A.M. (2011). Effects of progressive exercise during phase I cardiac rehabilitation on the heart rate variability of patients with acute myocardial infarction. *Disability and Rehabilitation, 33,* 835–842. doi:10.3109/09638288.2010.514016

Vollman, K.M. (2013). Understanding critically ill patients hemodynamic response to mobilization: Using the evidence to make it safe and feasible. *Critical Care Nursing Quarterly, 36,* 17–27. doi:10 .1097/CNQ.0b013e3182750767

Wieske, L., Dettling-Ihnenfeldt, D.S., Verhamme, C., Nollet, F., van Schaik, I.N., Schultz, M.J., … van der Schaaf, M. (2015). Impact of ICU-acquired weakness on post-ICU physical functioning: A follow-up study. *Critical Care, 19,* 196. doi:10.1186/s13054-015-0937-2

CHAPTER 16

Wounds and Critical Care

Brenda Freymiller, BSN, MBA, RN, CWON, CWS,
and William H. Tettelbach, MD, FACP, FIDSA, FUHM, CWS

Introduction

The skin is the largest organ of the body, using up to 30% of our total blood volume through its extensive capillary system (Wysocki, 2016). A continuing challenge for the oncology nurse is maintaining skin integrity and healing ability in the patient with cancer. Government regulations, patient and family satisfaction, and advancing technology add to care complexity, making the nurse's role more multifaceted. Patients with cancer who have open wounds can experience delays in cancer treatment because of the infection concerns that can accompany the effects of chemotherapy and radiation on the immune system. Appropriate identification of potential and actual skin problems and knowledge of available preventive and treatment options are essential to improving quality and decreasing mortality in this patient population.

Wounds and Critical Care

Skin as an Organ

The skin serves several vital functions, such as protection, thermoregulation, sensation, metabolism, and communication. The thickness of the skin can vary from just 0.5 mm in the tympanic membrane to 6 mm over the soles of the feet and palms of the hands (Wysocki, 2016). Like any other organ, the skin can fail because of critical or terminal illness (Delmore, Cox, Rolnitzky, Chu, & Stolfi, 2015).

Layers of the Skin

Epidermis

The skin comprises three main components. The outermost component, the epidermis, is the body's first line of defense. It is mainly composed of keratin, which protects the host through its resistance to changes in temperature and pH (Wysocki, 2016). The epidermis has five layers: stratum corneum, stratum lucidum, stratum granulosum, stratum spinosum, and the basal layer. The innermost layer, the basal layer, plays an important role in connecting the underlying components of the skin through rete ridges or dermal papillae. These ridges flatten as people age, putting them at higher risk for skin breakdown, especially skin tears. It takes about two or three weeks for the epidermis to replace itself through a continual process of differentiation from the basal layer (Nicol & Huether, 2010; Wysocki, 2016).

Dermis

The dermal layer is the thickest layer of the skin and comprises the papillary dermis and the reticular dermis. The papillary dermis contains the complementary structures that anchor the rete ridges of the epidermis to the dermal layer. The reticular dermis includes cutaneous blood vessels, collagen fibers, and elastin. These collagen and elastin proteins give the skin its strength and elasticity. Hair follicles, sweat glands, blood vessels, lymphatic vessels, and nerves are also located in the dermis (Nicol & Huether, 2010; Wysocki, 2016).

Hypodermis

Also known as the subcutaneous layer, this component of the skin contains adipose tissue and blood vessels. Its primary role is to connect the skin to its underlying structures (Wysocki, 2016).

Wound Assessment

Baseline wound assessment facilitates a basis to compare wound progress and deterioration over time. A thorough assessment includes location, shape, size, undermining, tunneling, wound bed characteristics, exudate, and surrounding tissue condition.

Location

Wound location needs to be specific to the anatomic body part and contain additional descriptors indicating right or left, medial or lateral, posterior or anterior, etc. This specific location information helps medical professionals to differentiate the wounds. Location can also give the nurse information about wound etiology. For example, pressure injuries are usually located over a bony prominence, moisture-associated skin damage (MASD) occurs in the perineal area or in skinfolds, and skin tears usually occur on the arms and lower legs (Bates-Jensen, 2016).

Size and Shape

Wound shape can tell a great deal of information about potential causes. For example, terminal pressure ulcers typically have a butterfly shape, ulcers that look punched out are usually from arterial disease, and rounder wounds can indicate pressure injury (Bates-Jensen, 2016).

Wound measurements give a better method of evaluating size changes over time. Terms such as *quarter sized* or *fifty-cent piece* are not considered effective ways to communicate wound dimensions. Measurements should be documented in centimeters or millimeters and illustrate the length, width, and depth of the wound. Literature supports using the clock method for linear measuring of the wound. To do this, imagine a clock over the patient, with 12 being the head and 6 being the feet. Length will be the measurement of the wound from the 12 to 6 positions, and width is the wound's measurement from the 9 to 3 positions (see Figure 16-1).

Depth is measured by placing a cotton-tipped applicator or measuring device into the deepest part of the wound and measuring up to the skin's edge (Bates-Jensen, 2016; Nix, 2016). Undermining and tunneling can occur because of infection or

Figure 16-1. Wound Measurement Using the Clock Method

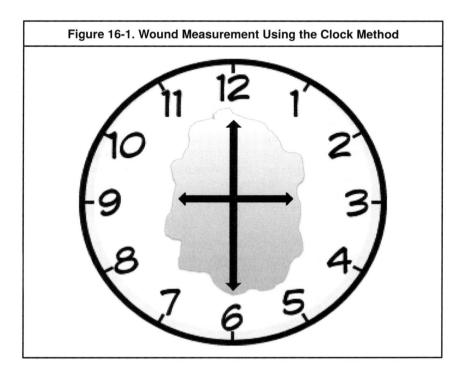

shearing forces. This presents as a tract or as a shelf underneath the intact skin of a wound edge. In some cases, tunneling can connect two separate wounds under a section of intact skin. Measurements should be done using the clock method (i.e., "tract at 6, measuring 2.5 cm," or "undermining from 10 to 2, measuring 1.5 cm"). Care should be taken when using cotton-tipped applicators for measuring tracts and undermining to ensure no particles are left behind. Wooden shaft applicators should not be used to measure undermining, given the risk of leaving splinters in the wound bed, tunnels, or undermining areas (Bates-Jensen, 2016; Nix, 2016).

Wound Bed

Healthy granulation tissue is pink to red in color with a bumpy appearance. Granulation tissue is a sign of healing. A wound that is pale pink and flat, dark red and friable, or has yellow or black necrotic tissue will not progress through the normal stages of healing, which could be caused by infection, pressure, nutritional deficiencies, poor circulation, edema, and other diseases (e.g., diabetes, renal failure, heart disease) (Grey, Enoch, & Harding, 2006).

The volume and characteristics of wound exudate are also important aspects of wound assessment. Serosanguinous drainage that decreases over time is a normal part of the healing process. Cloudy, green, yellow, or malodorous exudate can be a sign of infection or inflammation requiring treatment. The amount of drainage also helps the nurse to determine the best dressing for the wound to maintain a moist environment that does not cause maceration or make the wound bed too dry, both of which can inhibit healing (Bates-Jensen, 2016).

Periwound Skin

The condition of the skin surrounding the wound must be included as part of overall wound assessment. Initially after an injury, it is normal to see some redness or firmness to the area around the wound as part of the body's inflammatory process. Firmness, bogginess, crepitus, or redness that extends and persists several days after the injury are signs of impending further tissue damage caused by infection, continued pressure to the area, or edema (Bates-Jensen, 2016).

The Healing Process

The three classifications of wound closure include primary intention, secondary intention, and delayed closure. Primary closure occurs in wounds that have been approximated and stitched, such as surgical incisions. Secondary closure occurs in wounds that close without the use of closure devices, such as sutures or staples. Wounds that heal by secondary intention include burns, ulcers, and dehisced surgical incisions. Delayed closure occurs when a wound initially left open is later closed, such as surgical wounds or pressure injuries closed by muscle flap or grafting surgery (Grey et al., 2006; Nettina, 2014). Normal healing in acute injuries follows a three-phase process: inflammation, reconstruction, and maturation. Wounds such as pressure injuries and diabetic ulcers do not follow this normal healing cascade, creating a chronic wound. These wounds require special care to help navigate the healing process (Nettina, 2014).

Pressure Injuries

Prevalence and Cost

In 2008, the Centers for Medicare and Medicaid Services (CMS) announced a new payment policy aimed at improving safety in the hospital setting. The focus was to bring attention to a specific list of adverse conditions considered preventable, or "never events." Among the list of conditions identified, hospital-acquired stage III and IV pressure injuries were included as never events. Under the policy, hospitals would not be reimbursed for the cost of care related to treatment of the pressure injury, and many states would require facilities to report these never events to the U.S. Department of Health (CMS, 2008).

According to Lyder et al. (2012), a retrospective review of Medicare data from 2006 to 2007 revealed that 4.5% of patients admitted to the hospital acquired at least one new pressure injury. These patients also had a higher incidence of readmission or death within 30 days of discharge and a length of stay that was double of those who did not develop a pressure injury. Patients are at a higher risk of developing hospital-acquired pressure injuries in the intensive care unit, with prevalence rates noted from 8.8%–42% (Curry et al., 2012; VanGilder, Amlung, Harrison, & Meyer, 2009). Treatment cost for these injuries can range from $500–$70,000 per patient, with an annual cost of up to $11 billion (Padula et al., 2015).

Defining Pressure Injuries

The National Pressure Ulcer Advisory Panel (NPUAP, 2016) defines a pressure injury as the following:

> Localized damage to the skin and/or underlying soft tissue usually over a bony prominence or related to a medical or other device. The injury can present as intact skin or an open ulcer and may be painful. The injury occurs as a result of intense and/or prolonged pressure or pressure in combination with shear. The tolerance of soft issue for pressure and shear may also be affected by microclimate, nutrition, perfusion, co-morbidities and condition of the soft tissue. (para. 4)

This pressure and shear injury can occur with relatively low levels of sustained pressure that may lead to tissue ischemia. Considering that blood supply to the skin comprises a complex network of small capillaries, the amount of pressure needed to occlude and damage tissue in many cases can be minimal. Shearing is the force created with the sliding movement of skin and subcutaneous tissue while the underlying muscle and bone remain stationary. Internally, this creates a strain on the underlying tissues and vessels, creating ischemia and ultimately tissue death (Wounds International, 2010).

Pressure Injury Staging

Pressure injury staging was initially defined in 1975 to describe the level of tissue loss associated with a pressure-related wound. NPUAP has since expanded and further clarified six stages to assess and document the extent of tissue damage (see Figure 16-2).

Stage I

This stage is defined as intact skin with nonblanchable redness (i.e., the area does not lose redness with palpation) of a localized area, usually over a bony prominence. In people with darker pigment, this may appear as a different color than the surrounding skin. The area may be painful, indurated, soft, warm, or cool when compared to surrounding tissue.

Stage II

This stage is defined as a shallow, partial thickness loss of the dermis with a pink wound bed. This injury may also present as an intact or open serum or serosanguinous fluid-filled blister. Frequently, this category is inappropriately used to describe skin tears, tape injury, incontinence-associated dermatitis, maceration, or excoriation. These nonpressure-related wounds should be described using the terms *partial thickness* or *full thickness* skin loss.

Stage III

These injuries present as full thickness tissue loss. Tissue damage can extend to the subcutaneous fat; however, tendon, muscle, and bone are *not* exposed. Undermining and tunneling may be present because of shearing forces. Although slough may be visible in the wound bed, the injury may be staged if it does not obscure the depth of tissue loss.

Stage IV

This stage comprises full thickness tissue loss with exposed tendon, muscle, or bone. If the bone is palpable but not visible, the injury is considered stage IV. Undermining and tunneling are frequently present because of shear. With these injuries, slough and eschar may be present but should not obscure the depth of tissue loss.

Stage III and IV pressure injury depth may vary based on anatomic location. For example, at the ear, occiput, bridge of the nose, and malleolus, where no adipose tissue exists, these injuries can be much shallower than on the sacrum or heel.

Figure 16-2. Pressure Injury Stages

Stage I pressure injury	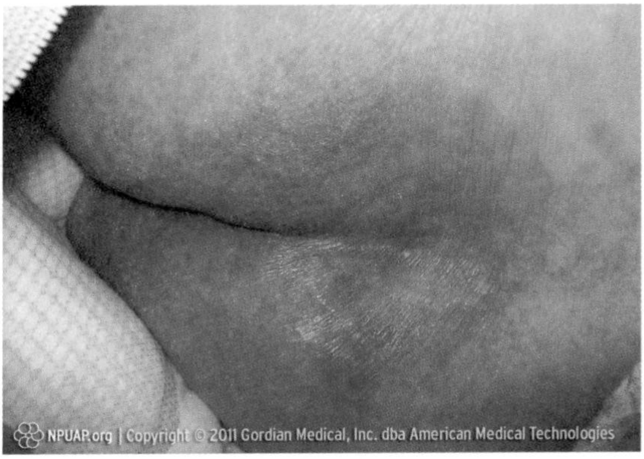
Stage II pressure injury	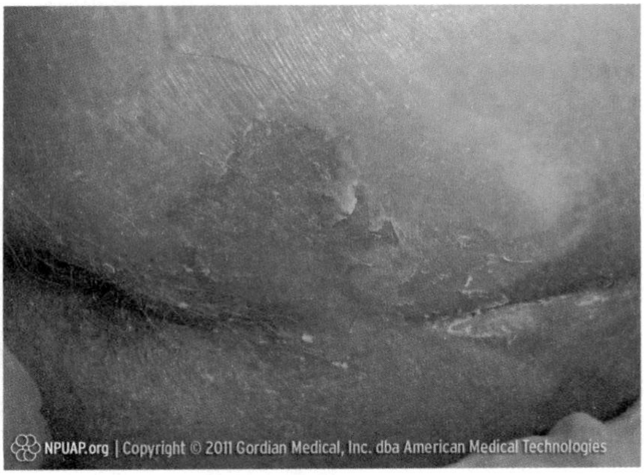
Stage III pressure injury	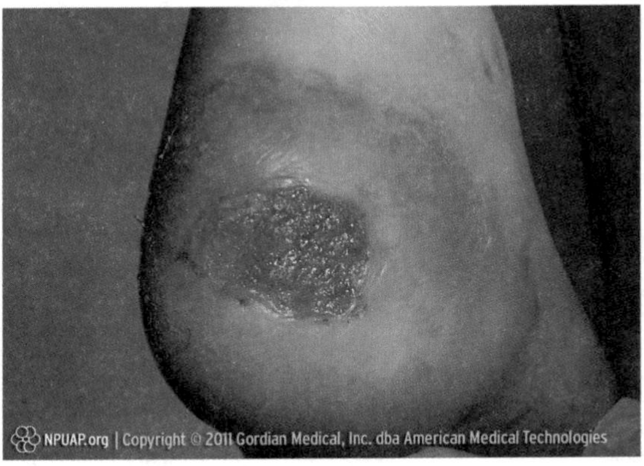

(Continued on next page)

Figure 16-2. Pressure Injury Stages (Continued)

Stage IV pressure injury	
Unstageable	
Deep tissue injury	

Note. Photos 1–3, 6 copyright 2011 by Gordian Medical, Inc. dba American Medical Technologies. Used with permission. Photos 4–5 copyright by Association for the Advancement of Wound Care (www.aawconline.org). Used with permission.

Unstageable

The unstageable stage comprises full thickness ulcers where the wound bed is completely covered in slough or eschar, making it impossible to determine the level of tissue damage. These ulcers typically are found to be stage III or IV pressure injuries once the necrotic tissue is removed.

Deep Tissue Injury

A deep tissue injury is an intact or nonintact area of the skin that has a persistent, nonblanchable purple or maroon area of localized tissue damage, usually over a bony prominence. This can present as blood-filled blisters caused by underlying tissue damage from friction or shearing forces. Assessment can include pain, mushiness, bogginess, warmness, or coolness in the affected area. The concern with this injury is the potential for rapid development to a stage III or IV pressure injury (NPUAP, 2016).

Other Types of Pressure Injuries

Mucosal Pressure Injuries

Mucous membranes line the mouth, gastrointestinal tract, nasal passages, urinary tract, and vaginal canal. The anatomy of the mucous membrane differs from the skin due to the lack of keratin in its outermost layer. These areas are subject to pressure-related injury, primarily from the use of medical devices, such as catheters, nasal cannulas, endotracheal tubes, and nasogastric tubes. Because of the differences in the mucosal tissue from that of the skin, these ulcers should not be staged and instead should be labeled as mucosal pressure injuries (NPUAP, 2012).

Device-Related Injuries

As healthcare technology has advanced, so too has pressure injury incidence related to the use of medical devices. It has been estimated that 10% of pressure injuries are the result of a medical device intended to help the patient (Cooper, 2013). Endotracheal tubes, tracheostomy ties, retention sutures, nasogastric tubes, oxygen tubing, continuous positive airway pressure therapy masks, and arterial line tubing are just some of the devices that create significant pressure injuries in areas not always associated with a bony prominence (see Figure 16-3). These injuries should be documented as medical device injuries and include the appropriate pressure injury stage (NPUAP, 2016).

End-of-Life Ulcers

The Kennedy Terminal Ulcer was first described in 1989 by a nurse practitioner who had noted rapidly progressing pressure ulcers that were occurring in

---

Figure 16-3. Devices Related to Pressure Injury Development

- Arterial line tubing
- Cervical collar
- Continuous positive airway pressure mask
- Endotracheal tubes
- Fecal containment devices
- Foley catheters
- IV tubing
- Nasal cannula
- Nasogastric tubes
- Pulse oximeter
- Retention sutures
- Sequential compression pumps
- Splints
- Tracheostomy ties

---

terminal patients in long-term care. These ulcers typically appear within hours or days of the patient's death; usually occur on the sacrum; have the shape of a pear, butterfly, or horseshoe; and range in color from red, black, or purple (Cooper, 2013). The onset is rapid, with staff usually noting their sudden appearance within a day or two. They can progress rapidly to partial and full thickness ulcers (Kennedy Terminal Ulcer, 2014).

Acute Skin Failure

Critically ill patients have a unique set of concerns related to the skin. This population represents the sickest patients, who typically have many comorbidities, are hemodynamically unstable, and have poor tissue perfusion and oxygenation from underlying cardiac, respiratory, and renal conditions. These patients are often older adults, sedated, nutritionally deficient, and mechanically ventilated. Mechanical ventilation creates its own risk for pressure injury development caused by head of the bed elevation between the 30°–45° recommended to decrease the risk of ventilator-associated pneumonia (Black, Berke, & Urzendowski, 2012; Haesler, 2014).

As more patients are surviving illnesses and injuries that would have resulted in death in the past, clinicians are questioning whether previously documented pressure injuries in the intensive care unit were in fact pressure injuries or a complication of what has become known as acute skin failure. Langemo and Brown (2006) defined acute skin failure as "an event in which skin and underlying tissue die due to hypoperfusion concurrent with severe dysfunction or failure of other organ systems" (p. 206). Patients with risk factors for multiorgan dysfunction syndrome, such as advanced age, chronic disease, tissue hypoperfusion, immunosuppression, and sepsis, are more likely to also experience failure of the largest organ, the skin (Delmore et al., 2015).

Another study on acute skin failure found that organ failure of two or more systems was a significant risk factor, with respiratory and renal organ failure being the most frequent. Other risk factors for patients with acute skin failure included albumin levels less than 3.5 mg/dl, suggesting a compromised nutritional status, generalized edema, ventilator use, and a mean arterial pressure less than 70 mm Hg (Curry et al., 2012).

Vasopressors are used in critical care to increase mean arterial pressure in patients with hypoxia and impaired tissue perfusion. These drugs constrict the blood vessels, shunting blood centrally to the vital organs to preserve them and creating a decrease in perfusion to the extremities and skin. Limited studies have suggested that vasopressors, such as norepinephrine and vasopressin, can increase the likelihood of skin breakdown (Cox & Roche, 2015).

Current literature has not clearly defined how to determine when or if acute skin failure is the only cause of skin breakdown, as pressure can also be a contributing factor. Experts recognize that not all pressure injuries are preventable. Although a consensus has not been reached, it is important for the intensive care nurse to be aware of the phenomena when assessing areas of breakdown and implementing preventive measures (Brindle, Creehan, Black, & Zimmerman, 2015).

Pressure Injury Prevention

Pressure injuries that develop during a patient's hospitalization can increase their length of stay fivefold (Haesler, 2014). For hospitals, this adds to the cost of care along with the resources needed to treat these injuries. With the introduction of the CMS payment policy, prevention of these injuries has become a priority.

Literature supports the development and implementation of a comprehensive pressure injury prevention program that consists of multiple strategies (Gray-Siracusa & Schrier, 2011; Padula et al., 2015). Strategies to consider include assessment of risk, skin and tissue assessment, preventive skin care, and use of preventive therapies and devices (Haesler, 2014).

Pressure Injury Risk Assessment

Several risk assessment tools have been developed to help the clinician identify when a patient may be at risk for pressure injury development. Risk assessments should be initially performed within eight hours of admission to the hospital and when a significant change in the patient's condition occurs (Haesler, 2014). Because of the potential for a rapid change in a patient's condition in the critical care arena, literature has suggested risk assessments be performed every 12 hours (Gray-Siracusa & Schrier, 2011).

In the United States, the Braden Scale for Predicting Pressure Sore Risk is the most commonly used tool for pressure injury risk assessment. It comprises six subscales that evaluate patients for sensory perception, moisture issues, level of activity, bed and chair mobility, nutrition, and friction and shear. A total score of 18 or lower suggests that the patient is at risk for developing a pressure injury (Agency for Healthcare Research and Quality, 2014). Specific interventions can be tied to the different subscales of the tool (see Figure 16-4).

Skin and Tissue Risk Assessment

Skin and tissue should also be assessed within the first eight hours of admission and every 12 hours following as part of an overall risk assessment (Haesler, 2014). The skin should be assessed for blanchable and nonblanchable erythema, skin temperature differences, edema, indurated or boggy areas, open lesions, and pain. Skin and tissue under and around medical devices should also be assessed twice daily for signs of injury. For edematous patients susceptible to fluid shifts, consider performing risk assessments, including skin assessments, more frequently (Haesler, 2014).

Preventive Skin Care

The skin needs to be healthy to perform its functions of protection, thermoregulation, sensation, metabolism, and communication. Factors such as illness, immobility, incontinence, nutritional deficiencies, and advanced age compromise the patient's ability to maintain optimal skin integrity (Lichterfeld et al., 2015).

Moisture

Keeping the skin clean and dry is the first step to maintaining integrity. Patients with weeping edema, urinary or fecal incontinence, and diaphoresis are at a higher risk for breakdown because of excess moisture and chemical irritants compromising the skin flora and strength (i.e., Braden subscore of 1 or 2). Mattresses and mattress overlays provide a microclimate function to alleviate the effects of moisture on the skin by creating a drying effect. Dry skin can also compromise integrity and place patients at a higher risk of breakdown (Haesler, 2014; Lichterfeld et al., 2015).

Bathing should occur daily with lukewarm water using pH-balanced skin cleansers and soft cleansing cloths. Patient should have moisturizer applied to dry skin areas (e.g., face, back) twice daily or more often if needed. Moisturizing lotions and creams should be avoided in moist skin areas, such as the axilla, skinfolds, under the breast, the groin, and between the toes. Fecal and urinary incontinence also increases the risk of skin breakdown (Haesler, 2014; Lichterfeld et al., 2015).

Figure 16-4. Braden Scale for Predicting Pressure Sore Risk

Patient's Name _____ Evaluator's Name _____ Date of Assessment _____

	1	2	3	4
SENSORY PERCEPTION ability to respond meaningfully to pressure-related discomfort	**1. Completely Limited** Unresponsive (does not moan, flinch, or grasp) to painful stimuli, due to diminished level of consciousness or sedation OR limited ability to feel pain over most of body.	**2. Very Limited** Responds only to painful stimuli. Cannot communicate discomfort except by moaning or restlessness OR has a sensory impairment which limits the ability to feel pain or discomfort over ½ of body.	**3. Slightly Limited** Responds to verbal commands, but cannot always communicate discomfort or the need to be turned OR has some sensory impairment which limits ability to feel pain or discomfort in 1 or 2 extremities.	**4. No Impairment** Responds to verbal commands. Has no sensory deficit which would limit ability to feel or voice pain or discomfort.
MOISTURE degree to which skin is exposed to moisture	**1. Constantly Moist** Skin is kept moist almost constantly by perspiration, urine, etc. Dampness is detected every time patient is moved or turned.	**2. Very Moist** Skin is often, but not always moist. Linen must be changed at least once a shift.	**3. Occasionally Moist** Skin is occasionally moist, requiring an extra linen change approximately once a day.	**4. Rarely Moist** Skin is usually dry; linen only requires changing at routine intervals.
ACTIVITY degree of physical activity	**1. Bedfast** Confined to bed.	**2. Chairfast** Ability to walk severely limited or non-existent. Cannot bear own weight and/or must be assisted into chair or wheelchair.	**3. Walks Occasionally** Walks occasionally during day, but for very short distances, with or without assistance. Spends majority of each shift in bed or chair.	**4. Walks Frequently** Walks outside room at least twice a day and inside room at least once every two hours during waking hours.
MOBILITY ability to change and control body position	**1. Completely Immobile** Does not make even slight changes in body or extremity position without assistance	**2. Very Limited** Makes occasional slight changes in body or extremity position but unable to make frequent or significant changes independently.	**3. Slightly Limited** Makes frequent though slight changes in body or extremity position independently.	**4. No Limitation** Makes major and frequent changes in position without assistance.
NUTRITION usual food intake pattern	**1. Very Poor** Never eats a complete meal. Rarely eats more than ⅓ of any food offered. Eats 2 servings or less of protein (meat or dairy products) per day. Takes fluids poorly. Does not take a liquid dietary supplement OR is NPO and/or maintained on clear liquids or IVs for more than 5 days.	**2. Probably Inadequate** Rarely eats a complete meal and generally eats only about ½ of any food offered. Protein intake includes only 3 servings of meat or dairy products per day. Occasionally will take a dietary supplement OR receives less than optimum amount of liquid diet or tube feeding.	**3. Adequate** Eats over half of most meals. Eats a total of 4 servings of protein (meat, dairy products) per day. Occasionally will refuse a meal, but will usually take a supplement when offered OR is on a tube feeding or TPN regimen which probably meets most of nutritional needs.	**4. Excellent** Eats most of every meal. Never refuses a meal. Usually eats a total of 4 or more servings of meat and dairy products. Occasionally eats between meals. Does not require supplementation.
FRICTION & SHEAR	**1. Problem** Requires moderate to maximum assistance in moving. Complete lifting without sliding against sheets is impossible. Frequently slides down in bed or chair, requiring frequent repositioning with maximum assistance. Spasticity, contractures or agitation leads to almost constant friction.	**2. Potential Problem** Moves feebly or requires minimum assistance. During a move skin probably slides to some extent against sheets, chair, restraints or other devices. Maintains relatively good position in chair or bed most of the time but occasionally slides down.	**3. No Apparent Problem** Moves in bed and in chair independently and has sufficient muscle strength to lift up completely during move. Maintains good position in bed or chair.	
				Total Score _____

NPO—nothing by mouth; TPN—total parenteral nutrition

Note. Copyright 1988 by Barbara Braden, PhD, RN, FAAN, and Nancy Bergstrom, PhD, RN, FAAN. Reprinted with permission.

Mobility

When a blanchable or nonblanchable area is noted during a skin assessment, efforts to keep the patient off that site should be implemented. These areas should not be massaged, as this could cause further damage to the already compromised tissue. Heels should be protected with a quality heel boot or elevated using cushions under the full length of the calves to prevent pressure on the Achilles tendon (Haesler, 2014).

For patients with a lower Braden subscore (1 or 2) for mobility, the use of a low air loss surface as part of the prevention plan can reduce the incidence of pressure injury development. These beds help lower the risk of injury caused by friction and shearing forces created with head of bed elevations greater than 30° (Black et al., 2012).

Turning frequency may vary based on the individual patient's tolerance to repositioning. Although critical care patients may experience problems tolerating movement, few cannot tolerate any turning schedule, and patients who have not been repositioned for prolonged periods are at greater risk of instability when a schedule is resumed. For those unable to tolerate a full turning schedule, small frequent shifts (i.e., every 30 minutes) can increase perfusion and may decrease risk of pressure injury development. The key is to make slow, small movements (15° for 15 seconds, then 30° for 15 seconds, then 45° for 15 seconds, etc.) while monitoring for changes.

A continuous lateral rotation therapy bed may also be useful in preventing the development of gravitational equilibrium. It is important to remember that these devices do not replace the need for repositioning. Brindle et al. (2013) suggested that patients unable to tolerate a full repositioning schedule be trialed with a slow, gradual turn, allowing for a 10-minute recovery time every eight hours to assess for the ability to resume a more frequent schedule (Haesler, 2014).

Prone positioning is used in the critical care setting for patients with acute pulmonary complications. Assessment of the face, breast, knees, toes, pelvis, penis, etc., needs to occur with each rotation (Haesler, 2014). Use of a protective thin foam dressing across the forehead, cheeks, chin, and between the nose and upper lip has been successfully used to decrease the shearing forces that occur from head gear used to secure the patient in specialty beds designed for prone positioning (Jackson, Verano, Fry, Rodriguez, & Russian, 2012).

Preventive Therapies and Devices

Elevated skin temperature, perspiration, edema, and incontinence can increase the risk for developing a pressure injury. These patients (Braden subscore of 1 or 2) may benefit from a microclimate surface to decrease the humidity of the skin and lower skin temperature. This is accomplished by moving air underneath the patient (Black et al., 2012; Haesler, 2014).

Medical companies have developed products to assist with patient turning and positioning. Three small studies using these products have shown a statistically significant difference in the number of pressure injuries developed when using a turn and position system (e.g., Prevalon®) compared to the standard of care with lift sheets and pillows. These devices consist of a special sheet that reduces the effects of friction and shearing forces when positioning the patient. Wedges are then placed to maintain the position (see Figure 16-5) (Flockhart, 2011; Powers, 2016; Way, 2014).

The use of prophylactic dressings has gained support as a preventive measure in recent years. Several studies have shown a decrease in pressure injury development with the use of multilayer dressings with a silicone adhesive on areas such as the sacrum and heels. These dressings can also be used under or around medical devices to pad and protect the skin and tissue. The silicone adhesive allows for removal and replacement of the same dressing to regularly assess the area. These dressings should be used as part of an overall prevention bundle and changed every three days or when soiled (Brindle & Wegelin, 2012; Haesler, 2014; Torra i Bou et al., 2009; Walsh et al., 2012).

Figure 16-5. Turn and Assist Position System

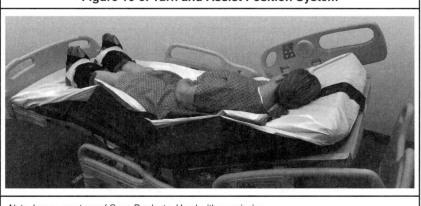

Note. Image courtesy of Sage Products. Used with permission.

Moisture-Associated Skin Damage

MASD is an inflammation and erosion of the skin caused by prolonged exposure to moisture. Sources of this moisture can be from urine, stool, perspiration, saliva, and wound drainage. High levels of moisture in the skin weaken the stratum corneum, which is further complicated by increased colonization of microorganisms, such as *Staphylococcus*, *Candida albicans*, and *Pseudomonas* species, along with friction and shearing forces, leading to further breakdown and potential pressure injury development. Literature has shown that patients with fecal incontinence are 22 times more likely to develop a pressure injury (Driver, 2007; Gray et al., 2011; Park & Kim, 2014).

The four common forms of MASD are incontinence-associated dermatitis (IAD), intertriginous dermatitis (ITD), periwound moisture-associated dermatitis, and peristomal moisture-associated dermatitis (Gray et al., 2011).

Incontinence-Associated Dermatitis

IAD is often confused with a pressure injury, as both stage I pressure injuries and mild to moderate IAD present as erythema of intact skin. A blanchability assessment of the area can assist in identification. A stage I pressure injury is defined as a nonblanchable area of redness, meaning that palpation does *not* cause the area to change color. IAD erythema *will* blanch (change color) with palpation and is associated with effluent or moist skin. A stage II pressure injury can also be confused with a more severe IAD with partial thickness skin loss (see Figure 16-6).

IAD assessment will typically reveal a less-defined border of erythema or skin loss, include a patient complaint of burning and itching, and commonly will be

---

Figure 16-6. Incontinence-Associated Dermatitis

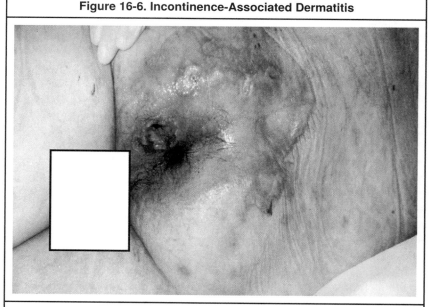

Note. Copyright by Association for the Advancement of Wound Care (www.aawconline.org). Used with permission.

found in the skinfolds where stool and urine can come in contact for extended periods. The nurse needs to consider the overall patient condition related to moisture and incontinence to help determine if lesions are related to pressure or IAD (Black et al., 2011; Doughty et al., 2012).

Prevention and care of IAD includes prompt cleansing of the skin after incontinence episodes with the use of a skin protectant. Moisturizers and moisture barriers containing zinc oxide, petrolatum, or polydimethylsiloxane help improve skin function and create a protective film on the skin designed to inhibit penetration of moisture from substances like stool and urine (Black et al., 2011; Doughty et al., 2012; Lichterfeld et al., 2015).

Studies have shown that gentle cleansing with disposable cloths and a pH-appropriate, no-rinse cleanser is effective at removing bacteria and protects the skin's moisture barrier better than using soap and water with towels. Many skin protectant products now contain both a moisturizer and a protectant in the form of a cream or wipe. These should be applied after cleansing and routinely as needed (Black et al., 2011; Brunner, Droegemueller, Rivers, & Deuser, 2012; Doughty et al., 2012).

Containment of urine or stool with a urinary catheter or fecal containment device may be appropriate in some cases. Although these devices can be effective, it is still possible to have stool or urine leakage onto the skin. Good skin care and cleansing will continue to be an important part of a care plan. As medical devices, these products can also put the patient at risk for mucosal and device-related pressure injuries. Risks and benefits need to be weighed before implementing these options (Black et al., 2011; Haesler, 2014). Bed surfaces and specialty mattress overlays with microclimate technology can help manage heat and humidity through evaporation. These surfaces use a pump that pushes air through small holes in the cushions of the mattress to create a continuous airflow, which can lower skin temperature and have a drying effect on the skin. These surfaces have been shown to be more effective than standard foam mattresses in reducing the risk of skin breakdown (Wounds International, 2010).

The number of linen layers and the type of absorptive underpads used are important factors to consider in the prevention of skin breakdown from moisture and pressure. Underpads should be breathable to allow transmission of moisture and reduce humidity of the skin (Wounds International, 2010). NPUAP guidelines recommend fewer layers of linens and underpads, as multiple layers have been shown to increase pressure, especially over the sacral area. For patients with moisture problems, the benefit of a mattress with microclimate features is decreased as layers of linen and underpads are added (Haesler, 2014; Williamson, 2009).

Intertriginous Dermatitis

ITD is defined as "an inflammatory dermatosis of opposing skin surfaces caused by moisture" (Black et al., 2011, p. 365). It commonly develops in skinfolds of the breasts, abdomen, and groin but can occur in any area where skin touches skin, such as the neck, back, and legs. It typically presents as an inflammatory process with linear lesions caused by skin-to-skin friction and prolonged moisture from perspiration. These lesions are painful, with patients also reporting burning, itching, and odor. Obese patients who suffer from higher levels of perspiration and skin pH are more likely to develop ITD. Uncontrolled diabetes and steroid or antibiotic use have also been identified as risk factors (Black et al., 2011; Doughty et al., 2012).

Organisms associated with ITD commonly contain fungal organisms, such as *Candida* species, but a recent study has shown that bacteria, such as *Pseudomonas aeruginosa*, *Escherichia coli*, methicillin-resistant *Staphylococcus aureus*, and vancomycin-resistant *Enterococcus*, have also been found in skinfolds. The increased burden of potentially pathogenic bacteria in an environment where moisture has weakened the stratum corneum increases the risk of cellulitis in these patients (Black et al., 2011).

Keeping the skin between folds clean and dry is the best defense. As with other skin care, a pH-balanced cleanser and a soft, disposable cloth should be used to cleanse and prevent the spread of bacteria. These areas are extremely painful to touch, so the skin should be dried by gently patting the area, fan drying, or using a hair dryer on a cool setting. Talcum- or cornstarch-based powders, antiperspirants, gauze, linens, and paper towels have been ineffective or do not have enough evidence to support use as a prevention or treatment. When indicated, antifungal agents may be used. It is important to ensure a light dusting of the product to avoid caking within the skinfold (Black et al., 2012). Commercially available wicking textile products placed between skinfolds have been shown to be an effective way to treat and prevent ITD (Kennedy-Evans, Smith, Viggiano, & Henn, 2007; Tessling, Freyberg, & Netsch, 2007).

Skin Tears

Definition and Risk

Skin tears were defined in 2011 by the International Skin Tear Advisory Panel (ISTAP) as "a wound caused by shear, friction, and/or blunt force resulting in separation of skin layers. A skin tear can be partial-thickness (separation of the epidermis from the dermis) or full-thickness (separation of both the epidermis and dermis from underlying structures)" (LeBlanc & Baranoski, 2011, p. 6). Skin tears occur most frequently on the arms, hands, and lower legs and are caused by blunt trauma from assistive devices, transfers, falls, and tape removal (Fleck, 2007; LeBlanc & Baranoski, 2011). They tend to be painful and can become infected if not properly treated (Bank & Nix, 2006).

Skin tears are very common in older adults because of the changes in skin layers that accompany aging. The skin becomes less elastic with decreased tensile strength and surface moisture because of dermal and subcutaneous tissue loss, thinning of the epidermis, and changes to serum composition (LeBlanc & Baranoski, 2011). The rete ridges that help anchor the epidermis to the dermis flatten, leading to decreased resistance to friction and shearing forces (Fleck, 2007; LeBlanc & Baranoski, 2011). Blood vessels also become more fragile, leading to bruising beneath the skin, or senile purpura, which presents as a purplish discoloration on the hands and forearms and accounts for 40% of skin tears (Ratliff & Fletcher, 2007).

Other risk factors include decreased sensory perception, altered nutrition, polypharmacy, incontinence, and cardiac, pulmonary, or vascular problems. Medications, such as antibacterials, antihypertensives, antineoplastic agents, diuretics, hypoglycemic agents, nonsteroidal anti-inflammatory drugs, and steroids, have been shown to adversely affect the skin and are commonly seen in the chronically or critically ill (LeBlanc et al., 2013). Because fall risk is strongly correlated with skin tear risk, skin tear prevention interventions should be part of a comprehensive fall risk program (Fleck, 2007; LeBlanc et al., 2013).

Prevention

Prevention is based on the basic principles of skin care. Cleansing with a pH-balanced cleanser and a moisturizer applied twice daily will hydrate the stratum corneum and increase its elasticity (Black et al., 2011; Doughty et al., 2012; Guenther et al., 2012; LeBlanc & Baranoski, 2011). It is also important to collaborate with a dietitian to optimize the patient's nutrition and maintain adequate hydration (LeBlanc & Baranoski, 2011).

Extremity protection is a key component of a skin tear prevention care plan. Minimizing the use of tape, using skin preps prior to applying tape, using non-tape methods to secure dressings when possible (e.g., self-adherent wraps, mesh netting, gauze), repositioning patients with turn sheets, and padding objects that could cause trauma when bumped should be measures implemented as part of the overall prevention plan (Bank & Nix, 2006; Fleck, 2007; LeBlanc & Baranoski, 2011).

Improper tape selection and removal can create skin tears and strip the epidermis, leaving a partial thickness wound. For this reason, higher adhesive tapes should be reserved only for securing critical medical devices, such as endotracheal tubes and vascular lines. Removal of these and any other tapes should be done carefully using adhesive remover products and a gentle, slow approach while supporting the skin immediately adjacent to the tape (Thayer, Rozenboom, & Baranoski, 2016).

Assessment and Treatment

ISTAP developed a decision algorithm that assists the clinician with assessment and treatment strategies for patients with skin tears (see Figure 16-7).

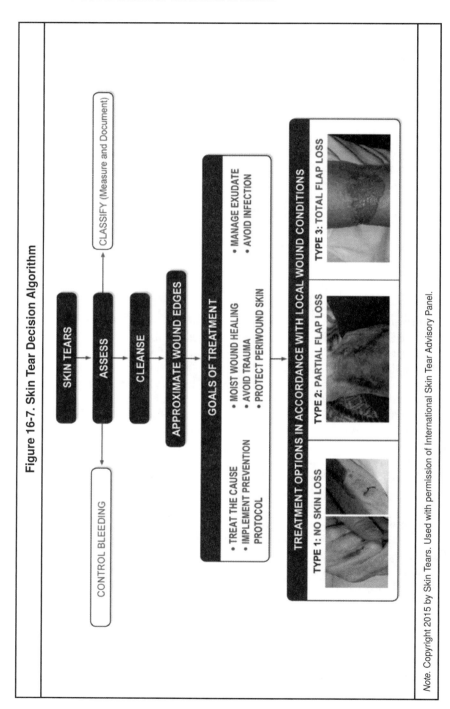

Figure 16-7. Skin Tear Decision Algorithm

Wound Cleansing and Dressing Selection

The first step in establishing a treatment plan for acute or chronic wounds is to remove the causative factors creating the wound. Unless the causes of the wound (e.g., pressure, incontinence, infection) have been addressed, topical treatments will not be effective in promoting healing. A common concept to remember when approaching treatment of wounds is to consider the "whole" person, not just the "hole" in the person.

Cleansing

Wound cleansing is the process of removing surface contaminants, remnants of previous dressings, and excess bacteria from the wound and periwound areas (Haesler, 2014). Wounds are most commonly cleansed with water or saline; however, other cleansers that contain surfactants and antimicrobials are also available. Skin cleansers designed for removing fecal material, povidone-iodine, chlorhexidine, acetic acid, and hydrogen peroxide can be used for short periods in infected or heavily soiled wounds. These products should not be used on a clean wound, as they are cytotoxic to granulating tissue (Bryant & Nix, 2016; Rodeheaver & Ratliff, 2007). Wounds with slough and necrotic tissue should be referred to a wound specialist for possible debridement.

Dressing Selection

A multitude of dressings are available for wound care. A clinician may be confused with this growing list of options when determining the optimal dressing for patients and their wounds. A basic understanding of dressing types and their uses is necessary when choosing a product (see Table 16-1) (Jaszarowski & Murphree, 2016). With an understanding of how different dressings work, the nurse can use a simple assessment tool to select an appropriate option (see Figure 16-8) (Jaszarowski & Murphree, 2016).

Nutrition

Nutrition has been recognized by clinicians for centuries as an important aspect of health, disease, and healing. A great deal of energy is needed to promote wound healing. Caloric requirements vary from patient to patient and are reached through the daily consumption of proteins, fats, and carbohydrates (Arnold & Barbul, 2006). Patients at risk for nutritional deficiencies should be referred to a registered dietitian within the first 48 hours of admission to the unit (Posthauer, Dorner, & Collins, 2010).

Metabolic rates can increase because of surgery, wounding, and sepsis, quickly consuming energy and putting further stress on an already nutritionally compromised patient. A patient with an uncomplicated abdominal surgery can expect an increase in metabolic rate of around 10% (Arnold & Barbul, 2006). Fever also increases metabolism by 10% for every 1°C above normal (Arnold & Barbul, 2006). When nutritional stores and intake are limited, an

Table 16-1. Dressing Selection		
Dressing Type	**Characteristics/Functions**	**Best Uses**
Foam	Moderately absorbent product made from polyurethane foam Comes with and without adhesive borders Comes in various thicknesses for different drainage amounts Allows for less frequent dressing changes (every 2–7 days) Does not typically need a cover dressing Can be used as a cover dressing	Thin foams for minimally exudating wounds Thick foams for moderate exudating wounds Padding for bony prominences Friction protection
Alginate or fiber	Made from soft woven fibers Highly absorptive Can be moistened with saline or water to hydrate dry wounds Allows for less frequent dressing changes (every 2–5 days) Needs a cover dressing	Used dry for higher exudate wounds Used moistened for dry wounds to promote a moist environment
Hydrocolloid	Occlusive adhesive dressing Manages light to moderate exudate Forms a gel; allows for less frequent dressing changes (every 2–5 days) Does not need a cover dressing	Wounds with low to moderate drainage Friction protection
Hydrogel	Maintains a moist wound environment Available in sheet dressings and gels Helps to moisten dry wounds Absorbs minimal drainage Helps reduce pain in some partial thickness wounds Cover dressing required with gel forms	Partial thickness wounds with minimal exudate
Transparent film	Waterproof but allows for transfer of oxygen and water vapor Helps maintain a moist wound environment Does not absorb drainage	Superficial wounds with minimal drainage Can be used to secure other dressings Friction protection

(Continued on next page)

Table 16-1. Dressing Selection *(Continued)*		
Dressing Type	**Characteristics/Functions**	**Best Uses**
Nonadherent contact layer	Provides a protective interface between the wound and cover dressings Allows drainage to transfer from the wound to the cover dressing Helps reduce pain with dressing changes Protects the wound and surrounding skin from trauma with dressing removal Requires a cover dressing	Wounds with low to high amounts of exudate

Note. Based on information from Jaszarowski & Murphree, 2016.

illness or injury can quickly catabolize and deplete the proteins, carbohydrates, and fats needed for the energy required to fight infection and promote healing (Arnold & Barbul, 2006).

Protein

Protein supplies nitrogen and amino acids, which help to create the enzymes, collagen, and antibodies needed for healing and a healthy immune system. When patients do not receive enough calories, the proteins from their diet, as well as their muscles, are used to produce energy (Posthauer et al., 2010). Protein loss caused by protein–calorie malnutrition is the most common malnutrition today. This deficit in protein affects the wound's tensile strength and the ability to fight infection (Arnold & Barbul, 2006).

Arginine and glutamine have been the most extensively studied amino acids in relation to wound healing. They have been found to promote collagen development and energy for cell development (Posthauer et al., 2010). Arginine supplementation in diabetics with wounds is thought to be especially important and has been shown to improve wound tissue strength (Arnold & Barbul, 2006).

Carbohydrates and Fats

Carbohydrates and fats are the primary source of energy for the body. Without sufficient carbohydrates, the body will convert protein to needed energy, creating muscle wasting and diminished subcutaneous tissue (Posthauer et al., 2010). Fats carry vitamins A, D, E, and K, provide padding for skin and bony prominences, and are a significant energy source (Posthauer et al., 2010). Deficiencies in essential fatty acids are seen most commonly in patients receiving total parenteral nutrition (TPN) for an extended period. Once started, TPN can facilitate a deficiency within 10 days of the start of treatment (Arnold & Barbul, 2006).

Figure 16-8. Tool for Wound Dressing Assessment

Cavity Wound Moderate to Large Exudate Deep and Wet	**Cavity Wound Minimum to No Exudate Deep and Dry**
Goals • Fill dead space • Absorb exudate • Maintain a moist environment • Support autolysis of necrotic tissue • Protect and insulate **Need:** absorptive filler and cover dressing **Fill the wound with** • Calcium alginate or fiber dressing • Cavity foam • Gauze **Cover with** • Foam dressing • Gauze	**Goals** • Fill dead space • Create a moist environment • Protect and insulate **Need:** hydrating filler and cover dressing **Fill the wound with** • Calcium alginate or fiber dressing (moistened) • Hydrogel with or without gauze **Cover with** • Foam dressing • Gauze with transparent film dressing
Shallow Wound Moderate to Large Exudate Shallow and Wet	**Shallow Wound Minimum to No Exudate Shallow and Dry**
Goals • Absorb exudate • Maintain a moist environment • Support autolysis of necrotic tissue • Protect and insulate • Protect the periwound skin **Need:** absorptive cover (sometimes filler) **Options** • Foam dressing • Calcium alginate or fiber dressing + cover • Nonadherent contact layer + cover	**Goals** • Create and maintain a moist wound environment • Protect and insulate **Need:** hydrating or moisture-retentive cover dressing **Options** • Hydrogel + cover • Hydrocolloid • Thin foam • Nonadherent contact layer + cover

Note. From "Wound Cleansing and Dressing Selection" (p. 142), by K.A. Jaszarowski and R.W. Murphree in D.B. Doughty and L.L. McNichol (Eds.), *Wound, Ostomy and Continence Nurses Society® Core Curriculum: Wound Management,* 2016, Philadelphia, PA: Wolters Kluwer Health/ Lippincott Williams & Wilkins. Copyright 2016 by Wound, Ostomy and Continence Nurses Society. Adapted with permission.

Micronutrition

The two vitamins most closely correlated with wound healing are water-soluble vitamin C and fat-soluble vitamin A. Vitamin C is essential in supporting collagen formation and angiogenesis. Deficiencies in vitamin C also decrease the host's resistance to infection. Supplementation above the recommended intake of 70–90 mg/day has not been shown to have a significant effect on wound healing (Arnold & Barbul, 2006; Ter Riet, Kessels, & Knipschild, 1995). Vitamin A is important to wound healing through its promotion of epithelialization and collagen formation. Although deficiencies of vitamin A are rare, supplementation in patients with chronic corticosteroid use can help reverse the anti-inflammatory effects of those medications (Ehrlich & Hunt, 1968). Other studies have shown improvement in healing with vitamin A supplementation in conditions such as diabetes and with postradiation treatment in patients with cancer (Levenson et al., 1984; Seifter et al., 1981; Weinzweig et al., 1990).

Zinc and vitamin D have also been correlated with skin and wound health. Deficiencies in zinc and vitamin D are more prevalent in older adults, diminishing the function of their immune systems (Aranow, 2011; National Institutes of Health, 2016). Studies have shown that even mild zinc and vitamin D deficiencies can have a negative effect on the immune system and connective tissue, while vitamin D has been related to autoimmune conditions, such as diabetes, multiple sclerosis, lupus, and inflammatory bowel disease (Aranow, 2011; National Institutes of Health, 2016).

Fluids

Optimal hydration is essential for all body functions. Up to 60% of an adult's weight comes from fluid stored in the intracellular, interstitial, and intravascular systems (Posthauer et al., 2010). For patients with wounds, maintaining appropriate hydration is critical for oxygen perfusion, delivery of important nutrients, and removal of waste (Posthauer et al., 2010). Patients with elevated temperature, diarrhea, and draining wounds need to be monitored for fluid replacement (Thomas et al., 2008).

Summary

Prevention and treatment of skin issues is an important part of care of acutely and chronically ill patients with cancer. Maintaining skin integrity through preventive measures saves patients from pain and potentially life-threatening infections and also may lower the total cost of care by reducing length of admission. Appropriate treatment early in the cascade of injury and healing improves outcomes and satisfaction. A wound care specialist can help to develop, direct, and assist with patient care, also leading to improved outcomes and decreased hospital length of stay.

References

Agency for Healthcare Research and Quality. (2014). Preventing pressure ulcers in hospitals. Retrieved from http://www.ahrq.gov/professionals/systems/hospital/pressureulcertoolkit/putool3.html#33

Aranow, C. (2011). Vitamin D and the immune system. *Journal of Investigative Medicine, 59*, 881–886.

Arnold, M., & Barbul, A. (2006). Nutrition and wound healing. *Plastic and Reconstructive Surgery, 117*(Suppl. 7), 42S–58S. doi:10.1097/01.prs.0000225432.17501.6c

Bank, D., & Nix, D. (2006). Preventing skin tears in a nursing and rehabilitation center: An interdisciplinary effort. *Ostomy/Wound Management, 52*(9), 38–40, 44, 46.

Bates-Jensen, B.M. (2016). Assessment of the patient with a wound. In D.B. Doughty & L.L. McNichol (Eds.), *Wound, Ostomy and Continence Nurses Society® core curriculum: Wound management* (pp. 38–68). Philadelphia, PA: Wolters Kluwer Health/Lippincott Williams & Wilkins.

Black, J.M., Berke, C., & Urzendowski, G. (2012). Pressure ulcer incidence and progression in critically ill subjects: Influence of low air loss mattress versus a powered air pressure redistribution mattress. *Journal of Wound, Ostomy and Continence Nursing, 39*, 267–273. doi:10.1097/WON.0b013e3182514c50

Black, J.M., Gray, M., Bliss, D.Z., Kennedy-Evans, K.L., Logan, S., Baharestani, M.M., ... Ratliff, C.R. (2011). MASD part 2: Incontinence-associated dermatitis and intertriginous dermatitis: A consensus. *Journal of Wound, Ostomy and Continence Nursing, 38*, 359–370. doi:10.1097/WON.0b013e31822272d9

Brindle, C.T., Creehan, S., Black, J.M., & Zimmerman, D. (2015). The VCU pressure ulcer summit: Collaboration to operationalize hospital-acquired pressure ulcer prevention best practice recommendations. *Journal of Wound, Ostomy and Continence Nursing, 42*, 331–337. doi:10.1097/WON.0000000000000151

Brindle, C.T., Malhotra, R., O'Rourke, S., Currie, L., Chadwik, D., Falls, P., ... Creehan, S. (2013). Turning and repositioning the critically ill patient with hemodynamic instability: A literature review and consensus recommendations. *Journal of Wound, Ostomy and Continence Nursing, 40*, 254–267. doi:10.1097/WON.0b013e318290448f

Brindle, C.T., & Wegelin, J.A. (2012). Reduction of sacral pressure ulcers in the intensive care unit using a silicone border foam dressing. *Journal of Wound, Ostomy and Continence Nursing, 39*, 133–142.

Brunner, M., Droegemueller, C., Rivers, S., & Deuser, W.E. (2012). Prevention of incontinence-related skin breakdown for acute and critical care patients: Comparison of two products. *Urologic Nursing, 32*, 214–219.

Bryant, R.A., & Nix, D.P. (2016). Principles of wound healing and topical management. In R.A. Bryant & D.P. Nix (Eds.), *Acute and chronic wounds: Current management concepts* (5th ed., pp. 306–324). Philadelphia, PA: Elsevier.

Centers for Medicare and Medicaid Services. (2008). CMS improves patient safety for Medicare and Medicaid by addressing never events. Retrieved from https://www.cms.gov/Newsroom/MediaReleaseDatabase/Fact-sheets/2008-Fact-sheets-items/2008-08-042.html

Cooper, K.L. (2013). Evidence-based prevention of pressure ulcers in the intensive care unit. *Critical Care Nurse, 33*, 57–66. doi:10.4037/ccn2013985

Cox, J., & Roche, S. (2015). Vasopressors and development of pressure ulcers in adult critical care patients. *American Journal of Critical Care, 24*, 501–510. doi:10.4037/ajcc2015123

Curry, K., Kutash, M., Chambers, T., Evans, A., Holt, M., & Purcell, S. (2012). A prospective, descriptive study of characteristics associated with skin failure in critically ill adults. *Ostomy/Wound Management, 58*(5), 36–43.

Delmore, B., Cox, J., Rolnitzky, L., Chu, A., & Stolfi, A. (2015). Differentiating a pressure ulcer from acute skin failure in the adult critical care patient. *Advances in Skin and Wound Care, 28*, 514–524. doi:10.1097/01.ASW.0000471876.11836.dc

Doughty, D.B., Junkin, J., Kurz, P., Selekof, J., Gray, M., Fader, M., ... Logan, S. (2012). Incontinence-associated dermatitis: Consensus statements, evidence-based guidelines for prevention and treatment, and current challenges. *Journal of Wound, Ostomy and Continence Nursing, 39*, 303–315. doi:10.1097/WON.0b013e3182549118

Driver, D.S. (2007). Perineal dermatitis in critical care patients. *Critical Care Nurse, 27*, 42–46.

Ehrlich, H.P., & Hunt, T.K. (1968). Effects of cortisone and vitamin A on wound healing. *Annals of Surgery, 167,* 324–328. doi:10.1097/00000658-196803000-00004

Fleck, C.A. (2007). Preventing and treating skin tears. *Advances in Skin and Wound Care, 20,* 315–321. doi:10.1097/01.ASW.0000276416.91750.d4

Flockhart, L. (2011, November). *Use of a repositioning system in postoperative cardiovascular ICU patients results in a 63% reduction in facility-acquired sacral pressure ulcers.* Retrieved from https://sage-products.co.uk/wp-content/uploads/2015/08/Flockhart_15098.pdf

Gray, M., Black, J.M., Baharestani, M.M., Bliss, D.Z., Colwell, J.C., Goldberg, M., ... Ratliff, C.R. (2011). Moisture-associated skin damage. *Journal of Wound, Ostomy and Continence Nursing, 38,* 233–241. doi:10.1097/WON.0b013e318215f798

Gray-Siracusa, K., & Schrier, L. (2011). Use of an intervention bundle to eliminate pressure ulcers in critical care. *Journal of Nursing Care Quality, 26,* 216–225. doi:10.1097/NCQ.0b013e31820e11be

Grey, J.E., Enoch, S., & Harding, K.G. (2006). Wound assessment. *BMJ, 332,* 285–288. doi:10.1136/bmj.332.7536.285

Guenther, L., Lynde, C.W., Andriessen, A., Barankin, B., Goldstein, E., Skotnicki, S.P., ... Sloan, K. (2012). Pathway to dry skin prevention and treatment. *Journal of Cutaneous Medicine and Surgery, 16,* 23–31. doi:10.1177/120347541201600106

Haesler, E. (Ed.). (2014). *Prevention and treatment of pressure ulcers: Clinical practice guideline* (2nd ed.). Osbourne Park, Australia: Cambridge Media.

Jackson, M.E., Verano, J.X., Fry, J.E., Rodriguez, A.P., & Russian, C. (2012). Skin preparation process for the prevention of skin breakdown in patients who are intubated and treated with Roto-Prone. *Respiratory Care, 57,* 311–314. doi:10.4187/respcare.01235

Jaszarowski, K.A., & Murphree, R.W. (2016). Wound cleansing and dressing selection. In D.B. Doughty & L.L. McNichol (Eds.), *Wound, Ostomy and Continence Nurses Society® core curriculum: Wound management* (pp. 131–144). Philadelphia, PA: Wolters Kluwer Health/Lippincott Williams & Wilkins.

Kennedy Terminal Ulcer. (2014). Understanding the Kennedy Terminal Ulcer. Retrieved from http://www.kennedyterminalulcer.com

Kennedy-Evans, K., Smith, D., Viggiano, B., & Henn, T. (2007). Multisite feasibility study using a new textile with silver for management of skin conditions located in skinfolds: 1431. *Journal of Wound, Ostomy and Continence Nursing, 34*(Suppl. 3), S68. doi:10.1097/01.WON.0000271039.01843.16

Langemo, D.K., & Brown, G. (2006). Skin fails too: Acute, chronic, and end-stage skin failure. *Advances in Skin and Wound Care, 19,* 206–212. doi:10.1097/00129334-200605000-00014

LeBlanc, K., & Baranoski, S. (2011). Skin tears: State of the science: Consensus statements for the prevention, prediction, assessment, and treatment of skin tears. *Advances in Skin and Wound Care, 24*(Suppl. 9), 2–15. doi:10.1097/01.ASW.0000405316.99011.95

LeBlanc, K., Baranoski, S., Christensen, D., Langemo, D., Sammon, M., Edwards, K., ... Regan, M. (2013). International Skin Tear Advisory Panel: A tool kit to aid in the prevention, assessment, and treatment of skin tears using a simplified classification system. *Advances in Skin and Wound Care, 26,* 459–476. doi:10.1097/01.ASW.0000434056.04071.68

Levenson, S.M., Gruber, C.A., Rettura, G., Gruber, D.K., Demetriou, A.A., & Seifter, E. (1984). Supplemental vitamin A prevents the acute radiation-induced defect in wound healing. *Annals of Surgery, 200,* 494–512. doi:10.1097/00000658-198410000-00011

Lichterfeld, A., Hauss, A., Surber, C., Peters, T., Blume-Petavi, U., & Kottner, J. (2015). Evidence-based skin care: A systematic literature review and the development of a basic skin care algorithm. *Journal of Wound, Ostomy and Continence Nursing, 42,* 501–524. doi:10.1097/WON.0000000000000162

Lyder, C.H., Want, Y., Metersky, M., Curry, M., Kliman, R., Verzier, N.R., & Hunt, D.R. (2012). Hospital-acquired pressure ulcers: Results from the National Medicare Patient Safety Monitoring System study. *Journal of the American Geriatrics Society, 60,* 1603–1608. doi:10.1111/j.1532-5415.2012.04106.x

National Institutes of Health. (2016). Zinc: Fact sheet for health professionals. Retrieved from https://ods.od.nih.gov/factsheets/Zinc-HealthProfessional

National Pressure Ulcer Advisory Panel. (2012). *Mucosal pressure ulcers: An NPUAP position statement.* Retrieved from http://www.npuap.org/wp-content/uploads/2012/03/Mucosal_Pressure _Ulcer_Position_Statement_final.pdf

National Pressure Ulcer Advisory Panel. (2016). NPUAP pressure injury stages. Retrieved from http://www.npuap.org/resources/educational-and-clinical-resources/npuap-pressure-injury-stages

Nettina, S.M. (Ed.). (2014). *Lippincott manual of nursing practice* (10th ed.). Philadelphia, PA: Wolters Kluwer Health/Lippincott Williams & Wilkins.

Nicol, N.H., & Huether, S.E. (2010). Structure, function, and disorders of the integument. In K.L. McCance, S.E. Huether, V.L. Brashers, & N.S. Rote (Eds.), *Pathophysiology: The biologic basis for disease in adults and children* (6th ed., pp. 1644–1679). Maryland Heights, MO: Elsevier Mosby.

Nix, D.P. (2016). Skin and wound inspection and assessment. In R.A. Bryant & D.P. Nix (Eds.), *Acute and chronic wounds: Current management concepts* (5th ed., pp. 109–123). Philadelphia, PA: Elsevier.

Padula, W.V., Makic, M.B.F., Mishra, M.K., Campbell, J.D., Wald, H.L., & Valuck, R.J. (2015). Comparative effectiveness of quality improvement interventions for pressure ulcer prevention in academic medical centers in the United States. *Joint Commission Journal on Quality and Patient Safety, 41,* 246–256. doi:10.1016/s1553-7250(15)41034-7

Park, K.H., & Kim, K.S. (2014). Effect of a structure skin care regimen on patients with fecal incontinence: A comparison cohort study. *Journal of Wound, Ostomy and Continence Nursing, 41,* 161–167. doi:10.1097/WON.0000000000000005

Posthauer, M.E., Dorner, B., & Collins, N. (2010). Nutrition: A critical component of wound healing. *Advances in Skin and Wound Care, 23,* 560–572. doi:10.1097/01.ASW.0000391185.81963.e5

Powers, J. (2016). Two methods for turning and positioning and the effect on pressure ulcer development: A comparison cohort study. *Journal of Wound, Ostomy and Continence Nursing, 43,* 46–50. doi:10.1097/WON.0000000000000198

Ratliff, C.R., & Fletcher, K.R. (2007). Skin tears: A review of the evidence to support prevention and treatment. *Ostomy/Wound Management, 53*(3), 32–40.

Rodeheaver, G.T., & Ratliff, C.R. (2007). Wound cleansing, wound irrigation, wound disinfection. In D.I. Krasner, G.T. Rodeheaver, & R.G. Sibbald (Eds.), *Chronic wound care: A clinical source book for healthcare professionals* (4th ed., pp. 331–342). Malvern, PA: HMP Communications.

Seifter, E., Rettura, G., Padawer, J., Stratford, F., Kambosos, D., & Levenson, S.M. (1981). Impaired wound healing in streptozotocin diabetes: Prevention by supplemental vitamin A. *Annals of Surgery, 194,* 42–50. doi:10.1097/00000658-198107000-00008

Ter Riet, G., Kessels, A.G.H., & Knipschild, P.G. (1995). Randomized clinical trial of ascorbic acid in the treatment of pressure ulcers. *Journal of Clinical Epidemiology, 48,* 1453–1460. doi:10.1016 /0895-4356(95)00053-4

Tessling, J., Freyberg, J., & Netsch, D. (2007). Moisture management challenges for the WOC nurse: 1367. *Journal of Wound, Ostomy and Continence Nursing, 34*(Suppl. 3), S54. doi:10.1097 /01.won.0000270997.78971.d2

Thayer, D.M., Rozenboom, B., & Baranoski, S. (2016). "Top-down" injuries: Prevention and management of moisture-associated skin damage (MASD), medical adhesive–related skin injury (MARSI), and skin tears. In D.B. Doughty & L.L. McNichol (Eds.), *Wound, Ostomy and Continence Nurses Society® core curriculum: Wound management* (pp. 281–321). Philadelphia, PA: Wolters Kluwer Health/Lippincott Williams & Wilkins.

Thomas, D.R., Cote, T.R., Lawhorne, L., Levenson, S.A., Rubenstein, L.Z., Smith, D.A., … Morley, J.E. (2008). Understanding clinical dehydration and its treatment. *Journal of the American Medical Directors Association, 9,* 292–301. doi:10.1016/j.jamda.2008.03.006

Torra i Bou, J.E., Rueda López, J., Camañes, G., Herrero Narváez, E., Blanco, J., Ballesté Torralba, J., … Soriano, J.V. (2009). Preventing pressure ulcers on the heel: A Canadian cost study. *Dermatology Nursing, 21,* 268–272.

VanGilder, C., Amlung, S., Harrison, P., & Meyer, S. (2009). Results of the 2008–2009 International Pressure Ulcer Prevalence Survey and a 3-year, acute care, unit-specific analysis. *Ostomy/Wound Management, 55*(11), 39–45.

Walsh, N.S., Blanck, A.W., Smith, L., Cross, M., Andersson, L., & Polito, C. (2012). Use of a sacral silicone border foam dressing as one component of a pressure ulcer prevention program in an intensive care unit setting. *Journal of Wound, Ostomy and Continence Nursing, 39,* 146–149. doi:10.1097/WON.0b013e3182435579

Way, H. (2014). *Safe patient handling initiative results in reduction in injuries and improved patient outcomes for pressure ulcer prevention.* Retrieved from https://sageproducts.com/wp-content/uploads/Heather-Way-SPH-Poster-2014_22280.pdf

Weinzweig, J., Levenson, S.M., Rettura, G., Weinzweig, N., Mendecki, J., Chang, T.H., & Seifter, E. (1990). Supplemental vitamin A prevents the tumor-induced defect in wound healing. *Annals of Surgery, 211,* 269–276.

Williamson, R. (2009). Impact of linen layers to interface pressure and skin microclimate [Abstract]. *Journal of Wound, Ostomy and Continence Nursing, 36*(Suppl. 3), S62.

Wounds International. (2010). *International review: Pressure ulcer prevention: Pressure, shear, friction and microclimate in context.* Retrieved from http://www.woundsinternational.com/media/issues/300/files/content_8925.pdf

Wysocki, A.B. (2016). Anatomy and physiology of skin and soft tissue. In R.A. Bryant & D.P. Nix (Eds.), *Acute and chronic wounds: Current management concepts* (5th ed., pp. 40–62). Philadelphia, PA: Elsevier.

CHAPTER 17

Pharmacology

Anthony T. Gerlach, PharmD, BCPS, FCCP, FCCM

Introduction

Critically ill patients with cancer pose unique challenges when admitted to the intensive care unit (ICU). Although these patients are often admitted with similar problems as the general population (e.g., sepsis), physiologic responses and pharmacologic therapy may be altered. An understanding of pharmacokinetic, pharmacodynamic, and pharmacologic changes in this population can help clinicians maximize drug therapy.

Pharmacokinetics and Pharmacodynamics

Pharmacokinetics

Pharmacokinetics is the process of drug absorption, distribution (movement), and elimination through the body. The main pharmacokinetic parameters are bioavailability, volume of distribution (VD), clearance, and half-life (Bauer, 2014). Alterations in these parameters may occur in critically ill patients, including those with cancer. Some are easier to overcome, such as decreased bioavailability, when suitable IV formulations are readily available.

Bioavailability

Bioavailability is the percentage of a drug that reaches the systemic circulation of a patient (Brundage & Mann, 2017; Shargel, Yu, & Wu-Pong, 2012). Although most commonly attributed to enteral medications, it also applies to subcutaneous injections. A drug with 100% or nearly 100% bioavailability reaches similar concentrations in the body when administered orally or intravenously. Factors that can affect bioavailability include absorption, change in gastrointestinal transit time, and first-pass metabolism. *First-pass effect* is the term used to describe a drug that is metabolized by the gut wall or liver before reaching the systemic circulation (Brundage & Mann, 2017; Shargel et al., 2012). Drugs with significant first-pass metabolism have decreased bioavailability and different dosing intravenously than orally. Metoprolol and labetalol are drugs with a significant first-pass effect. Changes in absorption can be caused by drug properties and different drug formulations. For example, the absorption of itraconazole tablets is different than the oral solution. Decreased gastrointestinal motility can also affect absorption, especially in the presence of ileus. Although sublingual, rectal, transdermal, and subcutaneous administration may overcome some absorption problems, these routes have disadvantages, such as unpredictable serum concentrations. In patients with shock receiving vasopressor therapy to maintain blood pressure, transdermal absorption is decreased. On the other hand, tacrolimus has a significant first-pass effect that is bypassed with sublingual administration; therefore, using sublingual administration may increase concentrations.

Volume of Distribution

VD describes how a drug is distributed in the body (Bauer, 2014; Brundage & Mann, 2017; Shargel et al., 2012). Measured in liters, VD corresponds to the lipophilicity (fat solubility) and protein binding of a drug. Factors that affect VD include age, total body water, intestinal permeability, and acid–base disturbances. Only an unbound drug exerts a pharmacologic effect. Some drugs are highly protein bound, such as phenytoin to albumin. In critically ill patients, albumin concentrations are often decreased, resulting in potentially inaccurate total phenytoin concentration measurements (Brundage & Mann, 2017). An alternative method is to measure the free concentrations of phenytoin. Drugs with small VD, such as vasoactive catecholamines, are distributed only to plasma and do not cross into tissues. Aminoglycosides also have small VD and are distributed in body water. This should be considered when dosing aminoglycosides in critically ill patients receiving significant fluid resuscitation. Drugs with large VD often have significant tissue distribution. Amiodarone has a VD of approximately 60 L/kg because it is very lipid soluble (Andreasen, Agerbaek, Bjerregaard, & Gøtzsche, 1981); therefore, it is quickly removed from the plasma where it exerts its antiarrhythmic effect. This may explain why a continuous infusion is needed for those naïve to it. Midazolam is also a drug that has a large VD because of lipophilicity, which allows it to cross the blood–brain barrier and have a quick onset of action. With bolus use, such as for conscious sedation, midazolam has a quick offset, but prolonged infusions may cause the drug to accumulate in fat tissue, resulting in a prolonged duration of action. Loading doses are used to quickly achieve a therapeutic concentration and are predominantly based on the VD of a specific drug. Loading doses are the same in renal or hepatic dysfunction, typically 20 mcg/kg. This should be halved in those with renal insufficiency because of altered protein binding (Shammas & Dickstein, 1988).

Clearance

Clearance is the pharmacokinetic term for drug elimination (Bauer, 2014; Brundage & Mann, 2017; Shargel et al., 2012). The main routes of drug clearance are renal and hepatic, and other routes include reticuloendothelial clearance, biliary excretion, and plasma enzymes. Hepatically cleared drugs are typically glucuronidated or oxidized through the cytochrome P450 enzyme system. Biliary cleared drugs are eliminated unchanged through the bile. Clearance is measured as volume divided by time (V/T), usually liters or milliliters divided by hour (L/hr). Total body clearance is the sum of all the ways that a drug is eliminated from the body and includes zero-order, first-order, and nonlinear or Michaelis-Menten clearance. In zero-order, drug clearance is fixed, and only a certain amount can be removed at a time, allowing for additional drug accumulation. Ethanol is a classic example of a drug with zero-order clearance. Most drugs have first-order or linear kinetics, where the clearance increases proportionally with drug concentrations. A hyperbolic curve characterizes nonlinear clearance. Phenytoin has a nonlinear clearance and is linear at low concentrations and saturable at higher concentrations. Small changes in concentration can cause a significant change in clearance. Renal and hepatic clearances are the main routes of elimination, and changes in their function need to be considered when determining dosing in critically ill patients with cancer. For example, drugs with renal elimination will need to be dose reduced in patients with acute kidney injury.

Half-Life

The half-life of a drug is the time it takes for the drug concentration to decrease by half. Half-life ($T_{1/2}$) is represented by the equation $T_{1/2} = (0.693 \times VD/\text{clearance})$ (Bauer, 2014) and is directly proportional to VD and inversely proportional to clearance. In other words, a drug with a large VD will have a longer half-life. For example, amiodarone has a 60 L/kg VD and a half-life of approximately 60 days. Conversely, drugs with fast clearances have a short half-life. The vasoactive catecholamines, such as norepinephrine or epinephrine, are eliminated by plasma enzymes and have very short half-lives of 2–5 minutes (Zaritsky, 1994). Generally, it takes 5 half-lives to be at a steady state concentration and approximately 3.3 half-lives to be at 90% steady state concentration (Bauer, 2014). For example, early methadone use has shown to improve outcomes in critically ill burn patients, but because of its long half-life (24–72 hours), it should not be titrated every day, as it could accumulate (Jones et al., 2013). Dose adjustments should be made every three to five days.

Pharmacodynamics

Pharmacodynamics is the relationship between drug concentration and pharmacologic response, or what the drug does to the body (Bauer, 2014; Brundage & Mann, 2017). Pharmacokinetics and pharmacodynamics are closely related, making it difficult to distinguish between the two. For example, resistance to loop diuretics (e.g., furosemide) is the result of changes in either pharmacodynamics or pharmacokinetics (Cody & Pickworth, 1994). Furosemide works inside the nephron at the loop of Henle (Cody & Pickworth, 1994) and is secreted into the nephron by active transport via the organic acid pathway. This only occurs above a threshold concentration. Once it is secreted into the nephron, it can cause diuresis. In critically ill patients with increased total body fluid, significant gut edema can cause a delay in absorption with enteral furosemide. Although the concentration over time, also known as area under the curve, does not change, a decrease in peak or maximal concentration can occur. A possible consequence is that the threshold concentration needed to reach the nephron is not achieved; therefore, diuresis does not occur. This is the pharmacokinetic reason for diuretic resistance, which can be overcome by administering IV furosemide. In patients with chronic furosemide use, there also can be a pharmacodynamic reason for resistance. In these patients, distal tubules may increase sodium and water reabsorption, and increasing the dose of furosemide or the use of an IV route does not produce increased diuresis. This can be overcome by concomitant use of a thiazide diuretic to block sodium reabsorption in the distal tubule.

Pharmacodynamic effects often describe the relationship between a drug and its receptor that produces a pharmacologic response (Bauer, 2014); therefore, the effect may lag the interaction between the drug binding to its receptor and pharmacokinetics. For example, the sedative dexmedetomidine is an alpha-2a agonist that produces cooperative sedation without causing respiratory depression because of its ability to lower norepinephrine concentration in the locus coeruleus (Gerlach & Dasta, 2007). Dexmedetomidine has a half-life of 2–3 hours, and a loading infusion is recommended, although studies have determined its use does not increase onset of action, which correlates with its pharmacodynamics (Gerlach, Murphy, & Dasta, 2009). Dexmedetomidine binds to alpha-2a receptors on the presynaptic neuron and blocks norepinephrine reuptake, which initially results in increased norepinephrine concentrations. Norepinephrine is rapidly metabolized by the plasma enzymes carboxy-O-methyl transaminases and monoamine oxidases with a half-life of 2–5 minutes (Zaritsky, 1994); therefore, it will take 4–5 half-lives (20 minutes) to decrease norepinephrine concentrations for the onset of dexmedetomidine (Gerlach & Dasta, 2007; Gerlach et al., 2009). Initially, the level of dexmedetomidine concentration does not matter, as dexmedetomidine does not metabolize norepinephrine. The pharmacodynamic effect is needed for sedation to occur.

As pharmacokinetics and pharmacodynamics are interrelated, many sophisticated models are used for the development of drug-dosing regimens (Meibohm & Derendorf, 1997). These models are increasingly being used outside of drug development to maximize efficacy, most notably with antimicrobial therapy (Nielsen & Friberg, 2013), and to describe the effect-time course from a fixed dose of a drug and extrapolate it to existing data with the goal of maximizing a drug-induced effect or a change in a physiologic parameter (Meibohm & Derendorf, 1997). Efficacy is difficult to quantify in complex, critically ill patients because surrogates are often used and are constantly changing. For example, one would expect changes in heart rate or blood pressure to be used as a surrogate for dexmedetomidine because of their ability to decrease norepinephrine concentrations. However, blood pressure would not be a good surrogate for dexmedetomidine because the drug loses its selectivity for the alpha-2a receptor, a vasodilator, and binds to the alpha-2b receptor, a vasoconstrictor, with increased concentration; therefore, dexmedetomidine can cause both hypotension and hypertension. Various parameters also affect heart rate other than norepinephrine, making it a poor surrogate of dexmedetomidine in the critically ill patient.

Fluid Resuscitation

Fluid resuscitation is often a first-line therapy for critically ill patients (Dellinger et al., 2013). Fluids are broken into crystalloids (e.g., normal saline) and colloids (e.g., albumin). Crystalloids can be isotonic, hypotonic, or hypertonic (Waikar & Winkelmayer, 2012). Most crystalloids are isotonic, including 0.9% saline (normal saline) and balanced salt solutions (Ringer's lactate electrolyte A solution). Normal saline contains 154 mEq/L of both sodium and chloride and an average pH of 5 (see Table 17-1) (Yunos et al., 2011). Balanced salt solutions are more physiologic, contain less sodium and chloride, and have more physiologic pH. Typically, hypotonic resuscitation is not recommended because of iatrogenic hyponatremia and the potential for hypernatremia without close monitoring (Waikar & Winkelmayer, 2012). Recent studies have demonstrated that critically patients who developed hypochloremia had worse outcomes, but it is unknown if the use of balanced salt solutions could improve these outcomes (Neyra et al., 2015; Tani, Morimatsu, Takatsu, & Morita, 2012).

Colloids are broken into 5% albumin, 25% albumin, dextran, and the hetastarches (Annane et al., 2013). Dextran and the hetastarches are limited to about a liter in adults and are not commonly used in the ICU because of the risk of platelet dysfunction. Albumin is the main colloid used for resuscitation. Two recent trials have attempted to determine the best practice between colloid and crystalloid use. The SAFE trial compared 4% albumin against normal saline in 6,997 critically ill patients and found no significant difference in 28-day mortality (Finfer et al., 2004). Similar findings were reported in the CRISTAL trial, when 2,857 patients were randomized to colloids (gelatins, dextran, or albumin 4% or 20%) or crystalloids (saline or Ringer's lactate solution) (Annane et al., 2013).

Vasopressors

Vasopressors typically are the next step for resuscitation after IV fluid, especially in septic patients (Dellinger et al., 2013). Vasopressors are vasoactive cate-

Table 17-1. Comparison of Crystalloid Solutions and Albumin

Name	Normal Saline	Lactated Ringer's	Electrolyte A	Albumin (5%)	Albumin (25%)
pH (range)	5 (4.5–7)	6.5 (6–7)	7.4 (6.5–8)	6.4–7.4	6.4–7.4
Sodium (Na) (mEq)	154	130	140	130–160	130–160
Chlorine (Cl) (mEq)	154	109	98	130–160	130–160
Potassium (K) (mEq)	0	4	5	0	0
Magnesium (Mg) (mEq)	0	0	3	0	0
Acetate (mEq)	0	0	27	0	0
Gluconate (mEq)	0	0	28	0	0
Calcium (Ca) (mEq)	0	3	0	0	0
Lactate (mEq)	0	28	0	0	0
Osmolarity (mOsm/L)	308	273	294	285	285

Note. Based on information from Yunos et al., 2011.

cholamines, such as norepinephrine, epinephrine, dopamine, and phenylephrine, and noncatecholamines, such as vasopressin. In recent years, norepinephrine has become the predominant vasopressor used in ICUs (Dellinger et al., 2013).

Vasoactive catecholamines work by activating the alpha-1 receptors that cause smooth muscle in the vasculature to contract and increase blood pressure (see Tables 17-2 and 17-3). Norepinephrine and epinephrine work to activate alpha and beta receptors, while dopamine activates dopamine, alpha, and beta receptors. Phenylephrine works only on alpha receptors. Adverse effects are based on the mechanism of action for each drug. Norepinephrine, epinephrine, and dopamine can cause hypertension, tachycardia, atrial fibrillation, ventricular tachycardia, hyperglycemia, and ischemia, including tissue necrosis if extravasated. Dopamine can also decrease peristalsis and gastrointestinal motility. Compared to norepinephrine, dopamine is associated with worse outcomes, especially in patients with car-

Table 17-2. Location and Action of Receptors Controlling Blood Pressure		
Receptor	Location	Action
Alpha-1	Blood vessels	Constriction
Alpha-2	Presynaptic neuron Bladder	Negative feedback Constriction
Beta-1	Heart Blood vessels	Chronotropy/inotropy Dilation
Beta-2	Lungs	Dilation
Dopamine-1	Mesenteric blood vessels	Dilation
Dopamine-2	Systemic blood vessels	Constriction
Vasopressin	Blood vessels	Constriction
Note. Based on information from Holmes et al., 2014; Marino, 2014.		

diogenic shock (De Backer et al., 2010). Phenylephrine can cause ischemia, hypertension, and arrhythmias but at a lesser rate than the other catecholamines, as it does not activate beta receptors to cause tachycardia. The binding of these catecholamines may be affected by acidosis, and their effectiveness may be decreased at low pH. Because these agents work on vascular smooth muscle, where actin needs to bind to myosin, they are optimal with normal serum ionized calcium levels.

Although it leads to similar results, vasopressin typically is the second-line agent in resuscitation, as it has a different mechanism of action than the catecholamines (Dellinger et al., 2013; Holmes, Patel, Russell, & Walley, 2001). Vasopressin stimulates vasopressin receptors. It has similar adverse effects as phenylephrine and is typically dosed as a continuous infusion at 0.01–0.04 units/min (Dellinger et al., 2013). A dosage greater than 0.04 units/min typically is not used because of increased risk of myocardial infarction (mesenteric or peripheral ischemia). Vasopressin also differs from the catecholamines because it has a longer half-life of 15–20 minutes and is less dependent on pH (Holmes et al., 2001).

Inotropes

Inotropes are used to increase cardiac output. The two main inotropes are dobutamine and milrinone (Annane et al., 2013). Dobutamine is a beta-agonist and works to stimulate beta receptors, resulting in an increased intracellular calcium concentration caused by an increase in cyclic adenosine monophosphate production. This allows myocardial actin to bind to myosin and increases cardiac

Table 17-3. Vasopressors		
Drug/Dose	**Receptor Agonist**	**Action**
Epinephrine • 0.5–50 mcg/min • 0.05–1 mcg/kg/min	Alpha-1, alpha-2, beta-1, beta-2	Chronotropy/inotropy Vasoconstriction
Norepinephrine • 0.5–100 mcg/min • 0.05–3 mcg/kg/min	Alpha-1, alpha-2, beta-1, beta-2	Chronotropy/inotropy Vasoconstriction
Phenylephrine • 0.5–9 mcg/kg/min	Alpha-1, alpha-2	Vasoconstriction
Vasopressin • 0.01–0.04 units/min	Vasopressin	Vasoconstriction
Dopamine • 1–5 mcg/kg/min • 5–10 mcg/kg/min • 10–20 mcg/kg/min	Dopamine-1, dopamine-2 Beta-1, beta-2 Alpha-1, alpha-2	Natriuresis Chronotropy/inotropy Vasoconstriction

Note. Based on information from Holmes et al., 2014; Marino, 2014.

contractility. Dobutamine also increases heart rate through vasodilation of arterial smooth muscle. It is administered by a continuous infusion of 2–20 mcg/kg/min, although no more than 5 mcg/kg/min is usually administered (Zaritsky, 1994). Dobutamine is a catecholamine that has a short half-life of 2–5 minutes and is metabolized by plasma enzymes. Milrinone is a phosphodiesterase inhibitor that prevents the breakdown of cyclic adenosine monophosphate in the myocardium and nitric oxide. As a result, it also can decrease blood pressure and improve inotropy. Milrinone is eliminated renally and has a half-life of 2.5 hours in those with normal renal function. It can be given as a loading infusion up to 50 mcg/kg over 10 minutes, although most do not recommend this because of risk of hypotension (Zaritsky, 1994). The maintenance dosage is 0.125–0.75 mcg/kg/min, although dosages above 0.5 mcg/kg/min should also be used with caution because of risk of hypotension (Zaritsky, 1994).

Analgesics and Sedatives

The Society of Critical Care Medicine Pain, Agitation, and Delirium Clinical Practice Guidelines recommend an "analgesia first" approach for the treatment of any agitated critically ill patient (Barr et al., 2013). These guidelines recommend the use of validated sedation scales, pain assessment scores in nonverbal patients, and delirium screens. They also suggest protocols with minimal sedation and that patients use medications as needed versus continuous infusion because of the risk of prolonged mechanical ventilation.

Opiates

Opiates are mainstays in the ICU (Barr et al., 2013). They work as mu-receptor agents to treat nociceptive pain, increase sedation, decrease respiratory drive, and reduce gastric motility. Unlike other analgesics, such as nonsteroidal anti-inflammatory drugs, opiates do not have a ceiling effect; however, higher dosages can depress the respiratory drive, making careful titration a constant need. In addition, no tolerance exists to the constipation effect of opiates.

Opiates include three classes of agents: phenanthrenes, phenylpiperidines, and diphenylheptanes (Gutstein & Akil, 2001).

Phenanthrenes include morphine, codeine, hydromorphone, oxycodone, oxymorphone, and hydrocodone. Morphine and hydromorphone are commonly used and available in parenteral formulations. They have similar effects when in equianalgesic dosages, except hydromorphone causes less histamine release (Barr et al., 2013). Although morphine and hydromorphone are glucuronidated via the liver, morphine has active metabolites that are renally eliminated. Morphine can accumulate in renal and hepatic failure. For patients who are allergic to the phenanthrenes, a drug from another class can be substituted.

Phenylpiperidines include meperidine, fentanyl, and remifentanil. Meperidine is not commonly used because of accumulation of normeperidine, which is eliminated renally and decreases seizure threshold. Fentanyl is commonly used and can be administered through IV, transmucosal, or transdermal routes. It has no active metabolites, is eliminated hepatically, and can accumulate in adipose tissue. Remifentanil is an ultra-short-acting fentanyl derivative eliminated by plasma hydrolysis and does not accumulate. It has a short half-life of 10–20 minutes and should only be administered as a continuous infusion (Battershill & Keating, 2006).

Methadone is the only diphenylheptane and has a dual mechanism of action, working as both a mu receptor and an N-methyl-D-aspartate agonist. Methadone has a long half-life of 24–72 hours and an onset of 2–6 hours (Jones et al., 2013). It should not be titrated daily or used for acute pain.

Sedatives

Sedatives are often used in patients who are agitated despite adequate analgesic therapy (Barr et al., 2013). Common sedatives include propofol, benzodiazepines, and dexmedetomidine.

Propofol

Propofol is a sedative-hypnotic agent that produces sedation without analgesia. Although the mechanism of action is not fully understood, propofol works as a gamma-aminobutyric acid (GABA) agonist, a major inhibitory neurotransmitter. Propofol is very lipid (fat) soluble and only available in 10% lipid emulsion. As a result, bottles and IV lines should be changed every 12 hours because of the potential for infectious complication with the lipid emulsions (Marik, 2004). It also can produce hypotension, bradycardia, decreased cardiac output, and respiratory depression. Because of its high lipid solubility, propofol has a quick onset of 1–2 minutes, readily crossing the blood–brain barrier (Barr et al., 2013). It is typically dosed as a continuous infusion from 5–75 mcg/kg/min or 0.5–5 g/kg/hr (Barr et al., 2013). With short use, propofol has a quick onset, but because of lipid solubility, it can accumulate with prolonged use and have a half-life of more than 50 hours (Barr et al., 2013). Although propofol is considered safe and effective, a condition termed *propofol-related infusion syndrome* can be manifested by metabolic acidosis, bradyarrhythmias, and progressive myocardial failure. This syndrome has been described in those with prolonged high-dose propofol use (greater than 83 mcg/kg/min or 5 g/kg/hr) (Roberts et al., 2009). Treatment includes prompt recognition and discontinuation of the sedative.

Benzodiazepines

Benzodiazepines are also GABA agonists (Barr et al., 2013). They work by binding to benzodiazepine receptors on the alpha units of the GABA receptors. This augments the effect of the body's natural GABA, unlike other sedatives such as barbiturates. Effects of benzodiazepines include sedation, hypnosis, respiratory depression, retrograde amnesia, muscle relaxation, and seizure therapy. Benzodiazepines commonly used in the ICU include midazolam, lorazepam, and diazepam to a lesser extent. Midazolam and diazepam are both highly lipid soluble, metabolized in the liver by the cytochrome P450 enzyme system, and have a quick onset of action of 2–5 minutes (Barr et al., 2013). Both have renally eliminated active metabolites. Midazolam has a half-life of 3–11 hours, and diazepam has a half-life of 20–120 hours (Barr et al., 2013). Both can accumulate in adipose tissue and in patients with renal or hepatic failure. Lorazepam is glucuronidated in the liver and does not have any active metabolites. It is less lipid soluble than midazolam and diazepam; therefore, it has a longer onset of action of 15–20 minutes with a half-life of 4–15 hours (Barr et al., 2013).

Dexmedetomidine

Unlike propofol and benzodiazepines, dexmedetomidine does not work on the GABA receptors (Gerlach & Dasta, 2007). It is an alpha-1 agonist that produces light or "cooperative" sedation without causing respiratory depression. Dexmedetomidine can produce hemodynamic effects, including hypotension, hypertension, and bradycardia. It is glucuronidated by the liver and has a half-life of 2–3 hours in both healthy volunteers and critically ill patients. Although a loading dose is recommended, it is not usually administered (Gerlach et al., 2009). The maintenance dose is typically 0.2–1.5 mcg/kg/hr (Gerlach et al., 2009).

Neuromuscular Blocking Agents

Neuromuscular blocking agents are used to facilitate procedures, such as endotracheal intubation, and as continuous infusions in critically ill patients (Murray et al., 2002). These agents are divided into depolarizing agents and nondepolarizing agents and work on nicotinic receptors at the neuromuscular junction (Murray et al., 2002). Acetylcholine binds to these receptors and opens a sodium-potassium ATPase, causing an influx of sodium into the cell and an efflux of potassium out of the cell, resulting in depolarization and muscle contraction. Succinylcholine is the only available depolarizing agent, and it binds to the nicotinic receptor and mimics the action of acetylcholine with a longer duration of 5–10 minutes (Marino, 2014). The net result is a contraction followed by paralysis, as the muscle cell cannot repolarize. A potential for hyperkalemia exists, especially in those who have a baseline hyperkalemia or abnormal muscle end plates from the mechanism of action. Succinylcholine is only used as a bolus and never a continuous infusion because of the risk of fatal arrhythmias from hyperkalemia. As succinylcholine mimics acetylcholine, it has a quick onset of action of 30–60 seconds. It is eliminated by pseudocholinesterase in the blood and has a duration of 5–10 minutes. Succinylcholine is dosed as 1–1.5 mg/kg by IV push and may be given intramuscularly if needed (Marino, 2014).

Nondepolarizing neuromuscular blocking agents work as competitive antagonists of acetylcholine; therefore, they have a slower onset of action (1–3 minutes) compared to succinylcholine (Murray et al., 2002). Unlike succinylcholine, nondepolarizing neuromuscular blocking agents do not activate the nicotinic receptors and will not cause hyperkalemia. These agents are divided into two classes, the aminosteroid compounds and the benzylisoquinoliniums. The aminosteroid agents share the same ring structure as steroids, and as a result, they may not produce adequate paralysis when used in patients receiving high-dose steroids. Pancuronium, rocuronium, and vecuronium are aminosteroids. These agents have both renal and hepatic metabolism and can accumulate in renal or hepatic insufficiency. Atracurium and cisatracurium are benzylisoquinoliniums and are eliminated by plasma hydrolysis and Hofmann elimination. These agents are preferred in patients with hepatic or renal insufficiency, as they will not accumulate. All nondepolarizing neuromuscular blocking agents are associated with arthralgias, myalgias, muscle weakness, and global motor deficit. Pancuronium is associated with tachycardia caused by effects on the vagus nerve. Atracurium is associated with a histamine release, and it may be less with cisatracurium. Because these agents work only on skeletal muscle, associated orders to provide adequate sedation, amnesia, and analgesia are needed with continuous infusions of neuromuscular blockers. Likewise, patients should have eye lubrication, range of motion, venous thromboembolism, and stress ulceration prophylaxis.

Anticoagulants

Parenteral Anticoagulants

Heparin, low-molecular-weight heparins (LMWHs; dalteparin and enoxaparin), and pentasaccharides (fondaparinux) are used for prevention and treatment of thromboembolism in the ICU (Hirsh & Raschke, 2004). These agents are indirect thrombin inhibitors because they bind to antithrombin III to exert the anticoagulant effect. Heparin is monitored by activated partial thromboplastin time or antifactor Xa assay levels. LMWHs can only be monitored by antifactor Xa. Heparin is a very large molecule and eliminated via the reticuloendothelial system. Its VD is best estimated by total blood volume and explains why critically ill patients who are obese or morbidly obese require higher dosages of therapeutic heparin (Gerlach et al., 2013). LMWHs and fondaparinux are administered subcutaneously with higher dosages for treatment of venous thromboembolism than for prophylaxis (Hirsh & Raschke, 2004). These drugs are eliminated renally because they are smaller in size than heparin. These agents may accumulate in patients with renal insufficiency and lead to bleeding complications.

Oral Anticoagulants

Until recently, the only oral anticoagulant in the United States was warfarin, a vitamin K antagonist that inhibits production of vitamin K–dependent clotting factors II, VII, IX, and X. The effects of warfarin are monitored by the international normalized ratio (INR) and can be reversed with use of fresh frozen plasma and vitamin K. Because of pharmacokinetic and pharmacodynamic interactions, warfarin is a complex drug to use in the ICU. Now, new anticoagulants have been introduced in the United States, such as an oral direct thrombin inhibitor called dabigatran etexilate and three antifactor Xa inhibitors: apixaban, edoxaban, and rivaroxaban (Mekaj, Mekaj, Duci, & Miftari, 2015).

Dabigatran etexilate cannot be chewed or crushed, which limits its use in the ICU. Currently, monitoring of these agents is problematic, as no substantive laboratory markers exist and all are eliminated between 25%–50% unchanged in the urine (Mekaj et al., 2015). Reversal agents for the antifactor Xa inhibitors are currently in phase III trials, while idarucizumab was recently approved to reverse dabigatran etexilate (Mekaj et al., 2015). Clinical studies excluded use in patients with creatinine clearance less than 30 ml/min.

Until more studies and better monitoring tests are available, these anticoagulants should be used with extreme caution in patients with renal insufficiency (Mekaj et al., 2015).

Histamine-2 Antagonists and Proton Pump Inhibitors

Clinically significant gastrointestinal bleeding was once common in ICU patients but has decreased significantly with the use of acid suppression agents, including histamine-2 antagonists and proton pump inhibitors (Dellinger et al., 2013). Proton pump inhibitors have a relatively short half-life of 2–3 hours but bind to the proton pump and allow for daily dosing for prophylaxis of bleeding. Main risk factors for bleeding include mechanical ventilation for more than 48 hours, coagulopathy defined as a platelet count less than 50,000/mm³, INR greater than 1.5 in those not receiving warfarin, or activated partial thromboplastin time greater than two times the upper limit of normal in those not receiving heparin or direct thrombin inhibitors (Cook et al., 1994). The risk of clinically important bleeding without one of these risk factors is very low and estimated to be 0.2% (95% confidence interval [0.02%, 0.5%]) (Cook et al., 1994). Acid secretion serves as protection against *Clostridium difficile* infections. Studies have suggested that the use of acid suppression, especially twice-daily proton pump inhibitors, increases the rate of this infection (Marik, Vasu, Hirani, & Pachinburavan, 2010). The use of these agents should be assessed for risks and benefits every day, as up to 52% of non-ICU patients received stress ulcer prophylaxis (Janicki & Stewart, 2007; Marik et al., 2010).

Summary

Drug therapy in the critical care of patients with cancer is complex, as changes in pharmacokinetics and pharmacodynamics can affect therapy. Basic knowledge of these studies will help to maximize efficacy and minimize adverse effects. Alterations in pharmacokinetics and pharmacodynamics can be multifactorial and constantly changing. As a result, the use of alternative dosing methods may be required to optimize drug therapy.

References

Andreasen, F., Agerbaek, H., Bjerregaard, P., & Gøtzsche, H. (1981). Pharmacokinetics of amiodarone after intravenous and oral administration. *European Journal of Clinical Pharmacology, 19,* 293–299. doi:10.1007/BF00562807

Annane, D., Siami, S., Jaber, S., Martin, C., Elatrous, S., Declère, A.D., ... Chevret, S. (2013). Effects of fluid resuscitation with colloids vs crystalloids on mortality in critically ill patients presenting with hypovolemic shock: The CRISTAL randomized trial. *JAMA, 310,* 1809–1817. doi:10.1001/jama.2013.280502

Barr, J., Fraser, G.L., Puntillo, K., Ely, E.W., Gélinas, C., Dasta, J.F., ... Jaeschke, R. (2013). Clinical practice guidelines for the management of pain, agitation, and delirium in adult patients in the intensive care unit. *Critical Care Medicine, 41,* 263–306. doi:10.1097/CCM .0b013e3182783b72

Battershill, A.J., & Keating, G.M. (2006). Remifentanil: A review of its analgesic and sedative use in the intensive care unit. *Drugs, 66,* 365–385. doi:10.2165/00003495-200666030-00013

Bauer, L.A. (Ed.). (2014). *Applied clinical pharmacokinetics* (3rd ed.). New York, NY: McGraw-Hill Education.

Brundage, R.C., & Mann, H.J. (2017). General principles of pharmacokinetics and pharmacodynamics. In J.-L. Vincent, E. Abraham, F.A. Moore, P.M. Kochanek, & M.P. Fink (Eds.), *Textbook of critical care* (7th ed., pp. 1062–1070). Philadelphia, PA: Elsevier.

Cody, R.J., & Pickworth, K.K. (1994). Approaches to diuretic therapy and electrolyte imbalance in congestive heart failure. *Cardiology Clinics, 12,* 37–50.

Cook, D.J., Fuller, H.D., Guyatt, G.H., Marshall, J.C., Leasa, D., Hall, R., ... Willan, A. (1994). Risk factors for gastrointestinal bleeding in critically ill patients. *New England Journal of Medicine, 330,* 377–381. doi:10.1056/NEJM199402103300601

De Backer, D., Biston, P., Devriendt, J., Madl, C., Chochrad, D., Aldecoa, C., ... Vincent, J.-L. (2010). Comparison of dopamine and norepinephrine in the treatment of shock. *New England Journal of Medicine, 362,* 779–789. doi:10.1056/NEJMoa0907118

Dellinger, R.P., Levy, M.M., Rhodes, A., Annane, D., Gerlach, H., Opal, S.M., ... Moreno, R. (2013). Surviving Sepsis Campaign: International guidelines for management of severe sepsis and septic shock: 2012. *Critical Care Medicine, 41,* 580–637. doi:10.1097/CCM.0b013e31827e83af

Finfer, S., Bellomo, R., Boyce, N., French, J., Myburgh, J., & Norton, R. (2004). A comparison of albumin and saline for fluid resuscitation in the intensive care unit. *New England Journal of Medicine, 350,* 2247–2256. doi:10.1056/NEJMoa040232

Gerlach, A.T., & Dasta, J.F. (2007). Dexmedetomidine: An updated review. *Annals of Pharmacotherapy, 41,* 245–252. doi:10.1345/aph.1H314

Gerlach, A.T., Folino, J., Morris, B.N., Murphy, C.V., Stawicki, S.P., & Cook, C.H. (2013). Comparison of heparin dosing based on actual body weight in non-obese, obese and morbidly obese critically ill patients. *International Journal of Critical Illness and Injury Science, 3,* 195–199. doi:10 .4103/2229-5151.119200

Gerlach, A.T., Murphy, C.V., & Dasta, J.F. (2009). An updated focused review of dexmedetomidine in adults. *Annals of Pharmacotherapy, 43,* 2064–2074. doi:10.1345/aph.1M310

Gutstein, H.B., & Akil, H. (2001). Opioid analgesics. In J.G. Hardman, L.E. Limbird, & A.G. Gilman (Eds.), *Goodman and Gillman's the pharmacological basis of therapeutics* (10th ed., pp. 569–621). New York, NY: McGraw-Hill Education.

Hirsh, J., & Raschke, R. (2004). Heparin and low-molecular-weight heparin: The Seventh ACCP Conference on Antithrombotic and Thrombolytic Therapy. *Chest, 126*(Suppl. 3), 188S–203S. doi:10.1378/chest.126.3_suppl.188S

Holmes, C.L., Patel, B.M., Russell, J.A., & Walley, K.R. (2001). Physiology of vasopressin relevant to management of septic shock. *Chest, 120,* 989–1002. doi:10.1378/chest.120.3.989

Janicki, T., & Stewart, S. (2007). Stress-ulcer prophylaxis for general medical patients: A review of the evidence. *Journal of Hospital Medicine, 2,* 86–92. doi:10.1002/jhm.177

Jones, G.M., Porter, K., Coffey, R., Miller, S.F., Cook, C.H., Whitmill, M.L., & Murphy, C.V. (2013). Impact of early methadone initiation in critically injured burn patients: A pilot study. *Journal of Burn Care and Research, 34,* 342–348. doi:10.1097/BCR.0b013e3182642c27

Marik, P.E. (2004). Propofol: Therapeutic indications and side-effects. *Current Pharmaceutical Design, 10,* 3639–3649. doi:10.2174/1381612043382846

Marik, P.E., Vasu, T., Hirani, A., & Pachinburavan, M. (2010). Stress ulcer prophylaxis in the new millennium: A systematic review and meta-analysis. *Critical Care Medicine, 38,* 2222–2228. doi:10.1097/CCM.0b013e3181f17adf

Marino, P.L. (Ed.). (2014). *Marino's the ICU book* (4th ed.). Philadelphia, PA: Wolters Kluwer Health/Lippincott Williams & Wilkins.

Meibohm, B., & Derendorf, H. (1997). Basic concepts of pharmacokinetic/pharmacodynamic (PK/PD) modelling. *International Journal of Clinical Pharmacology and Therapeutics, 35,* 401–413.

Mekaj, Y.H., Mekaj, A.Y., Duci, S.B., & Miftari, E.I. (2015). New oral anticoagulants: Their advantages and disadvantages compared with vitamin K antagonists in the prevention and treatment of patients with thromboembolic events. *Therapeutics and Clinical Risk Management, 11,* 967–977. doi:10.2147/TCRM.S84210

Murray, M.J., Cowen, J., DeBlock, H., Erstad, B., Gray, A.W., Jr., Tescher, A.N., ... Lumb, P.D. (2002). Clinical practice guidelines for sustained neuromuscular blockade in the adult critically ill patient. *Critical Care Medicine, 30,* 142–156. doi:10.1097/00003246-200201000-00021

Neyra, J.A., Canepa-Escaro, F., Li, X., Manllo, J., Adams-Huet, B., Yee, J., & Yessayan, L. (2015). Association of hyperchloremia with hospital mortality in critically ill septic patients. *Critical Care Medicine, 43,* 1938–1944. doi:10.1097/CCM.0000000000001161

Nielsen, E.I., & Friberg, L.E. (2013). Pharmacokinetic-pharmacodynamic modeling of antibacterial drugs. *Pharmacological Reviews, 65,* 1053–1090. doi:10.1124/pr.111.005769

Roberts, R.J., Barletta, J.F., Fong, J.J., Schumaker, G., Kuper, P.J., Papadopoulos, S., ... Devlin, J.W. (2009). Incidence of propofol-related infusion syndrome in critically ill adults: A prospective, multicenter study. *Critical Care, 13,* R169. doi:10.1186/cc8145

Shammas, F.V., & Dickstein, K. (1988). Clinical pharmacokinetics in heart failure: An updated review. *Clinical Pharmacokinetics, 15,* 94–113. doi:10.2165/00003088-198815020-00002

Shargel, L., Yu, A., & Wu-Pong, S. (Eds.). (2012). *Applied biopharmaceutics and pharmacokinetics* (6th ed.). New York, NY: McGraw-Hill Education.

Tani, M., Morimatsu, H., Takatsu, F., & Morita, K. (2012). The incidence and prognostic value of hypochloremia in critically ill patients. *Scientific World Journal, 2012,* 474185. doi:10.1100/2012/474185

Waikar, S.S., & Winkelmayer, W.C. (2012). Saving the kidneys by sparing intravenous chloride? *JAMA, 308,* 1583–1585. doi:10.1001/jama.2012.14076

Yunos, N.M., Kim, I.B., Bellomo, R., Bailey, M., Ho, L., Story, D., ... Hart, G.K. (2011). The biochemical effects of restricting chloride-rich fluids in intensive care. *Critical Care Medicine, 39,* 2419–2424. doi:10.1097/CCM.0b013e31822571e5

Zaritsky, A.L. (1994). Catecholamines, inotropic medications, and vasopressor agents. In B. Chernow & D.C. Brater (Eds.), *The pharmacologic approach to the critically ill patient* (3rd ed., pp. 387–404). Philadelphia, PA: Williams & Wilkins.

CHAPTER 18

Vascular Access

Cynthia Chernecky, PhD, RN, AOCN®, FAAN,
and Denise Macklin, BSN, RN, VA-BC

Introduction

A vascular access device allows clinicians to connect to their patients' vascular system for multiple therapeutic interventions (Macklin & Chernecky, 2004). Vascular access is used for chemotherapy administration, laboratory blood samples, blood product administration, nutritional support, IV fluids, medications, and withdrawal of fluid through the abdomen (ascites) or lungs (effusion) (Chernecky & Berger, 2013; Chernecky & Murphy-Ende, 2009). Therapeutic intervention via vascular access is used for molecular targeted therapy, genetic therapy, molecular major pathway control, nanotechnology, and immunotherapy. In the intensive care unit (ICU), although peripheral catheters still exist, the primary IV vascular access method is through a central venous catheter (CVC). The higher flow rate of blood in the superior vena cava ensures hemodilution, protecting the vein wall from alkaline or acidic infusates, such as those with a pH less than 5 (e.g., ciprofloxacin, dopamine, dobutamine, etoposide, gentamicin, mitoxantrone, morphine sulfate, paclitaxel, potassium chloride, promethazine, vancomycin, vinorelbine) or greater than 9 (e.g., acyclovir, amphotericin, ampicillin, 5-fluorouracil, ganciclovir, phenobarbital, phenytoin, trimethoprim-sulfamethoxazole). The corrosive nature of fluids that are hypotonic, or below 250 mOsm/L (e.g., 0.45% NaCl/normal saline [NS], 0.33% NS, 0.2% NS, 2.5% D5W), or hypertonic, or above 600 mOsm/L (e.g., 3% NS, 5% NS, D10W, D20W, D50W, total parenteral nutrition [TPN]), is irritating to the vein wall.

With the complex nature of therapeutic regimens, age differences in patient populations (Chernecky, Macklin, & Blackburn, 2015), and the severity of illness of an ICU patient with cancer (Bagshaw et al., 2009), it is common for a patient to have multiple CVCs and an arterial catheter (catheter tip in an artery). CVCs have their distal tip placed in the lower third of the superior vena cava or at the cavo-atrial junction. CVCs are commonly categorized by the intended length of stay and include short-term catheters (less than 30 days), intermediate catheters (30–42 days), and long-term catheters (greater than 42 days). Each of these devices has its own risks and benefits, advantages and disadvantages, and special care and maintenance requirements. Many patients with cancer have long-term catheters inserted early in treatment for long-term chemotherapy and to save their veins for future use. In the ICU, patients will have this long-term catheter, but because of treatment complexity, they may also have a short-term CVC, intermediate CVC, and/or a peripheral IV.

Central Venous Catheter Characteristics

All CVCs have some commonalities, which can be divided into materials, configuration, and coatings. Materials include polyurethane and silicone. Polyurethane is very strong and can be stiff or soft. It has a thin wall by design and becomes softer as it is thinned. The stiffer the catheter, the harsher it is on the vein lining, leading to increased rates of thrombosis. Silicone catheters are soft and flexible and have increased strength because of thicker walls. This means that the inner diameter is smaller when compared to a polyurethane catheter of the same guage. The gauge size (circumference) directly affects blood flow around the catheter (vein catheter/ratio). It is this ratio that directly influences venous thrombosis. One size does not fit every vein. CVCs are configured with single, double, triple, or quadruple lumens. Lumens are either open ended or may have a distal or a proximal valve. Valves remain closed when not in use. This configuration prevents physiologically occurring reflux (e.g., with patient respirations). Multilumen catheters have staggered internal openings with lumens of different gauges, allowing for multiple interventions to concurrently occur. CVC coatings have been available for more than 20 years and can be bonded or impregnated. Antibiotics (e.g., minocycline, rifampin), antithrombotic heparin, and antiseptics (e.g., chlorhexidine [CHG], silver) are the most common coatings. Theoretically, coatings ease the common complications associated with CVCs: infection and thrombosis. Research varies on their success; however, the Centers for Disease Control and Prevention (CDC) recommended coatings in patients at high risk for infection, a history of multiple infections, and with dialysis catheters that will remain in place longer than two weeks (O'Grady et al., 2002).

Principles of Flow

A common troubleshooting problem with a patient's CVC is related to achieving the prescribed flow rate. A patient may have multichannel large-volume infusion pumps, a small-volume pump (e.g., patient-controlled analgesia), and be on a ventilator. A pressure gradient between the IV bag and the vein is necessary for flow to occur. The gradient depends on static pressure (height of the solution, patient activity, and patient's blood pressure) and dynamic pressure (resistance generated by the fluid flowing through the IV system [flow rate]).

Force is applied by the infusion pump and the thumb, as with IV pushes and the intervention of flushing. It is this force that provides the dynamic pressure required to overcome resistance.

Resistance within the fluid pathway is related to the pathway length, the internal diameter, and the viscosity of the administered fluid. As resistance in the fluid pathway rises or falls, the dynamic pressure also rises and falls. The infusion pump detects the resistance and sounds an occlusion alarm when a specific pump pressure limit is reached. An occlusion alarm is a notification that resistance has risen in the fluid pathway, not that the IV catheter or tubing is occluded. It can be frustrating when a pump occlusion alarm occurs, especially when the catheter flushes clear. This occurs because the force applied to the syringe plunger is greater than the force being applied by the pump. The key to successful troubleshooting is to identify the cause of the resistance. The longer the catheter or thicker the infusate, the greater the resistance.

Changes in the internal diameter (distance from one inside edge of the catheter lumen to the opposite inside edge) have the greatest influence on flow rate. Catheters may have the same gauge (catheter circumference) but have different internal diameters. Tubing is another area to assess. Macrobore tubing has a large internal diameter, whereas microbore tubing has a small internal diameter. If the catheter radius is doubled, the flow rate increases by a factor of 16; however, a 19% decrease in the radius reduces the flow rate by half. A roller clamp works by either decreasing the internal diameter (tightening the clamp) or increasing the internal diameter (loosening the clamp) of the tubing. A partially closed clamp will increase resistance, resulting in an increase in dynamic pressure and possibly causing an occlusion alarm over time. The location of the smallest internal diameter of the tubing or catheter identifies the greatest resistor.

Catheter Types

Short-term CVCs (e.g., percutaneous, nontunneled) commonly are configured with three lumens (e.g., triple-lumen catheter) and can be valved or open tipped. The lumens are staggered and have two 18-gauge lumens (medial, proximal internal lumen) and one 16-gauge lumen (distal internal lumen). The external pigtails are labeled and are often color coded for gauge. Typically, the distal lumen is used for hemodynamic monitoring, high-volume fluids, or blood samples. The medial is used for TPN, lipids, and medications. The proximal is used for blood sampling, IV fluids, blood product administration, IV push, and piggyback medications. These catheters are inserted at the bedside, are economical, and can be easily removed. With 80,000 catheter-related bloodstream infections (CRBSIs) occurring yearly in ICUs (Srinivasan et al., 2011), these catheters pose a serious risk to the immune-suppressed patient with cancer. In addition, the catheter is stiffer than long-term catheters and can cause vein wall damage and potential vein thrombosis. Dialysis catheters and pulmonary artery catheters are also short-term CVCs. Dialysis catheters are only used for short-term hemodialysis. These catheters are very large (13- to 16-gauge), which makes them difficult to stabilize and maintain an occlusive dressing.

The pulmonary artery catheter, or Swan-Ganz catheter, is inserted into a central vein (subclavian or jugular) and advanced until the tip is placed in the pulmonary artery. The catheter is 110 cm long, is heparin coated, and commonly has four lumens, which are attached to hemodynamic monitoring equipment that measures arterial pressure. A balloon surrounds the distal end of the catheter, allowing it to "float" through the right atrium and ventricle and into the pulmonary artery. Once the balloon is inflated, it maintains the correct position of the catheter and measures pressure from the left side of the heart. The Swan-Ganz product has an additional connector that allows infusions through the introducer sheath. A Swan-Ganz catheter is used mostly in neuro-oncology and with cardiac problems to monitor shock, blood flow, cardiac output, and fluid status. Main complications include pneumothorax, arrhythmia, line sepsis, and pulmonary artery rupture.

Intermediate CVCs for use up to six weeks, such as the Hohn®, are single-lumen (4–5 Fr) or double-lumen (7 Fr) soft silicone catheters that include a soft silver-impregnated cuff, which is inserted into the subclavian vein at the bedside or in interventional radiology. This type of catheter is a good choice for immunocompromised patients who have experienced infections with other CVCs. Because it is made of silicone, this catheter has a smaller internal diameter than a polyurethane catheter of the same guage.

Long-term CVCs include tunneled (e.g., Broviac®, Hickman®), implanted (e.g., ports), and peripherally inserted central catheters (PICCs). Tunneled catheters can be open ended, proximal or distal valve, and come in single-, double-, or multilumen configurations. These catheters are commonly used in pediatrics and with adults who require daily treatments. Patients will have both a catheter entrance and exit site, and the catheter tunnel under the skin will be sore and bruised after insertion. Implanted catheters, or ports, have a reservoir that can be made of plastic, stainless steel, or titanium; be high or low profile; and have a single- or double-lumen configuration. A septum covers the reservoir; varies in thickness, diameter, and density; and can be either domed or recessed. The catheter comes either attached to the reservoir or is attached at the time of placement and can be open ended or with a proximal or distal valve. Only Huber needles should be used to access the port, as they do not core the silicone septum. One should *never* use a regular needle to access a port, as it creates a permanent hole, allowing leaks to occur and requiring port replacement. A PICC is inserted using ultrasonography into the cephalic or basilic (preferred site) veins in the upper arm. PICCs can be single, double, or triple lumen and can be open ended or with a proximal or distal valve. This type of catheter has the greatest length, and the most common side effect after insertion is phlebitis. A small-gauge silicone PICC requires a pump to achieve a flow rate. PICCs are inappropriate for renal-impaired patients or those with renal failure, as their veins need to be preserved for the fistulas needed for dialysis.

Central Venous Catheter Care and Maintenance

Care and maintenance of CVCs is the sole responsibility of the bedside RN. The goal of care is to provide required therapies with no complications for the duration of the patient's stay. Because the patient with cancer often has altered immunity, low blood counts with multiple CVCs, and a myriad of treatments, accomplishing this goal can be very challenging. Generally, two pathways need to be protected: the extraluminal catheter tract and the intraluminal fluid pathway. The two major complications associated with care and maintenance are CRBSIs and occlusions.

Handwashing is the primary critical practice intervention within vascular access care. One-third of CRBSIs are caused by isolates found on healthcare workers' hands (Cherifi et al., 2013). Healthcare practitioners should note that during handwashing, the thumbs are most often missed (Taylor, 1978), and using foam requires a minimum of two dollops and 20 seconds of friction. Handwashing should be completed both before donning gloves and after glove removal. See www.steris.com for more information.

Extraluminal Catheter Tract

It is well understood that a biofilm colony is the causative agent of CRBSIs. Biofilm is an aggregation of microbial cells attached to a surface and enclosed in a matrix of primarily polysaccharide material, often referred to as "slime." Any free-floating (planktonic) bacteria can attach to a solid surface. When several such organisms are in proximity, a biofilm can form (Donlan, 2002). The amount of biofilm formation depends on the number of bacteria, the presence of fibrin on the catheter wall, and the flow rate of the fluid through the catheter (Donlan, 2001). It is now understood that *Staphylococcus epidermidis* adheres only to fibronectin, and *Staphylococcus aureus* adheres to fibronectin, fibrinogen, laminin, and gram-negative bacteria (e.g., *Pseudomonas aeruginosa, Klebsiella, Enterobacter*) (Donlan & Costerton, 2002). Because a vascular access device is placed in a vein, a hospitable biofilm formation environment is guaranteed. A biofilm colony is extremely difficult to eradicate, making the best plan of action to prevent its occurrence. This requires minimizing bacteria entry into the bloodstream and minimizing the habitat source (fibrin buildup) from forming on the catheter wall.

Skin Integrity

    Skin varies with age, comorbidities (e.g., cancer, cardiac dysfunction, diabetes, hypertension, renal failure), hydration status, and therapeutic regimens (e.g., steroids, chemotherapy, nonsteroidal anti-inflammatory drugs). Approximately 80% of transient microflora live in the first five layers of the skin and repopulate the skin's surface within 18 hours (Menyhay & Maki, 2006; Ryder, 2006). Skin flora type and pervasiveness vary on the body area, with the lowest levels on dry areas (e.g., arms, legs) and the highest levels (including fungi) on the sebum-rich areas (e.g., groin, armpits, skinfolds [abdomen, chest]). Skin flora is the most common source of CRBSIs (Bashir, Olson, & Walters, 2012).

    The insertion site creates a direct catheter/vein link to skin surface bacteria, and the body's inflammatory response to a puncture is the development of edema and serosanguineous fluid secretion. The edema can result in an enlargement of the puncture site. The enlarged moist puncture site, particularly the femoral site (Marik, Flemmer, & Harrison, 2012), provides the perfect environment for bacterial migration down the extraluminal pathway. An increased laboratory value of international normalized ratio may exacerbate bleeding around the puncture site (Carino, Tsapenko, & Sweeney, 2012). The vein intimal layer promotes platelet adherence to damage on the vein wall and is followed by thrombus formation to promote healing. The "healing" thrombus just inside the puncture site provides the ideal site for fibrin/fibronectin bacteria to colonize and form biofilm. In fact, the most colonized area of a CVC is the proximal end (Nahum et al., 2002). The healing response occurs where the indwelling catheter damages the vein wall. The body's response to foreign objects is a platelet and leukocyte coating that occurs within minutes of device placement. The patient produces small pistoning motions with respiration and change of position that move the catheter in and out of the puncture site, enhancing an entry point for bacteria. These bacteria can build a biofilm colony. Catheter material and poor catheter-to-vein ratio may increase the incidence of thrombin formation.

Dressings

    Dressing management is dependent on catheter securement, with jugular and femoral sites being the most difficult. CDC noted avoiding the use of the femoral vein for central venous access in adult patients as a category 1A recommendation—

the strongest backed by clinical evidence (Miller & O'Grady, 2012). If the femoral site must be used, dressing management can be extremely difficult and requires frequent attention and special products. Transparent dressings vary in moisture vapor transmission rate (MVTR). The higher the MVTR (e.g., Opsite 3000™), the more skin moisture can move through the dressing. Diaphoresis may be a common problem for patients with cancer in the ICU, and it may be advantageous to use a dressing with the highest MVTR. Newer transparent dressings are impregnated with silver, CHG, or both to aid in bacterial destruction. For dressings to accomplish site protection, they must always be dry and completely intact. This includes all dressings, such as those on arterial lines (A-lines) and pulmonary artery catheters (Swan-Ganz). Although easy and quick, reinforcing less-intact dressings is extremely problematic. This seals bacteria into the site and forms a terrarium-like effect, allowing bacteria to thrive.

Changing dressings based on the day of the week should be absolutely avoided and instead based on continued patient assessment. A sterile technique must be maintained throughout the dressing change procedure, making meticulous attention to each step very important. Dressing changes can be time consuming, but skin damage can be disastrous. Adhesive removal pads (e.g., PDI®, Dynarex®, Medline) can be the best solution. Catheter manipulation should be done very carefully during the cleaning process. Damage to the insertion site increases the habitat for bacterial anchoring. The effect of CHG/isopropyl alcohol skin preparations is negated in the presence of blood, so all exudate and dry blood should be thoroughly removed first with half-strength hydrogen peroxide and sterile cotton swabs. CHG's disinfection activity requires a dry time, which may take two minutes or more. The skin is cleaned either up and down or across using friction. Fanning, blowing (increases bacteria), or blotting the area decreases bacterial kill. CDC strongly advises against routinely applying antimicrobial ointment to any insertion site, as this practice can cause insertion site maceration and promote fungal growth (Miller & O'Grady, 2012). CHG-impregnated discs (e.g., Biopatch®, Tegaderm™) or CHG gel dressing (e.g., 3M™), should be applied, as this will maintain significantly lower counts than skin prepped with CHG-containing skin antiseptic alone; remember, microflora cannot be totally eradicated (Bashir et al., 2012). Using a skin protectant prior to dressing application is important. This protectant must be allowed to completely dry prior to dressing application and should be applied to a wide enough area to include any window-pane taping of the dressing.

Intraluminal Fluid Pathway

Catheter manipulations are the primary cause of bacterial migration into the intraluminal pathway. Intraluminal protection depends on two simple yet often haphazardly performed or overlooked practices: septum surface disinfection and flushing. These activities exemplify how vascular access product knowledge, especially of connector products, influences outcome. Swabbing procedures vary in time and disinfectant type. Time recommendations for swabbing the hub vary from 3 to 30 seconds (Richardson, 2006). Disinfectants include alcohol alone or a combination of CHG and alcohol. Research has confirmed that complete bacterial eradication of some IV connectors' septum surfaces is difficult and may not be achievable at high rates in the clinical setting (Menyhay & Maki, 2006). Currently, nursing research has shown that positive connectors have been associated with increased bloodstream infections (Chernecky & Macklin, 2014; Chernecky & Waller, 2010; Jarvis, 2010; Rupp et al., 2007). These connections are also under U.S. Food and Drug Administration (2010) investigation for possibly causing deaths. Today, alcohol caps applied to connector septums are common in some institutions, and research shows their effectiveness (Wright et al., 2013). These caps bathe the entry continuously with alcohol. When the caps are removed for vascular access, they need to be discarded. Additional swabbing should take place before each access. A drying time of 2–3 minutes should occur, and then a new cap should be applied.

Flushing is the only strategy for minimizing fibrin adhesion to the intraluminal surfaces and preventing drug precipitates as precursors to CRBSI and catheter occlusion. Some medications, such as norepinephrine, dopamine, and dobutamine, promote biofilm formation of *Staphylococcus epidermidis* (Frank & Patel, 2008). Several medications are incompatible with others because of precipitation, including aminoglycosides (e.g., amikacin, gentamicin, neomycin, streptomycin, tobramycin), diazepam, digitalis glycosides, pentobarbital, phenytoin, secobarbital, sodium bicarbonate, and theophylline (see Table 18-1).

The connector and catheter should be flushed using a 10 ml syringe (20 ml after a blood draw) of 0.9% NS (Earhart, 2014). Steady flush is best because it minimizes bacterial catheter wall adhesion (Donlan, 2002). This flushing intervention requires active attention, as it is an opportunity to assess the absence or presence of resistance in the fluid pathway. Fibrin can build up on the internal lumen surface; or the tip, referred to as a fibrin tail (can flush but unable to withdraw blood); and on the outside of the catheter, which can lead to a mural thrombus. Some patients with cancer (e.g., lung, gynecologic) are at greater risk of thrombosis. If resistance is felt, avoid the instinct to apply more force; rather, stop, and then reassess. For example, with a PICC, intermittent occlusion can occur when upper arm muscles are flexed; however, deep vein thrombosis may also cause the PICC to be occluded. It is imperative to know what type of connector is being used (i.e., positive, negative, or neutral) (Chernecky, Macklin, Casella, & Jarvis, 2009). Determining the connector type can be difficult, as it is not always noted on the connector package. If the connector is positive (reflux on connection), the clamp must be opened before syringe access. With a negative connector (reflux with disconnection), the syringe must be connected first and then the clamp opened. With a positive connector, the syringe must be disconnected (pulled out of the connector) and then the clamp closed. With a negative connector, the clamp must be closed and then the syringe disconnected from the connector. When implemented correctly, these actions minimize blood

Table 18-1. Common IV Incompatibilities/Precipitates in Oncology

Medication	Incompatible Products
Cefazolin (Ancef®)	Cefoxitin (Mefoxin®)
Ceftriaxone (Rocephin®)	Calcium products (e.g., Ringer's lactate, total parenteral nutrition)
Ciprofloxacin (Cipro®)	Acyclovir (Zovirax®), ampicillin-sulbactam (Unasyn®), cefepime (Maxipime®), clindamycin (Cleocin®), dexamethasone (Decadron®)
Dexamethasone	Calcium gluconate, ciprofloxacin, diphenhydramine (Benadryl®)
Dextrose in water (5%)	Ampicillin (Amoxil®), daptomycin (Cubicin®), phenytoin (Dilantin®)
Diphenhydramine	Ampicillin, cefazolin, cefoxitin, ceftazidime (Fortaz®), dexamethasone
Dobutamine hydrochloride (Dobutrex®)	Acyclovir, ampicillin, cefazolin, cefoxitin, dexamethasone
Dopamine hydrochloride (Intropin®)	Acyclovir, ampicillin, cefazolin
Doxorubicin (Adriamycin®)	Furosemide (Lasix®), heparin (Cohen et al., 1985)
Famotidine (Pepcid®)	Azithromycin (Zithromax®)
Furosemide	Doxorubicin, droperidol (Inapsine®), levofloxacin (Levaquin®), metoclopramide (Reglan®), vinblastine (Velban®), vincristine (Oncovin®)
Heparin	Amikin (Amikacin®), amiodarone (Cordarone®), ciprofloxacin, mitoxantrone (Novantrone®)
Ondansetron (Zofran®)	Alkaline environments (e.g., sodium bicarbonate, potassium chloride)
Phenytoin	Dextrose solutions (Phenytoin can be given with normal saline.)
0.9% sodium chloride (normal saline)	Amiodarone, ampicillin (infuse within 6 hours of mixing), amphotericin B, diazepam (Valium®), doxorubicin hydrochloride liposome (Doxil®), erythromycin lactobionate, fluconazole (Diflucan®), granulocyte macrophage–colony-stimulating factor (Sargramostim®), interleukin, oxaliplatin (Eloxatin®), theophylline

Note. Based on information from Barton-Burke et al., 2001; Vijayakumar et al., 2014.

reflux and the potential for occlusions and infections. Neutral connectors have no specific pattern of care required to minimize reflux. Final heparin flushes remain a controversial topic, but research over the past 30 years has shown them to be no more effective than NS alone in preventing occlusion. Heparin is a protein and has been demonstrated to stimulate *Staphylococcus aureus* biofilm formation (Schallom, Prentice, Sona, Micek, & Skrupky, 2012).

When accessing a port for flushing on a patient in the ICU, place the needle tip up (bevel up) and toward the shoulder in a chest port. This will increase removal of debris when flushing (Guiffant, Durussel, Flaud, Vigier, & Merckx, 2012). Obtain a blood return and flush prior to giving any IV push medication, and then flush again after giving the medication. If a partial occlusion is identified, instill alteplase (e.g., Cathflo®) 2 mg in 2 ml. Leave for 30 minutes and reassess for a blood return. If no blood return, assess again in 90 minutes. If still no blood return, repeat the process, including new drug instillation. If a blood return is not achieved, contact the physician, and do *not* use the catheter (Macklin, 2010).

Blood sampling from CVCs often is a primary ICU nursing responsibility. It is important when drawing blood samples that the clinician achieves success the first time. Repeated sampling from erroneous results or contamination increases catheter manipulations and exposes the intraluminal pathway to numerous blood episodes, increasing the potential for habitat growth, microorganism anchoring, and sepsis. With CVCs, the syringe is the most consistently successful method of blood specimen collection because the withdrawal pressure can be more easily controlled. Blood is aspirated into a syringe, which is then attached to a transfer device (e.g., Vacutainer® tube). The preset vacuum in each tube will withdraw blood from the syringe and fill it with the correct volume. The vacuum pressure is exerted on the syringe and not the soft catheter. It is important to note that less pressure is exerted with a small syringe during withdrawal (the opposite of flushing). For example, if using a 10 ml syringe and having difficulty withdrawing an adequate volume, switch to the next smaller syringe (5 ml) for increased success (Macklin, 2010). The draw order of color tubes is crucial in preventing erroneous results from additive crossover and/or dilution potential (see Table 18-2).

If citrate tube draws (e.g., coagulation tests) are the first or only tube drawn, the clinician *must* get a discard tube (with no additives) to remove air and tissue fluid from the blood collection set; otherwise, the process invalidates the blood-to-additive ratio.

Summary

Extensive knowledge is needed for safe and effective care of a vascular access device in critical and acute care patients with cancer (see Table 18-3).

All aspects of care and maintenance take time and directly influence the treatment and patient. Assessment knowledge includes vascular access history, therapeutic needs, patient preference, and potential discharge care and maintenance. Expertise and research associated with products, catheter insertion, catheter tip location (vein, artery, cavity, epidural, hepatic), and nursing care and maintenance are paramount to avoid major problems that affect cost, mortality, and quality of life. A useful research tool is the Healthcare and Technology Synergy Framework, which includes the major variables of patient, product, and practice (Chernecky, Zadinsky, Macklin, & Maeve, 2013). An understanding of the physics of flow and differences in CVCs is imperative to help educate patients and implement effective care and maintenance. Knowledge of care associated with intraluminal and extraluminal fluid pathways is related to patient outcomes. It is the bedside RN's knowledge and implementation of vascular access care and maintenance that will make a difference in patient outcomes.

Table 18-2. Laboratory Blood Withdrawal Sequence

Tube Top Color (Additives in Tube)	Uses
Yellow	Blood cultures
Light blue (buffered sodium citrate)	Coagulation studies, such as prothrombin time, partial thromboplastin time, fibrinogen, D-dimer
Royal blue (EDTA)	Toxicology, metals, nutrition, antibody screening, copper, zinc, trace elements
Red or pink	Serology, blood bank, type and screening, cross-match
Gold/tiger top/serum separator tube (gel separator tube)	Chemistry panels, hepatitis, routine blood donor screening
Bright green (sodium heparin)	Alpha-fetoprotein blood cultures, HLA-B27, chromosome studies
Light green (lithium heparin)	Troponin, metabolic panel, lipids, liver panel, ammonia (ice), HIV rapid antibody
Dark green (lithium)	Ionized calcium (not part of blood gas), ammonia (ice)
Lavender (EDTA)	Hematology, complete blood count, platelets, sedimentation rate, G6PD, HgbA1C, CD4
White (partial thromboplastin time T gel)	Antibody screening, copper, zinc, trace elements
Gray (Na⁺ fluoride or K⁺ oxalate)	Glucose, lactate (lactic acid)

Note. Based on information from Becton, Dickinson and Company, 2002; UC Davis Health, n.d.

Table 18-3. Vascular Access Problems and Interventions

Problem	Causes	Signs and Symptoms	Interventions
Occlusion: Mechanical	Catheters are placed medially in clavicle first rib space. Malposition can happen at any time.	Inability to flush and/or obtain blood return. A change in arm position allows blood to be obtained and/or catheter flushed. Ringing in ear, rushing sound, headache, pain in shoulder	X-ray the patient's arm, which must remain at patient's side. Other positions may correct the compression. If occlusion is diagnosed, the catheter is removed. X-ray and reposition
Occlusion: Medication, precipitation	Improper or missing flushing. Higher precipitate values include potassium, calcium phosphate, phenytoin, lorazepam, lipids, total parenteral nutrition, and aminophylline.	Loss of patency	Flush between each drug using SAS method (saline, administer medication, saline). Consult pharmacist, who may recommend nonfibrinolytic agent.
Occlusion: Thrombotic	Fibrin is a cause. Patients at high risk include those with diabetes, cancer, trauma, atrial fibrillation, and chronic inactivity.	Inability to flush and/or withdraw from central venous catheter (CVC). Edema at or around entry site (Cornock, 1996), erythema (Cornock, 1996), edema of arm, neck, and/or face, with associated pain, tingling or numbness (Cornock, 1996; Kayley, 1997), distension of neck veins and/or peripheral vessels. Catheter occlusion (Krzywda, 1999)	Alteplase administration

(Continued on next page)

Table 18-3. Vascular Access Problems and Interventions *(Continued)*

Problem	Causes	Signs and Symptoms	Interventions
Hematoma (blood outside of blood vessel) at site	Trauma of blood vessel wall, thrombocytopenia, anticoagulant medications	Irritation, swelling, inflammation, dark area at puncture site	Rest, ice, compression, elevation
Exudate at site	Pistoning of catheter in and out of the site due to movement, lack of anchoring, infection, disseminated intravascular coagulation, thrombocytopenia	Oozing of fluid from insertion site	Culture insertion site after cleaning with normal saline, as pus is just dead white blood cells and needs to be removed before culturing Possible removal of device IV antibiotics Do not use ointments at site, as they can grow bacteria.
Catheter migration	Tip of catheter migration out of superior vena cava due to power injection, push-pause flushing, severe vomiting, suctioning	Loss of blood return, discomfort in upper arm, neck, or chest during infusions, exposure length externally increased	Do not use CVC, notify physician immediately, and prepare for interventional radiology and chest x-ray interventions.
Catheter damage: External	Improper care, hemostats	Leaking during flushing	Peripherally inserted central catheters (PICCs) and tunneled catheters may be able to be repaired. Clamp exposed catheter below the hole.
Phlebitis: Chemical	Chemical common with peripheral IV (PIV) solutions that are acidic or alkaline or have a high or low osmolarity	Red streak along the vein path above the catheter tip location (not insertion site); warmth, tenderness, burning, or itchiness; swelling	Consider CVC.

(Continued on next page)

Table 18-3. Vascular Access Problems and Interventions *(Continued)*

Problem	Causes	Signs and Symptoms	Interventions
Phlebitis: Mechanical	Common with PIVs and PICCs due to trauma to the vein during insertion or using a vascular access device or PIV that is too big for the vein-to-catheter ratio	Red streak over catheter, warm, tenderness, itchiness	Change PIV. For PICCs, first apply heat to affected arm and then a cold pack to affected arm. Elevate arm and limit its use. If venous thrombosis is present, anticoagulation may be necessary.
Catheter-related bloodstream infection	Biofilm formation Bacterial entry via intraluminal or extraluminal pathways	Pyrexia, rigor after flushing; generally feeling unwell, hypotension, tachycardia, and shock Positive blood cultures (peripheral and central)	Full barrier precautions with insertion Bundle approach to care Meticulous disinfection practices with all aspects of care Minimization of catheter manipulations Proper flushing for type of connectors used (positive, negative, neutral)
Embolism: Catheter, fibrin, or air	Catheter fracture Forceful flushing to overcome resistance Lack of occlusive dressing after CVC removal	Anxiety, pallor, cyanosis, shortness of breath (SOB), rapid weak pulse, hypotension, chest pain, loss of consciousness	Place patient on left side and prepare for surgical removal and cardiac catheterization. Prepare for diagnostic linogram, ultrasound, chest x-ray, and/or venography.

(Continued on next page)

Table 18-3. Vascular Access Problems and Interventions *(Continued)*

Problem	Causes	Signs and Symptoms	Interventions
Pneumo-thorax: Can also occur after chest tube removal	Insertion attempt of CVC; incidence varies between 1% and 6.6% (Kusminsky, 2007). The experience of the physician inserting the CVC is important, as procedures done by physicians who have performed ≥ 50 catheterizations are half as likely to result in pneumothorax (Bernard & Stahl, 1971).	Increased sudden respiratory rate, SOB, respiratory distress, tachycardia, reduced oxygen saturation levels, hypotension	Chest tube insertion: Monitor vital signs, especially respiratory rate and lung sounds every 5 minutes for 3 times and then 10 minutes one time after CVC insertion.

References

Bagshaw, S.M., Webb, S.A.R., Delaney, A., George, C., Pilcher, D., Hart, G.K., & Bellomo, R. (2009). Very old patients admitted to intensive care in Australia and New Zealand: A multicentre cohort analysis. *Critical Care, 13,* R45. doi:10.1186/cc7768

Barton-Burke, M., Wilkes, G.M., & Ingwersen, K. (2001). *Cancer chemotherapy: A nursing process approach.* Burlington, MA: Jones & Bartlett Learning.

Bashir, M.H., Olson, L.K.M., & Walters, S.-A. (2012). Suppression of regrowth of normal skin flora under chlorhexidine gluconate dressings applied to chlorhexidine gluconate-prepped skin. *American Journal of Infection Control, 40,* 344–348. doi:10.1016/j.ajic.2011.03.030

Becton, Dickinson and Company. (2002). Order of draw for multiple tube collections: Designed for your safety. Retrieved from http://www.bd.com/resource.aspx?IDX=1157

Bernard, R.W., & Stahl, W.M. (1971). Subclavian vein catheterizations: A prospective study: I. Noninfectious complications. *Annals of Surgery, 173,* 184–190. doi:10.1097/00000658-197102000-00002

Carino, G.P., Tsapenko, A.V., & Sweeney, J.D. (2012). Central line placement in patients with and without prophylactic plasma. *Journal of Critical Care, 27,* 529.e9–529.e13. doi:10.1016/j.jcrc.2011.12.016

Cherifi, S., Mascart, G., Dediste, A., Hallin, M., Gerard., M., Lambert, M.-L., & Byl, B. (2013). Variations in catheter-related bloodstream infections rates based on local practices. *Antimicrobial Resistance and Infection Control, 1,* 10. doi:10.1186/2047-2994-2-10

Chernecky, C., & Berger, B. (2013). *Laboratory tests and diagnostic procedures* (6th ed.). St. Louis, MO: Elsevier Saunders.

Chernecky, C., & Macklin, D. (2014). The role of IV needleless connectors and IV complication management and prevention. *Advances in Research, 2,* 195–206. doi:10.9734/AIR/2014/8475

Chernecky, C., Macklin, D., & Blackburn, P. (2015). Catheter-related bloodstream infections (CR-BSI) in geriatric patients in intensive care units. *Critical Care Nursing Quarterly, 38,* 280–292. doi:10.1097/CNQ.0000000000000076

Chernecky, C., Macklin, D., Casella, L., & Jarvis, E. (2009). Caring for patients with cancer through nursing knowledge of IV connectors. *Clinical Journal of Oncology Nursing, 13,* 630–633. doi:10 .1188/09.CJON.630-633

Chernecky, C., & Murphy-Ende, K. (2009). *Acute care oncology nursing* (2nd ed.). St. Louis, MO: Elsevier Saunders.

Chernecky, C., & Waller, J. (2010). Comparison of bacterial CFUs in five intravenous connectors. *Clinical Nursing Research: An International Journal, 19,* 416–428. doi:10.1177/1054773810375110

Chernecky, C., Zadinsky, J., Macklin, D., & Maeve, M.K. (2013). The healthcare and technology synergy (HATS) framework for comparative effectiveness research as part of evidence-based practice in vascular access. *Journal of the Association for Vascular Access, 18,* 169–174. doi:10.1016 /j.java.2013.05.001

Cohen, M.H., Johnston-Early, A., Hood, M.A., McKenzie, M., Citron, M.L., Jaffe, N., & Krasnow, S.H. (1985). Drug precipitation within IV tubing: A potential hazard of chemotherapy administration. *Cancer Treatment Reports, 69,* 1325–1326.

Cornock, M. (1996). Making sense of central venous catheters. *Nursing Times, 92*(49), 30–31.

Donlan, R.M. (2001). Biofilms and device-associated infections. *Emerging Infectious Diseases, 7,* 277–280. doi:10.3201/eid0702.010226

Donlan, R.M. (2002). Biofilms: Microbial life on surfaces. *Emerging Infectious Diseases, 8,* 881–890. doi:10.3201/eid0809.020063

Donlan, R.M., & Costerton, J.W. (2002). Biofilms: Survival mechanisms of clinically relevant microorganisms. *Clinical Microbiology Reviews, 15,* 167–193. doi:10.1128/CMR.15.2.167-193.2002

Earhart, A. (2014). Providing optimal care for patients with central catheters. *American Nurse Today, 9*(5), 22–26.

Frank, K.L., & Patel, R. (2008). Intravenously administered pharmaceuticals impact biofilm formation and detachment of *Staphylococcus lugdunensis* and other staphylococci. *Diagnostic Microbiology and Infectious Disease, 60,* 9–16. doi:10.1016/j.diagmicrobio.2007.07.008

Guiffant, G., Durussel, J.J., Flaud, P., Vigier, J.P., & Merckx, J. (2012). Flushing ports of totally implantable venous access devices, and impact of the Huber point needle bevel orientation: Experimental tests and numerical computation. *Journal of Medical Devices: Evidence and Research, 5,* 31–37. doi:10.2147/MDER.S30029

Jarvis, W.R. (2010). Choosing the best design for intravenous needleless connectors to prevent bloodstream infections. *Infection Control Today, 14*(8), 1–2.

Kayley, J. (1997). Skin-tunnelled cuffed catheters. *Community Nurse, 3*(5), 21–22.

Krzywda, E.A. (1999). Predisposing factors, prevention, and management of central venous catheter occlusions. *Journal of Intravenous Nursing, 22*(Suppl. 6), S11–S17.

Kusminsky, R.E. (2007). Complications of central venous catheterization. *Journal of the American College of Surgeons, 204,* 681–696. doi:10.1016/j.jamcollsurg.2007.01.039

Macklin, D. (2010). Catheter management. *Seminars in Oncology Nursing, 26,* 113–120. doi:10.1016 /j.soncn.2010.02.002

Macklin, D., & Chernecky, C. (2004). *Real World Nursing Survival Guide: IV therapy.* Philadelphia, PA: Saunders.

Marik, P.E., Flemmer, M., & Harrison, W. (2012). The risk of catheter-related bloodstream infection with femoral venous catheters as compared to subclavian and internal jugular venous catheters: A systematic review of the literature and meta-analysis. *Critical Care Medicine, 40,* 2479–2485. doi:10.1097/CCM.0b013e318255d9bc

Menyhay, S.Z., & Maki, D.G. (2006). Disinfection of needleless catheter connectors and access ports with alcohol may not prevent microbial entry: The promise of a novel antiseptic-barrier cap. *Infection Control and Hospital Epidemiology, 27,* 3–7. doi:10.1086/500280

Miller, D.L., & O'Grady, N.P. (2012). Guidelines for the prevention of intravascular catheter-related infections: Recommendations relevant to interventional radiology for venous catheter placement and maintenance. *Journal of Vascular and Interventional Radiology, 23,* 997–1007. doi:10.1016 /j.jvir.2012.04.023

Nahum, E., Levy, I., Katz, J., Samra, Z., Ashkenazi, S., Ben-Ari, J., ... Dagan, O. (2002). Efficacy of subcutaneous tunneling for prevention of bacterial colonization of femoral central venous catheters in critically ill children. *Pediatric Infectious Disease Journal, 21,* 1000–1004. doi:10.1097 /00006454-200211000-00005

O'Grady, N.P., Alexander, M., Dellinger, E.P., Gerberding, J.L., Heard, S.O., Maki, D.G., ... Weinstein, R.A. (2002). Guidelines for the prevention of intravascular catheter-related infections. *Morbidity and Mortality Weekly Report, 51,* 1–26.

Richardson, D. (2006). Vascular access nursing practice, standards of care, and strategies to prevent infection: A review of skin cleansing agents and dressing materials (Part I of a 3-part series). *Journal of the Association of Vascular Access, 11,* 215–221. doi:10.2309/java.11-4-14

Rupp, M.E., Sholtz, L.A., Jourdan, D.R., Marion, N.D., Tyner, L.K., Fey, P.D., ... Anderson, J.R. (2007). Outbreak of bloodstream infection temporally associated with the use of an intravascular needleless valve. *Clinical Infectious Diseases, 44,* 1408–1414. doi:10.1086/517538

Ryder, M. (2006). Evidence-based practice in the management of vascular access devices for home parenteral nutrition therapy. *Journal of Parenteral and Enteral Nutrition, 30*(Suppl. 1), S82–S93. doi:10.1177/0148607106030051S82

Schallom, M.E., Prentice, D., Sona, C., Micek, S.T., & Skrupky, L.P. (2012). Heparin or 0.9% sodium chloride to maintain central venous catheter patency: A randomized trial. *Critical Care Medicine, 40,* 1820–1826. doi:10.1097/CCM.0b013e31824e11b4

Srinivasan, A., Wise, M., Bell, M., Cardo, D., Edwards, J., Fridkin, S., ... Pollock, D. (2011). Vital signs: Central line-associated blood stream infections: United States, 2001, 2008, and 2009. *Morbidity and Mortality Weekly Report, 60,* 243–248.

Taylor, L.J. (1978). An evaluation of handwashing techniques. *Nursing Times, 74,* 54–55.

UC Davis Health. (n.d.). Central line blood draw. Retrieved from http://ucdmc.ucdavis.edu/cppn /resources/clinical_skills_refresher/central_line_blood_draw

U.S. Food and Drug Administration. (2010). *Letter to infection control practitioners regarding positive displacement needleless connectors, July 2010.* Retrieved from http://www.fda.gov/Medical Devices/Safety/AlertsandNotices/ucm220459.htm

Vijayakumar, A., Sharon, E.V., Teena, J., Nobil, S., & Nazeer, I. (2014). A clinical study on drug-related problems associated with intravenous drug administration. *Journal of Basic and Clinical Pharmacy, 5,* 49–53. doi:10.4103/0976-0105.134984

Wright, M.-O., Tropp, J., Schora, D.M., Dillon-Grant, M., Peterson, K., Boehm, S., ... Peterson, L.R. (2013). Continuous passive disinfection of catheter hubs prevents contamination and bloodstream infection. *American Journal of Infection Control, 41,* 33–38. doi:10.1016/j.ajic.2012 .05.030

CHAPTER 19

Transitions in Care

Christine Hull, RN, MSN, OCN®

Introduction

For a significant portion of the 20th century, patients with cancer had narrow treatment options, often relying on overpowering therapies with high mortality rates and limited life-prolonging care in the intensive and critical care settings. Furthermore, complications from cancer and its treatment were exceedingly difficult to manage. Moving patients with cancer to a higher level of care was uncommon because of grave prognoses and the improbability of clinical improvement in an inpatient intensive care unit (ICU).

With recent advances in research and the development of antineoplastic agents, patients with cancer are living longer and with an improved quality of life (Buchheidt, Hummel, Engelich, & Hehlmann, 2004; Gutierrez & Pastores, 2009). With further advancement of targeted therapies and personalized medicine, cancer ultimately will change from a chronic to a curable illness (von Bergwelt-Baildon, Hallek, Shimabukuro-Vornhagen, & Kochanek, 2010).

Many patients are able to receive cancer treatment on an outpatient basis and only require an inpatient admission for supportive management. Additionally, when patients are admitted to the hospital, their length of stay is longer, which equates to an inevitable need for critical care support (Wigmore, Farquhar-Smith, & Lawson, 2013). Regardless of treatment setting, when patients with cancer become critically ill from complications of cancer or its treatment, the goal should be to optimize survival and ensure the highest quality of life, especially in patients with no curative option who are undergoing palliative treatment. To address this goal, it is necessary for a transfer or transition of care to occur from the ambulatory outpatient or inpatient medical-surgical setting to the critical care setting. This allows patients to receive the specialized supportive care that only practitioners trained in critical care can provide, which can make the difference in reversing life-threatening conditions and achieving positive outcomes.

The Meaning of Transition

The term *transition* is defined as "a passage from one state, stage, subject, or a change of place to another" or as "a movement, development, or evolution from one form, stage, or style to another" ("Transition," n.d.). Ludin, Arbon, and Parker (2013) described transition as both a process and an outcome. Nurses in the inpatient medical-surgical setting may consider only the process, or the physical movement of a patient to a higher level of care, not recognizing that this is just one component of transition (Ludin et al., 2013). It is during this situational transition that critically ill patients are particularly vulnerable, as the potential exists for fragmented care. An acute awareness of patient needs is imperative to increase the probability of surviving a life-threatening complication, such as an oncologic emergency or sepsis (Ludin et al., 2013). Early recognition of symptoms related to complications and deteriorating physiologic condition increases the chances of a timely move to the critical care setting, the initiation of critical care interventions, and patient condition stabilization.

The Time Has Come

The transition of patients with cancer to the critical care setting is addressed when initial signs and symptoms of clinical deterioration are recognized. Some early signs include tachypnea, tachycardia, transient hypotension, marbling, oliguria, decreasing oxygen saturation, and impaired consciousness (Azoulay, 2014). According to Pattison, Ashley, Farquhar-Smith, Roskelly, and O'Gara (2010), "Delayed recognition of unwell or at-risk patients contributed to late referral to critical care services or outreach" (p. 1670). For neutropenic patients, the only sign of early sepsis may be a low-grade temperature that quickly increases to 104°F (40°C) or higher. Studies have argued that early recognition of symptoms is just one factor that contributes to better outcomes in critically ill patients with cancer, with other factors including screening and improvements in antimicrobial, cytotoxic, and biologic agents (Andréjak et al., 2011; Anisoglou et al., 2013). The screening process involves several different factors. For example, a patient's performance status and number of comorbidities contribute to higher mortality, such as cardiovascular, respiratory, or renal dysfunction (Rosolem et al., 2012). Good performance status has a clear connection to improved prognosis and has a greater influence on outcome than any other factor. For example, if patients already have sepsis or acute respiratory distress syndrome on admission, their mortality risk increases. The intensivist in the ICU is primarily concerned with cure; however, it is important to remember that the focus of cure may not be on the cancer itself but rather the complications it has produced (Wigmore et al., 2013).

Ethical Responsibilities

Because of the expense of lengthy ICU stays, a prejudice has existed against providing aggressive treatment and critical care to patients with cancer. Williams et al. (2004) detailed a hospital with admissions for sepsis that represented 4.9% of all hospitalizations for patients with cancer; however, these admissions expended 14% of the cost of care. In terms of positive clinical outcomes, it was without merit, as demonstrated by the increasing incidence of positive outcomes resulting from ICU admissions for patients who did *not* have widespread metastatic disease.

This negative view of treating critically ill patients with cancer in the ICU has recently changed (Farquhar-Smith & Wigmore, 2008). Studies have confirmed that the mortality rate for these patients has declined in the past decade from 75%–85% to 40%–55% (Aygencel, Turkoglu, Sucak, & Benekli, 2014; Azoulay, 2014; Thiery, Darmon, & Azoulay, 2007). Furthermore, current data fail to justify the denial of critical care interventions to patients with cancer who have two or fewer comorbidities, partly because of these improved mortality rates.

Souza-Dantas, Salluh, and Soares (2011) demonstrated that neutropenia as a single risk factor did not result in increased mortality in critically ill patients with cancer admitted to the ICU. This defied conventional wisdom that sending a neutropenic, immunocompromised patient into a busy critical care area could result in sepsis and death; however, patients with prolonged neutropenia, such as those with hematologic cancers or recipients of hematopoietic stem cell transplantation (HSCT), did not fare as well as patients with short-term neutropenia, such as those with solid-tumor disease. Buchheidt et al. (2004) defined the different classifications of neutropenia as low risk, lasting five or fewer days; intermediate risk, lasting from six to nine days; and high risk, lasting more than nine days.

An ICU admission should not be denied based on individual factors such as cancer diagnosis or age. An interprofessional team should evaluate each case to determine the best action for each patient. Azoulay et al. (2011) suggested allowing three to five days in the ICU for all treatments to be administered prior to making an informed decision on continuation of care based on the patient's clinical response (Schönfeld & Timsit, 2008). Kostakou, Rovina, Kyriakopoulou, Koulouris, and Koutsoukou (2014) and Soubani, Shehada, Chen, and Smith

(2014) proposed the use of an ICU trial in the treatment of critically ill patients with cancer. Patient evaluation after the administration window should be interprofessional with a reevaluation of treatments goals (Soubani et al., 2014). When the focus of care shifts from cure to comfort, Hartjes (2015) suggested that palliative care for symptom management can be addressed before admission to the critical care setting, especially as cancer incidence is expected to rise 45% by 2030.

Admitting Diagnoses and Complications

Acute respiratory failure (ARF), often associated with an infectious process, is the predominant reason for admission of a critically ill patient with cancer to the ICU (Gutierrez & Pastores, 2009). Patients with cancer are at a tremendous risk of developing ARF of infectious etiology because of the immunosuppressive characteristics of anticancer agents, the cancer itself (the infiltration of the lungs by cancerous cells), and drug toxicities (Azoulay, 2014). Pneumonia is a frequently encountered infectious cause of ARF, resulting in a transition to critical care (Gutierrez & Pastores, 2009). The mortality and prognosis of ARF are dependent on the cause (Gutierrez & Pastores, 2009). Other infectious processes involve commonly occurring *Candida*, pulmonary fungal invasions such as aspergillosis, and mucormycosis, which results in increased mortality, especially in patients with hematologic cancers and HSCT recipients (Sipsas & Kontoyiannis, 2012). With the introduction of multiple new antineoplastic agents that target the immune system and the use of steroids to combat the inflammatory response, more infections are likely to occur (Kelly, 2008; Staudinger & Pène, 2014). The immediate initiation of broad-spectrum antibiotics is critical in the treatment of unconfirmed infections after the collection of cultures. Once the infective species is confirmed, the initiation of antifungals and targeted antibiotics is paramount, as mortality increases with delay (Sipsas & Kontoyiannis, 2012).

Other admitting diagnoses for critically ill patients with cancer include but are not limited to acute lung injury, acute respiratory distress, surgical oncologic emergencies (e.g., gastrointestinal tract obstruction), and oncologic emergencies (e.g., tumor lysis syndrome, sepsis, cardiac tamponade) (Bosscher, van Leeuwen, & Hoekstra, 2014; Wilson & Berns, 2014). With cardiac tamponade, an indirect relationship exists between the speed of fluid accumulation in the pericardial sac and the volume needed to cause symptoms such as shortness of breath or chest pain. For example, the faster the fluid accumulates, the smaller the volume needed for the patient to become symptomatic; otherwise, with a slow fluid accumulation, the pericardial sac could accommodate up to 2 L of fluid prior to symptom onset (Perri et al., 2015). Patients with cancer also may be admitted to the ICU for the prevention, recognition, or management of one or more oncologic emergencies (Kaplow, 2014).

Noninvasive and Mechanical Ventilation

Noninvasive ventilation (NIV), such as continuous positive airway pressure, and mechanical ventilation (MV), such as intubation, encourage positive outcomes for critically ill patients with cancer with ARF as a predominant presenting diagnosis. The consensus is that critically ill patients with cancer fare better with NIV, as "it may be possible to keep the airway defense mechanisms intact and preserve swallowing function" (Nava & Cuomo, 2004, p. 92); however, the mortality rate has decreased for those using MV in the past two decades (Azoulay, 2014). MV is not preferred for artificial ventilation because of the risk of ventilator-associated pneumonia resulting from intubation (Nava & Cuomo, 2004). Azoulay (2014) noted that it is important to consider both interventions if patients are on chemotherapy for either cure or palliation, can provide consent to the procedure, and are mobile (not bedbound). This is a departure from previous standards of care but is substantiated by studies confirming improved survival rates (Azoulay, 2014).

Potential Pitfalls During Transition

The transition process is facilitated by the interprofessional team using an emergency or rapid response system designed to move patients to the critical care setting quickly and effectively. Despite the system's fluidity, potential pitfalls cannot be overlooked. To better understand these pitfalls, it is critical to first understand the concept of an interhospital transfer. An interhospital transfer involves sending a critically ill patient by ambulance or helicopter to a facility better equipped to address their needs (Dunn, Gwinnutt, & Gray, 2007). This may occur when a patient is admitted to a small community hospital, is diagnosed with a hematologic malignancy (e.g., acute lymphocytic leukemia, acute myelocytic leukemia), and then needs an interhospital transfer to receive immediate induction chemotherapy at a larger facility with personnel trained in the care of patients with hematologic disorders. If the focus is an internal transfer from the medical or oncology unit to the ICU, specific considerations need to be followed to ensure safe patient transfer.

Three potential pitfalls during the transition process include poor communication, equipment failure, and the human factor. Poor communication may lead to inappropriate care and results in incorrect or vague clinical information given to the healthcare team, including the ICU receiving the patient. This lack of communication fails to provide reassurance to anxious and frightened family members of the patient, who have been thrust into an uncertain situation. It is paramount that communication between all parties is maintained at all stages of transition—before departure, during the physical transfer, and on arrival to the

ICU (Dunn et al., 2007). Additionally, it is recommended that the patient's family is notified of any impending or completed emergent transfers as soon as possible to provide an update on clinical status and assure them that everything is being done to ensure the patient's survival and symptom management. This will provide comfort and peace of mind to family members, especially if they were not present at the time of the patient's clinical deterioration and were unable to witness the care provided by the healthcare team. If possible, it is also helpful to provide the family with the patient's new location and room number, the contact information for the ICU, and the name of a staff member who can accompany them to the ICU waiting area. If the primary nurse for the patient is unable to provide family notification and supplemental support, then the charge nurse or unit leader may take over that responsibility, enabling the primary nurse to participate in the patient's care, give a handoff report to the ICU, and transfer the patient.

With advances in technology, equipment failure is often not considered a potential pitfall but can have a detrimental effect on the transition process. Very few manual mechanisms are used in the clinical care setting, though two significant tools include the stethoscope and sphygmomanometer. Clinicians need to be aware of the possibility of power failure of vital equipment caused by a depleted or critically low battery supply. For example, the cardiac monitor used during patient transport is also an automated external defibrillator (AED) as well as a telemetry device. This device is essential for all monitored transports of patients to critical care areas where a higher level of care is to be provided. Lethal outcomes may result if the AED battery were to fail during transport, making it essential that these lifesaving devices always have functional batteries.

The human factor is the final potential pitfall in patient transport. Gillman et al. (2006) demonstrated that the most significant error in the transfer of a patient to the operating room prior to the ICU was the discovery of an incorrect patient ID bracelet. They also identified a significant number of transfer delays to the ICU because of unavailable beds, inadequate staffing, and workload (Gillman et al., 2006). With increased awareness of these potential pitfalls, healthcare providers can take preventive measures and thus improve patient outcomes.

Summary

The transition of care of the critically ill patient with cancer to the ICU is in a state of change and progress. As the incidence of cancer and cancer-related complications increases, this population will also increase. The challenge moving forward is to apply some of the concepts discussed in this chapter consistently to patients who do not have widespread metastatic disease and have a good probability of benefiting from critical care intervention. Ideally, these decisions should also involve an interprofessional team and include discussion of care goals with the patient and family. Despite these statistics, clinicians are obligated to provide the best possible care based on the evidence (Divatia, 2007). Future research into improving the care and outcomes of patients requiring critical care intervention will guarantee that.

References

Andréjak, C., Terzi, N., Thielen, S., Bergot, E., Zalcman, G., Charbonneau, P., & Jounieaux, V. (2011). Admission of advanced lung cancer patients to intensive care unit: A retrospective study of 76 patients. *BMC Cancer, 11,* 159. doi:10.1186/1471-2407-11-159

Anisoglou, S., Asteriou, C., Barbetakis, N., Kakolyris, S., Anastasiadou, G., & Pneumatikos, I. (2013). Outcome of lung cancer patients admitted to the intensive care unit with acute respiratory failure. *Hippokratia, 17,* 60–63.

Aygencel, G., Turkoglu, M., Sucak, G.T., & Benekli, M. (2014). Prognostic factors in critically ill cancer patients admitted to the intensive care unit. *Journal of Critical Care, 29,* 618–626. doi:10.1016/j.jcrc.2014.01.014

Azoulay, E. (2014). A new standard of care for critically ill patients with cancer. *Chest, 146,* 241–244. doi:10.1378/chest.14-0620

Azoulay, E., Soares, M., Darmon, M., Benoit, D., Pastores, S., & Afessa, B. (2011). Intensive care of the cancer patient: Recent achievements and remaining challenges. *Annals of Intensive Care, 1,* 5. doi:10.1186/2110-5820-1-5

Bosscher, M.R.F., van Leeuwen, B.L., & Hoekstra, H.J. (2014). Surgical emergencies in oncology. *Cancer Treatment Reviews, 40,* 1028–1036. doi:10.1016/j.ctrv.2014.05.005

Buchheidt, D., Hummel, M., Engelich, G., & Hehlmann, R. (2004). Management of infections in critically ill neutropenic patients. *Journal of Critical Care, 19,* 165–173. doi:10.1016/j.jcrc.2004.07.007

Divatia, J.V. (2007). Critical care for cancer patients. *Indian Journal of Critical Care Medicine, 11,* 1–3. doi:10.4103/0972-5229.32429

Dunn, M.J.G., Gwinnutt, C.L., & Gray, A.J. (2007). Critical care in the emergency department: Patient transfer. *Emergency Medicine Journal, 24,* 40–44. doi:10.1136/emj.2006.042044

Farquhar-Smith, W.P., & Wigmore, T. (2008). Outcomes for cancer patients in critical care. *Trends in Anaesthesia and Critical Care, 19,* 91–95. doi:10.1016/j.cacc.2008.01.003

Gillman, L., Leslie, G., Williams, T., Fawcett, K., Bell, R., & McGibbon, V. (2006). Adverse events experienced while transferring the critically ill patient from the emergency department to the intensive care unit. *Emergency Medicine Journal, 23,* 858–861. doi:10.1136/emj.2006.037697

Gutierrez, C., & Pastores, S.M. (2009, December 5). When should the cancer patient get an ICU bed? *Critical Connections.* Retrieved from http://www.sccm.org/Communications/Critical-Connections/Archives/Pages/When-Should-the-Cancer-Patient-Get-an-ICU-Bed.aspx

Hartjes, T.M. (2015). Making the case for palliative care in critical care. *Critical Care Nursing Clinics of North America, 27,* 289–295. doi:10.1016/j.cnc.2015.05.004

Kaplow, R. (2014). Oncologic issues in the older adult in critical care. *Critical Care Nursing Clinics of North America, 26,* 147–154. doi:10.1016/j.ccell.2013.09.007

Kelly, P. (2008). The cancer critical care paradox. *Current Anaesthesia and Critical Care, 19,* 96–104. doi:10.1016/j.cacc.2008.01.002

Kostakou, E., Rovina, N., Kyriakopoulou, M., Koulouris, N.G., & Koutsoukou, A. (2014). Critically ill cancer patient in intensive care unit: Issues that arise. *Journal of Critical Care, 29,* 817–822. doi:10.1016/j.jcrc.2014.04.007

Ludin, S.M., Arbon, P., & Parker, S. (2013). Patients' transition in the intensive care units: Concept analysis. *Intensive and Critical Care Nursing, 29,* 187–192. doi:10.1016/j.iccn.2013.02.001

Nava, S., & Cuomo, A.M. (2004). Acute respiratory failure in the cancer patient: The role of non-invasive mechanical ventilation. *Critical Reviews in Oncology/Hematology, 51,* 91–103.

Pattison, N., Ashley, S., Farquhar-Smith, P., Roskelly, L., & O'Gara, G. (2010). Thirty-day mortality in critical care outreach patients with cancer: An investigative study of predictive factors related to outreach referral episodes. *Resuscitation, 81,* 1670–1675. doi:10.1016/j.resuscitation.2010.07.007

Perri, T., Lantsberg, D., Ben-Baruch, G., Beiner, M.E., Jakobson-Setton, A., & Korach, J. (2015). Malignant pericardial effusion in ovarian malignancy: A treatable oncologic emergency. *Journal of Emergency Medicine, 49,* 281–283. doi:10.1016/j.jemermed.2015.04.024

Rosolem, M.M., Rabello, L.S.C.F., Lisboa, T., Caruso, P., Costa, R.T., Leal, J.V.R., ... Soares, M. (2012). Critically ill patients with cancer and sepsis: Clinical course and prognostic factors. *Journal of Critical Care, 27,* 301–307. doi:10.1016/j.jcrc.2011.06.014

Schönfeld, N., & Timsit, J.-F. (2008). Overcoming a stigma: The lung cancer patient in the intensive care unit. *European Respiratory Journal, 31,* 3–5. doi:10.1183/09031936.00126307

Sipsas, N.V., & Kontoyiannis, D.P. (2012). Invasive fungal infections in patients with cancer in the intensive care unit. *International Journal of Antimicrobial Agents, 39,* 464–471. doi:10.1016/j.ijantimicag.2011.11.017

Soubani, A.O., Shehada, E., Chen, W., & Smith, D. (2014). The outcome of cancer patients with acute respiratory distress syndrome. *Journal of Critical Care, 29,* 183.e7–183.e12. doi:10.1016/j.jcrc.2013.10.011

Souza-Dantas, V.C., Salluh, J.I.F., & Soares, M. (2011). Impact of neutropenia on the outcomes of critically ill patients with cancer: A matched case-control study. *Annals of Oncology, 22,* 2094–2100. doi:10.1093/annonc/mdq711

Staudinger, T., & Pène, F. (2014). Current insights into severe sepsis in cancer patients. *Revista Brasileira de Terapia Intensiva, 26,* 335–338. doi:10.5935/0103-507X.20140051

Thiery, G., Darmon, M., & Azoulay, E. (2007). Deciding intensive care unit-admission for critically ill cancer patients. *Indian Journal of Critical Care Medicine, 11,* 12–18. doi:10.4103/0972-5229.32431

Transition. (n.d.). In *Merriam-Webster's online dictionary* (11th ed.). Retrieved from http://www.merriam-webster.com/dictionary/transition

von Bergwelt-Baildon, M., Hallek, M.J., Shimabukuro-Vornhagen, A.A., & Kochanek, M. (2010). CCC meets ICU: Redefining the role of critical care of cancer patients. *BMC Cancer, 10,* 612. doi:10.1186/1471-2407-10-612

Wigmore, T.J., Farquhar-Smith, P., & Lawson, A. (2013). Intensive care for the cancer patient: Unique clinical and ethical challenges and outcome prediction in the critically ill cancer patient. *Best Practice and Research Clinical Anaesthesiology, 27,* 527–543. doi:10.1016/j.bpa.2013.10.002

Williams, M.D., Braun, L.A., Cooper, L.M., Johnston, J., Weiss, R.V., Qualy, R.L., & Linde-Zwirble, W. (2004). Hospitalized cancer patients with severe sepsis: Analysis of incidence, mortality, and associated costs of care. *Critical Care, 8,* R291–R298. doi:10.1186/cc2893

Wilson, F.P., & Berns, J.S. (2014). Tumor lysis syndrome: New challenges and recent advances. *Advances in Chronic Kidney Disease, 21,* 18–26. doi:10.1053/j.ackd.2013.07.001

CHAPTER 20

Palliative Care in the Intensive Care Unit

Kathleen Blazoff, RN, ANP-BC, ACHPN

Introduction

The World Health Organization (n.d.) defines palliative care as "an approach that improves the quality of life of patients and their families facing the problem[s] associated with life-threatening illness, through the prevention and relief of suffering by means of early identification and impeccable assessment and treatment of pain and other problems, physical, psychosocial and spiritual" (para. 1). Palliative care is an interprofessional approach to supportive care and is appropriate at any age and during any stage of serious illness. It can be provided at the same time as disease treatment to help maintain quality of life.

The most aggressive care is given in the intensive care unit (ICU). Patients with cancer are admitted to the ICU for a variety of reasons. Following hematopoietic stem cell transplantation, patients can develop acute renal failure and require mechanical ventilation, and those presenting with metastatic cancer can require ICU admission. These patients have a high mortality rate (Groeger & Aurora, 2001; Lecuyer et al., 2007; Soares et al., 2010). Despite advances in the management of cancer and its therapies in the ICU, studies have shown that patients requiring ICU admission overall have a worse prognosis (Darmon & Azoulay, 2009). Risks of mortality and severe morbidity are high, and almost all ICU patients have palliative care needs (Freedman, 2017).

Historically, palliative care, critical care, and oncology care specialists have not collaborated on patient care (Billings & Keeley, 2006; Laird, 2015; Perrin & Kazanowski, 2015; Von Roenn, Voltz, & Serrie, 2013; White & Luce, 2004). In the past, critical care and oncology specialists have regarded palliative care as strictly end-of-life or hospice care (Cherny & Catane, 2003;

DeCato et al., 2013); however, evidence has shown that palliative care can benefit the patient and family, improve quality of life, and potentially improve survival (Temel et al., 2010). Curative and palliative care should be congruently provided. The primary role of palliative care is to reduce symptom burden for patients and their families. A prognosis should not limit interventions for symptom burden of disease, communication of treatment goals, timely and appropriate transition of care, and alignment of treatment and therapy goals, values, and preferences (Nelson et al., 2011). The palliative care team can also help alleviate caregiver stress.

This chapter will review important aspects of palliative care for patients with cancer in critical care situations. Topics will include screening for palliative care, management of symptoms (e.g., nausea and vomiting, pain), functions of family meetings, advance directives, cultural aspects, spiritual and psychosocial needs, and end-of-life care.

Identifying Palliative Care Needs

Unfortunately, clinicians, especially those in the ICU, typically do not use specified criteria to determine the need for a palliative care consultation. Use of criteria may help clinicians determine the potential benefits of a consultation and can draw attention to patients and families in need of specialist care. Evidence suggests that palliative care needs are not consistently recognized or addressed and that opportunities exist to improve palliative care in ICUs; however, a key concern of specified criteria use is that it might engender dissatisfaction, distrust, or resistance from primary physicians or teams, as they may prefer complete authority and discretion on referrals. In general, the following are key indicators for a palliative care consultation in the ICU (Nelson et al., 2011):

- Physical symptoms are difficult to control, despite usual treatment approaches.
- Patients/surrogates wish to explore non-ICU supportive care options (e.g., hospice services).
- Staff have questions about appropriateness of life-sustaining therapies in the setting of advanced chronic illnesses.
- Complex family dynamics, including cultural or spiritual issues, affect decisions concerning life-sustaining treatments.
- Disagreements exist between staff or staff and patients/surrogates about prognosis and/or life-sustaining treatments.
- Patients are more frequently being readmitted to the ICU within a given time frame.

Screening or trigger tools should be individualized based on the needs of the patient and staff on specific units and trigger a palliative care team consult. For example, an 800-bed community hospital developed a palliative care trigger tool after screening more than 1,500 patients (Hicks & Distefano, 2011). It identified screening criteria, including the following:

- Change of code status to "do not resuscitate"
- Conflict concerning stopping or starting life-prolonging treatment (e.g., dialysis, chemotherapy)
- Need for goals of care or code status discussion and/or surrogate or proxy distressed regarding decision making
- Prescence of uncontrolled symptoms (e.g., pain, nausea, dyspnea, insomnia, fatigue, weight loss) that affect quality of life
- Marked decrease in functional status or activities of daily living (ADL) in past 60 days
- Consideration for percutaneous endoscopic gastrostomy tube placement
- Admitted from extended-care facility with inability to perform ADL or chronic care needs

Other screening tools may include a trigger criterion of stage IV cancer with one or more comorbidities (Hicks & Distefano, 2011).

Symptom Management

Pain

Healthcare professionals have an ethical mandate to provide comfort to their patients (Brennan, Carr, & Cousins, 2007). Despite advances in pain assessment and management, hospitalized patients continue to report inadequate pain management (Bernhofer, 2011). Tips for adequate pain management are included in Figure 20-1.

A patient's report of pain is still the most valid source for pain management. This becomes more challenging when patients are unable to report pain level. Benzodiazepines are commonly used to sedate patients; however, they may become too sedated and unable to report or respond to pain. Propofol or neuromuscular blocking agents may limit patients' ability to express pain or may mask visible

---

Figure 20-1. Pain Management Tips in the Intensive Care Unit

- Healthcare professionals should be patient advocates for effective pain control.
- Most critically ill patients experience pain during an intensive care unit stay.
- Obtaining a pain history is essential for proper cancer pain management.
- Healthcare professionals should assume that pain is present, especially when the patient cannot self-report or when subjective measures of pain conflict.
- Early recognition and assessment of pain is most effective in controlling and managing pain.
- If any signs of patient pain exist, analgesics should be given prior to sedative agents, especially with agents that possess little or no analgesic effect.

Note. Based on information from Barr et al., 2013; Erstad et al., 2009.

behavioral signs of pain. These agents do not provide analgesic properties, and any outward signs of pain disappear with their use.

For patients unable to self-report pain because of illness, a pain assessment tool becomes necessary. Despite strong evidence that documentation of pain assessments improves pain management and decreases pain, no one pain assessment instrument has been universally recommended. Stites (2013) published a review of objective pain measures used in the critically ill.

The Behavioral Pain Scale (BPS) was developed to quantify pain in sedated, mechanically ventilated patients (Puntillo, Smith, Arai, & Stotts, 2008). The BPS comprises three observational items: facial expressions, upper limb movements, and compliance with mechanical ventilation. These items are scored from 1–4. Scores range from 3 (no pain) to 12 (maximum pain) (Puntillo et al., 2008).

The Critical-Care Pain Observation Tool has four domains for assessment: facial expressions, movement, muscle tension, and ventilator compliance. Each domain is scored 0–2 for a total of 8, with 0 meaning no pain and 8 meaning maximum pain. This tool is useful in both deeply sedated and moderately sedated patients (Ahlers, van der Veen, van Dijk, Tibboel, & Knibbe, 2010).

Evidence shows both tools to be reliable and valid in nonverbal critically ill adults. These assessment tools should be routinely completed.

Although these tools can be useful, obtaining a thorough pain history on admission is the most important intervention tool, as many patients with cancer are already using narcotics or other medications to control pain. The healthcare team should obtain a complete pain history from the patient's family, including any previous medical history of pain and pain medication use (Mularski, 2004).

Pain can be classified as somatic, visceral, or neuropathic. Somatic pain (nociceptive) is usually well localized and described as dull, achy, throbbing, or sore. This is the most common type of pain for patients with cancer (Moryl, Carver, & Foley, 2010). Possible causes include bone metastases, fractures, immobility, and injury to deep musculoskeletal structures. Treatment options include nonsteroidal anti-inflammatory drugs (NSAIDs), steroids, muscle relaxants, opioids, and radiation. Visceral pain is usually poorly localized and is described as cramping, gnawing, colicky, pressure, distension, and deep. Possible causes include bowel obstruction, venous occlusion, ischemia, liver metastases, ascites, and pancreatitis. Treatment options include opioids and NSAIDs. Neuropathic pain is described as burning, numb, tingling, radiating, rocking, "on fire," or shock-like pain. Possible causes include nerve involvement by tumor, postherpetic neuralgia, diabetic neuropathy, chemotherapy-induced neuropathy, poststroke pain, postradiation plexopathies, and phantom pain. Treatment options include anticonvulsants, local anesthetics, antidepressants, benzodiazepines, opioids, steroids, and nerve blocks.

Many analgesics and modalities must be administered to critically ill adults. Choosing the best medication and method of delivery depends on the patient's body composition, development of tolerance, and the adverse effect profiles of various opioids or other pain modalities. Continuous infusions of opioids, such as morphine, hydromorphone, and fentanyl, are commonly used in the ICU, allowing for titration of the drug to a level of analgesic effectiveness and for maintenance of steady plasma levels within a therapeutic range. Intermittent opioid boluses are used for breakthrough pain.

Nonpharmacologic interventions can also be considered in the ICU, including distraction (e.g., music, humor), relaxation, and massage. These interventions are low cost, easy to provide, and safe (Czarnecki et al., 2011; Gélinas, Arbour, Michaud, Robar, & Côté, 2012).

Procedural Pain

A patient can experience many diagnostic and treatment procedures in critical care settings, including central, arterial, or peripheral line placement, bone marrow biopsy, nasogastric or oral tube placement, tracheal or endotracheal suctioning, paracentesis, wound debridement, chemotherapy, and/or hemodialysis. Despite their prevalence, routine procedures continue to cause pain in ICU patients (Delgado-Guay, Parsons, Li, Palmer, & Bruera, 2009; Siffleet, Young, Nikoletti, & Shaw, 2007). Nurses should be aware of this pain during procedures and offer guidance to assist in appropriate pain management (Elliott, 2005; Freire, Afessa, Cawley, Phelps, & Bridges, 2002). Patients scheduled for procedures should be offered additional pain medication prior to transport.

Besides adequate pain relief, other goals for procedural pain management include the patient experiencing minimal or no anxiety and fear related to the procedure, being able to cooperate during the procedure, and having a safe recovery from the effects of the procedure. Understanding pain management during the procedure is essential to the patient plan of care. Nurses need to advocate for the patient, who may be unable to express pain or discomfort before, during, or after the procedure (Siffleet et al., 2007).

Dyspnea

The American Thoracic Society defines dyspnea as "a subjective experience of breathing discomfort that consists of qualitatively distinct sensations that vary in intensity" (Parshall et al., 2012, p. 436) and recommends evaluating dyspnea by assessing the intensity of the distinct sensations, the degree of distress involved, and its burden on ADL. Distinct sensations of breathing discomfort are defined as effort/work, chest tightness, and air hunger (the feeling of not getting enough oxygen). It is important to understand the differences between dyspnea and tachypnea. Tachypnea is a rapid respiratory rate only and does not include the other aspects included with dyspnea. The medical team must ask if patients have discomfort with breathing to assess for dyspnea. Dyspnea assessment in the ICU is challenging because patients are often sedated, on assisted support (e.g., a ventilator), or cannot self-report.

Like pain, dyspnea should be rated by the patient to establish a baseline (Mahler & O'Donnell, 2014). Multiple assessment tools have been developed, including the Borg Scale (Kendrick, Baxi, & Smith, 2000) and the visual analog scale (Gift, 1989; Tanaka, Akechi, Okuyama, Nishiwaki, & Uchitomi, 2000). Newer scales, such as the Dyspnea-12, include the physical and affective aspects of dyspnea (Yorke, Moosavi, Shuldham, & Jones, 2010). No comparative trials have demonstrated superior performance of one scale over another. The Respiratory Distress Observation Scale (RDOS) is designed for patients unable to self-report (Campbell, Templin, & Walch, 2010). RDOS provides needed information to assist in symptom treatment. The scale measures heart rate per minute, respiratory rate per minute, restlessness, nonpurposeful movements, paradoxical breathing patterns, accessory muscle use, grunting at end expiration, nasal flaring, and look of fear. The scoring is simple and takes less than five minutes to complete. Comatose patients are unlikely to demonstrate respiratory distress. Brain-dead patients will not show respiratory distress, cough, gag reflexes, or spontaneous breaths.

The best treatment of dyspnea is to treat its underlying cause. If this is not possible, both nonpharmacologic and pharmacologic methods are used. Nonpharmacologic treatments include positioning (i.e., sitting upright and supported by pillows or leaning over the bedside table), using a fan, and receiving oxygen. Relaxation techniques may also be helpful, such as massage and pursed-lip breathing. Opioids are the drugs of choice for dyspnea, with early use improving quality of life.

Nausea and Vomiting

Although often simultaneously occurring, nausea and vomiting are two distinct symptoms. Nausea is subjective and is a feeling of queasiness with the inclination to vomit. Vomiting is the forceful expulsion of gastric contents from the mouth or nose. Symptoms are subjective and can negatively affect a patient's hospitalization, treatment plan, and quality of life. Critically ill patients frequently experience nausea and vomiting related to underlying diseases, procedures, and medical interventions (i.e., medication, enteral feeding, and surgery). The nurse needs to perform a subjective assessment that explores the patient's perception and symptom impact to develop a comprehensive plan of care. Unfortunately, little evidence exists to guide assessment of nausea, vomiting, and diarrhea in critically ill nonverbal patients. Understanding the disease processes, medical treatments, and pathophysiology of these symptoms will assist the critical care nurse in anticipating symptoms and developing a proactive plan to alleviate symptom-associated discomfort (Makic, 2011).

An understanding of the principles of emesis control for the patient with cancer is vital (National Comprehensive Cancer Network® [NCCN®], 2017). Knowledge of pathophysiology and a thorough assessment become crucial in providing management of nausea and vomiting. As knowledge is currently limited, more research is needed to develop valid and reliable tools for nausea and vomiting, especially for nonverbal patients; however, several tools currently exist, all of which are self-reported symptoms (Brearley, Clements, & Molassiotis, 2008). These include the visual analog scale, the Morrow Assessment of Nausea and Emesis, the Rhodes Index of Nausea and Vomiting–Form 2, and the Functional Living Index–Emesis. Clinicians need to be skilled in assessment and recognition of potential and real-time triggers that may cause nausea and vomiting. Behavioral cues for nonverbal or cognitively impaired patients can help clinicians recognize distressing symptoms (Wood, Chapman, & Eilers, 2011).

Treatment interventions may be used simultaneously to optimize symptom relief. Pharmacologic agents block neurotransmitters (e.g., dopamine, serotonin, neurokinin-1) that stimulate symptoms. No single agent blocks all receptor types. When the healthcare provider is deciding on an antiemetic agent to administer, factors include an evaluation of the etiology or trigger for the symptoms, agent onset and duration of action, and adverse effects (e.g., sedation). Often, a combination of antiemetic agents is needed for patients with significant nausea and vomiting for adequate symptom management (Makic, 2011). Figure 20-2 details the pharmacologic agents used to treat nausea and vomiting.

Nonpharmacologic therapies include diet modification, environmental and psychological strategies, and complementary therapies. These therapies may be forgotten and difficult to perform in a critical care setting. Self-care strategies should be used if the patient can participate. Alternative therapies, such as music therapy and aromatherapy, have shown effectiveness.

Figure 20-2. Pharmacologic Agents to Treat Nausea and Vomiting

Anticholinergic Agents
• Scopolamine

Antihistamines
• Cyclizine
• Dimenhydrinate
• Diphenhydramine

Benzodiazepines
• Diazepam
• Lorazepam

Butyrophenones
• Haloperidol

Cannabinoids
• Dronabinol
• Nabilone

Corticosteroids
• Dexamethasone

5-HT$_3$ Receptor Antagonists (Serotonin Antagonists)
• Dolasetron
• Granisetron
• Ondansetron
• Palonosetron

Neurokinin Receptor Antagonists
• Aprepitant

Opioid Receptor Antagonists
• Chlorpromazine
• Phenothiazine agents
• Prochlorperazine

Prokinetic Agents
• Domperidone
• Metoclopramide

Miscellaneous
• Compazine
• Droperidol

Note. Based on information from Makic, 2011.

Tipton et al. (2007) developed a resource that summarizes evidence-based interventions for the effective management of chemotherapy-induced nausea and vomiting. These interventions can be used as treatment templates and to reduce symptom burden. It is important to use all available resources, including specific guidelines from NCCN, the Center to Advance Palliative Care, the American Society of Clinical Oncology, and the Multinational Association of Supportive Care in Cancer.

The Family Meeting

The family meeting is the cornerstone procedure in palliative medicine and is coordinated by the interprofessional team (Palliative Care Network of Wisconsin, n.d.). Its function in the ICU is to establish goals for critically ill patients. Interprofessional team meetings educate patients and families about the disease process and therapy options and how to make decisions about treatment goals. This reduces patient burden and distress during hospitalization (Nolen & Warren, 2014). When communication deficits occur, problems usually follow (Nelson et al., 2011). Nelson, Mulkerin, Adams, and Pronovost (2006) emphasized the importance of nurse involvement in family meetings. The critical care nurse understands a patient's current condition, has a relationship with the family, and has a continuous presence at the bedside. This nurse can provide continuity to the family, ensuring that communication and decisions are consistent within the team. Because the critical care nurse gives direct care to the patient and witnesses interactions between the family and the patient, the nurse's input and support is invaluable in a family meeting. Patients with cancer and their families have a trusting relationship with their oncologist, and involving them in the family meeting may be important (Gay, Pronovost, Bassett, & Nelson, 2009; Hillen, de Haes, & Smets, 2011).

The VALUE communication technique improves the communication process between ICU clinicians and family members during end-of-life conferences. VALUE is a tool that encompasses the following principles and action statements (Lautrette et al., 2007):
• Value family statements.
• Acknowledge family emotions.
• Listen to the family.
• Understand the patient as a person through the family.
• Elicit family questions.

In a study conducted with 126 dying patients in a French ICU, researchers compared standardized care and the VALUE intervention. Family members who received the intervention had a significantly lower symptom prevalence of posttraumatic stress disorder, anxiety, and depression (Lautrette et al., 2007).

Providing accurate, clear medical information about a patient's status, prognosis, and treatment options provides support for the family during the decision-making process. A key component of the family meeting is the discussion concerning a patient's advance directive and wishes. The advance directive may assist the family in making difficult decisions. If a decision is made to forgo life-sustaining therapies in an ICU setting, all therapies should be evaluated and discussed, including mechanical ventilation, blood products, hemodialysis, vasopressors, artificial feeding (total parenteral nutrition), and chest compressions. A clear treatment plan, education, and support should be provided to the family. Accurate documentation and communication with the ICU team and attending physician should be included. Lack of communication and documentation can interfere with the plan of care (Hudson, Quinn, O'Hanlon, & Aranda, 2008; Kirchhoff, Song, & Kehl, 2004; Quill, 2000).

Spirituality

The National Consensus Project for Quality Palliative Care (2013) recognized spirituality as one of eight domains of quality palliative care. Addressing patients' spiritual care needs is fundamental to palliative care. It is important for the critical care nurse to provide spiritual care through deep listening, bearing witness, and compassion. Challenges exist in finding time to be able to provide aspects of spiritual care and recognizing when to consult a spiritual care provider to assist in complicated spiritual issues, such as the fear and loneliness experienced with serious illness. The FICA tool (faith and belief, importance, community, address in care) has been found to be reliable and useful for detecting spiritual distress in the ICU setting. This can be used by the patient or family when the patient is nonverbal or critically ill and can assist in developing palliative care interventions (Borneman, Ferrell, & Puchalski, 2010; Puchalski, 2004; Puchalski, Lunsford, Harris, & Miller, 2006). The ICU nurse can incorporate this tool or parts of it in a patient assessment and can discuss results with the palliative care team and/or spiritual care provider. Studies have shown that spiritual care interventions can maintain quality of life, such as the therapeutic communication exercises of reflective listening, compassionate care, open-ended questions, life review, and presence to help decrease anxiety and distress (Piderman et al., 2014).

A board-certified spiritual care provider can offer individualized counseling, guidance, and emotional support to help alleviate distress.

End-of-Life Care

It is estimated that withholding or withdrawing life support occurs in 67%–84% of ICU deaths (Kostakou, Rovina, Kyriakopoulou, Koulouris, & Koutsoukou, 2014). The decision to remove life-sustaining therapies occurs when death is believed to be inevitable, despite aggressive interventions. The American College of Physicians supports the right of a competent patient to refuse life-sustaining and life-prolonging therapy (Snyder, 2012). Critical care organizations as well as the Ethical and Religious Directives for Catholic Health Care Services support patient autonomy regarding withholding or withdrawing therapies (Szalados, 2007; U.S. Conference of Catholic Bishops, 2010).

When the decision has been made to remove ventilator support, methods of mechanical ventilation withdrawal and analgesic and sedative needs should be considered. Two methods of ventilator withdrawal exist: immediate extubation and terminal weaning. Patient comfort should dictate the extubation method. In immediate extubation, the endotracheal tube is removed after suctioning. Humidified air or oxygen is given to prevent the airway from drying. This is the preferred choice to relieve discomfort if the patient is conscious, the volume of secretions is low, and the airway is unlikely to be compromised after extubation. Negative aspects include noisy breathing and dyspnea, which may be distressing to the family (Truog et al., 2008).

In the terminal weaning method, the first steps include decreasing the ventilatory rate, oxygen levels, and positive end-expiratory pressure (PEEP). This process may be carried out over periods of as little as 30–60 minutes. If the patient survives, the endotracheal tube can be removed with ongoing symptomatic and comfort care. Occasionally, the endotracheal tube may be left in place to ensure patency of the upper airway, such as in angioedema, and a T-bar can be placed. Terminal weaning allows titration of drugs to control symptoms and maintains airway for suctioning if necessary. The hope is that the patient will not develop upper airway obstruction, will have a longer time between ventilator withdrawal, and the process will prevent death. The patient's family may feel less moral burden because the method appears less active (Campbell, 2007).

Prior to either terminal weaning or immediate extubation, the patient needs to be assessed for the need for analgesics or anxiety-reducing medications. Consensus guidelines on the provision of analgesia and sedation for dying ICU patients support the titration of analgesics and sedatives based on the patient's request or observable signs of distress. The guidelines stress that no maximum dose of opioids or sedatives exist, especially considering that many ICU patients receive high doses of these drugs during their ICU stay. Anticipatory dosing, as opposed to reactive dosing, is recommended by some to avoid patient discomfort and distress (Truog et al., 2008). No one specific protocol exists for withdrawal of mechanical ventilation, but the following sequence should be considered (Truog et al., 2008):

• Anticipate and prevent distress.
  – Educate the patient and family on the process. Reassure them that the primary goal is the patient's comfort. Include education on discontinuing therapies that are not conducive to comfort, such as vasopressors, tubes, restraints, laboratory tests, and x-rays.
  – Refer to spiritual care and social work.
  – Consider premedication with analgesics or sedatives prior to extubation.

- Optimize the airway.
  - Administer breathing treatment if indicated.
  - Suction out the mouth, hypopharynx, and endotracheal tube (see Table 20-1).
  - Consider pretreatment with muscarinic receptor blockers (i.e., anticholinergic drugs). No evidence-based guidelines exist, but current standard-of-care guidelines use these agents.
- Ventilator withdrawal: Consider terminal weaning versus immediate extubation.
- A comfort protocol is initiated based on the patient's comfort and distress.
  - This protocol should include opioids, sedatives, and anticholinergics.
  - Nonpharmacologic therapies include performing oral care, turning for comfort, and using a fan.
  - Observe the patient (and not the monitor) for signs of distress.
- Consult hospice for continued care.

Table 20-1. Excessive Secretion Management			
Drug	Route	Starting Dose	Onset
Scopolamine	Patch	1.5 mg patch	12–24 hr to steady state
Glycopyrrolate	PO	1 mg	30 min
	IV or subcutaneous	0.2 mg	1 min
Atropine sulfate	IV or subcutaneous	0.1 mg	1 min
	Sublingual	1 gtt (1% ophthalmic solution)	30 min

Note. Based on information from Ohio Hospice and Palliative Care Organization, 2001; Wildiers & Menten, 2002.

Case Study

N.G. is a 79-year-old man of Chinese descent who was admitted to the ICU after reporting abdominal pain. A computed tomography scan revealed a mass in the colon causing obstruction. N.G. was taken to the operating room for debulking surgery. During the surgery, it was noted that the patient had an intestinal perforation. The area was washed out and the tumor was removed.

The pathology revealed adenocarcinoma, and N.G. was diagnosed with stage IV colon cancer with metastatic disease in the liver. He has been to the operating room two additional times since his original surgery for wound washout. The bedside RN urged the palliative care team for a consultation from an intensivist and the surgeon.

Socially, the patient is a chemical engineering professor and actively teaching. He and his wife travel extensively and both were in good health prior to this diagnosis. He does not smoke or drink alcohol and practices Buddhism. N.G. and his wife had a relationship with a monk, who died about two years ago. They do not practice at a specific chapel. They have two educated sons living out of state.

Currently, N.G. has multiple drains and an open wound. He is on three different antibiotics for peritonitis and on and off vasopressors for blood pressure support. N.G. is sedated on a ventilator with a setting of 40% (fraction of inspired oxygen) and 8 PEEP with a versed drip. He is on continuous renal replacement therapy (CRRT) to gently reduce his fluid excess and is receiving morphine as needed for pain. N.G. is unable to have a feeding tube placed because of abdominal surgeries and is on total parenteral nutrition. His condition is critical.

His wife visits the hospital about eight hours per day but spends only a few minutes at a time in the patient's room. His sons and daughter-in-law rotate their time at the bedside. N.G. does not have a written advance directive, and his resuscitation plan is full code. The patient's wife speaks English but her primary language is Chinese. The sons speak and understand English.

The palliative care team is consulted to help support the patient and family with complex decision making. The patient has been on the ventilator for 13 days. It is time for discussions regarding a tracheotomy and a third washout of the open wound. The oncology surgeon, Dr. L, is supporting moving forward with a tracheostomy, but the patient's wife is questioning whether this would be beneficial given N.G.'s disease process. She is anxious and has difficulty expressing her opinions to her sons and confides in the bedside RN. The patient's sons are noncommittal and have a high respect for the surgical team.

A family meeting is arranged with the sons, Dr. L, the bedside RN, and the palliative care team, which includes a nurse practitioner, social worker, and hospital chaplain. One of the patient's sons cannot be there in person, so a conference call is arranged. N.G.'s wife refuses to participate, stating she is fine with whatever they decide.

The surgeon discusses either a tracheostomy with wound washout or a washout with a delayed tracheostomy of a few days. The palliative care team discusses the overall prognosis and diagnosis, reviews the patient's status with help from the bedside nurse, and educates the family about the tracheostomy, living in a long-term acute care facility with ventilator support, the prognosis, and treatment recommendations.

On investigation, it is revealed that the patient's family has a hard time making decisions, as N.G. has always been the primary decision maker. Also, because the family practices Buddhism, they believe in the premise of doing no harm. They feel a wrong decision would poorly reflect on their family. They have not made the time to meditate or reflect on N.G.'s life or to speak with him because of his sedation and critical situation. N.G.'s wife again confides in the bedside RN, saying, "I do not want to live like this." Despite this feeling, she believes N.G. should make the decisions about his life. The family decides to proceed with another wound washout in the hope that N.G. can become well enough to make his own decisions. They agree to hold off on the tracheostomy for now.

The spiritual care provider recommends the family go to the chapel to meditate. They also contact a local temple to provide guidance. The social worker provides the family with an advance directive written in Chinese and English to assist with decision making. Another family meeting is scheduled in three days to readdress the need for tracheostomy and continued life support.

On day 17, the patient has a fourth washout and the wound is cleaned but remains open. He continues CRRT and his ventilator settings are increased to FiO_2 of 50% with a PEEP of 10 cm H_2O. He continues the CRRT and now is on a morphine drip. The day prior, the ICU team tried to reduce his sedation and pain medication because the family wanted to see if he would become more lucid; however, he became more agitated.

Since the meeting, the patient's family has been able to meditate and reflect. They also reviewed the advance directive. The palliative care team, the bedside nurse, Dr. L, and the intensivist meet with the family to review the patient's overall status. Dr. L discusses the tracheostomy and reviews the disease process and a possible long-term plan. The palliative care team reviews terminal extubation and comfort measures. Discussion is centered around the patient's wishes. The patient's wife, with support from the bedside RN, verbalizes her feelings about the patient's wishes, which should not include undue suffering and being on a ventilator for an extended period. She is not in favor of a tracheostomy. She expresses that N.G.'s prognosis is poor, even after the tracheotomy, and that she does not want him to suffer anymore. Her sons acknowledge their mother but continue to struggle with decision making. The family discusses more in private.

The palliative care team remains and answers more questions about removing life-sustaining therapies. The family is concerned about suffering but is reassured regarding the patient's desired comfort. The family decides to not proceed with tracheostomy and honors N.G.'s wishes. A plan is implemented for palliative removal of the ventilator. The goals of care become comfort and a natural death. Hospice is consulted for continued care.

Summary

Palliative care helps reduce symptom burden for patients and families. A palliative care team can provide leadership and guidance when establishing treatment goals. Medical science has given the healthcare field remarkable power to ease the suffering and pain associated with cancer. Healthcare professionals have a responsibility to ensure that patients have quality of life *and* quality of dying on their journey (Gawande, 2015).

References

Ahlers, S.J.G.M., van der Veen, A.M., van Dijk, M., Tibboel, D., & Knibbe, C.A. (2010). The use of the behavioral pain scale to assess pain in conscious sedated patients. *Anesthesia and Analgesia, 110,* 127–133. doi:10.1213/ANE.0b013e3181c3119e

Barr, J., Fraser, G.L., Puntillo, K., Ely, E.W., Gélinas, C., Dasta, J.F., ... Jaeschke, R. (2013). Clinical practice guidelines for the management of pain, agitation, and delirium in adult patients in the intensive care unit. *Critical Care Medicine, 41,* 263–306. doi:10.1097/CCM.0b013e3182783b72

Bernhofer, E.A. (2011). Ethics: Ethics and pain management in hospitalized patients. *Online Journal of Issues in Nursing, 17.* Retrieved from http://www.nursingworld.org/MainMenuCategories/ANAMarketplace/ANAPeriodicals/OJIN/Columns/Ethics/Ethics-and-Pain-Management-.html

Billings, J.A., & Keeley, A. (2006). Merging cultures: Palliative care specialists in the medical intensive care unit. *Critical Care Medicine, 34*(Suppl. 1), S388–S393. doi:10.1097/01.CCM.0000237346.11218.42

Borneman, T., Ferrell, B., & Puchalski, C.M. (2010). Evaluation of the FICA Tool for spiritual assessment. *Journal of Pain and Symptom Management, 40,* 163–173. doi:10.1016/j.jpainsymman.2009.12.019

Brearley, S.G., Clements, C.V., & Molassiotis, A. (2008). A review of patient self-report tools for chemotherapy-induced nausea and vomiting. *Supportive Care in Cancer, 16,* 1213–1229. doi:10.1007/s00520-008-0428-y

Brennan, F., Carr, D.B., & Cousins, M. (2007). Pain management: A fundamental human right. *Anesthesia and Analgesia, 105,* 205–221.

Campbell, M.L. (2007). How to withdraw mechanical ventilation: A systematic review of the literature. *AACN Advanced Critical Care, 18,* 397–403. doi:10.4037/15597768-2007-4008

Campbell, M.L., & Templin, T., & Walch, J. (2010). A respiratory distress observation scale for patients unable to self-report dyspnea. *Journal of Palliative Medicine, 13,* 285–290. doi:10.1089/jpm.2009.0229

Cherny, N.I., & Catane, R. (2003). Attitudes of medical oncologists toward palliative care for patients with advanced and incurable cancer: Report on a survey by the European Society of Medical Oncology taskforce on palliative and supportive care. *Cancer, 98,* 2502–2510. doi:10.1002/cncr.11815

Czarnecki, M.L., Turner, H.N., Collins, P.M., Doellman, D., Wrona, S., & Reynolds, J. (2011). Procedural pain management: A position statement with clinical practice recommendations. *Pain Management Nursing, 12,* 95–111. doi:10.1016/j.pmn.2011.02.003

Darmon, M., & Azoulay, E. (2009). Critical care management of cancer patients: Cause for optimism and need for objectivity. *Current Opinion in Oncology, 21,* 318–326. doi:10.1097/CCO.0b013e32832b68b6

DeCato, T.W., Engelberg, R.A., Downey, L., Nielsen, E.L., Treece, P.D., Back, A.L., ... Curtis, J.R. (2013). Hospital variation and temporal trends in palliative and end-of-life care in the ICU. *Critical Care Medicine, 41,* 1405–1411. doi:10.1097/CCM.0b013e318287f289

Delgado-Guay, M.O., Parsons, H.A., Li, Z., Palmer, L.J., & Bruera, E. (2009). Symptom distress, interventions, and outcomes of intensive care unit cancer patients referred to a palliative care consult team. *Cancer, 115,* 437–448. doi:10.1002/cncr.24017

Elliott, D. (2005). Discomfort and factual recollection in intensive care unit patients. *Australian Critical Care, 18,* 43–44. doi:10.1016/S1036-7314(05)80023-2

Erstad, B.L., Puntillo, K., Gilbert, H.C., Grap, M.J., Li, D., Medina, J., ... Sessler, C.N. (2009). Pain management principles in the critically ill. *Chest, 135,* 1075–1086. doi:10.1378/chest.08-2264

Freedman, N. (2017, March 2). Prognosis of cancer patients in the intensive care unit [Literature review current through August 2017]. Retrieved from http://www.uptodate.com/contents/prognosis-of-cancer-patients-in-the-intensive-care-unit

Freire, A.X., Afessa, B., Cawley, P., Phelps, S., & Bridges, L. (2002). Characteristics associated with analgesia ordering in the intensive care unit and relationships with outcome. *Critical Care Medicine, 30*, 2468–2472. doi:10.1097/00003246-200211000-00011

Gawande, A. (2015). *Being mortal: Medicine and what matters in the end.* New York, NY: Henry Holt and Company.

Gay, E.B., Pronovost, P.J., Bassett, R.D., & Nelson, J.E. (2009). The intensive care unit family meeting: Making it happen. *Journal of Critical Care, 24*, 629.e1–629.e12. doi:10.1016/j.jcrc.2008.10.003

Gélinas, C., Arbour, C., Michaud, C., Robar, L., & Côté, J. (2012). Patients and ICU nurses' perspectives of non-pharmacological interventions for pain management. *Nursing in Critical Care, 18*, 307–318. doi:10.1111/j.1478-5153.2012.00531.x

Gift, A.G. (1989). Validation of a vertical visual analogue scale as a measure of clinical dyspnea. *Rehabilitation Nursing, 14*, 323–325. doi:10.1002/j.2048-7940.1989.tb01129.x

Groeger, J.S., & Aurora, R.N. (2001). Intensive care, mechanical ventilation, dialysis, and cardiopulmonary resuscitation. *Critical Care Clinics, 17*, 791–803. doi:10.1016/S0749-0704(05)70208-6

Hicks, M., Distefano, E., Davis, M., Merriman, M., & McKenna, E. (2011). No patient left behind: Universal screening for palliative care needs (526). *Journal of Pain and Symptom Management, 41*, 268. doi:10.1016/j.jpainsymman.2010.10.174

Hillen, M.A., de Haes, H.C.J.M., & Smets, E.M.A. (2011). Cancer patients' trust in their physician—A review. *Psycho-Oncology, 20*, 227–241. doi:10.1002/pon.1745

Hudson, P., Quinn, K., O'Hanlon, B., & Aranda, S. (2008). Family meetings in palliative care: Multidisciplinary clinical practice guidelines. *BMC Palliative Care, 7*, 12. doi:10.1186/1472-684X-7-12

Kendrick, K.R., Baxi, S.C., & Smith, R.M. (2000). Usefulness of the modified 0–10 Borg scale in assessing the degree of dyspnea in patients with COPD and asthma. *Journal of Emergency Nursing, 26*, 216–222. doi:10.1016/S0099-1767(00)90093-X

Kirchhoff, K.T., Song, M.-K., & Kehl, K. (2004). Caring for the family of the critically ill patient. *Critical Care Clinics, 20*, 453–466. doi:10.1016/j.ccc.2004.03.009

Kostakou, E., Rovina, N., Kyriakopoulou, M., Koulouris, N.G., & Koutsoukou, A. (2014). Critically ill cancer patient in intensive care unit: Issues that arise. *Journal of Critical Care, 29*, 817–822. doi:10.1016/j.jcrc.2014.04.007

Laird, B.J.A. (2015). Barriers to the delivery of palliative care. In N. Cherny, M. Fallon, S. Kassa, R. Portenoy, & D.C. Currow (Eds.), *Oxford textbook of palliative medicine* (5th ed., pp. 105–111). New York, NY: Oxford University Press.

Lautrette, A., Darmon, M., Megarbane, B., Joly, L.M., Chevret, S., Adrie, C., ... Azoulay, E. (2007). A communication strategy and brochure for relatives of patients dying in the ICU. *New England Journal of Medicine, 356*, 469–478. doi:10.1056/NEJMx070030

Lecuyer, L., Chevret, S., Thiery, G., Darmon, M., Schlemmer, B., & Azoulay, E. (2007). The ICU trial: A new admission policy for cancer patients requiring mechanical ventilation. *Critical Care Medicine, 35*, 808–814. doi:10.1097/01.CCM.0000256846.27192.7A

Mahler, D.A., & O'Donnell, D.E. (2014). Neurobiology of dyspnea: An overview. In D.A. Mahler & D.E. O'Donnell (Eds.), *Dyspnea: Mechanisms, measurement, and management* (3rd ed., pp. 3–10). Boca Raton, FL: CRC Press.

Makic, M.B.F. (2011). Management of nausea, vomiting, and diarrhea during critical illness. *AACN Advanced Critical Care, 22*, 265–274. doi:10.1097/NCI.0b013e3182248a2b

Moryl, N., Carver, A.C., & Foley, K.M. (2010). Management of cancer pain. In W.K. Hong, R.C. Bast Jr., W.N. Hait, D.W. Kufe, R.E. Pollock, R.R. Weichselbaum, ... E. Frei III (Eds.), *Holland-Frei cancer medicine* (8th ed., pp. 863–880). Shelton, CT: People's Medical Publishing House.

Mularski, R.A. (2004). Pain management in the intensive care unit. *Critical Care Clinics, 20*, 381–401. doi:10.1016/j.ccc.2004.03.010

National Comprehensive Cancer Network. (2017). *NCCN Clinical Practice Guidelines in Oncology (NCCN Guidelines®): Acute myeloid leukemia* [v.2.2017]. Retrieved from https://www.nccn.org/professionals/physician_gls/pdf/antiemesis.pdf

National Consensus Project for Quality Palliative Care. (2013). Clinical practice guidelines for quality palliative care (3rd ed.). Retrieved from http://keyweb24.com/nchpc/wp-content/uploads/2017/04/NCP_Clinical_Practice_Guidelines_3rd_Edition.pdf

Nelson, J.E., Mulkerin, C.M., Adams, L.L., & Pronovost, P.J. (2006). Improving comfort and communication in the ICU: A practical new tool for palliative care performance measurement and feedback. *BMJ Quality and Safety, 115,* 264–271. doi:10.1136/qshc.2005.017707

Nelson, J.E., Puntillo, K.A., Pronovost, P.J., Walker, A.S., McAdam, J.L., Ilaoa, D., & Penrod, J. (2011). In their own words: Patients and families define high-quality palliative care in the intensive care unit. *Critical Care Medicine, 38,* 808–818.

Nolen, K.B., & Warren, N.A. (2014). Meeting the needs of family members of ICU patients. *Critical Care Nursing Quarterly, 37,* 393–406. doi:10.1097/CNQ.0000000000000040

Ohio Hospice and Palliative Care Organization. (2001). *Palliative care pocket consultant* (2nd ed.). Dubuque, IA: Kendall Hunt Publishing.

Palliative Care Network of Wisconsin. (n.d.). Fast facts and concepts. Retrieved from https://www.mypcnow.org/fast-facts

Parshall, M.B., Schwartzstein, R.M., Adams, L., Banzett, R.B., Manning, H.L., Bourbeau, J., … O'Donnell, D.E. (2012). An official American Thoracic Society statement: Update on the mechanisms, assessment, and management of dyspnea. *American Journal of Respiratory and Critical Care Medicine, 185,* 435–452. doi:10.1164/rccm.201111-2042st

Perrin, K.O., & Kazanowski, M. (2015). Overcoming barriers to palliative care consultation. *Critical Care Nurse, 35,* 44–52. doi:10.4037/ccn2015357

Piderman, K.M., Johnson, M.E., Frost, M.H., Atherton, P.J., Satele, D.V., Clark, M.M., … Rummans, T.A. (2014). Spiritual quality of life in advanced cancer patients receiving radiation therapy. *Psycho-Oncology, 23,* 216–221. doi:10.1002/pon.3390

Puchalski, C.M. (2004). Spirituality in health: The role of spirituality in critical care. *Critical Care Clinics, 20,* 487–504. doi:10.1016/j.ccc.2004.03.007

Puchalski, C.M., Lunsford, B., Harris, M.H., & Miller, R.T. (2006). Interdisciplinary spiritual care for seriously ill and dying patients. *Cancer Journal, 12,* 398–416. doi:10.1097/00130404-200609000-00009

Puntillo, K.A., Smith, D., Arai, S., & Stotts, N. (2008). Critical care nurses provide their perspectives of patients' symptoms in intensive care units. *Heart and Lung, 37,* 466–475. doi:10.1016/j.hrtlng.2008.02.002

Quill, T.E. (2000). Initiating end-of-life discussions with seriously ill patients. *JAMA, 284,* 2502–2507. doi:10.1001/jama.284.19.2502

Siffleet, J., Young, J., Nikoletti, S., & Shaw, T. (2007). Patients' self-report of procedural pain in the intensive care unit. *Journal of Clinical Nursing, 16,* 2142–2148. doi:10.1111/j.1365-2702.2006.01840.x

Snyder, L. (2012). American College of Physicians Ethics manual: Sixth edition. *Annals of Internal Medicine, 156,* 73–104. doi:10.7326/0003-4819-156-1-201201031-00001

Soares, M., Caruso, P., Silva, E., Teles, J.M.M., Lobo, S.M.A., Friedman, G., … Salluh, J.I.F. (2010). Characteristics and outcomes of patients with cancer requiring admission to intensive care units: A prospective multicenter study. *Critical Care Medicine, 38,* 9–15. doi:10.1097/CCM.0b013e3181c0349e

Stites, M. (2013). Observational pain scales in critically ill adults. *Critical Care Nurse, 33,* 68–78. doi:10.4037/ccn2013804

Szalados, J.E. (2007). Discontinuation of mechanical ventilation at end-of-life: The ethical and legal boundaries of physician conduct in termination of life support. *Critical Care Clinics, 23,* 317–337. doi:10.1016/j.ccc.2006.12.006

Tanaka, K.T., Akechi, T., Okuyama, T., Nishiwaki, Y., & Uchitomi, Y. (2000). Development and validation of the cancer dyspnoea scale: A multidimensional, brief, self-rating scale. *British Journal of Cancer, 82,* 800–805. doi:10.1054/bjoc.1999.1002

Temel, J.S., Greer, J.A., Muzikansky, A., Gallagher, E.R., Admane, S., Jackson, V.A., … Lynch, T.J. (2010). Early palliative care for patients with metastatic non–small-cell lung cancer. *New England Journal of Medicine, 363,* 733–742. doi:10.1056/NEJMoa1000678

Tipton, J.M., McDaniel, R.W., Barbour, L., Johnston, M.P., Kayne, M., LeRoy, P., & Ripple, M.L. (2007). Putting evidence into practice: Evidence-based interventions to prevent, manage, and treat chemotherapy-induced nausea and vomiting. *Clinical Journal of Oncology Nursing, 11,* 69–78. doi:10.1188/07.CJON.69-78

Truog, R.D., Campbell, M.L., Curtis, J.R., Haas, C.E., Luce, J.M., Rubenfeld, G.D., … Kaufman, D.C. (2008). Recommendations for end-of-life care in the intensive care unit: A consensus statement by the American Academy of Critical Care Medicine. *Critical Care Medicine, 36,* 953–963. doi:10.1097/CCM.0B013E3181659096

U.S. Conference of Catholic Bishops. (2010). *Ethical and religious directives for catholic health care services* (5th ed.). Washington, DC: Author.

Von Roenn, J.H., Voltz, R., & Serrie, A. (2013). Barriers and approaches to the successful integration of palliative care and oncology practice. *Journal of the National Comprehensive Cancer Network, 11*(Suppl. 1), S11–S16.

White, D.B., & Luce, J.M. (2004). Palliative care in the intensive care unit: Barriers, advances, and unmet needs. *Critical Care Clinics, 20,* 329–343. doi:10.1016/j.ccc.2004.03.003

Wildiers, H., & Menten, J. (2002). Death rattle: Prevalence, prevention and treatment. *Journal of Pain and Symptom Management, 23,* 310–317.

Wood, J.M., Chapman, K., & Eilers, J. (2011). Tools for assessing nausea, vomiting, and retching: A literature review [Online exclusive]. *Cancer Nursing, 34,* E14–E24. doi:10.1097/NCC .0b013e3181e2cd79

World Health Organization. (n.d.). WHO definition of palliative care. Retrieved from http://www .who.int/cancer/palliative/definition/en

Yorke, J., Moosavi, S.H., Shuldham, C., & Jones, P.W. (2010). Quantification of dyspnea using descriptors: Development and initial testing of the dyspnoea-12. *BMJ Thorax, 65,* 21–26. doi:10 .1136/thx.2009.118521

CHAPTER 21

The Older Adult With Cancer in the Intensive Care Unit

Meghan Routt, MSN, ANP/GNP-BC, AOCNP®

Introduction

Cancer is considered a disease of aging. As the population increases worldwide, so too will cancer incidence. The U.S. Census Bureau projects that the number of adults aged 65 and older will double by 2030, contributing to a 45% increase in the number of people with cancer (U.S. Department of Commerce Census Bureau, n.d.). Aging is the most significant risk factor of the development of cancer (Lichtman, Hurria, & Jacobsen, 2014). Adults aged 65 years and older comprise 54% of all patients with cancer and 69.5% of all cancer deaths (Howlader et al., 2017). The National Comprehensive Cancer Network® (NCCN®, 2017) developed guidelines for the care of older adults with cancer, focusing on preserving quality of life and advocating that age should not be the driving force of treatment decisions.

Patients with cancer will most likely require admission to an intensive care unit (ICU) at some point. In fact, older adults currently comprise almost 50% of all ICU admissions in the United States (Baldwin et al., 2014). It is vital that ICU nurses understand the physiologic differences in the older adult population and know the specific geriatric syndromes that can play a role in morbidity and mortality in the ICU.

Physiology

Older adults do not present with the same signs and symptoms of illness as their younger counterparts. This older population is unable to mount the same metabolic and hemodynamic response to illness and present atypically with severe illness (Walker, Spivak, & Sebastian, 2014). For example, in the case of infection, white blood count and temperature may be normal, and the presenting sign could be altered mental status. Additionally, the organ systems in older adults change as part of the aging process, placing them at risk for pulmonary edema, acute congestive heart failure, pneumonia, gastric ulcers, and acute kidney injury.

Neurologic Changes

Brain size and cerebellar perfusion decrease with age; intelligence does not. *Dementia* is a general term that describes a group of symptoms, such as memory loss, impaired judgment, and impaired language (Alzheimer's Foundation of America, 2017). It is chronic in nature and develops over a long period of time. Prevalence of dementia has been estimated from 10%–18% in older adults (Walker et al., 2014). Patients with dementia are more likely to develop delirium, which can complicate how they are assessed and managed in the ICU (Lee et al., 2008). Delirium is an acute and temporary change in attention and can include disorientation, memory impairment, and perceptual disturbances (Balas et al., 2012). Depression and anxiety are common in older adults with dementia, often presenting as apathy, delusions, hallucinations, and agitation. These behaviors occur independently of delirium; however, they can be just as deleterious to the patient in the ICU. Because of decreased cerebellar perfusion, it is important that the patient maintains appropriate oxygenation to prevent neurologic insult (Walker et al., 2014).

Delirium in older adults in the ICU is associated with poor outcomes, including longer hospital stays, higher costs, increased mortality, greater use of sedation and physical restraints, functional decline, new institutionalization, and new onset of cognitive impairment (Balas et al., 2012). Risk factors for developing delirium in this population include dementia, administration of benzodiazepines before ICU admission, elevated serum creatinine levels, and low arterial pH (Balas et al., 2012). Treatment of delirium in the ICU typically includes antipsychotic medications. These medications have questionable safety and efficacy in the older adult and may exacerbate the delirium (Balas et al., 2012). The most effective treatment of delirium is recognition, removal, and reversal of its underlying causes in the ICU (Balas et al., 2012).

Cardiovascular Changes

With age, changes occur throughout the entire cardiovascular system. The heart becomes stiff from a buildup of amyloid in the myocardium and plaque in the arteries, leading to decreased cardiac output and increased afterload, which puts more stress on the heart in hypovolemic states (Walker et al., 2014). Because of this stiffening and the gradual failure of the heart, older adults are more at risk for developing bilateral lower extremity and pulmonary edema.

Pulmonary Changes

Atrophy of the respiratory muscles and increased chest wall compliance can lead to a less effective cough and decrease patients' maximal inspiratory and expiratory force by up to 50% (Walker et al., 2014). Diminished cough and pulmonary function can make an older adult more vulnerable to infections as well as complications from pleural effusions and pulmonary edema.

The mortality rate for older adults in the ICU is five times higher than for their younger counterparts (Walker et al., 2014). Older age is also strongly related to the mortality of ventilated ICU patients (Farfel, Franca, Sitta, Filho, & Carvalho, 2009). It is estimated that 300,000 patients require invasive mechanical ventilation longer than four days in the United States each year. Approximately 3%–7% of unweaned individuals remain seriously ill and require mechanical ventilation for longer than 21 days (Frengley, Sansone, Shakya, & Kaner, 2014). In a study examining the impact of increasing age on clinical outcomes of older adults who required prolonged mechanical ventilation, the likelihood of being weaned from the ventilator progressively declined as age increased (Frengley et al., 2014). This study highlighted the importance of early weaning of older adults off the ventilator to prevent increasing levels of morbidity and mortality.

Pneumonia prevention is critical in this population and can be easily implemented. Incentive spirometry is the best mechanism for pulmonary hygiene and promotes a stronger cough, prevents atelectasis, and encourages maximal lung expansion. In addition to incentive spirometry, older adults should get both the PCV13 and PPSV23 pneumonia vaccinations (Centers for Disease Control and Prevention, 2016). Early mobility in the ICU is also crucial to minimizing the risk of pneumonia.

Influenza causes more than 220,000 hospitalizations and 3,000–49,000 deaths annually in the United States, with the most morbidity and mortality occurring in older adults (Arriola et al., 2015). A recent study evaluated older adults hospitalized with influenza during the 2012–2013 season and found that those aged 50–65 years and vaccinated against influenza were more likely to be discharged earlier from the ICU than those who were not vaccinated (Arriola et al., 2015). Similar results were found in adults aged 65–75 years but were statistically insignificant. This study emphasized the importance of influenza vaccination in older adults.

Renal Changes

Kidney function decreases with age. By age 80, renal size decreases overall by 30% and renal blood flow by 50% (Walker et al., 2014). Glomerular filtration rate, which is a more accurate measurement of kidney function than creatinine alone, decreases with age and is typically lower in women (Walko & McLeod, 2014). This increases the risk of electrolyte abnormality and changes the efficacy and overall pharmacokinetics of water-soluble medications (Kilari & Mohile, 2012). Nephrotoxic medications should be used with caution in this population, and patients should be assessed frequently for dehydration. Table 21-1 presents some of the most common nephrotoxic medications.

Table 21-1. Common Nephrotoxic Medications	
Medication	**Mechanism of Nephrotoxicity**
Acyclovir	Acute kidney injury by crystal precipitation in the renal tubules with high-dose IV use
Aminoglycoside antibiotics	Preferential accumulation of drug in cortical tubular cells, leading to tubular cytotoxicity
Amphotericin B	Alterations in cell membrane permeability, causing acute tubular necrosis and tubular dysfunction; renal vasoconstriction
Angiotensin-converting enzyme inhibitors and angiotensin II receptor blockers	Arteriolar constriction, leading to increased intraglomerular pressure
Antiretroviral drugs	Acute kidney injury from direct toxicity to tubular cells, leading to acute tubular necrosis
Bisphosphonates	Segmental glomerulosclerosis and acute tubular necrosis with high dose
Calcineurin inhibitors	Acute toxicity related to altered renal hemodynamics and secondary to afferent arteriolar vasoconstriction
Chemotherapy agents	
• Cisplatin	Direct cellular toxicity to the proximal tubules
• Ifosfamide	Proximal tubular dysfunction, resulting in Fanconi-like syndrome or tubular cell death
• Methotrexate	Crystallization in renal tubules as well as direct tubular toxicity, resulting in acute tubular necrosis. Leucovorin can prevent systemic toxicity.
Ciprofloxacin	Acute interstitial nephritis and crystalluria
Foscarnet	Acute tubular necrosis and significant electrolyte abnormalities
Lithium	Nephrogenic diabetes insipidus
Nonsteroidal anti-inflammatory drugs	Prostaglandin inhibition
Proton pump inhibitors	Acute interstitial nephritis
Radiocontrast agents	Intense renal afferent vasoconstriction, leading to renal medullary hypoxia and acute tubular necrosis

(Continued on next page)

Table 21-1. Common Nephrotoxic Medications *(Continued)*	
Medication	**Mechanism of Nephrotoxicity**
Sulfa-based antibiotics	Acute interstitial nephritis
Vancomycin	Acute tubular necrosis
Vascular endothelial growth factor inhibitors (monoclonal antibodies)	Vascular development inhibition

Note. Based on information from Pazhayattil & Shirali, 2014.

Symptomatic urinary tract infections and bacteriuria are common in older adults. The major risk factors for urinary tract infection are female sex, functional impairment, and the use of indwelling urethral catheters (Nicolle, 2016). Older adults living in long-term care facilities are more likely to have asymptomatic bacteriuria than their community-dwelling counterparts. In fact, symptomatic urinary tract infections are the second most frequent infection in these residents (Nicolle, 2016). The change in vaginal pH and flora is believed to contribute to higher urinary tract infection incidence in women, and prostate hypertrophy is the most important contributor to urinary tract infections in men.

Clinical presentation of infections in older adults is the same as in their younger counterparts and includes urinary frequency, urgency, dysuria, nocturia, suprapubic discomfort, and sometimes hematuria. Altered mental status also can be an indication of urinary tract infection in older adults; however, other underlying patient factors confound it. Falls have not been found to be associated with bacteriuria (Nicolle, 2016). Treatment is not indicated for asymptomatic bacteriuria in older populations, and when it is indicated, it should be directed by urine culture because of high rates of antibiotic resistance (Nicolle, 2016).

Geriatric Syndromes

Geriatric syndromes describe clinical conditions in older adults that do not fit specific disease categories (Inouye, Studenski, Tinetti, & Kuchel, 2007). These syndromes have several common features, such as high prevalence in older adults, especially frail older adults; a negative effect on quality of life; and substantial disability. The chief complaint is multifactorial and does not represent the specific pathologic condition underlying the change in health status (Inouye et al., 2007). The most common geriatric syndromes in older adults with cancer include polypharmacy, frailty, and failure to thrive. These syndromes contribute to morbidity and mortality in older adult patients, reduced quality of life, and increased healthcare costs.

Polypharmacy

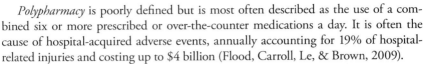

Polypharmacy is poorly defined but is most often described as the use of a combined six or more prescribed or over-the-counter medications a day. It is often the cause of hospital-acquired adverse events, annually accounting for 19% of hospital-related injuries and costing up to $4 billion (Flood, Carroll, Le, & Brown, 2009).

Polypharmacy is common in older adult patients with cancer. One reason for this is the number of specialists involved in this population's care, including cardiologists, pulmonologists, primary care providers, surgeons, medical oncologists, radiation oncologists, and endocrinologists. The Joint Commission (2017) has mandated medication reconciliation at each provider encounter to reduce medication errors caused by omissions, duplications, dosing errors, or drug interactions. Polypharmacy also occurs when a medication is prescribed to combat a side effect of another medication.

Older adults do not metabolize medications the same as their younger counterparts. Table 21-2 lists the most common pharmacokinetic changes in older adults. These changes can result in high or low blood levels of medications, which can lead to toxicity or inadequate treatment of diseases (Sera & McPherson, 2012).

Table 21-2. Pharmacokinetic Changes in Older Adults	
Process	**Effect on Drug Disposition**
Absorption	Reduced intestinal absorption of agents requiring active transport (iron, calcium, vitamin B_{12}) Reduced first-pass metabolism Increased absorption of high-clearance drugs (labetalol, nifedipine, verapamil) Decreased absorption of drugs from prodrugs (enalapril)
Distribution	Altered free fraction of some drugs due to low albumin (naproxen, phenytoin, warfarin) Altered volume of distribution Decreased volume of distribution in hydrophilic drugs (digoxin, morphine) Increased volume of distribution in lipophilic drugs (diazepam, amitriptyline) Increased permeability of blood–brain barrier (verapamil)
Metabolism	Delayed metabolism of high-clearance drugs (benzodiazepines, propranolol, indomethacin)
Excretion	Increased half-life for water-soluble drugs, which is due to impaired kidney function in older adults
Note. Based on information from Sera & McPherson, 2012.	

Older adults, especially those in the ICU, may have difficulty swallowing. If this problem persists, medications need to be able to be crushed and given via naso-gastric tube or intravenously. Not all medications are able to be crushed, nor have the same bioavailability intravenously.

Potentially inappropriate medication (PIM) usage and polypharmacy in older adults with cancer often occur concurrently. PIMs have been associated with adverse drug events, falls, fractures, delirium, lower scores on health-related quality of life, hospitalization, and mortality. The Beers Criteria for Potentially Inappropriate Medication Use in Older Adults (or Beers List) is a clinical tool used to assist providers in identifying PIM and improving medication safety (American Geriatrics Society, 2015). It offers three categories of medications: PIM, PIM due to drug–disease or drug–syndrome interactions that may exacerbate the disease or syndrome, and PIM to be used with caution in older adults. The Beers List identifies 14 drug categories to be avoided in older adult patients. Some top drug categories include:

- Anticholinergics (e.g., chlorpheniramine, cyproheptadine, diphenhydramine)
- Anti-infectives
- Antispasmodics
- Benzodiazepines

For a complete listing of all drug categories, rationales, and recommendations, see American Geriatrics Society, 2015.

Older adult patients with cancer need to have ongoing medication reconciliation to remove medications no longer indicated or to substitute in another medication for a PIM.

STOPP/START is another screening tool used for PIM assessment (O'Mahony et al., 2015). It differs from the Beers List in that it also identifies potential prescribing omissions. Studies have shown that STOPP/START significantly improves medication appropriateness and maintains this effect when used at a single point during hospitalization (O'Mahony et al., 2015).

Frailty

The concept of frailty is pervasive in the literature. It is most often defined as "a biologic syndrome of decreased reserve and resistance to stress, as a result from physiologic multi-system decline" (Kristjansson, Farinella, Gaskell, & Audisio, 2009, p. 499). Frailty by itself can predict morbidity and mortality (Baldwin et al., 2014). Key markers of frailty in the older adult include decline in lean body mass, endurance, strength, balance, and activity (Kristjansson et al., 2009). Although these markers identify physiologic aspects of frailty, it is also important to highlight its psychosocial consequences. Frail patients often require assistance in performing activities of daily living. This dependence on others can be difficult and decrease motivation and confidence. In an Australian study of 89,754 people older than age 45, the major cause of emotional distress was disability, which can be attributed to frailty (Banks et al., 2010). ICU survival has been strongly correlated to level of frailty at admission (Zeng et al., 2015). Recent literature of older ICU survivors who required mechanical ventilation indicated that many of these patients will develop new deficits after their critical illness resolves, necessitating admission to skilled nursing facilities or even extended or long-term care facilities (Baldwin et al., 2014).

Older Adult Failure to Thrive

Older adult failure to thrive has been described as the regression or inability to maintain body weight and as a component of functional decline (Rocchiccioli & Sanford, 2009). It is not a normal part of aging or a result of chronic diseases. Preventive measures need to be implemented, such as basic skin care and positioning, fall prevention, and exercise and range-of-motion activities, to avoid contractures and loss of muscle mass and strength (Murray & Sullivan, 2006).

Unanticipated functional decline can herald disease and impending mortality; however, a steep and sudden drop in functional abilities should not be taken as the anticipated course of chronic disease (Robertson & Montagnini, 2004). It requires investigation for reversible or treatable causes. Egbert (1996) proposed the 11 "Ds" as potential causes of failure to thrive: disease, dementia, delirium, drinking of alcohol, drug use, dysphagia, deafness or other sensory deficits, depression, desertion or isolation, destitution or poverty, and despair. Risk factors of older adult failure to thrive include losing the ability to make independent decisions, loneliness, role loss, feelings of shame and worthlessness, and presence of chronic disease (Rocchiccioli & Sanford, 2009). Early recognition may lead to better supportive treatments before the patient suffers an advanced level of deterioration. It is important to note that older adult patients in the ICU may have underlying failure to thrive and can have higher rates of morbidity and mortality (Rocchiccioli & Sanford, 2009).

Summary

As the worldwide population ages at an exponential rate, so too will the number of cancer diagnoses increase. At one time limited to surgery and a few antineoplastic medications, cancer treatment now has grown to include radiation therapy, biologic therapy, and immunotherapy. Treatment in the 21st century has become complex, but age should not be considered a contraindication to receiving therapy. ICU nurses need to be aware of the unique needs of older adult patients with cancer to successfully care for this population.

References

Alzheimer's Foundation of America. (2017). About dementia. Retrieved from http://www.alzfdn.org /AboutDementia/definition.html

American Geriatrics Society. (2015). American Geriatrics Society 2015 updated Beers Criteria for potentially inappropriate medication use in older adults. *Journal of the American Geriatrics Society, 63,* 2227–2246. doi:10.1111/jgs.13702

Arriola, C.S., Anderson, E.J., Baumbach, J., Bennett, N., Bohm, S., Hill, M., … Chaves, S.S. (2015). Does influenza vaccination modify influenza severity? Data on older adults hospitalized with influenza during the 2012-2013 season in the United States. *Journal of Infectious Diseases, 212,* 1200–1208. doi:10.1093/infdis/jiv200

Balas, M.C., Rice, M., Chaperon, C., Smith, H., Disbot, M., & Fuchs, B. (2012). Management of delirium in critically ill older adults. *Critical Care Nurse, 32,* 15–26. doi:10.4037/ccn2012480

Baldwin, M.R., Reid, M.C., Westlake, A.A., Rowe, J.W., Granieri, E.C., Wunsch, H., … Lederer, D.J. (2014). The feasibility of measuring frailty to predict disability and mortality in older medical intensive care unit survivors. *Journal of Critical Care, 29,* 401–408. doi:10.1016/j.jcrc.2013 .12.019

Banks, E., Byles, J.E., Gibson, R.E., Rodgers, B., Latz, I.K., Robinson, I.A., … Jorm, L.R. (2010). Is psychological distress in people living with cancer related to the fact of diagnosis, current treatment or level of disability? Findings from a large Australian study. *Medical Journal of Australia, 193*(Suppl. 5), S62–S67.

Centers for Disease Control and Prevention. (2016). Adults: Protect yourself with pneumococcal vaccines. Retrieved from https://www.cdc.gov/features/adult-pneumococcal

Egbert, A.M. (1996). The dwindles: Failure to thrive in older patients. *Nutrition Reviews, 54,* S25– S30. doi:10.1111/j.1753-4887.1996.tb03783.x

Farfel, J.M., Franca, S.A., Sitta, M.D.C., Filho, W.J., & Carvalho, C.R.R. (2009). Age, invasive ventilatory support and outcomes in elderly patients admitted to intensive care units. *Age and Ageing, 38,* 515–520. doi:10.1093/ageing/afp119

Flood, K.L., Carroll, M.B., Le, C.V., & Brown, C.J. (2009). Polypharmacy in hospitalized older adult cancer patients: Experience from a prospective, observational study of an oncology-acute care for elders unit. *American Journal of Geriatric Pharmacotherapy, 7,* 151–158. doi:10.1016 /j.amjopharm.2009.05.002

Frengley, J.D., Sansone, G.R., Shakya, K., & Kaner, R.J. (2014). Prolonged mechanical ventilation in 540 seriously ill older adults: Effects of increasing age on clinical outcomes and survival. *Journal of the American Geriatrics Society, 62,* 1–9. doi:10.1111/jgs.12597

Howlader, N., Noone, A.M., Krapcho, M., Miller, D., Bishop, K., Kosary, C.L., … Cronin, K.A. (Eds.). (2017). *SEER cancer statistics review, 1975–2014.* Retrieved from http://seer.cancer.gov /csr/1975_2014

Inouye, S.K., Studenski, S., Tinetti, M.E., & Kuchel, G.A. (2007). Geriatric syndromes: Clinical, research, and policy implications of a core geriatric concept. *Journal of the American Geriatrics Society, 55,* 780–791. doi:10.1111/j.1532-5415.2007.01156.x

Joint Commission. (2017). National Patient Safety Goals®. Retrieved from http://www .jointcommission.org/assets/1/6/HAP_NPSG_Chapter_2014.pdf

Kilari, D., & Mohile, S.G. (2012). Management of cancer in the older adult. *Clinics in Geriatric Medicine, 28,* 33–49. doi:10.1016/j.cger.2011.10.003

Kristjansson, S.R., Farinella, E., Gaskell, S., & Audisio, R.A. (2009). Surgical risk and post-operative complications in older unfit cancer patients. *Cancer Treatment Reviews, 35,* 499–502. doi:10 .1016/j.ctrv.2009.04.004

Lee, H.B., DeLoatch, C.J., Seong-Jin, C., Rosenberg, P., Mears, S.C., & Sieber, F.E. (2008). Detection and management of pre-existing cognitive impairment and associated behavioral symptoms in the intensive care unit. *Critical Care Clinics, 24,* 723–726. doi:10.1016/j.ccc.2008.05.006

Lichtman, S.M., Hurria, A., & Jacobsen, P.B. (2014). Geriatric oncology: An overview. *Journal of Clinical Oncology, 32*, 2521–2522. doi:10.1200/JCO.2014.57.4822

Murray, J., & Sullivan, P.A. (2006). Frail elders and the failure to thrive. *ASHA Leader, 11*, 14–16. doi:10.1044/leader.FTR5.11142006.14

National Comprehensive Cancer Network. (2017). *NCCN Clinical Practice Guidelines in Oncology (NCCN Guidelines*®): Older adult oncology* [v.2.2017]. Retrieved from http://www.nccn.org/professionals/physician_gls/pdf/senior.pdf

Nicolle, L.E. (2016). Urinary tract infections in the older adult. *Clinics of Geriatric Medicine, 32*, 523–538. doi:10.1016/j.cger.2016.03.002

O'Mahony, D., O'Sullivan, D., Byrne, S., O'Connor, M.N., Ryan, C., & Gallagher, P. (2015). STOPP/START criteria for potentially inappropriate prescribing in older people: Version 2. *Age and Ageing, 44*, 213–218. doi:10.1093/ageing/afu145

Pazhayattil, G.S., & Shirali, A.C. (2014). Drug-induced impairment of renal function. *International Journal of Nephrology and Renovascular Disease, 7*, 457–468. doi:10.2147/IJNRD.S39747

Robertson, R.G., & Montagnini, M. (2004). Geriatric failure to thrive. *American Family Physician, 70*, 343–350.

Rocchiccioli, J.T., & Sanford, J.T. (2009). Revisiting geriatric failure to thrive: A complex and compelling clinical condition. *Journal of Gerontological Nursing, 35*, 18–24. doi:10.3928/00989134-20090101-08

Sera, L.C., & McPherson, M.L. (2012). Pharmacokinetics and pharmacodynamic changes associated with aging and implications for drug therapy. *Clinics of Geriatric Medicine, 28*, 273–286. doi:10.1016/j.cger.2012.01.007

U.S. Department of Commerce Census Bureau. (n.d.). Population projections: 2012 national population projections: Summary tables. Retrieved from http://www.census.gov/population/projections/data/national/2012/summarytables.html

Walker, M., Spivak, M., & Sebastian, M. (2014). The impact of aging physiology in critical care. *Critical Care Nursing Clinics of North America, 26*, 7–14. doi:10.1016/j.ccell.2013.09.005

Walko, C.M., & McLeod, H.L. (2014). Personalizing medicine in geriatric oncology. *Journal of Clinical Oncology, 32*, 2581–2586. doi:10.1200/JCO.2014.55.9047

Zeng, A., Song, X., Dong, J., Mitnitski, A., Liu, J., Guo, Z., & Rockwood, K. (2015). Mortality in relation to frailty in patients admitted to a specialized geriatric intensive care unit. *Journal of Gerontology Series A: Biological and Medical Sciences, 70*, 1586–1594. doi:10.1093/gerona/glv084

CHAPTER 22

Ethics Concepts, Complexities, and Controversies

Katherine A. Brown-Saltzman, MA, RN, Carol Pavlish, PhD, RN, FAAN, and Patricia Jakel, RN, MN, AOCN®

Introduction: Case Study—Part 1

K.C. is a 36-year-old woman of Asian descent with acute lymphoblastic leukemia who had a bone marrow transplant six weeks ago. Two weeks ago, she developed persistent graft-versus-host disease with significant gastrointestinal disturbances and skin inflammation and sloughing. She also experienced neurologic bleed, which left her with significant right-sided weakness. She is now in the intensive care unit (ICU) with sepsis and respiratory failure and is currently intubated and on two vasopressors. Prior to the transplant, she told her hematologist that she would do anything to live to raise her two children, an 8-year-old daughter and a 5-year-old son. Her husband died in a car accident when her youngest child was just one year old. Although she has a sister, Julia, and two sets of healthy grandparents, K.C. is committed to preventing further trauma to her children.
• What are the potential ethical questions from this scenario?
• How can K.C.'s autonomy be respected, given that she is no longer able to participate in the goals of treatment conversation?
• What more do you want to know as you care for this patient and her family?

In the context of daily practice, oncology nurses who care for critically ill patients and their families encounter multiple challenges, such as keeping pace with perpetual research advances, ethical dilemmas, and conflicts; assisting patients and families in considering numerous treatment choices in context of uncertain prognoses; and advocating within complex, fragmented, resource-limited healthcare systems. Within these challenges, nurses must not only consider evidence and standards based on scientific research but also incorporate knowledge of ethics rooted in professional obligations and codes of conduct. The development of trusting relationships is also essential. This highly intense work requires a unique blend of high-tech interventions, patient and family engagement, and compassionate, knowledgeable care providers.

Nurses must also consider moral dimensions of care and how to articulate ethical concerns, including value conflicts with pain management, resource use, informed consent, and end-of-life treatment decisions (Cheon, Coyle, Wiegand, & Welsh, 2015; Espinosa, Young, Symes, Haile, & Walsh, 2010; McLennon, Ulrich, Lasiter, Chamness, & Helft, 2013; Olsen, 2016; Pavlish, Brown-Saltzman, Hersh, Shirk, & Nudelman, 2011; Pavlish, Brown-Saltzman, Jakel, & Fine, 2014; Pavlish, Brown-Saltzman, Jakel, & Rounkle, 2012; Shepard, 2010). Research indicates that critical care and oncology nurses frequently encounter challenging ethical situations (Azoulay et al., 2009; Browning, 2013; Dodek et al., 2016; Epstein, 2012; Fassier & Azoulay, 2010; Hamric & Blackhall, 2007; McLeod, 2014; Pavlish et al., 2012; Piers et al., 2011; Shepard, 2010; Sirilla, 2014; Weinzimmer et al., 2014) and experience medium to high levels of moral distress (American Association of Critical-Care Nurses, n.d.; Mason et al., 2014; McAndrew, Leske, & Garcia, 2011; Whitehead, Herbertson, Hamric, Epstein, & Fisher, 2015).

Healthcare professionals, including nurses, report increasing pressure from patients, families, colleagues, and administrators to offer high-intensity treatments (Austin, 2012; Bosslet et al., 2015; Dzeng et al., 2015; Hamric & Blackhall, 2007; Pavlish, Brown-Saltzman, Dirksen, & Fine, 2015). Structural problems, such as unhealthy work environments, ineffective communication, and systemic gaps in care, can lead to ethical conflicts and mounting moral distress (Curtis & Vincent, 2010; Musto, Rodney, & Vanderheide, 2015; Oh & Gastmans, 2015; Rittenmeyer & Huffman, 2009; Sauerland, Marotta, Peinemann, Berndt, & Robichaux, 2014; Ulrich, Lavandero, Woods, & Early, 2014; Ulrich, Hamric, & Grady 2010; Varcoe, Pauly, Storch, Newton, & Makaroff, 2012; Wall, Austin, & Garros, 2015). These often raise concerns about patient safety and care quality (Balevre, Cassells, & Buzaianu, 2012; Cimiotti, Aiken, Sloane, & Wu, 2012; Dyrbye & Shanafelt, 2016; Kelly, Kutney-Lee, Lake, & Aiken, 2013; Maiden, Georges, & Connelly, 2011; Rainer, 2015; Silber et al., 2016).

With the use of a case study, this chapter presents information on ethics-related concepts and the current ethical considerations and controversies relevant to critical oncology care. Applying research findings from an ethnographic study, this text reveals the challenges that oncology nurses encounter, the spectrum of action responses, and specific recommendations for creating moral communities and collaborative practices for care that integrate robust ethical responsiveness. This chapter concludes with a case-based exercise that demonstrates how critical care and oncology nurses can take leadership roles in creating better systems of care for seriously ill patients and their families.

Ethics Concepts in Clinical Practice

Moral Dilemmas and Distress

Complex clinical situations often produce moral uncertainty or pose moral dilemmas (see Table 22-1). These perplexing experiences can be uncomfortable and build over time, contributing to moral distress and residue, which potentially threaten a nurse's moral integrity. In a study on difficult ethical situations, oncology nurses described encountering six ethics-related challenges in working toward their professional goals (see Figure 22-1).

Some challenges cannot be avoided. For example, oncology nurses will continue to experience competing obligations in complex healthcare systems. Additionally, the nature of critical oncology care requires nurses to assist patients and families in maintaining realistic hope under conditions of uncertain prognoses; however, system-level issues also exist. For example, nurses who experienced very

Table 22-1. Definitions of Moral Concepts

Concept	Definition
Moral dilemma	Experience that arises when two or more ethical principles (e.g., autonomy, beneficence, nonmaleficence, justice) or values conflict. More than one principle applies and good reasoning can support mutually inconsistent courses of action. Although very difficult, violating a principle is inevitable.
Moral distress	Moral distress is the response when people believe that they know the morally right course of action, but constraints make it impossible to pursue the desired course of action. It includes initial distress, reactive distress, and the crescendo effect. Initial distress involves the feelings of frustration, anger, and anxiety experienced when faced with institutional obstacles and conflicts about values. Reactive distress is the response when people do not act on their initial distress. It usually results in feelings of worthlessness and can lead to burnout. The crescendo effect is the accumulating impact of multiple episodes of moral distress over time.
Moral integrity	Moral integrity is the sense of wholeness and self-worth that results from having congruence between clearly defined values and actions.
Moral residue	Moral residue includes the lingering effects of moral distress.
Moral uncertainty	Moral uncertainty is a situation in which a person questions if an ethical dilemma exists or is unsure about what principles or values apply in an ethical conflict.

Note. Based on information from Epstein & Hamric, 2009; Hardingham, 2004; Jameton, 1984, 1993.

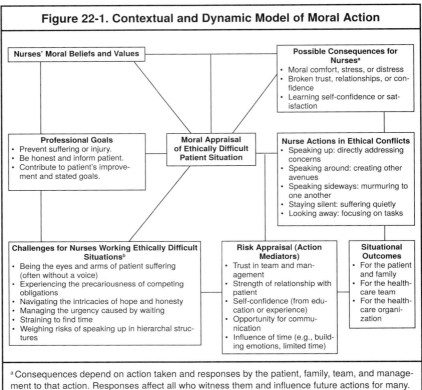

Figure 22-1. Contextual and Dynamic Model of Moral Action

Nurses' Moral Beliefs and Values		Possible Consequences for Nurses[a]

Possible Consequences for Nurses[a]
- Moral comfort, stress, or distress
- Broken trust, relationships, or confidence
- Learning self-confidence or satisfaction

Professional Goals
- Prevent suffering or injury.
- Be honest and inform patient.
- Contribute to patient's improvement and stated goals.

Moral Appraisal of Ethically Difficult Patient Situation

Nurse Actions in Ethical Conflicts
- Speaking up: directly addressing concerns
- Speaking around: creating other avenues
- Speaking sideways: murmuring to one another
- Staying silent: suffering quietly
- Looking away: focusing on tasks

Challenges for Nurses Working Ethically Difficult Situations[b]
- Being the eyes and arms of patient suffering (often without a voice)
- Experiencing the precariousness of competing obligations
- Navigating the intricacies of hope and honesty
- Managing the urgency caused by waiting
- Straining to find time
- Weighing risks of speaking up in hierarchal structures

Risk Appraisal (Action Mediators)
- Trust in team and management
- Strength of relationship with patient
- Self-confidence (from education or experience)
- Opportunity for communication
- Influence of time (e.g., building emotions, limited time)

Situational Outcomes
- For the patient and family
- For the healthcare team
- For the healthcare organization

[a] Consequences depend on action taken and responses by the patient, family, team, and management to that action. Responses affect all who witness them and influence future actions for many.

[b] Challenges are influenced by an individual's moral sensitivity and reasoning and by environmental factors such as relationships with colleagues and administrators.

Note. Lines indicate a relationship in both directions.

Note. Copyright 2012 by Carol Pavlish, Katherine Brown-Saltzman, and Patricia Jakel. Used with permission.

limited, if any, voice in the plan of care described the struggle of not only witnessing but also causing patient suffering when implementing questionably beneficial and potentially harm-inducing treatments. Nurses also described cultures of avoidance that led to crisis decision making and staffing patterns that undervalued a nurse's contributions to helping patients and families cope with critical illness or end of life. These challenges are modifiable. Descriptions of healthcare organizations as hierarchal power structures prevailed throughout the study and contributed to nurses' perceptions of increased risks of speaking up. Other conditions, such as relational conflict, divergent prognostication between the attending physician and consultants, inadequate support from nurse leaders, and moral uncertainty, also led to nurses' silence.

In contrast, an opportunity for team communication and self-confidence that emerged from ethics education, past clinical experiences, and a strong relationship with the patient tended to encourage nurses to ask questions about goals of care and participate in care planning, including family conferences and surrogate education (Pavlish et al., 2012).

To help meet the challenge of ethical decision making, various models have been proposed, most of which facilitate a clinician's capacity to make ethical choices (Cohen & Erickson, 2006). However, these models often focus on individual patient situations and fail to consider the ethical climate in which these situations occur. Ethical climate is largely based on the nature of relationships within an organization and relates to both responsibilities and power (Austin, 2012; Bruce, Weinzimmer, & Zimmerman, 2014; Dyrbye & Shanafelt, 2016; Foglia, Cohen, Pearlman, Bottrell, & Fox, 2013; Oh & Gastmans, 2015; Paradis et al., 2013; Rathert, May, & Chung, 2016; Rose, 2011; Varcoe, Pauly, Webster, & Storch, 2012). Climate also reflects a collection of individual values and beliefs about what comprises good clinical care. For example, a nurse's beliefs about appropriate and excellent care in a clinical situation may differ from what physicians or families believe.

In their unique position at the patient's bedside, nurses are amidst these multiple relationships and intersecting values and beliefs. Conceptualizing this as a position of strength expands opportunities for patient advocacy (Hamric, 2012; McLennon, Lasiter, et al., 2013); however, nurses' moral voices can be constrained within powerful medical, administrative, or family structures (Huffman & Rittenmeyer, 2012; Oh & Gastmans, 2015; Shannon, 2016). Because nursing practice is a morally relevant profession with its own code of ethics, nurses cannot abandon ethical obligations (American Nurses Association [ANA], 2015). Depending on individual attributes and work environments, nurses choose whether to vocalize their perspectives and act. Regrettably, some nurses silence their own moral appraisal of a situation to avoid conflict (Goethals, Gastmans, & de Casterlé, 2010; Pavlish, Brown-Saltzman, Hersh, Shirk, & Rounkle, 2011; Pavlish et al., 2012) or disengage from situations (Moss, Good, Gozal, Kleinpell, & Sessler, 2016; Varcoe et al., 2012). Others might experience enough moral distress that they leave their positions or the profession (Dodek et al., 2016; Huffman & Rittenmeyer, 2012; Whitehead et al., 2015).

The American Nurses Association Code of Ethics and Ethical Principles

ANA (2015) first developed a set of professional standards regarding ethical practice in 1950. The ANA Code of Ethics has since been revised numerous times to reflect societal needs and current healthcare contexts and practices. An in-depth look at these standards can be viewed at http://nursingworld.org/DocumentVault/Ethics-1/Code-of-Ethics-for-Nurses.html.

To further educate nurses on the nature of ethics and obligations, ANA defined the primary ethical principles that underlie the ANA Code of Ethics and guide nursing practice. To view these concepts, visit http://www.nursingworld.org/MainMenuCategories/EthicsStandards/Resources/Ethics-Definitions.pdf.

A Closer Look at Autonomy

Case Study—Part 2

During the past few weeks, K.C. has experienced progressive complications and expressed profound discouragement and weariness. She told her primary nurse that she was worn down from the long treatment course prior to the transplant and that the transplant itself seemed to have taken the last of her ability to fight. She also said she felt a core exhaustion, which she believed previewed her pending death, despite a slight improvement in her condition. Her intuition was strong that she, in fact, was going to die. K.C. described a dream of placing her two sleeping children into her sister's arms. The nurse tried to encourage her and offer reasons for hope, but the patient insisted that she believed she would die and to please make sure she did not suffer. K.C. shared that she had significant pain and was concerned that her parents continued to interfere when she asked for pain medication, saying she would become an addict and that she could not properly "fight" when the narcotics weakened her. K.C. also asked the nurse if she would be able to request assisted suicide if her condition further deteriorated.

- What would you say to this patient?
- When patients are receiving treatment, enduring side effects directly attributable to the provided therapy, can they change their minds?
- Did K.C. have the capacity to make decisions at the time she had this conversation with the nurse?
- Could the nurse have done anything differently to address the patient's suffering?
- How would you approach the pain issue? How would you intervene with the patient's parents, who are discouraging the use of opioids? Do potential underlying cultural issues need to be addressed?
- Can a surrogate decision maker refuse pain medication for a patient?
- What would you say to this patient concerning assisted suicide?

Respecting a patient's right to make decisions is a fundamental principle of patient care. Because its importance in health care has escalated in the past 20 years, autonomy requires careful consideration. Common questions concerning autonomy include the limits of advance decision making, a patient's capacity to make decisions, a surrogate's role in respecting autonomy, and the controversial question of whether healthcare professionals have the right to overrule patient preferences.

First, despite the drive for individuals to engage in advance care planning, thorny issues still exist. For example, directives with checkboxes too simplistic for multifaceted choices and limited patient conversations with surrogates and healthcare providers can lead to multiple interpretations of meaning. The common belief that advance directives always overrule what physicians deem medically appropriate treatment can also create misperceptions and role confusion. Additionally, advance care planning requires patients to make future decisions when they cannot fully appreciate the implications of living with treatment burdens or the resilience needed to adapt to these burdens. Making sure that patients have all the information needed to make informed choices and that they understand the nuances of treatment choices during advance care planning is very challenging and rarely accomplished. Although advance directives are one puzzle piece, they are not an absolute answer to honoring patient autonomy.

Second, patient capacity to make decisions is far more complicated than most clinicians appreciate. Unfortunately, this capacity is often presumed or dismissed without careful, in-depth assessment. To meet capacity requirements, patients must be able to understand information about treatment choices, appreciate the specifics and consequences of treatment options, cognitively and coherently manage the information, and ultimately communicate rationale for their choice (Ganzini, Volicer, Nelson, Fox, & Derse, 2005). Because ICU nurses are in such close proximity to patients, they are in key positions to assess, document, and inform the clinical team about patient capacity. Decisional capacity in critical illness can wax and wane. For example, a patient's level of sedation, degree of hypoxia, or experience of emotional distress can affect capacity. Therefore, capacity cannot always be determined in one examination at a fixed point in time. Each ICU patient will present specific challenges to capacity assessment, such as the communication complexities that accompany fatigue or intubation, or cognitive functioning that is compromised by multiple medications, infection, or delirium. Healthcare teams must work together to fully evaluate capacity because patients cannot make a truly autonomous and informed decision without it.

Finally, many critically ill patients lack decisional capacity, which requires healthcare teams to rely on an appointed surrogate or family member to make decisions. Surrogate decision makers have the responsibility to move beyond their own values and desires and reflect on what the patient would choose if given the options. In the event a patient's specific preferences are completely unknown, the clinical team generally asks the surrogate to consider the patient's values or past choices as the basis for surrogate decisions. When even these are unknown, surrogate decision making requires weighing the best interest of the patient with a careful deliberation of the benefits and burdens of the treatment options.

In a sense, surrogates are held to an even higher standard in decision making than patients themselves, and red flags, such as adamancy, fear of shouldering the responsibility, addressing primarily their own needs, or not being able to understand the information, should call for the careful evaluation of the surrogate's ability to make decisions.

In the case of physical pain, surrogates' rights should be quite restricted. At times, families have conflicted interests, misinformation, fear, or significant blind spots when it comes to pain management and may attempt to compromise the best interest of the patient (adequate pain management) and established standards of care. For example, families may want the patient to be more interactive or may hope to forestall the dying process, despite research that demonstrates that appropriate opioid use does not accelerate death and may even prolong survival.

At times, families may even focus on addiction concerns that are no longer appropriate. Surrogates may also value suffering for religious or cultural reasons and emphasize what may have been the patient's aspiration in other circumstances. The concern is that patients who lack capacity and are in pain can no longer communicate their response in the context and immediacy of the pain. This is particularly troubling for clinicians caring for a dying patient, especially when escalating aggressive therapies have been entreated by a surrogate decision maker who is unaware of the nurse's ethical obligations of beneficence (to do only good) and nonmaleficence (to do no harm). At this point, the clinician now wrestles with nonbeneficial treatments, and more troubling, potentially harms the patient by adhering to the surrogate's wishes of withholding the essence of good care— alleviation of pain and symptoms at the end of life. Surrogates are obligated, just as clinicians, to act in a patient's best interest, and many ethicists advocate for appropriate pain and symptom management, even if that requires overriding the surrogate.

Another significant issue arises at this point in the case—the request of the nurse for future assisted suicide. Although a few states have passed legislation for assisted suicide, many broad ethical questions concerning the topic remain. Currently, professional ethical guidelines are clear that nurses should not participate in euthanasia or assisted suicide. The ANA (2015) Code of Ethics states, "The nurse should provide interventions to relieve pain and other symptoms in the dying patient consistent with palliative care practice standards and may not act with the sole intent to end life" (p. 3).

A request for assisted suicide or euthanasia by a patient is an opportunity to explore concerns and fears and reassure the patient that pain and symptoms can be addressed by explaining options such as palliative sedation for unresolved pain. Although it can have physical components of pain and symptoms, suffering is not limited to these aspects. Cassell (1999) described suffering as a "specific state of distress that occurs when the intactness or integrity of the person is threatened or disrupted" (p. 531). It is an intensely personal experience, which can be oriented either in the present or toward the future. It often has components of worry, fear, sadness, and anxiety, which might be directed to concerns such as feeling a loss of control, being a burden, feeling a loss of dignity, being abandoned, or facing the unknown (Cassell, 1999). Cassell addressed the physician's clumsiness and even lack of awareness of suffering by proposing that patients be asked directly about their suffering and that clinicians respond by seeking to know patients and their values, using intuition when exploring suffering, and then responding with trustworthiness, caring, and understanding. Despite truly valuing presence, many nurses still feel unskilled and inadequate in the face of suffering. An ethic of care does not necessitate mending the suffering. Instead, it asks nurses to move beyond their own fears, trusting that their connection to the other will deeply prevail and provide what is needed to nurture not only the patient's integrity and dignity but the nurse's as well.

Ethical Complexities

Case Study—Part 3

K.C. never appointed a durable power of attorney for health care or completed an advance directive, and family members are now experiencing disagreement. On the one hand, her parents want to pursue every possible treatment in hopes of recovery or prolonged life. On the other hand, Julia reports conversations she had with K.C. just prior to her deterioration, which indicated that her sister was weary of fighting. Julia believed she had to advocate for her sister, who had "suffered enough." Julia supported treatment withdrawal and wanted to focus on a peaceful death for her sister. Communication with the family was difficult. K.C.'s parents only spoke Mandarin. However, Julia was fluent in both Mandarin and English, so the team relied on Julia to translate, as language interpreters were often difficult to find.

- As you learn about the patient's situation, what are the red flags that indicate an increased risk for ethical conflicts?
- Are there concerns about using a family member as an interpreter?

Intersecting Moral Kaleidoscopes

An uncomfortable sense that things are not quite right frequently foreshadows an ethical dilemma. Besides their own discomforts, nurses identified five additional indicators of ethical concerns: interpersonal conflict, patient suffering, patient autonomy or rights violations, unrealistic expectations, and poor team communication (Pavlish, Brown-Saltzman, Hersh, Shirk, & Nudelman, 2011). In an online survey, physicians identified circumstances such as divergent care goals, inadequate communication, and low trust as risk factors for ethical dilemmas and conflicts (Pavlish, Brown-Saltzman, Dirksen, et al., 2015). Once these early signs appear, healthcare providers are faced with tough decisions on how to respond.

Rest (1994) offered a theoretical perspective of moral action, detailing four components to consider when making a moral decision (see Table 22-2). Each person has a unique blend of these four components, depending on individual beliefs, values, and assumptions, which are often shaped by past experiences, current cir-

Table 22-2. Four-Component Model of Moral Action

Interacting Components	Description
Moral sensitivity	Interpreting how people's well-being is affected by possible actions; degree of empathy
Moral judgment	Considering own responsibilities and action options; skill of moral reasoning
Moral motivation	Determining priority values and primary obligations; skill of value prioritizing
Moral character	Implementing what one believes is right; degree of confidence and courage

Note. Based on information from Rest, 1994.

cumstances (e.g., positions within social and organizational structures), and disciplinary preparation.

Ethical decision making in critical care situations is particularly complex because many individuals with different values must interact to create a cohesive plan. For example, imagine peering through a kaleidoscope. Multiple, colorful elements create a unique pattern. When the scope is turned, a new pattern emerges from the same components. Such is the case with unique moral perspectives. Each person has a unique kaleidoscopic pattern or view of the situation that determines the response. In each ethically complex situation, multiple kaleidoscopic patterns must intersect, often in an interdependent manner. Tensions arise when people assume others have the same perspectives; however, as the kaleidoscope reveals, even small shifts in position create different viewpoints. The silence that frequently surrounds ethically complex situations widens differences and compounds tension (Molloy et al., 2009; Pavlish, Brown-Saltzman, Fine, & Jakel, 2013).

Moral Disagreements

Intrapersonal and interpersonal moral disagreements and conflicts are among the most challenging situations faced by critically ill patients with cancer, their families, healthcare providers, and the healthcare system. Moral disagreements are defined as "differences in conceptions of the good or different beliefs about moral obligations and individual rights" (Pavlish et al., 2013, p. 271). The term *disagreement* originates from the Latin words *dis* and *ad gratum*, which together mean "apart or moving in different directions" ("Disagreement," n.d.). Moral disagreements occur when people believe they know what is morally right in a specific situation and make decisions based on fundamentally different beliefs or viewpoints.

Clinicians should expect moral disagreements in complex clinical situations because multiple actors and varying degrees of uncertainty are often involved. Generally, moral disagreements pertain to divergent views about treatment harms and benefits, ideological differences about the meaning of life, varying interpretations about moral rules or principles, and discrepancies in who or what is protected by moral rules (Gert, Culver, & Clouser, 2006). Moral disagreements are most frequently viewed as interpersonal experiences, although intrapersonal disagreements also occur and are experienced as moral uncertainty or ambiguity.

Ethical Conflicts

If individuals or systems avoid opportunities to consider or resolve moral disagreements, ethical conflicts often result. The term *conflict* is derived from the Latin word *confligere*, which means "to strike together" ("Conflict," n.d.). Barsky (2008) defined *conflict* as "a crisis in interaction, in which each party becomes wrapped in self-interest, fails to see the other side and feels victimized, hurt, or disempowered" (p. 166). Conflict emerges "when patients, surrogates, or clinicians perceive that their goals related to care and outcomes are being thwarted by the incompatible goals of others" (Edelstein, DeRenzo, Waetzig, Zelizer, & Mokwunye, 2009, p. 342). Represented by a clashing of important values, strong and sometimes troubling emotions often characterize ethical conflicts.

Contrary to common belief, most ethical conflicts do not just suddenly erupt. Instead, ethical conflicts frequently begin as unstated moral disagreements about a specific issue or from the belief that an issue has been unfairly managed (Edelstein et al., 2009). Delayed conversations about difficult decisions, inflexible moral positioning, and disrespect for alternative moral views are also associated with the progression of moral disagreements into ethical conflicts. Unchecked, these conflicts can quickly flame into contentious arguments and disruptive behaviors, which often complicate or impair communication and ethical reasoning and escalate the conflict (Agich, 2011).

Ethical conflicts are not inevitable but rather unfolding processes with root causes, which can be analyzed to proactively address common and often reoccurring conflicts. Sensitizing critical care clinicians to early warning signs of moral disagreements and then developing and testing collaborative strategies that address moral differences and interrupt the evolution of ethical conflicts could benefit patients, families, providers, and healthcare organizations.

Ethical Controversies in Clinical Practice

Case Study—Part 4

K.C.'s team was in ethical conflict as well. Her hematologist, Dr. M, felt obligated to respect the patient's clear wishes expressed at treatment onset. Dr. M knew that the patient had very good informed consent, believed she understood the side effects and risks of treatment, and agreed to the bone marrow transplant. More importantly, Dr. M recognized that the patient was a fighter. She acknowledged that the patient was very sick, yet stressed that K.C.'s leukemia had been cured and that recovery would occur in a matter of time. From the hematologist's perspective, it would be morally wrong to withdraw life support when the complications are directly attributable to the treatment. The intensivist caring for the patient stated that K.C.'s chance of recovery was less than 5%. K.C. was not responding well to the aggressive treatment and was on her way to multiorgan failure. They anticipated that she would soon need dialysis, as her renal failure was worsening, her bleeding was most likely secondary to disseminated intravascular coagulation, her pulmonary status had further deteriorated with her lungs whited out, her ventilator requirements were increasing, and a third pressor had been added. Although the intensivist admitted uncertainty about her prognosis, especially given K.C.'s age, he had seen enough of these cases over the years to know that she most likely would not make it. He did not want to get into a conflict with the hematologist, who was well respected in the institution, and figured it was best to let the scenario unfold until death was imminent. Multiple consultants on the case also disagreed on appropriate goals of care. The ICU nurses were increasingly uncomfortable with the conflict.

- The very nature of ethical issues and dilemmas is one of differing values and perspectives. What is the ethical issue facing the family and team in this case?
- As the nurse caring for the patient, describe one action you might take to begin resolving the ethical issue.
- List three risks that are apparent to different individuals in this situation and three potential benefits of working to resolve the concerns.
- Why might different members of the family and team have different perspectives on when treatment has become nonbeneficial, futile, or harmful?

Treatment Decision Making as Time Progresses

The moral obligation to assess and respect patient preferences makes this situation so complex; however, patient wishes are rarely frozen in time. Dresser (2014) addressed the "changing self" that occurs in illness, reflecting on her own cancer treatment decisions, which transitioned from adamant refusal of a feeding tube to eventual acceptance. Because disease trajectories unfold over time, patient interpretation of the meaning of illness, quality of life, and their tolerance for suffering can change. Families and healthcare professionals must in real time assess and consider patients' amended wishes for their goals of treatment. Unfortunately, as the disease progresses, capacity often becomes compromised and more difficult to judge. Depression and emotional despair can also cloud judgment, while not necessarily eliminating capacity; clinicians recognize its influence. Decision making that once appeared clear and unwavering is far easier to honor than a dramatic reversal or a waxing and waning decisional capacity.

Ethically, clinicians struggle and sometimes suffer with these ambiguities when providing the necessary decision-making guidance to patients and families. Rather than see these treatment decisions as absolute, when choosing lifesaving treatment (e.g., chemotherapy, bone marrow transplant) clinicians must evaluate if patients fully anticipate or appreciate what the disease and treatment burdens will mean to them.

Treatment decisions have multiple meanings to various stakeholders. For example, for some families, the decision to treat fosters hope and forestalls grief. For healthcare professionals, the decision to treat might represent an unspoken desire for success, to rescue or win the battle against a relentless disease. Treatment decisions can also reflect subtle, more furtive conflicts of interest, such as the rating of transplant services based on days of survival.

Prognosis Under Conditions of Uncertainty

The uncertainty that often accompanies prognostication in critical care situations can contribute to delays in initiating discussion about treatment preferences, code status, or goals of care. This wait-and-see perspective can lead to false expectations of patient recovery in family members, cause moral distress in clinicians, and fuel ethical conflicts (Borowske, 2012; Dzeng et al., 2015; Fassier & Azoulay, 2010). Evidence indicates that some physicians are uncertain what to say to families when the outcome is indeterminate or disputed and tend to avoid goals of care conversations (Durall, Zurakowski, & Wolfe, 2012; Keating et al., 2010). Families or patients who have difficulty accepting a poor prognosis can also be barriers to such dialogues (You et al., 2015). Nurses also report missed opportunities for discussion about end-of-life preferences (Boyd, Merkh, Rutledge, & Randall, 2011). In a study on factors that impact surrogate decision makers, researchers found that inconsistent or unclear information from care providers increased surrogate stress levels (Iverson et al., 2014). In different studies, families indicated they wanted to hear clinicians' views on prognosis, even under conditions of uncertainty (Apatira et al., 2008; Curtis & Vincent, 2010; Hinderer, Friedman, & Fins, 2015; Siegel, 2011). Not hearing news appeared to be more difficult for surrogates than hearing bad news. Researchers identified the importance of prognosis-related communication with patients and families and emphasized the nurse's role in facilitating these vital conversations (McLennon, Lasiter, et al., 2013; McLennon, Ulrich, Lasiter, et al., 2013). Transparent communication about uncertainty leads to a shared acceptance, which encourages patients and families to develop more realistic views of treatment outcomes.

Case Study—Part 5

K.C.'s condition continued to deteriorate. Her sister shared with the nurse her devastation that she could not find a way to protect K.C. from suffering and loss of dignity. Julia was exhausted herself, and when she could go home and managed to sleep, she awoke with nightmares about her sister. The patient's parents were adamant that everything be done to keep K.C. alive. Julia asked the nurse to help convince her parents that they needed to stop. In tears, she begged, "We at least have to find a way to not code her if her heart finally gives out."

- If you are the nurse meeting with Julia, what feelings are stirred in you?
- On a scale of 0–5 (0 = complete sense of powerlessness; 5 = full sense of empowerment approaching the issue), rate how you feel as you leave the room after this discussion.
- Reflect on what leads to your scoring of your effectiveness/ineffectiveness in this situation.
- What available resources would help you to address these issues?
- What is happening in your unit, your institution, and in greater society that would help address these issues? What is attributing to disregarding these concerns?
- What are the leadership responses?
- What policies might help resolve these issues?
- Nothing has been mentioned about the patient's two children. From an ethics of care perspective, are there interventions that you might consider?

Addressing Treatment Decisions and Nonbeneficial Treatment/Futility

More than 25 years ago, the first definition of futility surfaced in the medical literature. Physicians committed to ethics were seeing the harm that futile treatment caused and were struggling to describe it quantifiably. This was a critical need because prognostication by itself could not be predicated with absolute certainty. Leonard Schneiderman gathered a large interprofessional group together to review experiences and suggested the following definition: "When physicians conclude (either through personal experience, experiences shared with colleagues, or consideration of published empiric data) that in the last 100 cases a medical treatment has been useless, they should regard that treatment as futile" (Schneiderman, Jecker, & Jonsen, 1990, p. 949). Nine years later, Texas became the first state to pass legislation supporting physicians' clinical decision making in the unilateral withdrawal or withholding of futile treatment after due process, even if it was against the wishes of family members or surrogates.

Nonbeneficial treatment has been defined as "life-sustaining treatments delivered to patients who ultimately did not survive to hospital discharge, when treatment conflicts occurred in the adult ICU" (Gilmer et al., 2005, p. 962). Some physicians and their institutions began to limit futile treatment, developing policies where it was legislatively supported and translating the goals of medicine back into their practices, honoring best interest and the ethical principle of nonmaleficence. However, many institutions and teams today still respect patient or surrogate autonomy without limits, believing that autonomy trumps any harm incurred to the patient, family, professions, or society. It is essential that clinicians create the moral space and continue to engage in this discussion, and those that see the harmful treatment have a moral obligation to voice concern.

Ethics committees and ethics consultants (where available) can work within institutions to create environments where the norm is to integrate these conversations on an ongoing basis. Ethics committees and consultants can engage in policy development and ultimately provide a review of cases and offer recommendations. The concept of "it takes a village" is vital in this endeavor, with representation of many value perspectives, including cultural and religious beliefs. Committees that are diverse and interprofessional, even reaching beyond the walls of the institution to include nonprofessional community representation, are essential in creating healthcare environments that empower healthy debate, responsible and just decision making, and protection of the most vulnerable.

In the clinical case of K.C., one sees the many layers of differences and concerns. Uncertainty sets everyone on edge. The barriers unfold, including the effect of multiple consultants offering different perspectives without clarifying that one improvement does not make for a whole, the weight of a family in conflict, the nature of viewing a young person as being worthy of salvage at all costs, the past promises clinicians have made, and ultimately, the view of death as a failure. Although avoidance and inertia are often seen to be more convenient and less confrontational, the damages are significant. Poor outcomes, diminished communication, compromised quality of care and safety, and moral distress that creates disengagement of clinicians and the exiting of professionals become a domino effect that harms everyone.

In K.C.'s situation, with her parents and sister in conflict, each family member is mindful of a moral duty to stand by their loved one, making sure she is cared for. Their perspectives clash—the parents request aggressive treatment despite the burdens, while the sister attempts to protect her from further harm.

ICU nurses can work with the interprofessional team to encourage frequent and early communication with the family. Introducing an honest range of outcomes from the beginning of ICU admission helps some families balance realistic hope. However, the end-of-life literature is full of studies documenting the difficulty of this goal, with trust often being compromised right from the start. Surrogates highly doubt futility prognostication, with one study noting that 64% of decision makers did not believe a physician's prediction (Zier et al., 2009). Ultimately, healthcare teams must address situations that become conflictual; leaving relatives in this hostility can set families up for future dysfunctional states and complicated grief. This is particularly significant when children are involved. When teams maneuver away from placing decision making squarely in the hands of families and assume the responsibility of advocating for the best interest of the patient and establishing appropriate recommendations for goals of care, everyone wins; however, the effort needed to enact this difficult work can easily cause setbacks. Ethical dialogue is a process that, by its very nature, must advance over time and requires patience. The outcomes are rarely perfect, and resolutions are sometimes messy and wounding. Even then, healthcare teams must find conduits to move through in healthy ways. This requires continued conversation, review, respect, forgiveness, and commitment to patients, families, and the healthcare team. The nursing profession is obligated to these ethical mandates. Given the potential for harm, would one ask for anything less?

The Importance of Resilience in High-Intensity Environments

Critical care nurses are repeatedly immersed in stressful situations, such as competing demands on time, distressed patients and families, difficult treatment decisions, uncertain prognosis, intense resuscitations, and high mortality rates (Mealer, Burnham, Goode, Rothbaum, & Moss, 2010). These highly emotional situations can lead to post-traumatic stress disorder (PTSD), compassion fatigue, burnout, or elements of all three (see Table 22-3).

In a study by Mealer et al. (2014), 44% of ICU nurses scored positive for PTSD. Unfortunately, the consequences can be severe. Conditions such as burnout and compassion fatigue in health care are associated with increased staff turnover, absenteeism, poor coworker relationships, depersonalization, decreased patient satisfaction, and medical errors (Sundin, Hochwälder, & Lisspers, 2011; Vahey, Aiken, Sloane, Clarke, & Vargas, 2004).

Developing job-related resilience in high-intensity environments is essential for oncology and critical care nurses. Resilient coping allows nurses to effectively adapt in the face of adversity, trauma, tragedy, threats, or significant sources of stress. Characteristics of resiliency include self-control, self-sufficiency, creativity, optimism, adaptability, persistence, and humor (American Psychological Association [APA], n.d.). Individual qualities that promote resilience include optimism, the ability to ask others for support, faith, the belief that stress builds strength, and working toward personal goals (APA, n.d.; Charney, 2004). Contextual factors that contribute to the development of individual resilience include strong family bonds and supportive work environments (APA, n.d.). Raingruber and Wolf (2015) explored nurses' perceptions of factors that contribute to their resilience and found four themes: patient vulnerability and gratitude, spirituality associated with practice, use of compassion and prayer for self and others, and being present in their own lives and setting priorities accordingly.

Research shows that ICU nurses with high resilience have less PTSD, burnout syndrome, anxiety, and depression (Hoge, Austin, & Pollack, 2007; Mealer et al., 2012; Rushton, Batcheller, Schroeder, & Donohue, 2015). Fortunately, resilience can be learned. For example, Mealer et al. (2014) tested an innovative educational workshop for ICU nurses that included self-care topics, guided mindfulness, expres-

	Table 22-3. Comparison of Syndromes Common to Intensive Care Unit Nurses		
Characteristic	Post-Traumatic Stress Disorder	Compassion Fatigue	Burnout
Onset	Response to a traumatic event or trigger	Sudden, acute onset	Gradual over time
Symptoms	Detachment, difficulty sleeping and concentrating, anxiety, recurrent and distressing dreams	Gastrointestinal distress, headaches, sleep problems, not relating to others	Exhaustion, decreased morale, added coping demands, lack of perceived goal achievement
Causes	Trauma (likely cumulative), caring while patients suffer, futile care	Consequences of caring for suffering patients, very empathic toward others, inability to change course of painful scenario or moral distress	Response to work or environmental stressors (e.g., staffing, high patient acuity workload, inadequate supplies or resources)
Outcomes	Depression, anxiety, job dissatisfaction, leave nursing	Continues to work but is less empathic and objectives affects patient safety and patient satisfaction	Decreased empathy, withdrawal, may leave nursing or change position or transfer

Note. Based on information from Boyle, 2011; Mealer et al., 2010; Sansó et al., 2015.

sive writing, and event-triggered counseling. The authors concluded that resilience training in ICU nurses is both feasible and acceptable. Findings such as these indicate that promoting nurses' resilience should be a high priority for nursing leadership. APA offered 10 suggestions for building resilience (see Table 22-4).

Part of nurses' ethical obligation to patients is caring for themselves and each other (ANA, 2015). In part, Provision 5 states, "The nurse owes the same duties to self as to others, including the responsibility to promote health and safety, preserve wholeness of character and integrity, maintain competence, and continue personal and professional growth" (ANA, 2015, p. 19). Strategies such as balancing work with leisure activities and practicing mindfulness are specifically described as methods to mitigate compassion fatigue. Ultimately, the best way to reduce PTSD risk, compassion fatigue, and burnout is careful attention to and a deliberate plan for self-care.

Table 22-4. Ways for Intensive Care Unit Nurses to Build Resilience	
Suggestions	Behaviors
Make connections	Make connections with family, friends, or others. Accept help from those who care about you. Join civic groups or faith-based organizations. Assist others in time of need.
Avoid seeing crises as insurmountable problems	Change how you view stressful events. Look beyond the present to the future. Note when you are feeling better about difficult situations.
Accept that change is part of living life	Accept that some things cannot be changed and focus on the things you can alter.
Move toward your goals	Be realistic in setting goals. Do something regularly to move toward your goal. Even small accomplishments are important.
Take decisive action	Act rather than detaching from stressors and problems.
Look for opportunities for self-discovery	People often learn something about themselves in time of crisis or loss (e.g., relationships grow stronger, sense of strength grows, sense of self-worth grows, spirituality improves).
Nurture a positive view of yourself	Develop confidence in your ability to solve problems and trust in yourself to build resilience.
Keep things in perspective	Even when facing painful situations, try to avoid blowing the event out of proportion. Consider the stressful situation in a broader sense.
Maintain a hopeful outlook	An optimistic outlook enables you to expect that good things will happen in your life. Try visualizing what you want rather than worrying about what you fear.
Take care of yourself	Pay attention to your needs and feelings. Engage in activities that you like. Exercise regularly. Keep your mind and body primed by self-care.

Note. Based on information from American Psychological Association, n.d.

Summary

Critical care nurses are repeatedly immersed in stressful situations, such as competing demands on time, distressed patients and families, difficult treatment decisions, uncertain prognosis, intense resuscitations, and high mortality rates. As they care for patients with cancer, they play a significant role in creating ethics-enriched practice settings where all perspectives and voices need to be heard.

Proactive, team-based ethics dialogue and collaborative, shared decision making should form the core of critical care practice. K.C.'s situation is not unusual. These ethically difficult situations will continue to arise in complex healthcare systems. Rather than avoiding moral differences and disagreements, nurses and leadership need to raise questions and initiate innovative processes, such as regularly scheduled ethics rounds, and in high-risk situations, provide early assessment and engagement. Other programs would be valuable, such as interprofessional ethics education and team-based conflict transformation. Mitigating the moral distress that often results in ethically complex situations requires developing nurses' competencies in addressing frequently encountered ethical challenges and designing practice settings where moral responsibilities are discussed and openly respected. Ultimately, ethics conversations must become a routine part of care. Resiliency practices and the collective interprofessional building of a moral community will go a long way to diminish some of the potential harms. High-quality patient care depends on healthcare organizations that are equally committed to delivering evidence- and ethics-based health care for patients and providing team-based, ethically responsive work environments for healthcare professionals.

References

Agich, G.J. (2011). Defense mechanisms in ethics consultation. *HEC Forum, 23,* 269–279. doi:10 .1007/s10730-011-9165-6

American Association of Critical-Care Nurses. (n.d.). Resources for ethics/moral distress. Retrieved from https://www.aacn.org/clinical-resources/ethics-moral-distress

American Nurses Association. (2015). *Code of ethics for nurses with interpretive statements.* Retrieved from http://nursingworld.org/MainMenuCategories/EthicsStandards/CodeofEthicsforNurses /Code-of-Ethics-For-Nurses.html

American Psychological Association. (n.d.). *The road to resilience.* Retrieved from http://www.apa.org /helpcenter/road-resilience.aspx

Apatira, L., Boyd, E.A., Malvar, G., Evans, L.R., Luce, J.M., Lo, B., & White, D.B. (2008). Hope, truth, and preparing for death: Perspectives of surrogate decision makers. *Annals of Internal Medicine, 149,* 861–868.

Austin, W. (2012). Moral distress and the contemporary plight of health professionals. *HEC Forum, 24,* 27–38. doi:10.1007/s10730-012-9179-8

Azoulay, E., Timsit, J.-F., Sprung, C.L., Soares, M., Rusinová, K., Lafabrie, A., ... Schlemmer, B. (2009). Prevalence and factors of intensive care unit conflicts: The Conflicus study. *American Journal of Respiratory and Critical Care Medicine, 180,* 853–860. doi:10.1164/rccm.200810-1614OC

Balevre, P., Cassells, J., & Buzaianu, E. (2012). Professional nursing burnout and irrational thinking: A replication study. *Journal for Nurses in Staff Development, 28,* 2–8. doi:10.1097/NND .0b013e318240a65a

Barsky, A. (2008). A conflict resolution approach to teaching ethical decision making: Bridging conflicting values. *Journal of Jewish Communal Service, 83,* 164–169.

Borowske, D. (2012). Straddling the fence: ICU nurses advocating for hospice care. *Critical Care Nursing Clinics of North America, 24,* 105–116. doi:10.1016/j.ccell.2012.01.006

Bosslet, G., Pope, T.M., Rubenfeld, G.D., Lo, B., Truog, R.D., Rushton, C.H., ... White, D.B. (2015). An official ATS/AACN/ACCP/ESICM/SCCM policy statement: Responding to requests for potentially inappropriate treatments in intensive care units. *American Journal of Respiratory and Critical Care Medicine, 191,* 1318–1330. doi:10.1164/rccm.201505-0924ST

Boyd, D., Merkh, K., Rutledge, D.N., & Randall, V. (2011). Nurses' perceptions and experiences with end-of-life communication and care [Online exclusive]. *Oncology Nursing Forum, 38,* E229–E239. doi:10.1188/11.ONF.E229-E239

Boyle, D.A. (2011). Countering compassion fatigue: A requisite nursing agenda. *Online Journal of Issues in Nursing, 16,* Manuscript 2. doi:10.3912/OJIN.Vol16No01Man02

Browning, A.M. (2013). CNE article: Moral distress and psychological empowerment in critical care nurses caring for adults at end of life. *American Journal of Critical Care, 22,* 143–151. doi:10.4037/ajcc2013437

Bruce, C.R., Weinzimmer, S., & Zimmerman, J.L. (2014). Moral distress in the ICU. In J.-L. Vincent (Ed.), *Annual update in intensive care and emergency medicine* (pp. 723–734). New York, NY: Springer.

Cassell, E.J. (1999). Diagnosing suffering: A perspective. *Annals of Internal Medicine, 131,* 531–534. doi:10.7326/0003-4819-131-7-199910050-00009

Charney, D.S. (2004). Psychobiological mechanisms of resilience and vulnerability: Implications for successful adaptation to extreme stress. *American Journal of Psychiatry, 161,* 195–216. doi:10.1176/appi.ajp.161.2.195

Cheon, J., Coyle, N., Wiegand, D.L., & Welsh, S. (2015). Ethical issues experienced by hospice and palliative nurses. *Journal of Hospice and Palliative Nurses, 17,* 7–13. doi:10.1097/NJH.0000000000000129

Cimiotti, J., Aiken, L.H., Sloane, D.M., & Wu, E.S. (2012). Nurse staffing, burnout, and health-care-associated infections. *American Journal of Infection Control, 40,* 486–490. doi:10.1016/j.ajic.2012.02.029

Cohen, J.S., & Erickson, J.M. (2006). Ethical dilemmas and moral distress in oncology nursing practice. *Clinical Journal of Oncology Nursing, 10,* 775–780. doi:10.1188/06.CJON.775-780

Conflict. (n.d.). In *Online Etymology Dictionary.* Retrieved from http://www.etymonline.com/index.php?allowed_in_frame=0&search=conflict

Curtis, J.R., & Vincent, J.-L. (2010). Ethics and end-of-life care for adults in the intensive care unit. *Lancet, 376,* 1347–1353. doi:10.1016/S0140-6736(10)60143-2

Disagreement. (n.d.). In *Online Etymology Dictionary.* Retrieved from http://www.etymonline.com/index.php?term=disagreement

Dodek, P.M., Wong, H., Norena, M., Ayas, N., Reynolds, S.C., Keenan, S.P., ... Alden, L. (2016). Moral distress in intensive care unit professionals is associated with profession, age, and years of experience. *Journal of Critical Care, 31,* 178–182. doi:10.1016/j.jcrc.2015.10.011

Dresser, R. (2014). Treatment decisions and changing selves. *Journal of Medical Ethics, 41,* 975–976. doi:10.1136/medethics-2014-102237

Durall, A., Zurakowski, D., & Wolfe, J. (2012). Barriers to conducting advance care discussions for children with life-threatening conditions. *Pediatrics, 129,* e975–e982. doi:10.1542/peds.2011-2695

Dyrbye, L., & Shanafelt, T. (2016). A narrative review on burnout experienced by medical students and residents. *Medical Education, 50,* 132–149. doi:10.1111/medu.12927

Dzeng, E., Colaianni, A., Roland, M., Levine, D., Kelly, M.P., Barclay, S., & Smith, T.J. (2015). Moral distress amongst American physician trainees regarding futile treatments at the end of life: A qualitative study. *Journal of General Internal Medicine, 31,* 93–99. doi:10.1007/s11606-015-3505-1

Edelstein, L.M., DeRenzo, E.G., Waetzig, E., Zelizer, C., & Mokwunye, N. (2009). Communication and conflict management training for clinical bioethics committees. *HEC Forum, 21,* 341–349. doi:10.1007/s10730-009-9116-7

Epstein, E.G. (2012). Preventive ethics in the intensive care unit. *AACN Advanced Critical Care, 23,* 217–224. doi:10.1097/NCI.0b013e31824b3b9b

Epstein, E.G., & Hamric, A.B. (2009). Moral distress, moral residue, and the crescendo effect. *Journal of Clinical Ethics, 20,* 330–342.

Espinosa, L., Young, A., Symes, L., Haile, B., & Walsh, T. (2010). ICU nurses' experiences in providing terminal care. *Critical Care Nursing Quarterly, 33,* 273–281. doi:10.1097/CNQ .0b013e3181d91424

Fassier, T., & Azoulay, E. (2010). Conflicts and communication gaps in the intensive care unit. *Current Opinion in Critical Care, 16,* 654–665. doi:10.1097/MCC.0b013e32834044f0

Foglia, M.B., Cohen, J.H., Pearlman, R.A., Bottrell, M.M., & Fox, E. (2013). Perceptions of ethical leadership and the ethical environment and culture: IntegratedEthics staff survey data from the VA Health Care System. *American Journal of Bioethics Primary Research, 4,* 44–58.

Ganzini, L., Volicer, L., Nelson, W.A., Fox, E., & Derse, A.R. (2005). Ten myths about decision-making capacity. *Journal of the American Medical Directors Association, 6*(Suppl. 3), S100–S104. doi:10.1016/j.jamda.2005.03.040

Gert, B., Culver, C., & Clouser, K. (2006). *Bioethics: A systematic approach.* New York, NY: Oxford University Press.

Gilmer, T., Schneiderman, L.J., Teetzel, H., Blustein, J., Briggs, K., Cohn, F., … Young, E. (2005). The costs of nonbeneficial treatment in the intensive care setting. *Health Affairs, 24,* 961–971. doi:10.1377/hlthaff.24.4.961

Goethals, S., Gastmans, C., & de Casterlé, B.D. (2010). Nurses' ethical reasoning and behaviour: A literature review. *International Journal of Nursing Studies, 47,* 635–650. doi:10.1016/j.ijnurstu.2009.12.010

Hamric, A.B. (2012). Empirical research on moral distress: Issues, challenges, and opportunities. *HEC Forum, 24,* 30–49. doi:10.1007/s10730-012-9177-x

Hamric, A.B., & Blackhall, L.J. (2007). Nurse-physician perspectives on the care of dying patients in intensive care units: Collaboration, moral distress, and ethical climate. *Critical Care Medicine, 35,* 422–429. doi:10.1097/01.CCM.0000254722.50608.2D

Hardingham, L.B. (2004). Integrity and moral residue: Nurses as participants in a moral community. *Nursing Philosophy, 5,* 127–134.

Hinderer, K.A., Friedman, E., & Fins, J.J. (2015). Withdrawal of life-sustaining treatment: Patient and proxy agreement: A secondary analysis of "contracts, covenants, and advance care planning". *Dimensions of Critical Care Nursing, 34,* 91–99. doi:10.1097/DCC.0000000000000097

Hoge, E.A., Austin, E.D., & Pollack, M.H. (2007). Resilience: Research evidence and conceptual considerations for posttraumatic stress disorder. *Depression and Anxiety, 24,* 139–152.

Huffman, D.M., & Rittenmeyer, L. (2012). How professional nurses working in hospital environments experience moral distress: A systematic review. *Critical Care Nursing Clinics of North America, 24,* 91–100. doi:10.1016/j.ccell.2012.01.004

Iverson, E., Celious, A., Kennedy, C.R., Shehane, E., Eastman, A., Warren, V., & Freeman, B.D. (2014). Factors affecting stress experienced by surrogate decision-makers for critically ill patients: Implications for nursing practice. *Intensive and Critical Care Nursing, 30,* 77–85. doi:10.1016/j.iccn.2013.08.008

Jameton, A. (1984). *Nursing practice: The ethical issues.* Englewood Cliffs, NJ: Prentice-Hall.

Jameton, A. (1993). Dilemmas of moral distress: Moral responsibility and nursing practice. *AWHONN's Clinical Issues, 4,* 542–551.

Keating, N.L., Landrum, M.B., Rogers, S.O., Jr., Baum, S.K., Virnig, B.A., Huskamp, H.A., … Kahn, K.L. (2010). Physician factors associated with discussions about end-of-life care. *Cancer, 116,* 998–1006. doi:10.1002/cncr.24761

Kelly, D., Kutney-Lee, A., Lake, E.T., & Aiken, L.H. (2013). The critical care work environment and nurse-reported health care–associated infections. *American Journal of Critical Care, 22,* 482–488. doi:10.4037/ajcc2013298

Maiden, J., Georges, J.M., & Connelly, C.D. (2011). Moral distress, compassion fatigue, and perceptions about medication errors in certified critical care nurses. *Dimensions of Critical Care Nursing, 30,* 339–345. doi:10.1097/DCC.0b013e31822fab2a

Mason, V.M., Leslie, G., Clark, K., Lyons, P., Walke, E., Butler, C., & Griffin, M. (2014). Compassion fatigue, moral distress, and work engagement in surgical intensive care unit trauma nurses: A pilot study. *Dimensions in Critical Care Nursing, 33,* 215–225. doi:10.1097/DCC .0000000000000056

McAndrew, N.S., Leske, J.S., & Garcia, A. (2011). Influence of moral distress on the professional practice environment during prognostic conflict in critical care. *Journal of Trauma Nursing, 18,* 221–230. doi:10.1097/JTN.0b013e31823a4a12

McLennon, S.M., Lasiter, S., Miller, W.R., Amlin, K., Chamness, A.R., & Helft, P.R. (2013). Oncology nurses' experiences with prognosis-related communication with patients who have advanced cancer. *Nursing Outlook, 61,* 427–436. doi:10.1016/j.outlook.2012.12.001

McLennon, S.M., Ulrich, M., Lasiter, S., Chamness, A.R., & Helft, P.R. (2013). Oncology nurses narratives about ethical dilemmas and prognosis-related communication in advanced cancer patients. *Cancer Nursing, 36,* 114–121. doi:10.1097/NCC.0b013e31825f4dc8

McLeod, A. (2014). Nurses' views of the causes of ethical dilemmas during treatment cessation in the ICU: A qualitative study. *British Journal of Neuroscience Nursing, 10,* 131–137. doi:10.12968/bjnn.2014.10.3.131

Mealer, M., Burnham, E.L., Goode, C.J., Rothbaum, B., & Moss, M. (2010). The prevalence and impact of post traumatic stress and burnout syndrome in nurses. *Depression and Anxiety, 26,* 1118–1126. doi:10.1002/da.20631

Mealer, M., Conrad, D., Evans, J., Jooste, K., Solyntjes, J., Rothbaum, B., & Moss, M. (2014). Feasibility and acceptability of a resilience training program for intensive care unit nurses. *American Journal of Critical Care, 23,* e97–e105. doi:10.4037/ajcc2014747

Mealer, M., Jones, J., Newman, J., McFann, K.K., Rothbaum, B., & Moss, M. (2012). The presence of resilience is associated with a healthier psychological profile in intensive care unit (ICU) nurses: Results of a national survey. *International Journal of Nursing Studies, 49,* 292–299. doi:10.1016/j.ijnurstu.2011.09.015

Molloy, D., Hadjistavropoulos, T., McCarthy, R., Evans, R., Zakus, D., Park, I., ... Williams, J. (2009). Culture and organizational climate: Nurses' insights into their relationship with physicians. *Nursing Ethics, 16,* 719–733.

Moss, M., Good, V.S., Gozal, D., Kleinpell, R., & Sessler, C.N. (2016). An official Critical Care Societies collaborative statement: Burnout syndrome in critical care healthcare professionals: A call for action. *American Journal of Critical Care, 25,* 368–376. doi:10.4037/ajcc2016133

Musto, L.C., Rodney, P.A., & Vanderheide, R. (2015). Toward interventions to address moral distress: Navigating structure and agency. *Nursing Ethics, 22,* 91–102. doi:10.1177/0969733014534879

Oh, Y., & Gastmans, C. (2015). Moral distress experienced by nurses: A quantitative literature review. *Nursing Ethics, 22,* 15–31. doi:10.1177/0969733013502803

Olsen, D.P. (2016). Ethical practice with patients in pain. *American Journal of Nursing, 116*(1), 57–60. doi:10.1097/01.NAJ.0000476172.74165.1c

Paradis, E., Leslie, M., Gropper, M.A., Aboumatar, H.J., Kitto, S., & Reeves, S. (2013). Interprofessional care in intensive care settings and the factors that impact it: Results from a scoping review of ethnographic studies. *Journal of Critical Care, 28,* 1062–1067. doi:10.1016/j.jcrc.2013.05.015

Pavlish, C., Brown-Saltzman, K., Dirksen, K.M., & Fine, A. (2015). Physicians' perspectives on ethically challenging situations: Early identification and action. *American Journal of Bioethics: Empirical Bioethics, 6,* 28–40. doi:10.1080/23294515.2014.972527

Pavlish, C., Brown-Saltzman, K., Fine, A., & Jakel, P. (2013). Making the call: A proactive ethics framework. *HEC Forum, 25,* 269–283. doi:10.1007/s10730-013-9213-5

Pavlish, C., Brown-Saltzman, K., Hersh, M., Shirk, M., & Nudelman, O. (2011). Early indicators and risk factors for ethical issues in clinical practice. *Journal of Nursing Scholarship, 43,* 13–21. doi:10.1111/j.1547-5069.2010.01380.x

Pavlish, C., Brown-Saltzman, K., Hersh, M., Shirk, M., & Rounkle, A.-M. (2011). Nursing priorities, actions, and regrets for ethical situations in clinical practice. *Journal of Nursing Scholarship, 43,* 385–395. doi:10.1111/j.1547-5069.2011.01422.x

Pavlish, C., Brown-Saltzman, K., Jakel, P., & Fine, A. (2014). The nature of ethical conflicts and the meaning of moral community. *Oncology Nursing Forum, 41,* 130–140. doi:10.1188/14.ONF.130-140

Pavlish, C., Brown-Saltzman, K., Jakel, P., & Rounkle, A.-M. (2012). Nurses' responses to ethical challenges in oncology practice: An ethnographic study. *Clinical Journal of Oncology Nursing, 16,* 592–600. doi:10.1188/12.CJON.592-600

Piers, R.D., Azoulay, E., Ricou, B., Ganz, F.D., Decruyenaere, J., Max, A., … Benoit, D.D. (2011). Perceptions of appropriateness of care among European and Israeli intensive care unit nurses and physicians. *JAMA, 306,* 2694–2703. doi:10.1001/jama.2011.1888

Rainer, J. (2015). Speaking up: Factors and issues in nurses advocating for patients when patients are in jeopardy. *Journal of Nursing Care Quality, 30,* 53–62. doi:10.1097/NCQ.0000000000000081

Raingruber, B., & Wolf, T. (2015). Nurse perspectives regarding the meaningfulness of oncology nursing practice. *Clinical Journal of Oncology Nursing, 19,* 292–296. doi:10.1188/15.CJON.292-296

Rathert, C., May, D.R., & Chung, H.S. (2016). Nurse moral distress: A survey identifying predictors and potential interventions. *International Journal of Nursing Studies, 53,* 39–49. doi:10.1016/j.ijnurstu.2015.10.007

Rest, J. (1994). Background: Theory and research. In J. Rest & D. Narvaez (Eds.), *Moral development in the professions: Psychology and applied ethics* (pp. 1–26). Hillsdale, NJ: Lawrence Erlbaum Associates.

Rittenmeyer, L., & Huffman, D.M. (2009). How professional nurses working in hospital environments experience moral distress: A systematic review. *JBI Library of Systematic Reviews, 7,* 1234–1291. doi:10.11124/01938924-200907280-00001

Rose, L. (2011). Interprofessional collaboration in the ICU: How to define? *Nursing in Critical Care, 16,* 5–10. doi:10.1111/j.1478-5153.2010.00398.x

Rushton, C.H., Batcheller, J., Schroeder, K., & Donohue, P. (2015). Burnout and resilience among nurses practicing in high-intensity settings. *American Journal of Critical Care, 24,* 412–420. doi:10.4037/ajcc2015291

Sansó, N., Galiana, L., Oliver, A., Pascual, A., Sinclair, S., & Benito, E. (2015). Palliative care professionals' inner life: Exploring the relationships among awareness, self-care, and compassion satisfaction and fatigue, burnout, and coping with death. *Journal of Pain and Symptom Management, 50,* 200–207. doi:10.1016/j.jpainsymman.2015.02.013

Sauerland, J., Marotta, K., Peinemann, M.A., Berndt, A., & Robichaux, C. (2014). Assessing and addressing moral distress and ethical climate, part 1. *Dimensions of Critical Care Nursing, 33,* 234–245. doi:10.1097/DCC.0000000000000050

Schneiderman, L.J., Jecker, N.S., & Jonsen, A.R. (1990). Medical futility: Its meaning and ethical implications. *Annals of Internal Medicine, 112,* 949–954. doi:10.7326/0003-4819-112-12-949

Shannon, S.E. (2016). The nurse as the patient's advocate: A contrarian view. *Hastings Center Report, 46*(Suppl. 1), S43–S47. doi:10.1002/hast.632

Shepard, A. (2010). Moral distress: A consequence of caring. *Clinical Journal of Oncology Nursing, 14,* 25–27. doi:10.1188/10.CJON.25-27

Siegel, M.D. (2011). End of life decision making and care of the dying patient (PCCSU Volume 25, Lesson 12). Retrieved from http://www.chestnet.org/Education/eLearning/e-Learning/End-of-Life-Decision-Making-and-Care-of-the-Dying-Patient

Silber, J.H., Rosenbaum, P.R., McHugh, M.D., Ludwig, J.M., Smith, H.L., Niknam, B.A., … Aiken, L.H. (2016). Comparison of the value of nursing work environments in hospitals across different levels of patient risk. *JAMA Surgery, 151,* 527–536. doi:10.1001/jamasurg.2015.4908

Sirilla, J. (2014). Moral distress in nurses providing direct care on inpatient oncology units. *Clinical Journal of Oncology Nursing, 18,* 536–541. doi:10.1188/14.CJON.536-541

Sundin, L., Hochwälder, J., & Lisspers, J. (2011). A longitudinal examination of generic and occupational specific job demands, and work-related social support associated with burnout among nurses in Sweden. *Work, 38,* 389–400. doi:10.3233/WOR-2011-1142

Ulrich, B.T., Lavandero, R., Woods, D., & Early, S. (2014). Critical care nurse work environments 2013: A status report. *Critical Care Nurse, 34,* 64–79. doi:10.4037/ccn2014731

Ulrich, C.M., Hamric, A.B., & Grady, C. (2010). Moral distress: A growing problem in the health professions? *Hastings Center Report, 40*(1), 20–22. doi:10.1353/hcr.0.0222

Vahey, D.C., Aiken, L.H., Sloane, D.M., Clarke, S.P., & Vargas, D. (2004). Nurse burnout and patient satisfaction. *Medical Care, 42*(Suppl. 2), II-57–II-66. doi:10.1097/01.mlr.0000109126 .50398.5a

Varcoe, C., Pauly, B., Storch, J., Newton, L., & Makaroff, K. (2012). Nurses' perceptions of and responses to morally distressing situations. *Nursing Ethics, 19,* 488–500. doi:10.1177 /0969733011436025

Varcoe, C., Pauly, B., Webster, G., & Storch, J. (2012). Moral distress: Tensions as springboards for action. *HEC Forum, 24,* 51–62. doi:10.1007/s10730-012-9180-2

Wall, S., Austin, W.J., & Garros, D. (2015). Organizational influences on health professionals' experiences of moral distress in PICUs. *HEC Forum, 28,* 53–67. doi:10.1007/s10730-015-9266-8

Weinzimmer, S., Miller, S.M., Zimmerman, J.L., Hooker, J., Isidro, S., & Bruce, C.R. (2014). Critical care nurses' moral distress in end-of-life decision making. *Journal of Nursing Education and Practice, 4,* 6–12. doi:10.5430/jnep.v4n6p6

Whitehead, P.B., Herbertson, R.K., Hamric, A.B., Epstein, E.G., & Fisher, J.M. (2015). Moral distress among healthcare professionals: Report of an institution-wide survey. *Journal of Nursing Scholarship, 47,* 117–125. doi:10.1111/jnu.12115

You, J.J., Downar, J., Fowler, R.A., Lamontagne, R., Ma, I.W., Jayaraman, D., … Heyland, D.K. (2015). Barriers to goals of care discussions with seriously ill hospitalized patients and their families: A multicenter survey of clinicians. *JAMA Internal Medicine, 175,* 549–556. doi:10.1001 /jamainternmed.2014.7732

Zier, L.S., Burack, J.H., Micco, G., Chipman, A.K., Frank, J.A., & White, D.B. (2009). Surrogate decision makers' responses to physicians' predictions of medical futility. *Chest, 136,* 110–117. doi:10.1378/chest.08-2753

Index

The letter f *after a page number indicates that relevant content appears in a figure; the letter* t, *in a table.*

A

ABCDEF bundle, 316–319, 317f
abdominal compartment syndrome (ACS)
  with gastrointestinal cancer, 159–161
  with pancreatic cancer, 113
abdominal distension
  with enteral nutrition, 329
  with intraperitoneal chemotherapy, 138t
abdominal pain with intraperitoneal chemotherapy, 138t
ABGs. *See* arterial blood gases (ABGs)
abiraterone acetate, cardiotoxicity of, 215
absolute lymphocyte count, 43t
absolute neutrophil count (ANC), 44t
  calculation of, 294, 294f
  grading of, 294, 294t
  in neutropenia, 294
  in neutropenic fever, 258
  with sepsis, 296, 299
acalculous cholecystitis, 58t
ACE inhibitors. *See* angiotensin-converting enzyme (ACE) inhibitors

acidity (pH) after thoracic surgery, 32–33, 33t
acidosis
  lactic, 183
  metabolic, 182–183
  renal tubular, 182–183
  after thoracic surgery, 33, 33t
Acinetobacter species, sepsis due to, 287, 288t
actinomycin D (dactinomycin), side effects of, 133t
activated protein C level, 46t
acute interstitial nephritis (AIN), 177t, 179
acute kidney injury (AKI)
  due to acute interstitial nephritis, 177t, 179
  causes of, 172
  due to contrast-induced nephropathy, 172
  defined, 171
  due to glomerular disease, 175t, 178
  hemodynamic, 173–174, 175t
  due to interstitial disease, 179
  with intra-abdominal hypertension, 160
  due to intrinsic renal disease, 174–179

  due to multiple myeloma, 172, 181–182
  due to nephrotoxic agents, 175t–177t
  nursing implications of, 171–172
  due to obstructive renal disease, 179–180
  overview of, 171–172
  renal replacement therapy for, 172, 187–188, 189t
  due to thrombotic microangiopathy, 174–178, 175t–176t
  due to tubular disease and acute tubular necrosis, 172, 178
  due to tumor lysis syndrome, 172, 180–181, 181f
  types of, 172–182
acute lung injury (ALI)
  with gastrointestinal cancer, 155
acute lymphoblastic leukemia (ALL)
  complications of, 56t
  cytogenetics of, 50t
  demographics of, 52t
  prognosis for, 51t
  treatment of, 55t

acute myeloid leukemia (AML)
complications of, 56t
cytogenetics of, 50t
demographics of, 52t
prognosis for, 51t
treatment of, 55t
acute pancreatitis (AP), 111–113
acute respiratory distress syndrome (ARDS)
enteral formulas for, 328
with gastrointestinal cancer, 155
due to hepatocellular carcinoma, 107
acute respiratory failure (ARF), 271
diagnostic studies for, 271–272
noninvasive ventilation for, 273–274
transitions in care for, 410
acute skin failure, 352–353
acute tubular necrosis (ATN), 172, 178
acyclovir, nephrotoxicity of, 436t
ADAMTS13, 46t
adenocarcinoma of lung, 24
adenomas, pituitary, 5–6, 6t
adenosine for dysrhythmias, 226t
adenosine triphosphate (ATP), 14–15
advance directives, 449
advanced neurologic monitoring, 1, 14–18
aging patients. See older adults
agitation. See pain, agitation, and delirium (PAD)
air leak after thoracic surgery, 30
AKI. See acute kidney injury (AKI)
albumin
concentrations of, 374

for fluid resuscitation, 377, 378t
in hepatocellular carcinoma, 109
alcohol caps with central venous catheters, 396
alginate dressing, 364t
alkalosis after thoracic surgery, 33, 33t
alkylating agents
cardiotoxicity of, 204–212
side effects of, 133t
ALL. See acute lymphoblastic leukemia (ALL)
allergic reactions with gynecologic cancer, 118t, 147–148
alveolar hemorrhage, diffuse, 81t
alveolar proteinosis, pulmonary, 87t
American Nurses Association (ANA) Code of Ethics, 447–448
amikacin, nephrotoxicity of, 176t
aminoglycosides
nephrotoxicity of, 176t, 436t
for sepsis, 301t
volume of distribution of, 374
aminosteroids, 383–384
amiodarone
for dysrhythmias, 226t
half-life of, 375
volume of distribution of, 374
AML. See acute myeloid leukemia (AML)
amphotericin B, nephrotoxicity of, 176t, 436t
anaerobic bacterial infection, 303f
analgesics, 381
for delirium, 317–318
in palliative care, 418–419
anaphylactic shock, 283
anaphylaxis with gynecologic cancer, 118t

anaplastic gliomas, 7
anastomotic leak with gastrointestinal cancer, 154–155
anastrozole, cardiotoxicity of, 215
ANC. See absolute neutrophil count (ANC)
anemia
aplastic, 70t
cardiovascular effects of, 203
due to chemotherapy for bone and soft tissue sarcomas, 165
hemolytic, 69, 70t
medication-induced, 91t
angiography, 199t
magnetic resonance, 12t
angiotensin-converting enzyme (ACE) inhibitors
for cardiomyopathy/heart failure, 232
for hypertension, 237
nephrotoxicity of, 175t, 436t
angiotensin receptor blockers (ARBs)
for cardiomyopathy/heart failure, 232
nephrotoxicity of, 436t
anion gap (AG) after thoracic surgery, 33
anorexia with gynecologic cancer, 118t, 144–145
anthracyclines, cardiotoxicity of, 167, 204, 212–213, 229–230
antibiotic agents
nephrotoxicity of, 177t
side effects of, 133t–134t
antibiotic therapy for sepsis, 299–302, 300f, 301t–302t, 303f
anticipatory nausea, 145
anticoagulants, 384–385
antidiuretic hormone (ADH), syndrome of inappropriate secretion of, 66t, 183, 248

antiemetic agents in palliative care, 421, 421*f*

antifungals for sepsis, 302*t*

antihypertensive agents, 237, 238*t*–239*t*

anti-inflammatory mediators in sepsis, 289

antimetabolites
cardiotoxicity of, 213
side effects of, 134*t*–135*t*

antineoplastic agents, hematologic/immunologic toxicity due to, 90–93, 91*t*–93*t*

antineoplastic medication–induced cardiotoxicity, 204–213, 205*t*–211*t*

antiphospholipid syndrome, 70*t*

antipsychotic medications, 314

antiretroviral drugs, nephrotoxicity of, 436*t*

antithrombin III, 46*t*

antivirals for sepsis, 302*t*

anxiety in older adults, 434

apixaban, 385

aplastic anemia, 70*t*

apoptosis, 9

ARDS. *See* acute respiratory distress syndrome (ARDS)

ARF. *See* acute respiratory failure (ARF)

arginine and wound healing, 365

aromatase inhibitors, cardiotoxicity of, 215

arrhythmias. *See* dysrhythmias

arterial blood gases (ABGs), 15
in respiratory failure, 272
hypoxic, 270
after thoracic surgery, 32–34, 33*t*, 34*t*

arterial oxygen saturation (SaO₂), 15
after thoracic surgery, 32

ascites with gynecologic cancer, 146

Aspergillus, sepsis due to, 288*t*

aspiration with gastrointestinal cancer, 155

assist-control ventilation (ACV), 278
after thoracic surgery, 31

assisted suicide, 450–451

astrocytoma, 7

atracurium, 384

atropine sulfate for excessive secretion management, 425*t*

atypical antipsychotics, 314

autonomy, 448–451

azotemia, prerenal, 173

B

bacteremia, 284*t*, 286–287

bacteriuria in older adults, 437

balanced salt solutions for fluid resuscitation, 377

base excess after thoracic surgery, 32

basophil(s), 292*f*, 293

B cells (B lymphocytes), 292*f*, 293

BCR-ABL, 50*t*, 51*t*

BCR-ABL tyrosine kinase inhibitors, 55*t*

Beck triad, 218

Beers Criteria for Potentially Inappropriate Medication Use in Older Adults (Beers List), 439

Behavioral Pain Scale (BPS) in palliative care, 418

benzodiazepines, 382

benzylisoquiniliniums, 384

beta-2 agonists for hyperkalemia, 254*t*

bevacizumab (Avastin)
cardiotoxicity of, 214
for lung cancer, 27
nephrotoxicity of, 175*t*
side effects of, 136*t*

bicarbonate (HCO₃) after thoracic surgery, 32, 33

bilevel positive airway pressure (BiPAP) after thoracic surgery, 32

biliary drains, 109, 111

biliary obstruction, 110

bilirubin, 42*t*

bilobectomy for lung cancer, 28

bioavailability, 373–374

biofilm, 393–394, 396

biologic therapy agents
cardiotoxicity of, 207*t*–208*t*, 213–214
side effects of, 136*t*–137*t*

BiPAP (bilevel positive airway pressure) after thoracic surgery, 32

biphasic positive airway pressure for acute respiratory failure, 273–274

bisphosphonates, nephrotoxicity of, 175*t*, 436*t*

bleeding, with hematologic disorders, 69–75

bleeding time, 45*t*

bleomycin (Blenoxane), side effects of, 133*t*

blood–brain barrier (BBB), 9–10

blood glucose level in sepsis, 296–297

blood-oxygen-level dependent (BOLD) MRI, 12*t*

blood pressure in pericardial disease, 219*t*

blood sampling from central venous catheters, 398, 399*t*

bloodstream infections, catheter-related, 392, 393–394, 402*t*

blood urea nitrogen (BUN), 296

B lymphocytes (B cells), 292*f*, 293

body image changes with gynecologic surgery, 131*t*

bone sarcomas, 163–168
chemotherapy side effects
with, 165–167
nursing implications of,
168
overview of, 163
pathophysiology of, 163–
164
radiation side effects with,
167
treatment of, 164–165
Borg Scale, 420
bowel obstruction with
gynecologic cancer, 143
bowel perforation with
gynecologic cancer, 143
brachytherapy for lung cancer, 25
Braden Scale for Predict-
ing Pressure Sore Risk,
354, 355f
brain function, monitor-
ing of. See brain mon-
itoring
brain injury
diagnosis of, 2, 4f
multimodal monitoring
for, 1, 14–18
symptom monitoring for,
1–4, 3f, 4f
therapy and treatment for,
19–20
treatment of, 3–5
brain metastases, 8–9
brain monitoring, 10–11
arterial blood gas for, 15
cerebral blood flow for,
18
cerebral cellular metabo-
lism and, 14–15
cerebral perfusion pressure
for, 17–18
continuous electroenceph-
alography for, 18
end-tidal carbon dioxide
for, 15–16
of intracranial pressure, 2,
3f, 17, 18
multimodal, 1, 14–18
near-infrared spectroscopy
for, 16–17

partial pressure of brain
tissue oxygen for, 16
pulse oximetry for, 15
symptoms in, 1–4, 3f, 4f
venous oxygen saturation
for, 16
brain natriuretic peptide
(BNP), serum levels of,
199t, 231–232
Brain Roadmap for delir-
ium, 314–316
brain tissue oxygen, partial
pressure of, 16
brain tumors
diagnosis of, 10–14, 12t
computed tomography
scan for, 11
electroencephalogram
for, 13–14
magnetic resonance
imaging for, 11–13,
12t
neurologic examination
in, 11
nursing history in,
10–11
positron-emission
tomography for, 13
gliomas as, 7–8
localization of, 2, 3f
meningiomas as, 6–7
metastatic, 8–9
pituitary adenomas as,
5–6, 6t
primary, 4–8
malignant, 7–8
nonmalignant, 5–7, 6t
symptoms of, 11
breast cancer metastatic to
brain, 8
bronchiolitis obliterans
organizing pneumo-
nia, 79t
bronchoplasty for lung cancer, 28
bronchoscopy for lung cancer, 25t
bronchospasm, 82t
burnout in high-intensity
environments, 458–459,
459t

C

calcineurin inhibitors,
nephrotoxicity of, 436t,
176t
calcitonin for hypercalcemia, 247t
calcium chloride for hyperkalemia, 254t
calcium gluconate for
hyperkalemia, 254t
CAM-ICU (Confusion
Assessment Method for
the Intensive Care Unit),
311, 312, 313f
camptothecins, side effects
of, 135t
Candida, sepsis due to, 287,
288t
capecitabine, cardiotoxicity
of, 213
capillary leak syndrome
(CLS), 173, 213–214
capnography for respiratory
failure, 272
carbapenems for sepsis, 301t
carbohydrate intake and
wound healing, 365
carbon dioxide (CO_2)
end-tidal, 15–16
partial pressure of. See partial pressure of carbon
dioxide ($PaCO_2$)
carbon dioxide (CO_2) monitoring, end tidal, for
respiratory failure, 272
carboplatin (Paraplatin),
side effects of, 133t
carcinomatosis, com-
plete cytoreduction with
heated intraperitoneal
chemotherapy for, 156–
161
cardiac arrhythmias. See
dysrhythmias
cardiac catheterization, 199t
cardiac complications. See
cardiovascular compli-
cations
cardiac computed tomogra-
phy, 200t

cardiac diagnostic tests, 197–198, 199t–201t
cardiac enzyme, 199t
cardiac injury, cancer-related, 197–217
cardiac magnetic resonance imaging, 198, 200t
cardiac metastases, 198
cardiac rhythm in pericardial disease, 219t
cardiac structures, cancer involvement of, 198–202
cardiac tamponade, 217–222, 260–261
    assessment of, 218–219, 219t–221t
    diagnosis of, 260
    malignant, 173
    nursing implications of, 260–261
    pathogenesis of, 217, 260
    risk factors for, 217–218
    signs and symptoms of, 260
    transitions in care for, 410
    treatment of, 221–222, 260
cardiac troponins, serum, 198, 199t
cardiogenic shock, 283
cardiomyopathy, 197, 229–233
    anthracycline-induced, 229–230
    with bone and soft tissue sarcomas, 167
    assessment of, 230–232, 231t
    cirrhotic, 106–107
    classification of, 229
    defined, 229
    dilated, 229
    ischemic, 229
    management of, 232–233, 233f
    nonischemic, 229
    pathogenesis of, 229
    restrictive (hypertrophic), 229
    risk factors for, 229–230
cardiorenal syndrome, 173

cardiotoxicity
    antineoplastic medication-induced, 204–213, 205t–211t
        of alkylating agents, 204–212
        of anthracyclines, 167, 204, 212–213, 229–230
        of antimetabolites, 213
        of taxanes, 213
        of hormonal agents, 207t, 215
        of immunotherapy agents, 207t–208t, 213–214
        of monoclonal antibodies, 207t–208t, 214
        radiation-induced, 215–217
        risk of, 196, 196t
        of targeted therapy, 209t–210t, 214–215
cardiovascular changes in older adults, 434
cardiovascular complications, 197–217
    epidemiology of, 195–196
    of gynecologic cancer, 142
    of hepatocellular carcinoma, 106–107
    risk of, 196, 196t
    after thoracic surgery, 30
cardiovascular critical care, 195–240
    for cardiovascular disorders, 217–240
    for complications, 197–217
    overview of, 195–197
cardiovascular disorders, 217–240
    and antineoplastic therapy, 198
    cardiomyopathy/heart failure as, 197, 229–233, 231t, 233t
    dysrhythmias as, 197, 222–229, 224t–228t
    hypertension as, 235–240, 238t–239t
    hypotension as, 233–235

pericardial disease as, 197, 217–222, 219t–221t
    preexisting, 203
cardiovascular effects of intra-abdominal hypertension, 160
cardiovascular emergencies, 260–261
cardiovascular support for sepsis, 299
cardiovascular system, non-specific demands on, 202–203
cast nephropathy, 172, 182
catheter(s), central venous. See central venous catheters (CVCs)
catheter damage with vascular access, 401t
catheter migration with vascular access, 401t
catheter-related bloodstream infections (CRBSIs), 392, 393–394, 402t
cation-exchange resins for hyperkalemia, 255t
ceiling lift for immobility, 338
central diabetes insipidus, 184
central line–associated bloodstream infection (CLABSI) with parenteral nutrition, 331
central venous catheters (CVCs), 389–403
    blood sampling from, 398, 399t
    care and maintenance of, 393
    characteristics of, 390
    coatings for, 390
    dressings for, 394–395
    extraluminal catheter tract with, 393–394
    indications for, 389
    intraluminal fluid pathway in, 395–398, 397t, 399t
    overview of, 389–390

peripherally inserted, 392–393
principles of flow and, 390–391
problems and interventions for, 398, 400t–403t
skin integrity with, 394
types of, 391–393
central venous pressure in pericardial disease, 219t
cephalosporins
nephrotoxicity of, 177t
for sepsis, 301t
cerebral blood flow, 18
cerebral cellular metabolism, 14–15
cerebral perfusion pressure (CPP), 17–18
cerebrospinal fluid (CSF)
drainage of, 3f
occlusion of flow of, 2
cervical cancer. See also gynecologic (GYN) cancers
treatment options for, 127t
cetuximab, cardiotoxicity of, 214
chair egress position for immobility, 338
chair position for immobility, 338
chemotherapy
and blood–brain barrier, 9–10
for bone and soft tissue sarcomas, 164
side effects of, 165–167
cardiotoxicity due to, 204–213, 205t–211t
for gynecologic cancer, 127t–129t, 129, 133t–137t, 138t
heated intraperitoneal, 156–161
gastrointestinal bleeding after, 156–159
intra-abdominal hypertension after, 159–161

small bowel perforation after, 159
intraperitoneal, 129, 138t
for lung cancer, 25–27
nephrotoxicity of, 436t
neurotoxic side effects of, 20
side effects of
with cholangiocarcinoma, 111
with gynecologic cancer, 129, 133t–137t, 138t
with hepatocellular carcinoma, 108–109
chemotherapy-related infections with gynecologic cancer, 141–142
chest discomfort in pericardial disease, 219t
chest x-ray
for cardiac injury, 198
for lung cancer, 25t
for pericardial disease, 221t
chlorhexidine (CHG) with central venous catheters, 390, 395
cholangiocarcinoma, 109–111
cholangiopancreatography, endoscopic retrograde, 105
cholangitis, 110–111
cholecystitis, acalculous, 58t
chronic lymphocytic leukemia (CLL)
demographics of, 52t
treatment of, 55t
chronic myeloid leukemia (CML)
cytogenetics of, 50t
demographics of, 52t
prognosis for, 51t
treatment of, 55t
ciprofloxacin, nephrotoxicity of, 436t
cirrhotic cardiomyopathy, 106–107
cisatracurium, 384
cisplatin (Platinol)
cardiotoxicity of, 204–212, 230

nephrotoxicity of, 176t, 436t
side effects of, 133t
clearance, 375
clotting tests, 46t–48t
coagulation
disseminated intravascular, 58t, 94
in sepsis, 289, 297
coagulopathy due to hepatocellular carcinoma, 108
cobalamin level, 40t
codeine, 381
Code of Ethics, 447–448
coenzyme Q10 for cardiomyopathy/heart failure, 232
cognitive impairment, radiation-induced, 19
colloids, 377, 378t
colony-stimulating factors (CSFs) for sepsis, 298
colorectal cancer, 153–161
adjuvant chemotherapy for, 153
complications of, 154–156
anastomotic leaks and sepsis as, 154–155
respiratory, 155–156
epidemiology of, 153
heated intraperitoneal chemotherapy for, 156–161
gastrointestinal bleeding after, 156–159
intra-abdominal hypertension after, 159–161
small bowel perforation after, 159
metastatic to brain, 8
overview of, 153–154
stereotactic body radiation therapy for, 153–154
surgery for, 153
Common Terminology Criteria for Adverse Events for gynecologic cancers, 117, 118t–124t
compassion fatigue, 458–459, 459t

complete metabolic panel (CMP), 296
computed tomography (CT)
  for brain injury, 2, 4*f*
  for brain tumor, 11
  cardiac, 200*t*
  for lung cancer, 25*t*
  for respiratory failure, 272
Confusion Assessment Method for the Intensive Care Unit (CAM-ICU), 311, 312, 313*f*
conivaptan for hyponatremia, 251*t*
constipation with gynecologic cancer, 119*t*, 145
continuous lateral rotation
  for immobility, 338
  for pressure injuries, 356
continuous mandatory ventilation after thoracic surgery, 31
continuous positive airway pressure (CPAP)
  for acute respiratory failure, 273
  after thoracic surgery, 32
  transition in care to, 411
continuous renal replacement therapy (CRRT), 182, 187, 188
contrast dye, nephrotoxicity of, 176*t*
contrast-induced nephropathy (CIN), 172
Coombs test, 42*t*
coronary artery ischemia or occlusion, 197, 202
corticotroph adenoma, 6, 6*t*
cough
  due to gynecologic cancer, 119*t*
  due to pericardial disease, 219*t*
CPAP. *See* continuous positive airway pressure (CPAP)
creatine phosphokinase, 199*t*
creatinine, 296

crescentic glomerulonephritis, 179
Critical-Care Pain Observation Tool in palliative care, 418
cryptogenic organizing pneumonia, 79*t*
crystalline amino acids (CAAs) in parenteral nutrition, 330
crystalloids, 377, 378*t*
CT. *See* computed tomography (CT)
Cushing syndrome, 6
CVCs. *See* central venous catheters (CVCs)
cyclophosphamide
  cardiotoxicity of, 212, 230
  nephrotoxicity of, 177*t*
  side effects of, 133*t*
cyclosporine, nephrotoxicity of, 176*t*
cystitis
  hemorrhagic, 60*t*
  due to chemotherapy for bone and soft tissue sarcomas, 167
  radiation-induced, 139*t*
cytokine(s) in sepsis, 289
cytokine release syndrome, 59*t*, 94–95

D

dabigatran etexilate, 385
dactinomycin (Cosmegen), side effects of, 133*t*
dalteparin, 384
dasatinib, nephrotoxicity of, 177*t*
daunorubicin, cardiotoxicity of, 229–230
D-dimer, 46*t*
dead space ventilation, 270
death and dying, 423–425, 425*t*. *See also* palliative care
decision making
  capacity for, 448–450
  changes over time in, 454–455

deep tissue injury, 350*f*, 351
dehydration with gynecologic cancer, 119*t*, 145
delayed wound closure, 346–347
delirium
  intensive care unit, 309–319
  analgesia and sedation for, 317–318
  assessment, prevention, and management of, 318
  clinical practice guidelines for, 311
  early mobility for, 318
  etiology of, 309–310
  family engagement and empowerment for, 319
  hyperactive, 310–311
  hypoactive, 311
  interprofessional care approach (ABCDEF bundle) for, 316–319, 317*f*
  management recommendations for, 312–314, 315*f*
  mixed, 311
  monitoring for, 311–312, 313*f*
  outcomes associated with, 311
  overview of, 309
  pain with, 316–317
  prevalence, 310
  risk factors for, 310, 310*f*
  script for interprofessional communication on, 314–316
  spontaneous awakening and breathing trials for, 317
  subtypes of, 309–311
  in older adults, 434
demeclocycline for hyponatremia, 250*t*
dementia in older adults, 434

dendritic cells, 292*f*, 293
denileukin diftitox, cardio-
    toxicity of, 213–214
denosumab for hypercalce-
    mia, 247*t*
depolarizing agents, 383
depression in older adults,
    434
dermal papillae, 344
dermatitis
    incontinence-associated,
        358–359, 358*f*
    intertriginous, 359–360
    radiation, with gyneco-
        logic cancer, 119*t*,
        139*t*
dermis, 344
device-related pressure inju-
    ries, 351, 352*f*
dexmedetomidine, 383
    pharmacodynamics of,
        376, 377
dexrazoxane for cardiomy-
    opathy/heart failure, 232
dextran for fluid resuscita-
    tion, 377
diabetes insipidus (DI), 184
diabetes mellitus, enteral
    formulas for, 328
dialysis
    catheters for, 392
    for hyperkalemia, 255*t*
    peritoneal, 187
    sustained low-efficiency,
        187, 188
diarrhea
    with enteral nutrition,
        329–330
    with gynecologic cancer,
        120*t*, 145
    radiation-induced, 140*t*
diastolic blood pressure
    (DBP), 234–235
diazepam, 382
diuretics for hyperkalemia,
    255*t*
dobutamine, 379–380
docetaxel
    cardiotoxicity of, 213
    for lung cancer, 26
    side effects of, 135*t*

dopamine, 379, 380*t*
doxorubicin
    cardiotoxicity of, 212,
        229–230
    side effects of, 134*t*
dressing(s)
    for central venous cathe-
        ters, 394–395
    for prevention of pressure
        injuries, 357
    selection of, 363,
        364*t*–365*t*, 366*f*
drug-dosing regimens, 376–
    377
dry mouth with gynecologic
    cancer, 120*t*
dyspnea
    with gynecologic cancer,
        120*t*
    with intraperitoneal che-
        motherapy, 138*t*
    palliative care for, 419–
        420
    in pericardial disease, 219*t*
Dyspnea-12 scale, 420
dysrhythmias, 197, 222–
    229
    assessment of, 223–225
    defined, 222
    management of, 225–229,
        226*t*–228*t*
    pathogenesis of, 222
    risk factors for, 223,
        224*t*–225*t*
    after thoracic surgery, 30
    unstable, 223

E

early mobility, 337–341
    for delirium, 318
    mobility teams for, 339–
        340
    progressive mobility for,
        338
    barriers and solutions
        to, 339
echocardiogram, 197,
    200*t*–201*t*
    in pericardial disease, 221*t*
edoxaban, 385

effect time course, 376–377
elderly. *See* older adults
electrocardiogram (ECG),
    197, 198, 200*t*
    in pericardial disease, 221*t*
electroencephalography
    (EEG)
    of brain tumor, 13–14
    continuous, 18
electrolyte(s), in parenteral
    nutrition, 330
electrolyte derangements,
    182–187
    hypercalcemia as, 185–187
    hyperkalemia as, 184–185
    hypernatremia as, 184
    hypocalcemia as, 187
    hypokalemia as, 185
    hypomagnesemia as, 185
    hyponatremia as, 183–184
    hypophosphatemia as, 185
    with intraperitoneal che-
        motherapy, 138*t*
    metabolic acidosis as,
        182–183
    with parenteral nutrition,
        332
elemental formulas for
    enteral nutrition, 327
embolism with vascular
    access, 402*t*
emergencies. *See* oncologic
    emergencies
emesis control in palliative
    care, 420–421
EN. *See* enteral nutrition
    (EN)
encephalopathy
    hepatic, 106
    ifosfamide-related, 166
encephalopathy syndrome,
    posterior reversible, 64*t*
end-of-life care, 423–425,
    425*t*. *See also* pallia-
    tive care
end-of-life ulcers, 351–352
endometrial cancer. *See also*
    gynecologic (GYN) can-
    cers
    treatment options for,
        128*t*

endoscopic retrograde cholangiopancreatography
(ERCP), 105
endothelial toxins, 289
endotracheal intubation
(ETT), 274–278
confirmation of, 277–278
contraindications to, 274
equipment and prepara-
tion for, 275–276
indications for, 274
medications for, 276
procedure for, 276–277
end-tidal carbon dioxide
(ETCO₂), 15–16, 272
engraftment syndrome, 59t,
94–95
enoxaparin, 384
enteral nutrition (EN), 326
with acute pancreatitis, 113
complications of, 328–330
formulas for, 327–328
indications for, 326
timing and route of, 326–
327
Enterobacter species, sepsis
due to, 288t
Enterococcus, sepsis due to,
288t
enterocolitis, neutrope-
nic, 68t
eosinophil(s), 292f, 293
epidermis, 344
epidural analgesia after thoracic surgery, 29
epinephrine, 378–379, 380t
half-life of, 375
epirubicin, cardiotoxicity of,
229–230
erythroblast, 292f
erythrocytes, 292f, 293
erythrocyte sedimentation
rate (ESR), 42t
Escherichia coli, sepsis due
to, 286, 287, 288t
esmolol for dysrhythmias,
227t
esophageal varices due to
complete cytoreduction
with heated intraperito-
neal chemotherapy, 158

esophagitis due to gynecologic cancer, 120t
ethanol clearance, 375
ethical climate, 447
ethical complexities, 451–
453, 452t
ethical conflicts, 453
and concerns about
patient safety and care
quality, 444
defined, 453
in high-intensity environments, 444, 458–459,
459t, 460t
and moral distress, 444,
445–447, 445t, 446t
over assisted suicide or
euthanasia, 450–451
on prognosis under con-
ditions of uncertainty,
455
sources of, 453
due to structural prob-
lems, 444
with surrogate decision
makers, 449–450
ethical controversies in clinical practice, 453–456
ethical decision making
complexity of, 452
models of, 447
ethical dialogue, 457–458
ethical responsibilities with
transitions in care, 409–
410
ethics, 443–461
ANA Code of, 447–448
autonomy in, 448–451
case study on, 443, 448,
451, 453–454, 455–
456
complexities in, 451–453,
452t
concepts in clinical practice of, 445–447, 445t,
446f
controversies over, 453–
456
in high-intensity environments, 444, 458–459,
459t, 460t

moral dilemmas and dis-
tress in, 444, 445–447,
445t, 446f
overview of, 443–444
and patient safety, 444
and quality of care, 444
structural problems and,
444
in transitions in care,
409–410
of nonbeneficial treat-
ment/futility, 456–458
value conflicts in, 444
ethics committees, 457
ethics consultants, 457
etoposide (VP-16, Toposar),
side effects of, 136t
euthanasia, 450–451
Ewing sarcoma, 164
exercise stress test, 198
exotoxins, 289
external beam therapy for
lung cancer, 25
external ventricular drain
(EVD), 2, 3f, 17
extrahepatic cholangiocarcinoma (ECC), 109
extraluminal catheter tract,
393–394
extubation from mechani-
cal ventilation, 279–280,
280t
exudate with vascular
access, 401t

F

failure to thrive in older
adults, 440
family empowerment for
delirium, 319
family meeting in palliative
care, 422–423
fatigue due to gynecologic
cancer, 121t
fat intake and wound healing, 365
febrile neutropenia, 258–
260
antimicrobial recommen-
dations for, 303f

due to gynecologic cancer, 121t
fentanyl, 381
in palliative care, 418–419
ferritin level, 40t
fever
due to gynecologic cancer, 121t
neutropenic, 258–260
antimicrobial recommendations for, 303f
due to gynecologic cancer, 121t
fiber dressing, 364t
fibrin degradation products (FDPs), 47t
fibrinogen level, 47t
fibrinolysis in sepsis, 289
FICA tool in palliative care, 423
filgrastim (Neupogen) for sepsis, 298
fine needle aspiration for lung cancer, 25t
first-order clearance, 375
first-pass effect, 374
reduced in hepatocellular carcinoma, 109
fistulas with gynecologic surgery, 130t
5-fluorouracil
cardiotoxicity of, 213, 230
flow rate, 390–391
fludrocortisone
for hyperkalemia, 255t
for hyponatremia, 250t
fluid-attenuated inversion recovery (FLAIR), 12, 12t
fluid intake and wound healing, 367
fluid restriction for hyponatremia, 250t
fluid resuscitation, 377, 378t
fluoroquinolones for sepsis, 301t
side effects of, 134t
flushing, 396–398, 397t
foam dressing, 364t
focal segmental glomerulosclerosis, 179

folate (folic acid) level, 40t
fondaparinux, 384
foscarnet, nephrotoxicity of, 436t
frailty in older adults, 439–440
full thickness skin loss, 348
fulvestrant, cardiotoxicity of, 215
Functional Classification of Heart Failure, 230–231
Functional Living Index–Emesis, 421
functional residual capacity (FRC), 271
functional MRI (fMRI), 12t
fungal infection, sepsis due to, 286, 287, 288t
antimicrobial recommendations for, 303f
furosemide
for hypercalcemia, 247t
pharmacodynamics of, 376
futile treatment, ethical concerns about, 456–458

G

gamma-aminobutyric acid (GABA) agonists, 382–383
gastric residual volumes (GRV) with enteral nutrition, 329
gastrointestinal (GI) bleeding
due to complete cytoreduction with heated intraperitoneal chemotherapy, 156–159
due to hepatocellular carcinoma, 107
gastrointestinal (GI) cancers, 153–161
complications of, 154–156
anastomotic leaks and sepsis as, 154–155
after complete cytoreduction with heated intraperitoneal chemotherapy, 156–161

respiratory, 155–156
heated intraperitoneal chemotherapy for, 156–161
gastrointestinal bleeding after, 156–159
intra-abdominal hypertension after, 159–161
small bowel perforation after, 159
metastatic to brain, 8
overview of, 153–154
gauge size, 390
G-CSF (granulocyte–colony-stimulating factor) for sepsis, 298
gemcitabine
for lung cancer, 26
nephrotoxicity of, 175t
side effects of, 135t
gentamicin, nephrotoxicity of, 176t
geriatric patients. See older adults
geriatric syndromes, 437
germ cell tumors. See also gynecologic (GYN) cancers
treatment options for, 128t–129t
gestational trophoblastic disease, 117. See also gynecologic (GYN) cancers
treatment options for, 128t–129t
glioblastoma multiforme (GBM), 7–8
gliomas, 7–8
glomerular disease, 179
glomerular filtration rate in older adults, 435
glomerulonephritis, crescentic, 179
glomerulosclerosis, focal segmental, 179
glutamine
in parenteral nutrition, 330–331
and wound healing, 365

glycopeptides for sepsis, 301*t*
glycopyrrolate for excessive secretion management, 425*t*
gonadotroph adenoma, 6*t*
granulation tissue, 346
granulocyte(s), 293
granulocyte–colony-stimulating factor (G-CSF) for sepsis, 298
granulocyte macrophage–colony-stimulating factor (GM-CSF) for sepsis, 298
gynecologic (GYN) cancers, 117–149
Common Terminology Criteria for Adverse Events for, 117, 118*t*–124*t*
complications of, 132–148
allergic and hypersensitivity reactions as, 118*t*, 147–148
anaphylaxis as, 118*t*
anorexia as, 118*t*
ascites as, 146
bowel obstruction/perforation as, 143
constipation as, 119*t*
cough as, 119*t*
dehydration as, 119*t*
diarrhea as, 120*t*
dry mouth as, 120*t*
dyspnea as, 120*t*
esophagitis as, 120*t*
fatigue as, 121*t*
febrile neutropenia as, 121*t*
fever as, 121*t*
gastrointestinal toxicity as, 145–146
headache as, 121*t*
hemorrhage as, 143
hepatotoxicity and renal toxicity as, 121*t*, 146–147
infection, 124*t*, 132–142
infusion-related reaction as, 122*t*
malnutrition as, 144–145
multiorgan failure as, 122*t*
nausea as, 122*t*
neurotoxicity as, 147
oral mucositis as, 122*t*
pain as, 123*t*, 147
proctitis as, 123*t*
pruritus as, 123*t*
pulmonary toxicity as, 144
radiation dermatitis as, 119*t*
seizure as, 123*t*
sepsis as, 123*t*
stroke and cardiac, 142
urinary frequency as, 124*t*
vaginal discharge as, 124*t*
vomiting as, 124*t*
epidemiology of, 125, 125*t*
factors associated with, 117–125
location of, 125, 126*f*
overview of, 117–126
resources for, 149, 149*t*
treatment modalities for, 125, 126–132, 127*t*–129*t*
chemotherapy as, 127*t*–129*t*, 129, 133*t*–137*t*, 138*t*
radiation therapy as, 127*t*–129*t*, 130–132, 139*t*–141*t*
surgery as, 127*t*–129*t*, 129, 130*t*–132*t*

H

half-life, 375
haptoglobin level, 42*t*
HCC. *See* hepatocellular carcinoma (HCC)
headache
due to brain tumor, 11
due to gynecologic cancer, 121*t*
healing of wound, 346–347
Healthcare and Technology Synergy Framework, 399
heart failure, 229–233
assessment of, 230–232, 231*t*
defined, 229
management of, 232–233, 233*f*
pathogenesis of, 229
risk factors for, 229–230
heart sounds in pericardial disease, 219*t*
heated intraperitoneal chemotherapy (HIPEC), 156–161
gastrointestinal bleeding after, 156–159
intra-abdominal hypertension after, 159–161
small bowel perforation after, 159
hematemesis due to complete cytoreduction with heated intraperitoneal chemotherapy, 156–158
hematocrit, 39*t*
hematologic disorders, 37–97
epidemiology of, 37
malignant
diagnostic tests for, 37–38, 39*t*–48*t*
nonmalignant hematologic disorders associated with, 69
nonrespiratory oncologic emergencies with, 57, 58*t*–68*t*
overview of, 49*t*–56*t*, 57
nonmalignant, 57–77
bleeding due to, 69–75
disseminated intravascular coagulation as, 58*t*, 94
engraftment syndrome as, 59*t*, 94–95
infection due to, 76–77
key features of, 69, 70*t*–74*t*
leukostasis as, 62*t*, 95–97

malignancies associated
with, 69
overview of, 57–69
thrombosis due to,
75–76
related to cancer treat-
ment, 90–94
medication-induced
toxicity as, 90–93,
91t–93t
radiation-induced, 94
respiratory complications
of, 77–78, 79t–89t
therapy for, 38–57
hematologic emergencies,
264–265, 265f
hematologic toxicity, 90–94
medication-induced,
90–93, 91t–93t
radiation-induced, 94
hematoma with vascular
access, 401t
hematopoiesis, 291–294,
292f, 294f, 294t
hematopoietic stem cell(s),
291
hematopoietic stem cell
transplantation (HSCT),
thrombotic microangiop-
athy due to, 174–177
hemodialysis, intermittent,
187, 188
hemodynamic resuscita-
tion with acute pancre-
atitis, 112
hemoglobin, 39t
mean corpuscular, 39t
hemoglobin concentration,
mean corpuscular, 39t
hemoglobin electrophore-
sis, 43t
hemoglobin stability, 47t
hemolytic anemia, 69, 70t
medication-induced, 91t
hemolytic uremic syndrome
(HUS), variant or atypi-
cal, 59t, 69
hemophagocytic lympho-
histiocytosis (HLH),
71t, 174
hemophilia, 71t

hemorrhage
diffuse alveolar, 81t
with gynecologic can-
cer, 143
intracerebral, 2, 4f
after thoracic surgery,
29–30
hemorrhagic cystitis, 60t
due to chemotherapy for
bone and soft tissue
sarcomas, 167
heparin, 384
hepatic encephalopathy,
106
hepatic veno-occlusive disease, 65t
hepatocellular carcinoma
(HCC), 105–109
cardiovascular complica-
tions of, 106–107
chemotherapy side effects
with, 108–109
coagulopathy due to, 108
gastrointestinal complications of, 107
hepatorenal syndrome due
to, 107
hyperlactatemia due to,
108
hypoglycemia due to, 108
infection due to, 108
liver failure due to, 106
neurologic complications
of, 106
nursing implications of,
109
pulmonary complications
of, 107
radiation side effects with,
109
risk factors for, 105–106
treatment for, 106
hepatojugular reflex in pericardial disease, 220t
hepatopulmonary syn-
drome, 107
hepatorenal syndrome, 107,
173
hepatotoxicity with gynecologic cancer, 121t, 146–
147

hetastarches for fluid resuscitation, 377
high-intensity environments
ethics in, 444
resilience in, 458–459,
459t, 460t
HIPEC. See heated intra-
peritoneal chemotherapy
(HIPEC)
histamine-2 antagonists,
385
Hodgkin lymphoma, 49t–
56t
additional clinical evaluation for, 53t
classification of, 49t
complications of, 56t
cytogenetics of, 50t
demographics of, 52t
description of, 49t
diagnosis of, 53t
key signs and symptoms
of, 54t
prognosis for, 51t
treatment of, 54t–55t
hormonal agents
cardiotoxicity of, 207t,
215
side effects of, 136t
host immunity, 9
hydrocodone, 381
hydrocolloid dressing, 364t
hydrogel dressing, 364t
hydromorphone, 381
in palliative care, 418–419
hyperammonemia syn-
drome, idiopathic, 61t
hypercalcemia, 185–187,
245–247
defined, 246
diagnosis of, 186, 246
epidemiology of, 185–
186, 245
with hematologic malig-
nancies and disor-
ders, 61t
nursing implications of,
247
pathophysiology of, 186,
245–246
severity of, 185

signs and symptoms of,
185, 186, 246, 246t
treatment of, 186–187,
246–247, 247t
hypercapnia in hypercarbic
respiratory failure, 270
hypercarbic respiratory failure, 270–271
hyperglycemia with paren-
teral nutrition, 331–332
hyperkalemia, 184–185,
253, 254t–255t
pseudo-, 253
hyperlactatemia due to hepatocellular carcinoma, 108
hypernatremia, 184
hyperphosphatemia, 258
hypersensitivity pulmonary
edema, 82t
hypersensitivity reactions
with gynecologic cancer,
118t, 147–148
hypertension, 235–240
assessment of, 237–238
epidemiology of, 235–236
intra-abdominal
with gastrointestinal
cancer, 159–161
with pancreatic can-
cer, 113
management of, 238–241,
239t–240t
pathogenesis of, 236
resistant (malignant),
237–240
risk factors for, 236
stage 1 vs. stage 2, 236
hypertonic saline for hyperkalemia, 254t
hypertonic solutions for
fluid resuscitation, 377
hyperuricemia, 258
hyperviscosity syndrome
(HVS), 264–265, 265t
hypocalcemia, 187
hypodermis, 344
hypoglycemia, 252
due to hepatocellular carcinoma, 108
hypokalemia, 185, 256–
257, 256t

hypomagnesemia, 185
hyponatremia, 183–184,
247–251
classification of, 249, 249t
defined, 247
diagnosis of, 249, 249t
diagnostic criteria for, 248
epidemiology of, 183, 247
euvolemic, 249, 249t,
250t–251t
grading of, 248
hypervolemic, 249, 249t,
250t–251t
hypovolemic, 249, 249t,
250t
nursing implications of,
249–251
pathophysiology of, 183,
247–248
severe, 251t
signs and symptoms of, 248
treatment of, 183–184,
249, 250t–251t
hypophosphatemia, 185
hypotension, 233–235
assessment of, 234–235
defined, 233–234
management of, 235
orthostatic, 234, 235
pathogenesis of, 233–234
risk factors for, 234
hypotonic solutions for
fluid resuscitation, 377
hypoventilation, 270
hypovolemic shock, 283
hypoxic respiratory failure,
269–270
hypercarbic, 270

I

idarubicin, cardiotoxicity of,
229–230
idiopathic hyperammone-
mia syndrome, 61t
ifosfamide (Ifex)
cardiotoxicity of, 212
encephalopathy related
to, 166
nephrotoxicity of, 176t,
177t, 436t

side effects of, 133t
imatinib, nephrotoxicity
of, 177t
immobility
complications of, 338
mobility teams for, 339–
340
progressive mobility for,
338
barriers and solutions
to, 339
immune-enhancing for-
mulas (IEFs) for enteral
nutrition, 328
immune thrombocytopenic
purpura (ITP), 69
immunologic disorders,
37–97
epidemiology of, 37
malignant
diagnostic tests for,
37–38, 39t–48t
nonmalignant hemato-
logic disorders asso-
ciated with, 69
nonrespiratory onco-
logic emergencies
with, 57, 58t–68t
overview of, 57
nonmalignant, 57–77
bleeding due to, 69–75
disseminated intravas-
cular coagulation as,
58t, 94
engraftment syndrome
as, 59t, 94–95
infection due to, 76–77
key features of, 69,
70t–74t
leukostasis as, 62t, 95–97
malignancies associated
with, 69
overview of, 57–69
thrombosis due to,
75–76
related to cancer treat-
ment, 90–94
medication-induced
toxicity as, 90–93,
91t–93t
radiation-induced, 94

respiratory complications
 of, 77–78, 79*t*–89*t*
therapy for, 38–57
immunologic toxicity,
 90–94
medication-induced,
 90–93, 91*t*–93*t*
radiation-induced, 94
immunosuppressive med-
 ications, hematologic/
 immunologic toxicity
 due to, 90–93, 91*t*–93*t*
immunotherapy agents
cardiotoxicity of,
 207*t*–208*t*, 213–214
for lung cancer, 27
incontinence-associated dermatitis (IAD), 358–359,
 358*f*
infection
catheter-related blood-
 stream, 392, 393–394,
 402*t*
due to gynecologic cancer,
 124*t*, 132–142
due to hepatocellular carcinoma, 108
with immunologic disor-
 ders, 76–77
with intraperitoneal che-
 motherapy, 138*t*
infectious emergencies,
 258–260
inflammation in sepsis,
 288–289
influenza in older adults, 435
infusion-related reaction
 due to gynecologic can-
 cer, 122*t*
inotropes, 379–380
insulin for hyperkalemia,
 254*t*
insulin-like growth factors
 (IGFs), 252
integrins, 9
Intensive Care Delirium
 Screening Checklist
 (ICDSC), 311, 312
intensive care unit (ICU)-
 acquired weakness (ICU-
 AW), 337

and complications of
 immobility, 338
mobility teams for, 339–
 340
progressive mobility for,
 338
barriers and solutions
 to, 339
intensive care unit (ICU)
 delirium. *See* delirium,
 intensive care unit
interferon alfa, cardiotoxicity of, 213
intermittent hemodialysis
 (IHD), 187, 188
international normalized
 ratio (INR), 384
interprofessional care
 approach for delirium,
 316–319, 317*f*
interprofessional communication on delirium, script
 for, 314–316
interstitial pneumonitis
 with pulmonary fibrosis,
 83*t*–84*t*
intertriginous dermatitis
 (ITD), 359–360
intra-abdominal hyperten-
 sion (IAH)
with gastrointestinal cancer, 159–161
with pancreatic cancer,
 113
intra-abdominal pressure
 (IAP), 159–161
intracerebral hemorrhage,
 2, 4*f*
intracranial pressure (ICP)
increased, 18, 263–264
monitoring of, 2, 3*f*, 17,
 18
intrahepatic cholangiocarcinoma (ICC), 109
intraluminal fluid pathway,
 395–398, 397*t*, 399*t*
intraperitoneal (IP) chemotherapy, 129, 138*t*
heated, 156–161
gastrointestinal bleeding
 after, 156–159

intra-abdominal hyper-
 tension after, 159–
 161
small bowel perforation
 after, 159
intrapulmonary shunt-
 ing, 270
intravenous fat emulsions
 (IVFE) in parenteral
 nutrition, 330
intubation. *See* endotracheal
 intubation (ETT)
irinotecan (Camptosar),
 side effects of, 135*t*
iron, serum, 41*t*
iron studies, 40*t*–41*t*
isotonic solutions for fluid
 resuscitation, 377

J

jugular venous distension
 (JVD) in pericardial disease, 220*t*
jugular venous pulsations
 (JVP) in pericardial disease, 220*t*

K

Kennedy Terminal Ulcer,
 351–352
kidney function in older
 adults, 435
kidney injury, acute. *See*
 acute kidney injury
 (AKI)
Klebsiella species, sepsis due
 to, 288*t*

L

labetalol for dysrhythmias,
 227*t*
lactate dehydrogenase
 (LDH), 43*t*
lactic acid in sepsis, 297
lactic acidosis, 183
large cell carcinoma of
 lung, 24
leukapheresis, 38–57

leukemia, 49t–56t, 57
additional clinical evaluation for, 53t
classification of, 49t
complications of, 56t
cytogenetics of, 50t
demographics of, 52t
description of, 49t
diagnosis of, 53t
key signs and symptoms
of, 54t
prognosis for, 51t
treatment of, 54t–55t
leukocytes, 293
leukoencephalopathy syn-
drome, posterior revers-
ible, 64t
leukopenia, medication-
induced, 92t
leukostasis, 62t, 95–97
acute kidney injury due
to, 174
with leukemia, 56t
pulmonary, 84t
level of consciousness
(LOC) with delirium,
311–312, 313
life support, withholding
or withdrawal of, 423–
425, 425t
linear clearance, 375
line infection, antimicrobial recommendations
for, 303f
lipopeptides for sepsis, 301t
liposomal doxorubicin
(Doxil), side effects of,
134t
lithium, nephrotoxicity of,
436t
liver failure due to hepatocellular carcinoma, 106
liver function
with intra-abdominal
hypertension, 159
with parenteral nutrition,
332
liver function tests (LFTs),
296
lobectomy for lung can-
cer, 28

loop diuretics, pharmacodynamics of, 376
lorazepam, 382
lower-extremity lymph-
edema with gynecologic
surgery, 131t
low-molecular-weight heparins (LMWHs), 384
lung cancer, 23–34
diagnosis and staging of,
24, 25t
epidemiology of, 23
metastatic to brain, 8, 9
non-small cell, 23, 24
postoperative care for,
28–34
for common complica-
tions, 29–30
pain management tech-
niques in, 29
ventilator management
in, 31–34, 33t, 34t
routine screening for, 24
small cell (oat cell), 23, 24
treatment of, 24–28
chemotherapy for,
25–27
immunotherapy for, 27
radiation therapy for,
24–25
surgery for, 27–28
targeted therapy for, 27
types of, 23–24
lung injury, acute, with
gastrointestinal can-
cer, 155
lung parenchyma–sparing
procedures, 28
lymphedema, lower-extremity,
with gynecologic sur-
gery, 131t
lymphocyte count, abso-
lute, 43t
lymphohistiocytosis, hemophagocytic, 71t, 174
lymphoid progenitor lin-
eage, 292f, 293
lymphoma, 49t–56t, 57
additional clinical evaluation for, 53t
classification of, 49t

complications of, 56t
cytogenetics of, 50t
demographics of, 52t
description of, 49t
diagnosis of, 53t
key signs and symptoms
of, 54t
prognosis for, 51t
treatment of, 54t–55t
lymphopenia, medication-
induced, 92t

M

macrobore tubing, 391
macrophage(s), 292f, 293
magnetic resonance angiography (MRA), 12t
magnetic resonance imag-
ing (MRI)
of brain injury, 2
of brain tumor, 11–13,
12t
cardiac, 198, 200t
functional, 12t
magnetic resonance spec-
troscopy (MRS), 12t, 13
malignant pericardial tamponade, 173
malignant spinal cord compression (MSCC), 262–
263
malnutrition
assessment of, 324
defined, 325, 325f
diagnosis of, 325, 325f
with gynecologic cancer,
144–145
interventions for, 326
enteral nutrition as,
327–330
parenteral nutrition as,
330–332
timing and route of,
326–327
nutrition care pathway for,
324–325
and wound healing, 365
mast cell, 292f
MDS. See myelodysplastic
syndrome (MDS)

mean arterial pressure (MAP), 234–235
and acute skin failure, 353
mean corpuscular hemoglobin, 39*t*
mean corpuscular hemoglobin concentration, 39*t*
mean corpuscular volume, 39*t*
mean platelet volume, 45*t*
mechanical ventilation (MV), 278–280
and delirium, 310
modes of, 278–279, 279*t*
of older adults, 435
terms associated with, 279, 279*t*
transition in care to, 411
weaning from, 279–280, 280*t*
terminal, 423–425, 425*t*
medication-induced hematologic/immunologic toxicity, 90–93, 91*t*–93*t*
megakaryoblast, 292*f*
megakaryocytes, 292*f*, 293
melanoma, metastatic to brain, 8
melena due to complete cytoreduction with heated intraperitoneal chemotherapy, 156–158
membranoproliferative disease, 179
membranous nephropathy, 179
meningiomas, 6–7
mental status in pericardial disease, 220*t*
meperidine, 381
metabolic acidosis, 182–183
after thoracic surgery, 33, 33*t*
metabolic alkalosis after thoracic surgery, 33, 33*t*
metabolic emergencies, 245–258
hypercalcemia as, 245–247, 246*t*, 247*t*
hyperkalemia as, 253, 254*t*–255*t*

hypoglycemia as, 252
hypokalemia as, 256–257, 256*t*
hyponatremia as, 247–251, 249*t*–251*t*
tumor lysis syndrome as, 257–258
metabolic rates and wound healing, 363–365
metabolic response to stress, 323–324
metastases to heart, 198
metastatic brain tumors, 8–9
metastatic cancer and blood–brain barrier, 9–10
methadone, 381
half-life of, 375
methicillin-resistant *S. aureus* (MRSA), sepsis due to, 288*t*, 303*f*
methotrexate
nephrotoxicity of, 436*t*
side effects of, 135*t*
methyl-guanine methyl transferase (*MGMT*) gene, 7–8
metoprolol for dysrhythmias, 228*t*
Michaelis-Menten clearance, 375
microangiopathy, thrombotic, 174–178, 175*t*–176*t*
microbore tubing, 391
micronutrition and wound healing, 366–367
midazolam, 382
volume of distribution of, 374
milrinone, 380
minimal change disease, 179
minute ventilation, 270
mitomycin (Mutamycin)
nephrotoxicity of, 175*t*
side effects of, 134*t*
mitoxantrone, cardiotoxicity of, 229–230
mobility
early. *See* early mobility and pressure injuries, 356

progressive, 338
barriers and solutions to, 339
mobility teams, 339–340
moisture and pressure injuries, 354
moisture-associated skin damage (MASD), 357–360
defined, 357
etiology and pathogenesis of, 357–358
incontinence-associated dermatitis as, 358–359, 358*f*
intertriginous dermatitis as, 359–360
moisture vapor transmission rate (MVTR), 395
monobactams for sepsis, 301*t*
monoblast, 292*f*
monoclonal antibodies
cardiotoxicity of, 207*t*–208*t*, 214
for lung cancer, 27
nephrotoxicity of, 437*t*
side effects of, 136*t*
monoclonal gammopathy of undetermined significance (MGUS), 49*t*, 51*t*, 53*t*, 54*t*
monocytes, 292*f*, 293
moral action
contextual and dynamic model of, 446*f*
theoretical perspective of, 451–452, 452*t*
moral character, 452*t*
moral concepts in clinical practice, 445–447, 445*t*, 446*f*
moral dilemmas, 444, 445–447, 445*t*, 446*f*
moral disagreements, 452–453
moral distress, 444, 445–447, 445*t*, 446*f*
moral integrity, 445*t*
moral judgment, 452*t*
moral motivation, 452*t*
moral residue, 445*t*

moral sensitivity, 452*t*
moral uncertainty, 445*t*
morphine, 381
  in palliative care, 418–419
Morrow Assessment of
  Nausea and Emesis, 421
M proteins, 53*t*
MRI. *See* magnetic reso-
  nance imaging (MRI)
mucosal pressure injuries,
  351
mucositis
  antimicrobial recommen-
    dations for, 303*f*
  due to chemotherapy for
    bone and soft tissue
    sarcomas, 166
  oral, due to gynecologic
    cancer, 122*t*
multigated acquisition
  (MUGA) scan, 197, 201*t*
multikinase inhibitors
  (MKIs), cardiotoxicity of,
  214–215
multilumen catheters, 390
multimodal brain monitor-
  ing, 1, 14–18
multiorgan dysfunction
  syndrome (MODS), 172,
  284*t*, 285
multiorgan failure due to
  gynecologic cancer, 122*t*
multiple myeloma, 49*t*–
  56*t*, 57
  acute kidney injury with,
    172, 181–182
  additional clinical evalua-
    tion for, 53*t*
  classification of, 49*t*
  complications of, 56*t*
  cytogenetics of, 50*t*
  demographics of, 52*t*
  description of, 49*t*
  diagnosis of, 53*t*
  key signs and symptoms
    of, 54*t*
  prognosis for, 51*t*
  treatment of, 54*t*–55*t*
multipluripotent stem cell,
  291
myeloblast, 292*f*

myelodysplastic syndrome
  (MDS), 49*t*–56*t*, 72*t*
  additional clinical evalua-
    tion for, 53*t*
  classification of, 49*t*
  complications of, 56*t*
  critical care implications
    of, 72*t*
  cytogenetics of, 50*t*
  demographics of, 52*t*
  description of, 49*t*, 72*t*
  diagnosis of, 53*t*
  key signs and symptoms
    of, 54*t*
  prognosis for, 51*t*
  therapy-related, 52*t*
  treatment of, 54*t*–55*t*
myelofibrosis, 72*t*
myeloid dendritic cells,
  292*f*, 293
myeloid progenitor lineage,
  292*f*, 293
myeloma
  multiple. *See* multiple
    myeloma
  smoldering, 49*t*
myeloma cast nephropathy,
  172, 182

N

natural killer cell, 292*f*, 293
nausea
  anticipatory, 145
  due to chemotherapy for
    bone and soft tissue
    sarcomas, 166
  with enteral nutrition,
    328–329
  with gynecologic cancer,
    122*t*, 145
  palliative care for, 420–
    422, 421*f*
near-infrared spectroscopy
  (NIRS), 16–17
nephritis, acute interstitial,
  177*t*, 179
nephrogenic diabetes insipidus, 184
nephropathy
  contrast-induced, 172

membranous, 179
  myeloma cast, 172, 182
  nephrotoxicity
  due to chemotherapy,
    175*t*–177*t*
  for bone and soft tissue
    sarcomas, 166–167
  in older adults, 435–437,
    436*t*–437*t*
neurocritical care monitoring. *See* brain monitoring
neurocritical care unit
  (NCCU), 3
neurogenic shock, 283
neurologic changes in older
  adults, 434
neurologic complications
  of hepatocellular carci-
    noma, 106
neurologic effects of intra-
  abdominal hyperten-
  sion, 160
neurologic emergencies,
  262–264
neurologic examination for
  brain tumor, 11
neurologic monitoring,
  advanced, 1, 14–18
neuromuscular blocking
  agents, 383–384
neuropathic pain, 418
neurotoxicity with gynecologic cancer, 147
neutropenia, 293–294,
  294*f*, 294*t*
  assessment criteria for,
    295–296
  due to chemotherapy for
    bone and soft tissue
    sarcomas, 165
  defined, 293
  febrile, 258–260
    antimicrobial recom-
      mendations for, 303*f*
    due to gynecologic can-
      cer, 121*t*
neutropenic enterocoli-
  tis, 68*t*
neutropenic fever, 258–260
  antimicrobial recommen-
    dations for, 303*f*

due to gynecologic cancer, 121*t*
neutropenic precautions for sepsis, 298
neutropenic sepsis, 283, 291, 293–294
antibiotic therapy for, 299–302, 300*f*, 301*t*–302*t*, 303*f*
nursing implications of, 302–303
neutrophil(s), 292*f*, 293
neutrophil count, absolute. *See* absolute neutrophil count (ANC)
NIV. *See* noninvasive ventilation (NIV)
nivolumab for lung cancer, 27
nociceptive pain, 418
nonadherent contact layer dressing, 365*f*
nonbeneficial treatment, ethical concerns about, 456–458
nondepolarizing agents, 383–384
non-Hodgkin lymphoma, 49*t*–56*t*
additional clinical evaluation for, 53*t*
classification of, 49*t*
complications of, 56*t*
cytogenetics of, 50*t*
demographics of, 52*t*
description of, 49*t*
diagnosis of, 53*t*
key signs and symptoms of, 54*t*
prognosis for, 51*t*
treatment of, 54*t*–55*t*
noninvasive positive-pressure ventilation (NIPPV) for acute respiratory failure, 273–274
noninvasive ventilation (NIV)
for acute respiratory failure, 273–274
after thoracic surgery, 32
transition in care to, 411

nonlinear clearance, 375
non-small cell lung cancer (NSCLC), 23, 24
chemotherapy for, 25, 26–27
nonsteroidal anti-inflammatory drugs (NSAIDs), nephrotoxicity of, 175*t*, 177*t*, 436*t*
norepinephrine, 378–379, 380*t*
half-life of, 375
normal saline
for fluid resuscitation, 377, 378*t*
for hypercalcemia, 247*t*
for hyponatremia, 250*t*
nutrition
with acute pancreatitis, 113
and wound healing, 363–365
nutritional assessment, 324, 325
nutritional status, 324
nutritional support, 323–332
diagnosis of malnutrition and, 325, 325*f*
enteral, 326
complications of, 328–330
formulas for, 327–328
indications for, 326
timing and route of, 326–327
interventions for, 326
and metabolic response to stress, 323–324
nutrition care pathway for, 324–325
overview of, 323
parenteral, 326
complications of, 331–332
formulas for, 330–331
indications for, 327
timing and route of, 327
nutrition care pathway, 324–325

nutrition screening, 325
nutrition studies, 40*t*–41*t*

O

oat cell carcinoma, 23, 24
obstructive renal disease, 179–180
occlusion, with vascular access, 400*t*
occlusion alarm, 391
older adults, 433–440
cardiovascular changes in, 434
demographics of, 433
failure to thrive in, 440
frailty in, 439–440
geriatric syndromes in, 437
neurologic changes in, 434
overview of, 433
physiology of, 433–437
polypharmacy in, 438–439, 438*t*
pulmonary changes in, 435
renal changes in, 435–437, 436*t*–437*t*
oncologic emergencies, 245–265
cardiovascular, 260–261
hematologic, 264–265, 265*f*
infectious, 258–260
metabolic, 245–258
hypercalcemia as, 245–247, 246*t*, 247*t*
hyperkalemia as, 253, 254*t*–255*t*
hypoglycemia as, 252
hypokalemia as, 256–257, 256*t*
hyponatremia as, 247–251, 249*t*–251*t*
tumor lysis syndrome as, 257–258
neurologic, 262–264
opioids, 381
in palliative care, 418–419
after thoracic surgery, 29
oral mucositis due to gynecologic cancer, 122*t*

orthostatic hypotension,
234, 235
osteosarcoma, 164
ovarian cancer. *See also*
gynecologic (GYN) can-
cers
treatment options for,
127*t*
oxazolidinones for sep-
sis, 301*t*
oxycodone, 381
oxygen (O$_2$), partial pressure of
arterial. *See* partial pressure of oxygen (PaO$_2$)
brain tissue, 16
oxygen saturation
arterial (SaO$_2$), 15
after thoracic surgery, 32
venous (SjvO$_2$), 16
oxymorphone, 381

P

paclitaxel
cardiotoxicity of, 213, 230
for lung cancer, 26
side effects of, 136*t*
PaCO$_2$. *See* partial pressure of carbon dioxide
(PaCO$_2$)
PAD. *See* pain, agitation,
and delirium (PAD)
pain, agitation, and delirium (PAD)
analgesia and sedation for,
317–318
and early mobility, 339
with gynecologic cancer,
123*t*, 147
interprofessional care
approach (ABCDEF
bundle) for, 316–319,
317*f*
management recommen-
dations for, 313
monitoring for, 311–312
neuropathic, 418
pain management for,
316–317
procedural, 419

script for interprofessional
communication on,
314–316
spontaneous awakening
and breathing trials
for, 317
somatic (nociceptive), 418
surrogate decision makers
and, 450
visceral, 418
pain assessment tool in palliative care, 418
pain management
in palliative care, 417–
419, 417*t*
after thoracic surgery, 29
palliative care, 415–427
benefits of, 416
case study on, 425–427
defined, 415
end-of-life care in, 423–
425, 425*t*
family meeting in, 422–
423
history of, 415–416
identifying need for, 416–
417
overview of, 415–416
and spirituality, 423
symptom management in,
417–422
for dyspnea, 419–420
for nausea and vomit-
ing, 420–422, 421*f*
for pain, 417–419, 417*f*
for procedural pain,
419
palliative surgical approach
for lung cancer, 27
pamidronate
for hypercalcemia, 247*t*
nephrotoxicity of, 175*t*
pancreatic cancer, 111–113
pancreatitis, 111–113
pancuronium, 384
PaO$_2$. *See* arterial partial pressure of oxygen
(PaO$_2$)
papillary dermis, 344
parathyroid hormone
(PTH), 186

parathyroid hormone–
related peptide (PTHrP),
186
paravertebral blocks after
thoracic surgery, 29
parenteral nutrition (PN),
326
complications of, 331–332
formulas for, 330–331
indications for, 327
timing and route of, 327
and wound healing, 365
partial pressure of brain tissue oxygen (PbtO$_2$), 16
partial pressure of carbon
dioxide (PaCO$_2$)
in hypercarbic respiratory
failure, 270
in hypoxic respiratory failure, 270
after thoracic surgery,
32, 33
partial thickness skin loss,
348
partial thromboplastin time
(PTT), 47*t*
passive range-of-motion
exercises for immobil-
ity, 338
patient-controlled analgesia
after thoracic surgery, 29
patient safety, 444
peak airway pressure, 279*t*
pegfilgrastim, for sepsis, 298
pembrolizumab for lung
cancer, 27
penicillins
nephrotoxicity of, 177*t*
for sepsis, 301*t*
pentasaccharides, 384
percutaneous transhepatic
cholangiography (PTC)
drainage, 109, 111
perfusion-weighted imaging
(PWI), 13
pericardial disease, 197,
217–222
assessment of, 218–219,
219*t*–221*t*
management of, 221–222
pathogenesis of, 217

risk factors for, 217–218
pericardial effusion, 217–
  222, 260–261
  assessment of, 218–219,
    219t–221t
  diagnosis of, 260
  with hematologic malig-
    nancies and disor-
    ders, 63t
  nursing implications of,
    260–261
  pathogenesis of, 217, 260
  risk factors for, 217–218
  signs and symptoms of,
    260
  treatment of, 221–222,
    260
pericardial tamponade,
  217–222, 260–261
  assessment of, 218–219,
    219t–221t
  diagnosis of, 260
  malignant, 173
  management of, 221–222,
    260
  nursing implications of,
    260–261
  pathogenesis of, 217, 260
  risk factors for, 217–218
  signs and symptoms of,
    260
pericardiocentesis, 221
pericarditis, 217–222
  assessment of, 218–219,
    219t–221t
  management of, 221–222
  pathogenesis of, 217
  risk factors for, 217–218
peri-engraftment syndrome,
  59t, 94–95
perioperative respiratory
  failure, 271
peripheral edema in pericardial disease, 220t
peripherally inserted central catheters (PICCs),
  392–393
peritoneal dialysis, 187
peritonitis, spontaneous
  bacterial, due to hepato-
    cellular carcinoma, 108

periwound, 346
pH after thoracic surgery,
  32–33, 33t
pharmacodynamics, 375–
  377
pharmacokinetics, 373–375
  in older adults, 438–439,
    438t
pharmacology, 373–386
  analgesics in, 381
  anticoagulants in, 384–385
  fluid resuscitation in, 377,
    378t
  histamine-2 antagonist
    in, 385
  inotropes in, 379–380
  neuromuscular blocking
    agents in, 383–384
  opiates in, 381
  pharmacodynamics in,
    375–377
  pharmacokinetics in, 373–
    375
  proton pump inhibitors
    in, 385
  sedatives in, 381–383
  vasopressors in, 378–379,
    379t, 380t
phenanthrenes, 381
phenylephrine, 379, 380t
phenylpiperidines, 381
phenytoin
  clearance of, 375
  concentrations of, 374
Philadelphia chromosome,
  50t, 51t
phlebitis with vascular
  access, 401t–402t
pilocytic astrocytoma, 7
pituitary adenomas, 5–6, 6t
pixel, 12t
plant alkaloids, side effects
  of, 135t–136t
plasma cell, 292f
plasmacytoma, solitary,
  49t, 54t
plasmapheresis, 38–57
plateau pressure, 279t
platelet(s), 292f
platelet autoantibody, 45t
platelet count, 45t

platelet tests, 45t
platelet volume, mean,
  45t
platinum-based chemother-
  apy for lung cancer, 26
pleural effusions, 85t–86t
  with gynecologic can-
    cer, 144
pluripotent stem cells, 291,
  292f
pneumonectomy
  for lung cancer, 28
  postpneumonectomy syn-
    drome after, 30
pneumonia
  bronchiolitis obliterans
    organizing (crypto-
      genic organizing), 79t
  with gastrointestinal can-
    cer, 155
  in older adults, 435
pneumonitis
  interstitial, with pulmo-
    nary fibrosis, 83t–84t
  radiation, 85t
pneumothorax with vascu-
  lar access, 403t
point of maximum impulse
  (PMI) in pericardial disease, 220t
polycythemia vera (PV), 73t
polymorphonuclear granu-
  locytes, 293
polypharmacy, 438–439,
  438t
porphyria, 73t
ports, 392
positive end-expiratory pressure (PEEP), 279t
positron-emission tomog-
  raphy (PET) of brain
  tumor, 13
posterior reversible encephalopathy syndrome, 64t
posterior reversible leu-
  koencephalopathy syn-
  drome, 64t
postpneumonectomy syn-
  drome, 30
post-traumatic stress disorder (PTSD) in high-

intensity environments, 458–459, 459t
potentially inappropriate medications (PIMs), 439
prerenal azotemia, 173
pressure control ventilation (PCV), 278–279
    after thoracic surgery, 32
pressure gradient, 391
pressure injuries, 347–357
    due to acute skin failure, 352–353
    defined, 347–348
    device-related, 351, 352f
    end-of-life, 351–352
    moisture and, 354
    mucosal, 351
    prevalence and cost of, 347
    prevention of, 353–357
        mobility in, 356
        preventive therapies and devices in, 356–357, 357f
        risk assessment in, 353–354, 355f
        skin care in, 354–356
    staging of, 348–351, 349f–350f
pressure support ventilation (PSV), 278–279
    after thoracic surgery, 32
primary intention, wound healing by, 346
procedural pain, palliative care for, 419
proctitis due to gynecologic cancer, 123t
prognosis under conditions of uncertainty, 455
progressive mobility, 338
    barriers and solutions to, 339
proinflammatory mediators in sepsis, 289
prolactinomas, 5, 6t
prone positioning and pressure injuries, 356
prophylactic dressings for prevention of pressure injuries, 357

propofol, 381–382
propofol-related infusion syndrome, 382
protein C level, activated, 46t
protein intake and wound healing, 365
proteinosis, pulmonary alveolar, 87t
prothrombin time, 47t
proton pump inhibitors, 385
    nephrotoxicity of, 436t
pruritus due to gynecologic cancer, 123t
pseudohyperkalemia, 253
Pseudomonas aeruginosa, sepsis due to, 286, 287, 288t
pulmonary alveolar proteinosis, 87t
pulmonary artery catheter, 392
pulmonary artery occlusion, 202
pulmonary changes in older adults, 435
pulmonary complications of hepatocellular carcinoma, 107
pulmonary edema hypersensitivity, 82t
    after thoracic surgery, 30
pulmonary embolism with gynecologic cancer, 130t, 144
pulmonary fibrosis
    with gynecologic cancer, 144
    interstitial pneumonitis with, 83t–84t
pulmonary function with intra-abdominal hypertension, 160
pulmonary support for sepsis, 299
pulmonary toxicity with gynecologic cancer, 144
pulse in pericardial disease, 220t
pulse oximetry, 15
    for respiratory failure, 272

purpura
    immune thrombocytopenic, 69
    thrombotic thrombocytopenic, 38, 69

Q

QT prolongation, 223, 224t–225t
quality of care, 444
quetiapine for delirium, 314
quick sepsis-related organ failure assessment (qSOFA), 285

R

radiation dermatitis with gynecologic cancer, 119t, 139t
radiation-induced cardiotoxicity, 215–217
radiation-induced hematologic/immunologic toxicity, 94
radiation-induced liver disease (RILD), 109
radiation pneumonitis, 85t
radiation-related infections with gynecologic cancer, 141–142
radiation therapy (RT)
    for bone and soft tissue sarcomas, 164
    side effects of, 167
    brain injury due to, 19
    for gynecologic cancer, 127t–129t, 130–132, 139t–141t
    for lung cancer, 23–25
    side effects of
        with bone and soft tissue sarcomas, 167
        with cholangiocarcinoma, 111
        with gynecologic cancer, 130–132, 139t–141t
        with hepatocellular carcinoma, 109

stereotactic body, for colorectal cancer, 153–154

radiocontrast agents, nephrotoxicity of, 437*t*

ramucirumab for lung cancer, 27

receptor activator of nuclear factor kappa-B ligand (RANKL), 61*t*

red blood cell (RBC) distribution width (RDW), 40*t*

red blood cell (RBC) morphology, 40*t*

red blood cell (RBC) studies, 39*t*–43*t*

refeeding syndrome in parenteral nutrition, 332

relaxation rates, 11, 12*t*

remifentanil, 381

renal artery obstruction, 173–174

renal changes in older adults, 435–437, 436*t*–437*t*

renal disease, 171–189
    glomerular, 178
    interstitial, 177*t*, 179
    intrinsic, 174–179
    with multiple myeloma, 172, 181–182
    obstructive, 179–180
    overview of, 171–172
    tubular, 178
    and tumor lysis syndrome, 172, 180–181, 181*f*
    types of, 172–182

renal failure, acute. *See* acute kidney injury (AKI)

renal formulas for enteral nutrition, 328

renal function with intraabdominal hypertension, 160

renal injury, acute. *See* acute kidney injury (AKI)

renal replacement therapy (RRT), 172, 187–188, 189*t*

renal toxicity with gynecologic cancer, 121*t*, 146–147

renal tubular acidosis (RTA), 182–183

renal vasoconstriction, 173–174

renal vein thrombosis, 174

repositioning and pressure injuries, 356, 357, 357*f*

resilience in high-intensity environments, 458–459, 459*t*, 460*t*

respiratory acidosis after thoracic surgery, 33, 33*t*

respiratory alkalosis after thoracic surgery, 33, 33*t*

respiratory complications
    of gastrointestinal cancer, 155–156
    of hematologic/immunologic disorders, 77–78, 79*t*–89*t*

Respiratory Distress Observation Scale (RDOS), 420

respiratory failure, 269–281
    acute, 271
    diagnostic studies for, 271–272
    noninvasive ventilation for, 273–274
    transitions in care for, 410
    causes of, 269–271
    clinical manifestations of, 271
    diagnostic studies for, 271–272
    endotracheal intubation for, 274–278
    mechanical ventilation for, 278–280, 279*t*, 280*t*
    noninvasive ventilation in, 273–274
    overview of, 269
    after thoracic surgery, 31–34, 33*t*, 34*t*
    type 1 (hypoxic), 269–270
    type 2 (hypercarbic), 270–271

type 3 (perioperative), 271

type 4 (shock), 271

respiratory treatment for acute pancreatitis, 112–113

rete ridges, 344

reticular dermis, 344

reticulocyte, 292*f*

reticulocyte count, 40*t*

Rhodes Index of Nausea and Vomiting–Form 2, 421

Richmond Agitation and Sedation Scale (RASS), 312

Riker Sedation-Agitation Scale (SAS), 312

Ringer's lactate electrolyte A solution for fluid resuscitation, 377, 378*t*

rituximab, cardiotoxicity of, 214

rivaroxaban, 385

rocuronium, 384

roller clamp, 391

S

sarcomas, bone and soft tissue, 163–168
    chemotherapy side effects with, 165–167
    nursing implications of, 168
    overview of, 163
    pathophysiology of, 163–164
    radiation side effects with, 167
    treatment of, 164–165

sargramostim, for sepsis, 298

scopolamine for excessive secretion management, 425*t*

secondary intention, wound healing by, 346

secretion management in end-of-life care, 425, 425*t*

Sedation-Agitation Scale (SAS), 312

sedatives, 381–383
    for delirium, 317–318
segmentectomy for lung
    cancer, 28
seizure(s)
    due to brain tumor, 11
    due to gynecologic can-
        cer, 123t
selectins, 9
sepsis, 283–304
    assessment criteria for,
        295–296
    defined, 284–285, 284t
    diagnostic evaluation of,
        296–297
    epidemiology of, 285–286
    etiology and risk factors
        for, 286–288, 286t,
        288t
    with gastrointestinal can-
        cer, 154–155
    due to gynecologic can-
        cer, 123t
    hematopoiesis and, 291–
        294, 292f, 294f, 294t
    neutropenic, 283, 291,
        293–294
        antibiotic therapy for,
            299–302, 300f,
            301t–302t, 303f
        nursing implications of,
            302–303
    nursing implications of,
        302–303
    overview of, 283
    pathophysiology of, 288–
        289, 290f
    severe, 284t, 285
    treatment management
        strategies for, 297–302
        antibiotic therapy as,
            299–302, 300f,
            301t–302t, 303f
        cardiovascular and pul-
            monary support as,
            299
        early goal-directed ther-
            apy as, 298–299
        prevention and early
            detection as, 297–
            298

vs. uncomplicated infec-
    tion, 296
sepsis care bundles, 298
sepsis-related organ failure
    assessment (SOFA), 285
sepsis syndrome, 284
sepsis triad, 288
septicemia, 284, 285
septic shock, 283, 284,
    284t, 285
septum surface disinfection,
    395–396
serum iron, 41t
sexuality with gynecologic
    surgery, 131t
shearing, 348
shock
    classification of, 283
    pathophysiology of, 283
    respiratory failure in, 271
    septic, 283, 284, 284t,
        285
sickle cell disease, 74t
sinusoidal obstruction syn-
    drome, 65t
sinus tachycardia, 223
skin
    functions of, 343
    layers of, 344
    as organ, 343
    thickness of, 343
skin breakdown with gyne-
    cologic surgery, 130t
skin cancer, metastatic to
    brain, 8
skin care, preventive, 354–
    356
skin damage, moisture-asso-
    ciated. See moisture-
    associated skin damage
    (MASD)
skin failure, acute, 352–353
skin infections, antimicro-
    bial recommendations
    for, 303f
skin tears, 360–361, 362f
sleeve resection for lung
    cancer, 28
small bowel perforation due
    to complete cytoreduc-
    tion with heated intra-

peritoneal chemother-
    apy, 159
small cell lung cancer
    (SCLC), 23, 24
    chemotherapy for, 26
small-molecule drugs for
    lung cancer, 27
small-molecule kinase
    inhibitor, side effects of,
    137t
smoldering myeloma, 49t
sodium, for hyponatremia,
    251t
sodium bicarbonate for
    hyperkalemia, 254t
sodium chloride tablets for
    hyponatremia, 250t
soft tissue infections, anti-
    microbial recommenda-
    tions for, 303f
soft tissue sarcomas, 163–
    168
    chemotherapy side effects
        with, 165–167
    nursing implications of,
        168
    overview of, 163
    pathophysiology of, 163–
        164
    radiation side effects with,
        167
    treatment of, 164–165
soluble transferrin receptor-
    ferritin ratio, 41t
somatic pain, 418
somatotroph adenoma,
    5–6, 6t
sorafenib, side effects of,
    108–109
specialized formulas for
    enteral nutrition, 327–
    328
spectroscopy
    magnetic resonance, 12t,
        13
    near-infrared, 16–17
spinal cord compression
    with hematologic malig-
        nancies and disor-
        ders, 66t
    malignant, 262–263

spirituality in palliative care, 423
spontaneous awakening trials (SATs) for delirium, 317
spontaneous bacterial peritonitis (SBP) due to hepatocellular carcinoma, 108
spontaneous breathing trials (SBTs), 279–280
for delirium, 317
spontaneous ventilation, 278–279
sputum cytology for lung cancer, 25*t*
squamous cell carcinoma of lung, 24
Staphylococcus aureus, sepsis due to, 286, 287, 288*t*
methicillin-resistant, 288*t*, 303*f*
Staphylococcus epidermidis
with central venous catheters, 393, 396
sepsis due to, 288*t*
statin for cardiomyopathy/heart failure, 232
stem cells, 291
stereotactic body radiation therapy (SBRT) for colorectal cancer, 153–154
steroids for hypercalcemia, 247*t*
STOPP/START screening tool, 439
Streptococcus pneumoniae, sepsis due to, 287, 288*t*
streptozotocin, nephrotoxicity of, 176*t*
stress, metabolic response to, 323–324
stroke, with gynecologic cancer, 142
subcutaneous layer, 344
succinylcholine, 383
suicide, assisted, 450–451
sulfa-based antibiotics, nephrotoxicity of, 437*t*
superior vena cava (SVC) syndrome, 261

surgery
for bone and soft tissue sarcomas, 164–165
for gynecologic cancer, 127*t*–129*t*, 129, 130*t*–132*t*
for lung cancer, 27–28
common complications after, 29–30
pain management techniques after, 29
postoperative care after, 28–34
ventilator management after, 31–34, 33*t*, 34*t*
surgery-related infections with gynecologic cancer, 141
surrogate decision makers, 449–450
sustained low-efficiency dialysis (SLED), 187, 188
swabbing with central venous catheters, 396
Swan-Ganz catheter, 392
symptom monitoring for brain injury, 1–4, 3*f,* 4*f*
synchronized intermittent mandatory ventilation (SIMV), 278
after thoracic surgery, 31
syndrome of inappropriate antidiuretic hormone secretion (SIADH), 66*t*, 183, 248
systemic analgesia after thoracic surgery, 29
systemic inflammatory response syndrome (SIRS), 284*t,* 285
systolic blood pressure (SBP), 234–235

T

T1, 11, 12*t*
T1-weighted sequence, 12, 12*t*
T2, 11, 12*t*

T2-weighted sequence, 12, 12*t*
tachycardia, sinus, 223
tacrolimus, nephrotoxicity of, 176*t*
tamoxifen (Nolvadex)
cardiotoxicity of, 215
side effects of, 136*t*
targeted therapy
cardiotoxicity of, 209*t*–210*t*, 214–215
for lung cancer, 27
taxanes, cardiotoxicity of, 213
tbo-filgrastim, for sepsis, 298
T cell(s) (T lymphocytes), 292*f,* 293
T-cell lymphoma, 50*t*
temsirolimus (Torisel), side effects of, 137*t*
terminal weaning, 423–425, 425*t*
thalassemia, 74*t*
therapeutic plasma exchange, 177–178
thoracic surgery for lung cancer, 27–28
common complications after, 29–30
pain management techniques after, 29
postoperative care after, 28–34
ventilator management after, 31–34, 33*t,* 34*t*
thrombin clotting time, 48*t*
thrombocytopenia
due to chemotherapy for bone and soft tissue sarcomas, 165–166
medication-induced, 93*t*
thrombocytopenic purpura
immune, 69
thrombotic, 38, 69
thromboplastin time, partial, 47*t*
thrombosis
with hematologic disorders, 75–76
with vascular access, 400*t*

thrombotic complications, 203
thrombotic microangiopathy (TMA), 174–178, 175*t*–176*t*
thrombotic thrombocytopenic purpura (TTP), 38, 69
tidal volume, 279*t*
tissue mast cell, 292*f*
T lymphocytes (T cells), 292*f*, 293
tobramycin, nephrotoxicity of, 176*t*
tolvaptan for hyponatremia, 251*t*
topotecan, side effects of, 135*t*
torsade de pointes, 223
total body clearance, 375
total iron-binding capacity (TIBC), 41*t*
total parenteral nutrition (TPN) and wound healing, 365
tracheobronchial obstruction, 88*t*
tracheoplasty for lung cancer, 28
transferrin level, 41*t*
transferrin saturation (TSAT), 41*t*
transitions in care, 407–413
    admitting diagnoses and complications with, 410
    defined, 408
    ethical responsibilities with, 409–410
    family notification of, 412
    history of, 407
    noninvasive and mechanical ventilation and, 411
    overview of, 407–408
    potential pitfalls during, 411–412
    recognition of need for, 408–409
transparent film dressing, 364*t*

trastuzumab, cardiotoxicity of, 214
treatment decisions, ethical concerns about, 456–458
troponins
    in pericardial disease, 221*t*
    serum cardiac, 198, 199*t*
tube feedings. See enteral nutrition (EN)
tubing, 391
tubular disease, 179
tumor lysis syndrome (TLS), 257–258
    and acute kidney injury, 172, 180–181, 181*f*
    diagnosis of, 258
    with hematologic malignancies and disorders, 67*t*
    with leukemia, 56*t*
    nursing implications of, 258
    pathophysiology of, 180, 257
    risk of, 180, 181*f*, 257
    signs and symptoms of, 257
    treatment of, 180–181, 258
turning frequency and pressure injuries, 356, 357, 357*f*
typhlitis, 68*t*
tyrosine kinase inhibitors (TKIs)
    cardiotoxicity of, 214–215
    nephrotoxicity of, 175*t*, 177*t*

U

ulcers, pressure. See pressure injuries
uncertainty, prognosis under conditions of, 455
upper gastrointestinal (UGI) hemorrhage due to complete cytoreduction with heated intraperitoneal chemotherapy, 156–158

urea for hyponatremia, 250*t*
urinary frequency
    due to gynecologic cancer, 124*t*
    with intraperitoneal chemotherapy, 138*t*
urinary tract infections in older adults, 437
urine output in pericardial disease, 220*t*
uterine cancer. See also gynecologic (GYN) cancers
    treatment options for, 128*t*

V

vaginal discharge due to gynecologic cancer, 124*t*
vaginal mucous membranes, radiation-induced changes in, 140*t*–141*t*
VALUE communication technique in palliative care, 422
value conflicts, 444
vancomycin, nephrotoxicity of, 176*t*, 437*t*
vascular access, 389–403
    blood sampling from, 398, 399*t*
    catheter care and maintenance for, 393
    catheter types for, 391–393
    characteristics of central venous catheters for, 390
    dressings for, 394–395
    extraluminal catheter tract with, 393–394
    indications for, 389
    intraluminal fluid pathway in, 395–398, 397*t*, 399*t*
    overview of, 389–390
    principles of flow and, 390–391
    problems and interventions for, 398, 400*t*–403*t*

skin integrity with, 394
vascular endothelial growth factor inhibitors, nephrotoxicity of, 175t, 437t
vascular leak syndrome, 173, 213–214
vasoactive catecholamines, 378–379, 379t, 380t
half-life of, 375
volume of distribution of, 374
vasogenic shock, 283
vasopressin, 379, 379t, 380t
vasopressors, 378–379, 379t, 380t
vecuronium, 384
vein/catheter ratio, 390
veno-occlusive disease, pulmonary, 89t
venous oxygen saturation (SjvO$_2$), 16
venous thromboses, 203
ventilation, mechanical. See mechanical ventilation (MV)
ventilation/perfusion mismatch, 270
ventilator management after thoracic surgery, 31–34, 33t, 34t
arterial blood gas interpretation and, 32–34, 33t, 34t
ventilator settings for, 31–32
ventilator settings after thoracic surgery, 31–32
arterial blood gas interpretation and, 32–34, 33t, 34t
pressure modes of, 32
volume modes of, 31
ventilator support, removal of, 423–425, 425t
verapamil for dysrhythmias, 228t
video-assisted thoracic surgery (VATS) for lung cancer, 28
vinca alkaloids, side effects of, 135t–136t

viral infection, antimicrobial recommendations for, 303f
visceral pain, 418
visual analog scale, 420, 421
vitamin(s), and wound healing, 366–367
vitamin A and wound healing, 366–367
vitamin B$_9$ level, 40t
vitamin B$_{12}$ level, 40t
vitamin C and wound healing, 366
vitamin D and wound healing, 367
volume of distribution (VD), 374
vomiting
due to chemotherapy for bone and soft tissue sarcomas, 166
with enteral nutrition, 328–329
with gynecologic cancer, 124t, 145
palliative care for, 420–422, 421f
voxel, 12t
VP-16 (etoposide), side effects of, 136t
vulvovaginal cancer. See also gynecologic (GYN) cancers
treatment options for, 128t

W

warfarin, 384–385
WBC. See white blood cell (WBC)
weakness, ICU-acquired. See intensive care unit (ICU)-acquired weakness (ICU-AW)
weaning from mechanical ventilation, 279–280, 280t
terminal, 423–425, 425t
wedge resection for lung cancer, 28

white blood cell (WBC) count, 44t, 294, 296
white blood cell (WBC) differential, 44t
white blood cell (WBC) studies, 43t–44t
wound(s), 343–367
assessment of, 344–346, 345f
chronic, 347
cleansing of, 363
color and appearance of, 346
and critical care, 343–344
depth of, 345–346
dressing selection for, 363, 364t–365t, 366f
and fluid intake, 367
healing process for, 346–347
location of, 344–345
measurement of, 345–346, 345f
and micronutrition, 366–367
due to moisture-associated skin damage, 357–360
incontinence-associated dermatitis as, 358–359, 358f
intertriginous dermatitis as, 359–360
and nutrition, 363–365
overview of, 343
pressure injuries as, 347–357
due to acute skin failure, 352–353
defined, 347–348
device-related, 351, 352f
end-of-life, 351–352
mucosal, 351
prevalence and cost of, 347
prevention of, 353–357, 355f, 357f
staging of, 348–351, 349f–350f

size and shape of, 345–
346, 345*f*
due to skin tears, 360–
361, 362*f*
wound bed, 346
wound cleansing, 363
wound closure, 346–347
wound dressing, selec-
tion of, 363, 364*t*–365*t*,
366*f*

wound exudate, 346
wound infection
due to gynecologic can-
cer, 124*t*
with gynecologic surgery,
130*t*

Z

zero-order clearance, 375

zinc
in parenteral nutrition,
330
and wound healing, 367
zoledronate (zoledronic
acid)
for hypercalcemia, 247*t*
nephrotoxicity of, 175*t*